CLINICAL MEDICAL ETHICS CASES AND READINGS

LOYOLA UNIVERSITY CHICAGO STRITCH SCHOOL OF MEDICINE MEDICAL HUMANITIES PROGRAM

By

David C. Thomasma, Ph.D.
The Fr. Michael I. English, S.J., Professor of Medical Ethics
Professor of Medicine and Philosophy
Director of the Medical Humanities Program

and

Patricia A. Marshall, Ph.D.
Associate Professor of Medicine
Associate Director of the Medical Humanities Program

With Special Assistance from:

Diane Kondratowicz, A.M., M.A.
Clinical Ethics Coordinator

C1995

UNIVERSITY PRESS OF AMERICA

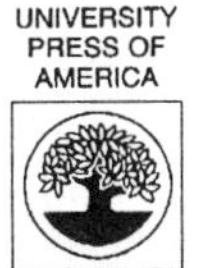

Lanham • New York • London

4720 Boston Way
Lanham, Maryland 20706

3 Henrietta Street
London WC2E 8LU England

Printed in the United States of America
British Cataloging in Publication Information Available

Library of Congress Cataloging-in-Publication Data

Thomasma, David C.
Clinical medical ethics : cases and readings : Loyola University of Chicago, Stritch School of Medicine, Medical Humanities Program / by David C. Thomasma and Patricia A. Marshall ; with special assistance from, Diane Kondratowicz.
p. cm.
Includes bibliographical references.
1. Medical ethics—Case studies. I. Marshall, Patricia A. II. Kondratowicz, Diane. III. Stritch School of Medicine. IV. Title.
[DNLM: 1. Ethics, Medical. 2. Curriculum. W 18 T463c 1994]
R724.T535 1994 174'.2—dc20
DNLM/DLC for Library of Congress 94–22890 CIP

ISBN 0–8191–9725–4 (pbk. : alk. paper)

The paper used in this publication meets the minimum requirements of American National Standard for Information Sciences—Permanence of Paper for Printed Library Materials, ANSI Z39.48–1984.

Dedication

This book is dedicated to our medical students at Loyola University Chicago Stritch School of Medicine.

TABLE OF CONTENTS

SECTION 3: **ISSUES IN PRACTICE**

ACKNOWLEDGEMENTS

Our gratitude extends to many people who have helped us complete this book. First and foremost we thank all of our faculty who have taught this course for over 20 years, first at the University of Tennessee Center for the Health Sciences since 1973, and then, starting in 1981, at Loyola University Chicago, Stritch School of Medicine. Many of the faculty, too numerous to name, actively helped us rewrite the cases in this book. Most cases occurred in our own health facilities or those with which we were associated, and came to our attention through the Ethics Consult Service. Diane Kondratowicz played a significant role in identifying articles to be used in conjunction with the cases. We thank her very much for that extensive review. Karin Dean, Administrative Secretary, and Doris Thomasma, Senior Secretary of the Medical Humanities Program, assisted us in piecing together each new year's improvements in the course (as we and our faculty rarely left the structure and content alone for more than one year), and Karin Dean offered many good suggestions for editing the text. Irene Zaura, Heather Unluata, Kathy Grevas, and Patricia M. Marschall, Secretaries, helped get the articles approved for publication and assisted assembling the book. All our secretaries were invaluable aides in caring for all the details. Travis Schwab, research assistant, finalized the formating details of each chapter, checking and retyping the references. His meticulous dedication to perfection and cheerful acceptance of responsibility was essential to the publication of this volume and is deeply appreciated. Finally we thank contributors to the Fr. Michael I. English, S.J. Chair of Medical Ethics, and the administrators of the medical school and the university for their support of the Medical Humanities Program that made this coursebook possible.

David C. Thomasma, Ph.D.
Patricia A. Marshall, Ph.D.

INTRODUCTION

Chapter 1

How to Use This Book

This course book is comprised of clinical cases, readings, and an ethical workup guide for resolving moral problems in patient care. The ethical workup guide was developed by David Thomasma in 1973 to guide students through a process of moral reasoning rather than teach them extensively about ethical theories. Typically, medical and nursing students have not had more than one ethics or medical ethics course in their undergraduate education; some have never had either course. The ethical workup guide introduces students to a model of moral reasoning which can be applied to difficult cases in patient care. This ethical workup guide is a heuristic device. As such, it represents one approach for resolving moral dilemmas in patient care. Other methods exist, and any can be substituted in this course for the workup provided here.

A cautionary note: there is a distinction between teaching ethics and teaching about ethics. The former, teaching ethics, has to do with teaching right from wrong, instilling in one's charges the virtues required by life and the profession. Teaching about ethics can pose moral dilemmas and puzzles, as in the cases presented in this book, for which there is no clear right or wrong answer. This latter exercise presupposes that the former work of teaching ethics has already occurred, such that the student may now pursue challenges to his or her own ethical synthesis.

The cases in this book are indexed in ten general categories. The categories cover the lifespan, moving from birth through pediatric, adult, and geriatric medicine. We also include cases from ordinary medical practice (so-called "non-dramatic cases") and cases that create dilemmas in medical entrepreneurship. The last category includes cases that require thinking about the physician-patient relationship in a broader social and political context. Since the focus of the course book is on clinical ethics, the cases are largely those found in the clinical practice of medicine. Hence the course profits from occasional supplemental cases such as those addressing genetic engineering, genetic manipulation of preembryos, or research ethics. We have included one multi-cultural case, but supplements from this important perspective will surely be required as well.

Space limited us in choosing appropriate readings. The readings found in this book meet three criteria: 1) They are judged helpful and understandable by the faculty and students; 2) They are current or provide more general background on issues; 3) They are chosen for general application to issues found in one or more of the cases, or one or more case categories. By no means are these all of the readings to be used for each case. Nor are these readings necessarily the "classic" readings in clinical or medical ethics. The latter can be found in standard reference textbooks. That is why students are asked in Step One of the Workup to research other papers and books. Furthermore, we typically supplement the readings in the book with others that are put on reserve in the library or sometimes distributed to students.

Depending on student contact hours, the course can be configured in various ways. At Loyola University Chicago, Stritch School of Medicine, the course is required of first year medical students. The course is scheduled for ten one and one-half hour sessions. There are approximately 130 students in the first year class. Students are assigned to eight sections comprised of 16 students. These sections are further divided into two small groups.

The heart and soul of the course is student group resolution of the cases using the ethical workup guide, case analyses, and the readings. One of the small group of students in a section (8 - 10 students) presents to their peers, another group of 8 - 10 students, under the tutelage and guidance of one or more faculty members. We try to have two faculty per each of the 8 course sections, one faculty from the humanities and one from medicine. The students resolve the case and develop their presentation outside of class time. The faculty function as guides for the use of the workup, consultants about the issues, and Socratic "provokers" of discussion for each of the points of the workup as the students make their way through the presentation.

In the past, we have put a particular spin on the use of the ethical workup guide by stressing only the first two steps during the first two student presentations, then four steps of the workup at the next two presentation sessions by students, and finally all six steps of the workup in the last four case presentations. This was done because an important goal of our course is to help the students become proficient at doing the research and thinking embodied in the workup guide. Be forewarned, though, that this strategy tends to place more emphasis on the workup guide than on the cases. Normally, however, each case is analyzed using all six steps. Near the end of the course, students must present a final case resolution to a "guest clinician," often the chairman of a department or our Dean, who evaluates their performance. They must also write a final paper, using the ethical workup guide, analyzing a case chosen by the faculty for its complexity.

We have found that only a one hour and a half introductory session is required for our course. This introduction provides information on the structure of the course, the physical location of the breakout rooms for the small groups, the division of students into small groups, and their subdivision into group A and group B for presentation purposes. Also presented is a general lecture on clinical ethics today. Currently this presentation explores the challenge of doing ethics in a post-modern, pluralistic society. Other introductory lectures are also possible. We have found that it is essential during the introductory sessions to provide students with an example of how to use the ethical workup. In the past, we have had faculty "role-play" the ethical resolution of a case, or we have had several faculty "walk through" the workup so that students understand how they are to cover specific topics during the workup and how they might present their collaborative thinking about the resolution of the case.

We sometimes have required notebooks of students, to keep track of their reading and their evaluations of the student presentations in their small group section, as well as a final examination detailing how their thinking has progressed during the course. We have also paused in the middle of the course to discuss ethical theory. A brief comparison sketch of competing ethical theories is provided in this book for that purpose. Sometimes we have used a pre- and post-test of students to evaluate how their thinking has matured during the course.

Students have been, from time to time, unable to reach a consensus about what to do in a case. In such instances, a "minority report" is filed by the dissenting students. Our experience has taught us that the students have the most difficulty with Step Six of the workup guide, since in that step they are to argue why one course of action is better than others, thus developing an ethical stance about the issue at stake in the case. The faculty must encourage students to develop reasons for their positions.

As noted above, the structure of the course is at the faculty's discretion. What follows is a brief presentation of our own objectives and the structure of the course, along with the overall objectives of our curriculum during four years of medical school training.

Chapter 2

Course Description

Class Schedule
The schedule for each year is distributed to students separately. The cases to be used each year are listed on this schedule. Refer to the cases in this book. Required reading material for each case is identified on the schedule. Required reading may not be limited to the articles found in this book. Supplemental articles will either be distributed to students or placed on reserve in the library.

The first class is a general session. All other classes are small group sessions with assigned faculty member(s).

Class One: Introduction

First 30 Minutes: Introduction to Course
45 Minutes: Introductory Lecture
Last 15 Minutes: Questions

Class Two: Ethical Workup Guide and Professional Ethics

Small Group Sessions conducted by the Faculty. (See Schedule and Faculty Assignments).

Classes Three to Ten: Small Group Sessions

Group A and Group B in each small group session alternate case presentations each week. Thus, one week Group A will make their presentation to Group B; the following week Group B presents to Group A (See Figure 1).

45 Minutes: Presentation of Case Resolution
45 Minutes: Class Discussion

Figure One

The Class is Divided Into Sections
Each section is divided into two sub-groups:

Group A	Group B
(8 students)	(8 students)

Goals of the Course

1. To introduce the student to a process of moral reasoning called an Ethical Workup.
2. To introduce the student to basic medical ethics problems through case analysis and reading.
3. To create an opportunity to resolve clinical ethical dilemmas through discussion with peers, class presentations, and final examination paper using the Ethical Workup.

Course Objectives

1. Each student, working in a small group with approximately eight other students, shall have the experience of resolving patient-care cases which raise ethical issues.
2. Each student, working in their small group, shall have the experience of presenting this case to another small group of eight peers.
3. Each student shall read the articles designated for each case.
4. Each student shall have the opportunity to present a case resolution to a guest clinician.
5. Each student shall resolve a case on his or her own, and prepare a written case resolution using the Ethical Workup. This is the final examination for the course.

Learning Objectives

At the end of this course, students will be able to conduct an ethical analysis of a moral dilemma in clinical care. Students will be able to:

1. Identify the medical facts of the case.
2. Identify social, professional, and personal values at risk.
3. Identify potential courses of action.
4. Choose a course of action that can be justified on medical and moral grounds.

Grading Policy

Our approach to grading has changed from year to year in an attempt to find effective, appropriate, and relevant solutions to student evaluation. One option is that students receive a grade of Honors, High Pass, Pass, or Fail. When we have used this policy, two-thirds of the grade is based on class participation and class presentation, and one-third of the grade is based on the written examination. When this approach is used, all students have an opportunity to earn a grade of Honors. Faculty will notify students if their participation, either attentive listening or discussion of the case, falls short of what is expected.

Another approach we have used consists of students receiving a Pass or Fail for the course with an option competing for High Pass or Honors if they complete the final written examination. Over the years we have found that, when this approach is used, approximately 75% of the class chose to write the cases analysis final examination.

The faculty for the course function as consultants for the small groups. Students are expected to consult with them when needed and to take advantage of any background materials in the library.

1. *Criteria for Class Presentation and Course Participation*

* Attend every class.
* Meet with small group outside of class to prepare for case presentation. Use steps in the Ethical Workup to guide the presentation.
* Participate in small group presentation of the case resolution. Each group member should be involved in presenting the case (e.g., rotate responsibilities--one person might present medical background, another person might present the relevant values, several people could present the final justification).
* Participate in general discussion of each case. All students must read every case and the required readings for the case.

2. *Specific criteria for skillful use of the Ethical Workup:*

* Read case and assigned materials.
* Research additional relevant information (e.g. medical facts, social and psychological information, financial information).

* Cite literature and demonstrate an understanding of the content of readings as they pertain to the case.
* Provide a thorough and complete description of plausible action plans or therapeutic goals in case resolution.
* Defend reasons for the course of action chosen (e.g., include reference to philosophical perspectives, philosophical principles, and professional obligations). See Figure 2.

3. *Criteria for Final Exam*
* Paper must be a minimum of 8 pages, including cover page and references.
* It must be typed, double spaced, on 8-1/2 X 11 paper.
* The student's name and address must be on the cover page.

4. *Criteria for Using the Ethical Workup Guide*
* Address each section of the Ethical Workup. Use sub-headings to delineate the sections in your paper.
* Present a thorough and concise description of the medical and social facts of the case.
* Present a full discussion of the values at risk in the case (patient, family, professional, society, etc.). Do not simply provide a "list" of the values.
* In paragraph form, discuss the primary value conflicts (e.g., patient autonomy vs. physician paternalism; social justice regarding allocation of scarce medical resources vs. a patient's autonomy/freedom to choose medical care).
* Identify several possible courses of action.
* Describe the course of action you have chosen.
* Incorporate an ethical justification for the recommended course of action, drawing on ethical perspectives (deontological, utilitarian, etc.; refer to specific ethical principles such as beneficence, non-maleficence, justice, and autonomy; refer to professional ethical responsibilities; make reference to the Hippocratic Oath and its meaning in the context of the case, if appropriate.)
* Incorporate relevant medical and bioethics literature in the discussion.
* Paper must cite at least eight references. Use the reference system and format of the *New England Journal of Medicine*. Use correct grammar and spelling.

5. *Criteria for Failing the Course*
* Student misses more than two sessions.
* Student is unprepared for and uninvolved in class presentation in discussion.
* The student fails the final exam.

Figure Two
Ethical Workup Guide - Descriptors of Grade Categories

	Fail	Pass	High Pass	Honors
Facts	Misrepresents the facts, misunderstands the facts, omits highly relevant facts, adds incorrect facts.	Accurately repeats factual data.	Accurately summarizes the data, adds additional factual information from previous personal education and experience.	Accurately summarizes, adds knowledge from previous personal education and experience, calls clinicians and/or uses the library for additional relevant information.
Values	Does not recognize values at risk in case, does not recognize the holders of those values.	Describes some of the principal values at risk and the holders of those values.	Identifies most of the values at risk and the holders of those values.	Provides a thorough description of values at risk and the holders of those values.
Primary Conflicts	Does not recognize principal conflicts.	Describes some of the principal conflicts.	Identifies most of the principal conflicts (e.g., patient autonomy vs physician paternalism; social justice vs individual freedom of choice).	Provides thorough description of principal conflicts. Correctly emphasizes most important conflict(s).
Courses of Action	Does not recognize possible courses of action, does not recognize some of the main values and principles that would be protected or infringed by the courses of action.	Describes some courses of action and the values and principles protected or infringed upon.	Identifies most of the possible courses of action, together with values and principles that would be protected or infringed upon.	Provides a thorough description of possible courses of action together with values and principles that would be protected or infringed upon. No reasonable options omitted.
Choice	Ambiguous or incomprehensible course of action, describes a course of action that does not address principle dilemma(s).	Minimal description of a course of action. No elaboration.	Identifies in greater detail a course of action.	Identifies a complete course of action. Addresses medical, social, professional elements of action, states who the agents are for decision-making and execution of action.
Defense	Offers no defense or an inappropriate defense.	States reason(s) for choosing course of action.	Identifies ethical theories applied to determine resolution of case, refers to at least some readings.	Identifies ethical theories applied to determine resolution of case, refers to readings, names competing possible resolutions with their possible defenses, states why chosen action and ethical reasoning were preferred in this case.

Chapter 3

Ethical Theory and Principles

There are many competing ethical theories and principles. In clinical medical ethics, the one goal of analysis is to balance these by deciding which is most important than others in a hierarchy of values, rights, interests, and concerns.

We have chosen just four theories out of many proposed throughout history, in order to present a comparison of the theories regarding the goal of conduct, the means to attain that goal, the construction of the good and the good life, and norms.

Background Reading

1. Graber GC. Basic theories in medical ethics, In: Monagle JF, Thomasma DC, *Medical Ethics: A Guide for Health Professionals*. Rockville, MD: Aspen Publishers, Inc., Chapter 37:462-475.

Study Guide for Major Ethical Thinkers

	Aristotle	Mill	Kant	Dewey
Goal: the	Happiness, all actions.	Happiness, goal of action.	A good will.	Happiness, goal of all action.
Means	The virtues reinforce natural tendencies toward happiness.	A calculus of pleasures and values justifies actions.	A good will is one which acts from duty.	Education and the cultivation of character.
Meanin g of the good	The good is happiness conceived as meshing with the common good.	Happiness is pleasure and the avoidance of pain.	Acts are done from duty if they are what reason requires.	Happiness is interest in those objects which secure the well being of all persons.
Norms	Actions should conform to the best human behavior as evidenced by scientific study of nature and psychology. Norms apply only generally and not absolutely.	Act always to maximize the benefit (good) which is pleasure. This is an absolute norm. Act always to maximize the sum of pleasure for all who will be affected by one's act. (Principle of Utility).	Categorical Imperative: Act always as if what you will do will become a universal law. Or, never treat persons merely as means only, but always as ends in themselves. Norms are absolute.	Actions should conform to the best character evidenced by scientific study, psychology, and society. Norms arise in context and are limited because our aims are limited.

Chapter 4

Ethical Workup Guide

The workup is an attempt to distill from the discipline of ethics an essential process of moral reasoning which can be applied to ethical dilemmas in patient care. Other heuristic devices are available as well. The workup itself should not be an object of extensive discussion, but rather the points towards which it guides the discussion of the case itself.

No attempt is made to force you to take one or another ethical position. Instead, you are asked to follow only one absolute: Come up with an ethically justifiable course of action for the patient that meshes with your professional duty to act in the best interest of the patient.

Step 1: What are the facts in the case? Be sure to research any medical facts not presented in the case, but possibly relevant to its outcome.

Step 2: What are the values at risk in the case? Describe all relevant values of the physicians, patients, housestaff, nurses, hospital administration, the institution, and society. This may not be an exhaustive listing of interests in the case.

Step 3: Determine the principal conflicts between values, professional norms, and between ethical axioms, rules and principles. Conflicts can occur among *prima facie* values, absolute values, norms, axioms, rules, and principles, and/or amongst each other. The primary conflict, in the final analysis, is the one you determine it to be. In determining this primary conflict, you should explain if you think principles and values are absolute and whether to be ethical means to act on principle, whether you hold that they are only at first glance, that is, *prima facie* absolute, and can yield to other important values and principles in the case.

Step 4: Determine possible courses of action, and which values and ethical principles each course of action would protect or infringe. At this step you will grapple with fundamental moral theory. Are you willing to seek a solution that is based on a single principle? Or are you willing to note that each decision you might make will place some values, principles, etc., at risk? Would you then be satisfied with being a utilitarian, that is, by protecting as many values and principles as possible in the case?

Step 5: Make a decision in the case. Decide upon a course of action for resolving the ethical dilemma.

Step 6: Defend this course of action. Why is "X " better than "Y"? In defending this course of action, ask whether consensus ethics is appropriate. Is doing what most think is right, necessarily right? Should the decision rest on a single value or principle? Instead should it protect as many values as possible? Or should it rest on the virtue of the caregivers or institutions in which it takes place?

***Respond to each of the following*:**

1. Were any values, principles, norms, axioms, rules weighted more heavily than others? If so, which values, principles, etc., were most important to protect and why? If not, was the case decided by protecting as may of the values in the case as possible?
2. Try to identify the type of moral reasoning applied in resolving the case (utilitarian, deontologic, virtue-ethic, care ethics, casuistic ethics, other) and state whether it was used because of your general preference in similar situations or because of its particular applicability to this specific case.
3. Universality test: Would you be willing that your decision and its reasons become universal law, and apply to every similar situation or to yourself? Is this test actually a valid way to determine what is ethical?
4. What role does society play in making this decision palatable? Can you imagine a different society and a different solution? Would the decision require you to change the political system or the way health care is delivered? Are social and political duties a feature of the nature of the profession and clinical judgment? Do you believe in cultural relativism?
5. How does this decision relate to others you have made in your life, in courses, and in actuality as a professional?

BACKGROUND READINGS:

1. Thomasma DC. Training in medical ethics: An ethical workup, *Forum on Medicine* 1978;I:33-36.
2. Siegler M. Decision-making strategy for clinical-ethical problems in medicine, *Archives of Internal Medicine* 1982;142:2178-2179.
3. Veatch RM. Medical ethics: Professional or universal? In: *The Patient-Physician Relation*. Bloomington, IN: Indiana University Press, 1992:16-32.

SUGGESTED READINGS:

1. Beauchamp TL, McCullough LB. *Medical Ethics: The Moral Responsibility of Physicians*. Englewood Cliffs, NJ: Prentice Hall, 1984.
2. Brody H. *The Healer's Power*. New Haven, CT: Yale University Press, 1993.
3. Pellegrino ED, Thomasma DC. *A Philosophical Basis of Medical Practice*. New York, NY: Oxford University Press, 1981.
5. Pellegrino ED, Thomasma DC. *The Virtues in Medical Practice*. New York, NY: Oxford University Press, 1993.
6. Pellegrino ED, Thomasma DC. *The Christian Virtues in Medicine*. Washington, DC: Georgetown University Press, 1995.
7. Veatch RM. *The Patient-Physician Relationship*. Bloomington, IN: Indiana University Press, 1993.

PRIMARY BASIC RESOURCES IN HEALTH CARE ETHICS

Basic Introductory Texts

1. Beauchamp TL, Childress JF. *Principles of Biomedical Ethics*. New York, NY: Oxford University Press, 4th ed., 1994.
2. Jonsen AR, Siegler M, Winslade WJ. *Clinical Ethics*. New York, NY: Macmillan

Publishers, 3rd ed., 1992.
3. Loewy EH. *Textbook of Medical Ethics.* New York, NY: Plenum, 1989.
4. Rachels J. *The Elements of Moral Philosophy*. New York, NY: Random House, 2nd ed., 1993.
5. Thomasma DC, Pellegrino ED. *For the Patient's Good: The Restoration of Beneficence in Health Care*. New York, NY: Oxford University Press, 1988.

Computer Listings

The Bioethics File
History of Medicine File
Medline/Bioethicsline
The Philosopher's Index

Encyclopedias

Encyclopedia Britannica
Dictionary of the History of Ideas
Encyclopedia of Philosophy
Encyclopedia of Ethics
Encyclopedia of Bioethics
Biolaw

Major Journals

Bioethics
Cambridge Quarterly of Healthcare Ethics
Ethics
Hastings Center Report
Journal of Clinical Ethics
Journal of Law, Medicine and Philosophy
Journal of Medical Ethics
Journal of Medical Humanities and Bioethics
Journal of Medicine and Philosophy
Kennedy Center Journal of Ethics
Medical Humanities Review
Philosophy and Public Affairs
Social Science and Medicine
Theoretical Medicine

SECTION 1

REPRODUCTIVE ISSUES

Chapter 5

Cases 1.0

Case 1.1: **THE ANGELA CARDER CASE**

A young woman, Angela Carder, now 27, had a 14-year bout with cancer. After a period of treatment, she went into remission.

She later decided to become pregnant. This decision was made against all medical advice, since the therapy she had received was considered possible high risk for normal fetal development. During her pregnancy, she was discovered to have terminal lung cancer, considered to be metastases from her original cancer or its treatment. From this point on her health deteriorated. Apparently there was no explicit discussion with her family about trying to save the fetus during her dying process. She was cared for at a major university medical center.

By the time the fetus was 24-weeks-old, Carder was clearly dying. She was placed on a respirator and given heavy sedation for her pain. At this point the hospital administration tried to communicate with her about her wishes regarding the fetus. This effort produced no consistent results. The mother at first refused to have a Caesarian because of the very high risk that she would die from it; she later relented, and then changed her mind again just before slipping into her final coma. Her doctor could not say for sure whether or not she wished to save her fetus. Her family felt that it was not appropriate to do so.

The gynecologists consulted noted that a child either born prematurely or taken by Caesarean at 24 weeks has about a 5% chance of living after one year, due to poorly developed lungs. But neonatal technology is continuing to develop at a rapid pace. Given the possible detrimental effects of the cancer care and Carder's dying process, however, the gynecologists recommended waiting until 28 weeks before trying to rescue the fetus. The earliest they could deliver the baby would be at 28 weeks without seriously harming the baby in the process. Since Carder will die before that time, this recommendation is, in effect, a statement that there should be no effort to try to save the fetus in this case.

But the hospital administration overrode this consulting recommendation, and the attending physician's support of the family decision not to proceed to try to save the fetus. The administration considered the hospital to have a duty to try to save the child in a dying mother, even if the prognosis for the survival of the child was very poor. They were concerned about their liability should they let the patient die without trying to save the fetus. This would be done by means of a Caesarean, even though Carder had never authorized this operation. The administration granted the risk to the mother would be fatal. Mrs. Carder would die from the Caesarean itself. But the possible chance to save the fetus outweighed that "risk," especially since Carder would die within 24 hours anyway from her disease process. The hospital sought a court order to save the baby.

Mrs. Carder's husband, other members of her family, and the doctors disagreed with this position, claiming that since the mother had not given consent to a Caesarean Section, the hospital had no right to force her to undergo this surgery, especially since the surgery itself would kill her. By performing such an unauthorized procedure, even if it were approved by a court, the hospital was failing to respect her autonomy and dignity as a human being. The family felt that the hospital had no right to interfere with the treatment plan as this was a private matter between the family and Carder's physician.

Although A.C.'s wishes were not specifically known at this moment, she had not conveyed a desire to have the baby by Cesarean section during her dying process at any time. Since no wishes were known, some people assumed that she had refused such surgery, and were in favor of going to court to get the approval to "rescue" the child.

This was the position of the hospital administration. Some fetuses survive after 24 weeks. The administration feared a lawsuit if it did not get some decision approved by the court. Some health professionals hearing about the case might later protest to the legal system if no effort were made to fulfill the responsibility of hospital's and the state's interest in preserving life (as happened in the infamous Clarence Hebert case in California, where 2 doctors were indicted for murder). The hospital administration planned to seek "declaratory relief from the Court to direct the hospital as to what it should do in terms of the fetus, whether to intervene and save its life." They were further in favor of trying to save the fetus, if possible, even if that meant bringing A.C. into the operating room against her wishes, or without them.

The attorney representing the hospital argued that "There are two lives in the balance, and the hospital should try to do the right thing." The administration was concerned that the patient might die from the operation, but felt that even though they "might shorten her life by a few hours," this risk was worth the benefit of possibly saving one of those two lives in the balance.

The family was naturally incensed, as were her doctors. They had assumed that an individual had a right to determine his or her own treatment. "Informed consent" for surgery, they argued, is "essential to recognize the dignity of the individual patient." The family and doctors refused to go along with the hospital administration plan regarding A.C.

They thought that no attempt would be made to rescue the fetus, and had specifically not asked her about such a rescue since she was dying. Furthermore, the family and physicians had embarked upon a course of treatment consistent with her previously expressed wishes, and felt entirely comfortable with allowing her to die without trying to have her give birth. They had not anticipated the need for more specific wishes, not having anticipated the strength of the worry of the hospital administration.

The family and physicians recognized that the hospital might be puzzled by the lack of specificity in A.C.'s wishes regarding the fetus, especially that "if she were to die, no intervention would be planned to save the fetus." However, puzzlement, concern, or abstract worrying about the legal meaning or application to this case of the, "state's interest in preserving life," do not justify intervening in the therapeutic plan of a family and the physician in regard to a currently dying and incompetent patient.

This case presents major difficulties in relation to health professional duties, women's rights, and fetal rights. Like cases regarding defective newborns, many other "interests" intervene when a pregnant woman and her fetus are at risk. Among them are pro-life interests, fetal rights groups, women's issue task forces, and many medical societies, including, in this case, the American Medical Association, the American College of Obstetricians and Gynecologists, and the county medical society.

Some groups argue that all life has a "right" to be born, or at least, to be given a chance to live. The lawyer for the medical center involved in this case argued that, "The state's compelling interest in fetal life was strong enough to justify 'handcuffing' a woman to the bed and forcing her to give birth."

The opposition argues either that a woman has a right to decide about her own body, including decisions over a fetus, or that doctors and patients ought to be "left alone" to make decisions on a case-by-case basis without court intervention.

The court granted the hospital's request. The case soon became a banner issue among many outside organizations representing views regarding women's rights, fetal rights, medical interests, and institutional and state duties. What are the ethical and legal protections of women who become pregnant? How far can the State go in intruding into the lives of such women, especially those who have become incompetent due to an accident or illness? Should this court order have been granted? Is it ever ethical to institute an action that will kill one human being (the Caesarean) to possibly save another (the fetus)? How does this differ from double-effect euthanasia, if at all?

If you were now arguing before an appeals court your medical ethics point of view on this case, what would it be?

Case 1.2: **CUSTODY AND STATUS OF FROZEN EMBRYOS**

The case in Tennessee of Junior and Mary Sue Davis shed national light on the problem of storing frozen embryos, and the language that ought to be used regarding their functional status.

News reports said that the couple "owned" seven frozen embryos, and that these were the "product" of his sperm and her eggs. At issue, according to Mary Sue's attorney, J. G. Christenberry, was "when or where do living cells require protection?" Does the sweat equity invested by Mary Sue in trying to become pregnant outweigh Junior's claim that becoming a father after a divorce would be a psychological and financial burden on him? Even though such frozen embryos have an uncertain legal status, infertility specialist Dr. Ray Kind testified in court that they should be preserved since they represent for someone "hope to be a parent." He said, "It would be wasteful and damaging to our profession if they were blatantly destroyed."[1]

Actually the tiny cells, together smaller than a grain of sugar, are properly called pre-embryos, since they as yet may not be individuals (but rather a community of cells each capable of becoming a single being)--but that is a point for later consideration. This said, a suggestion that the embryos just be thawed and allowed to die, was related directly to "taking someone off the respirator." John Robertson, a University of Texas law professor, taking the stand on Junior's behalf, argued that such beings should be treated with "special respect," but not accorded the respect due to a person under the law. He suggested they might be left to thaw. Christenberry compared this to removing a person from the respirator, and Robertson noted in response that the analogy was faulty. In the former instance, we do not deal with a legal person. In the latter, a legal person is involved.[2]

In December 1988, when nine embryos were created, two implanted and the other seven frozen, and stored in a Knoxville laboratory, the last thing the Davises were thinking was getting a divorce. Their marriage had been rocky throughout, but they thought that the combination of God's grace and the new technology might save their marriage by giving them a child. They had tried to adopt before, but were told there was little chance. Besides, the costs seemed astronomical. For the couple, fees ranging from $5,000 to $50,000 were unaffordable.

Junior had a very troubled childhood. When he was five, his mother had a nervous breakdown, his parents split up, and along with three of his brothers he was sent to an orphanage where he lived until he was 18. That experience convinced him that a child should not be raised without his parents.

Mrs. Davis detailed her five failed pregnancies and her six tries at *in vitro* fertilization. Each time, there were injections, blood tests, and egg retrieval. She thought her mental and physical pain gave her a greater stake in the survival of the embryos than her husband's. She argued in court that she should get "custody" of the embryos as she described herself as their "mother." She believed that the embryos were the "beginning of life." Mrs. Davis did not request that Junior support a child that might issue from implantation of the embryos. She was prepared to be a single mother.

Junior Davis believed that the embryos were "potential life," and that he should not be "raped of my reproductive rights." By this he meant that he did not want to be a father if divorced. In the court case, he did not want his wife or anyone else to use them (e.g., through an adoption program). He was not in favor of destroying the embryos either, as that would be "killing them."[3]

Blount County Circuit Court Judge W. Dale Young had to make the decision about the future of the embryos. No one knows exactly how long human embryos can survive after being frozen.

Case 1.3: **COCAINE ADDICTION AND MOTHERHOOD**

In the United States, 2.2 million individuals are addicted to cocaine, using it at least once a week. Five million women of childbearing age use illegal substances, with about 11% of the population abusing drugs during pregnancy. Cocaine abuse by young people has doubled in the past decade, with 17% of seniors in high school reporting use of the drug.

Cocaine is the number one illicit drug used by women of child-bearing age. The fetus of a cocaine dependent mother becomes addicted *in utero*. Congenital malformations, and developmental and learning disabilities may occur as a result of cocaine use. Although infants are often sent home from the nursery with the diagnosis of "normal;" neurological and developmental problems may emerge later.

Mary B. Johnson is 17 now. When she was 15, she gave birth to her son, Joey. Mary is a cocaine addict. When Mary was 11, an older brother introduced her to the drug by "free basing" some for her. He also introduced her to gang activities. He was killed one year ago in a gang fight. Since his death, Mary has desperately tried to avoid the gang members that have gotten her "in trouble," but peer pressure to stay involved in gang activities have defeated any steps to disassociate herself. She is now a willing and committed member of one of the city's most notorious gangs. Joey's father may be one of 5 young men who belong to the gang. Mary is unmarried.

Mary was born and raised in the ghetto. She lives with her grandmother, her mother having been killed by a boyfriend during a spat after "drinking all night." Mary is the eighth of nine children. No father is identified on the birth certificates of these children. Mary's grandmother raised 7 children; she lived on welfare all her life. The violent atmosphere in Mary's neighborhood, combined with personal family troubles and easy access to drugs, led Mary to find relief in cocaine. She now supports her addiction through prostitution activities.

Throughout her pregnancy with Joey, Mary used cocaine regularly. Joey, now two years old, was born prematurely at 31 weeks. Mary presented to the Emergency Room in premature labor. An examination in the E.R. revealed a tender uterus. The physician attending Mary suspected "abruptio placenta." An abdominal ultra sound confirmed this diagnosis. A monitor was placed on Mary's lower abdomen and revealed a fetal heart rate pattern consistent with fetal distress. Mary was taken to the birth center and delivery occurred by STAT cesarean section. Joey's apgar scores were 3 at 1 minute and 9 at five minutes. Resuscitation consisted of intermittent positive pressure ventilation by bag and mask for 3 minutes. Joey's response was excellent and by 5 minutes of life, he was alert, responsive, pink in room air, and in no distress. Examination in the nursery was unremarkable except for decreased head circumference and intrauterine growth retardation. Urine toxicology screening for both Joey and Mary were positive for cocaine.

During his stay in the NICU, Joey exhibited the symptoms of mild withdrawal syndrome. He was treated successfully with supportive care only. Over the course of his stay in the nursery, there was complete resolution of his symptoms from cocaine withdrawal.

In the days following Joey's birth, the doctors and nurses reviewed Joey's problems with Mary. She was told that he would need to be held for extended periods of time in order to calm him down. Mary, however, did not seem interested in caring for the infant in any way. Moreover, she said she had no intention of not using cocaine. When confronted with the effects of this drug on her and on Joey, Mary said that she was unable to stop her use of cocaine throughout her pregnancy. She knew a little bit about the drug, but she thought that the placenta would protect the baby from its effects. Mary denied the possibility of any long-lasting negative effects on Joey that could result from her cocaine use. When the caregivers pressed her further, she argued with them that cocaine was the only happiness she had in her life, and that she was simply not going to stop using it. As far as it is known, she is not protecting herself from any additional pregnancies.

After her release from the hospital, Mary no longer visited the infant despite repeated efforts on the part of the staff and unit social worker to persuade her to do so.

Does the fetus have a right to be protected from capricious mothers *in utero*? If so, how can we reconcile this right with the right of women to seek and obtain an abortion during the first trimester? Should Mary have been imprisoned during her pregnancy with Joey in order to protect him from passive addiction? If not, is it proper to ask society to pay for the consequences of her sociopathic and addictive behavior?

Case 1.4: ADOPTION AS SOLUTION?

A 32-year-old white mother brought in her 3-month-old son for a follow-up visit one week after hospitalization for an acute illness. The patient's symptoms were fully resolved, but the mother continued to ask the pediatrician, "Do you think he looks all right?"

Upon further questioning, the mother admitted to concerns that this child's father may not be her husband's. She had sexual intercourse with an African-American co-worker at a time consistent with this child's conception. Her white husband was unaware of this.

At this time. the child's physical exam was remarkable for skin pigmentation that was slightly darker than either parent, a lumbo-sacral mongolian spot, and no obvious black racial features.

Past history was remarkable for prolonged exaggerated physiologic jaundice. The work-up for this was repeatedly negative, but the mother had persisted that his color looked "funny." He had been hospitalized at 11 weeks for an acute illness and stayed for 6 days. Two pediatric staff members commented to the mother on the baby's "complexion" during hospitalization.

The child lived at home with his mother, her husband, and a four year old sibling. The family environment and the parent's relationship to this time was described by the mother as good.

At the time of this office visit, the mother was encouraged to disclose the full story to her husband. She had recently made the other alleged father aware of the situation. She was encouraged to initiate formal paternity testing and was also placed in contact with Social Service and Family Psychiatry.

After contacting Social Service and Psychiatry, the mother disclosed the full story to both potential fathers. Paternity testing was initiated and revealed that her co-worker was the biologic father.

The mother and her husband, with agreement from the biologic father, decided to place the child for adoption. This was accomplished through an adoption agency.

The mother and her husband are in family counseling. They have disclosed the truth to their own extended family members on both sides. They have chosen to tell neighbors, friends, and their four year old son that the baby died of SIDS.

Questions:

1. What is the role of the pediatrician and that of other healthcare providers in cases of adoption? Who is the physician's primary responsibility? E.g., is it the adopted child; the adoptive family?

2. What principles and values justify the disclosure or nondisclosure of information to adoptees? E.g., informed consent; child or adolescent's "right" to know; right to privacy.

3. Whose claims to information or the withholding of information hold priority? E.g., the adopted child or adolescent; biological parents; adoptive parents.

4. At what age should information be disclosed to adopted children or adolescents concerning their natural parents and background?

5. What possible adverse ramifications, if any, are there in disclosing to and withholding from adopted children and adolescents information about theirbiological parents and their background?

6. What can pediatricians and other health care providers do to serve the future needs of the child to be adopted and of the adoptive family?

Case 1.5: **CONFIDENTIALITY AND ADOLESCENT HEALTH CARE**

A 17-year-old woman (who said she was 18) was brought to the emergency room by her grandfather who is her legal guardian. The patient complained of severe constipation and pelvic pressure of one day's duration. The patient also complained of vaginal discharge. She had no other current symptoms, but admitted to a 20 pound weight gain over the past 4-5 months associated with increased appetite. The patient denied any other changes during that time, had remained physically active, attending high school and playing softball. The patient was not seeing a physician for any medical conditions.

Gynecological history was significant for irregular menses since menarche at age twelve. She only menstruated about every three months. Her periods lasted about ten days. Her last menstrual period had been approximately three months ago.

On entry physical examination it was found that the patient had just delivered an infant. (She was wearing loose clothing). The delivery was then completed by the obstetrics resident. The baby did not breathe spontaneously, so it was resuscitated. Plans were initiated to admit the patient to labor and delivery for delivery of the placenta and postpartum observation.

Upon further questioning, the patient denied knowing that she was pregnant. She stated she had sexual contact without contraception about eight or nine months ago and started on oral contraceptives shortly thereafter. She had always had irregular menses and continued to have occasional bleeding during the pregnancy.

The patient requested that her grandfather not be told of the situation. She said that her mother had her when she was fourteen years old and that her grandfather had suffered a heart attack when he found out she was pregnant. The nursing staff informed her that it would be difficult to hide especially when she would be admitted to the maternity ward. The patient said she felt too overwhelmed to talk to her grandfather now. She asked that he be told that she was alright and that she wanted to "tell him in her own way tomorrow."

The nurse told her it was not fair to send him home without telling and that she would not want her granddaughter to do that to her. The patient persisted with her request.

After the infant was taken from the room, the grandfather was brought in. When he asked what was going on, the nurse replied, "We are sorry, but we cannot give out any information. Your granddaughter has requested that we not tell you and since she is eighteen years old, we must honor that request."

The grandfather replied, surprised, "But she is only seventeen."

The nurse immediately responded, "Oh, then, she just had a baby." The patient began crying and apologizing to her grandfather, telling him that she had wanted to tell him in her own way.

This case raises the issue of whether or not the right to confidentiality in medical care is strictly age-dependent. Too, was the nurse correct in giving out the information to the grandfather without the patient's consent, or at least asking the patient again? In general, if adolescents are not to be protected by the same rules that govern adults, then who may decide whether or not to breach the confidentiality of a minor patient?

Case 1.6: **MULTIPLE GESTATIONS**

Phase One

A new patient presents seeking advice at 8 weeks gestation in her third pregnancy. Her previous health history is unremarkable. She conceived her first two pregnancies with *in vitro* fertilization (other treatments were tried and unsuccessful). They each resulted in a vaginal delivery at term of a normal infant, both of whom are thriving at home with the patient and her husband. The patient is seeking information and advice after the transfer of five embryos with her last ultrasound showing three fetuses each with strong regular fetal cardiac activity.

Questions

1. What is the obligation of physicians to patients in disclosing the risks of conceiving a high order multiple gestation?

2. Should a practitioner's incidence of multiple gestation be disclosed to the patient as part of the consent process? Some areas have already legislated this process.

3. Does the physician have an obligation to alter the number of embryos transferred based on a particular patient's risk of conceiving a high order multiple gestation?

Phase Two

The patient asks for information on selective pregnancy reduction. Her husband is not pleased with this request, but is willing to obtain this information. You discovered that he and his sibs are the result of a successful high order multiple gestation. The patient is concerned about her ability to carry a triplet pregnancy long enough to avoid the risk of mental handicap in the surviving fetuses. Her husband then asks about the experience at LUMC with high order multiple gestations.

Questions

1. Based on this information what counseling should a patient be given about selective pregnancy reduction?

2. How should this counseling differ in twin, triplet and quadruplet gestations or even greater gestations?

3. Does the concept of the greatest good for the greatest number of patients have any role in counseling such patients? (Consider the analogy of field triage in disaster and multiple trauma conditions.)

Phase Three
The patient decides to continue the triplet pregnancy after a much-heated discussion with her husband. At 26 weeks gestation she begins to experience the complication of preterm labor. She is treated with magnesium sulfate and the preterm labor is stopped. Her cervix is now 3 cm and completely effaced. Her physician now recommends prolonged hospitalization and bedrest. The fetuses continue to do well, but the mother becomes more distressed daily. She advises the staff that she will refuse further treatment for preterm labor with magnesium if it is recommended as she "can't go on any further--I can't stay in the hospital." Her husband visits daily, and pleads with her to continue treatment as long as she is in no known danger. He worries that refusal of treatment will place the fetuses in immediate danger. Several days later, the patient shares with you in confidence that she is worried about marital problems. The husband does not express these concerns, stating that he cares strongly for his wife and all five of his forthcoming children.

Questions

1. If the preterm labor returns how "forceful" should her physician be in recommending the magnesium sulfate to treat the preterm labor?

2. How much concern should be advanced for family dynamics in fertility counseling and intervention?

3. What is the role of the father?

Case 1.7: **FETAL TREATMENT**

Mrs. Egan is a 36-year-old mother of four who, during her last delivery, suffered a tear in the opening of the cervix. At that time, the physicians told her, should she want to have another child, she would need to have a "purse string" or cerclage operation, by which the cervix is sutured to give it sufficient structural strength so as to avoid a spontaneous abortion. Mrs. Egan declined, saying that she wished to have no further children and therefore did not need to have the operation.

Two years later the woman's physician finds that Mrs. Egan is again pregnant. The physician recommends that the woman have a cerclage operation, and the husband, Mr. Egan, concurs, insisting that he does not want the fetus aborted. The husband hopes it will be a son for whom he has long waited. The dispute continues into the fourth month of the pregnancy, at which point a sonogram shows that the fetus is a boy.

Mrs. Egan still refuses the cerclage operation, arguing that it is her right to have an abortion until the fetus is viable, and it should not concern anyone how she goes about getting it done, either by medical intervention or because of the structural weakness of her cervix.

Questions

1. Do you agree with Mrs. Egan's decision not to have her cervix surgically strengthened after the birth of her fourth daughter? If she really wished not to have any more children, should she have had her fallopian tubes tied off at that time?

2. What type of tensions are set up in the Egan family following the discovery that the wife is pregnant again? In their disagreement, is there evidence of good communication between Mr. and Mrs. Egan?

3. All people have personal rights, but whose rights take precedence in a case like this: the mother's, the father's, the sisters'? Who will speak out on behalf of the unborn child?

4. What might have encouraged Mrs. Egan to have the sonogram test to visualize the developing fetus within her? Does the knowledge that the baby is a boy instead of a girl have any bearing on her continued refusal for the cerclage operation?

5. What is Mrs. Egan's attitude toward abortion? Even if one is against an induced abortion of a seemingly healthy baby, is refusal to receive reasonable and routine medical treatment that is proven to help carry the fetus to term any less of an evil? That is, can one morally distinguish between active and passive abortion, analogous to active and passive euthanasia?

6. Discuss the individual feelings and family dynamics in this case following one of the many possible outcomes for Mrs. Egan: healthy baby delivered; genetically-diseased baby delivered; healthy baby aborted; genetically-diseased baby aborted.

Used with permission of Charles Webber, Ph.D.

Case 1.8: TERMINATION OF PREGNANCY: A DIFFICULT CHOICE

A.M. is a 19-year-old white female with a history of systemic lupus erythematosus (SLE) and diffuse proliferative lupus nephritis since 1984. During the 10 years she has had SLE, her medical care has been provided by the same physician; there is a strong patient-physician relationship. During the first six years of the disease most of the manifestations were extrarenal. In 1990, she had a severe exacerbation of lupus nephritis but responded well to six monthly infusions of cyclophosphamide. Following the intensive course of cyclophosphamide therapy, her disease was well controlled until about six months ago when she developed increasing proteinuria resulting in nephrotic syndrome. Because she developed perianal herpes infection and a herpetic skin lesion over her right anterior ankle, further intensive immunosuppression was postponed.

At a time when she demonstrated worsening lupus nephritis and was awaiting further intensive immunosuppressive therapy, she informed her physician that she was 7 weeks pregnant and wanted to continue the pregnancy. A.M.'s condition with active lupus and lupus nephritis places both her and her fetus at great risk. A.M.'s primary care physician and a consulting high risk obstetrician encouraged her to consider terminating pregnancy.

A.M. has overcome many social and medical problems. She was abandoned by her natural mother soon after birth and was raised by her paternal grandmother and her young father who was an alcoholic. At age 15, her father remarried and her stepmother assumed her grandmother's caregiving role. A.M. graduated from high school in 1992 and began attending community college; she withdrew during the first year because of physical limitations. About the same time, A.M. left home and moved in with her boyfriend. Her boyfriend supports her decision to continue the pregnancy.

Apart from the question of the morality of abortion, some other ethical problems are also presented by this case:

1. What is the role of the primary care physician who has enormous influence on a patient's decision-making in regard to abortion? How "coercive" should she be in urging A.M. to have an abortion?

2. What are the implications for the patient-physician relationship if a physician uses her influence to encourage a patient to make a decision that goes against the patient's values, beliefs, and wishes?

3. Even if one is against abortion in general, can abortion be justified at least on the grounds of potential damage to the fetus?

4. What reproductive "right" do we possess when exercizing it may harm the fetus, or, in this case, burden future caregivers if the mother should die?

5. To what extent are individuals conceived and born in the context of being valued and wanted by their parents, and should this "extrinsic" value have an impact on the abortion question?

6. Are medical values important enough in this case to override personal and even religious values?

7. If a high risk pregnancy is brought to term after warnings from health professionals, should insurance or a national health plan pay for the consequences?

Case 1.9: CROSS-CULTURAL ISSUES IN BIOETHICS: TO CIRCUMCISE OR NOT?

A family practice physician, Dr. Jones, was involved with a maternal/child health project funded by the World Health Organization. Her participation in the project included six months at a clinic located in a rural village about 100 miles from Cairo.

Dr. Jones was familiar with the common practice of female circumcision in certain Middle Eastern and African countries. She knew that as many as 80 million women have undergone tradition female surgeries, including clitoridectomy, excision of the labia minora, and infibulation. These operations are not medically required; they are performed for ritual, traditional, or religious reasons. The procedure is usually done on young girls; the age varies depending upon the local custom. Girls and women may experience physical problems subsequent to the circumcision. Problems include severe infection, hemorrhage, fistulae, ascending pelvic and renal infections, infertility, and increased female mortality.

Dr. Jones anticipated that she would treat women and girls with medical problems caused by circumcision. She was right. Although she had tried to prepare herself for this eventuality, Dr. Jones was surprised by her feelings of repulsion and frustration when she encountered the physical complications of circumcision, particularly in the young girls. Dr. Jones had always considered herself to be "liberal" in her acceptance of cultural traditions different from the Anglo western "mainstream." She tried her best to justify the practice of circumcision, in her own mind, based on its significance for the social survival of women in the village.

During her stay in the village, Dr. Jones became friends with a woman who acted as a research assistant for the project; her nickname was "Mosha." Dr. Jones was impressed by Mosha's abilities on the project and her insightful views about the community. One day, Mosha asked Dr. Jones for her advice about something that was troubling her. Mosha said that it was time to consider circumcision for her eight year old daughter. Mosha's sisters, her husband, and her husband's female relatives were urging her to go ahead with the procedure. Mosha herself had been circumcised, as had the majority of the women in the village. It was the custom. However, since her involvement as a local staff worker with World Health Organization projects over the last several years, Mosha had begun to have a change of mind about female circumcision. She was reluctant to have her daughter undergo the procedure, knowing the pain it would cause her and the risk of ongoing medical complications. On the other hand, Mosha knew that her daughter faced the possibility of being socially stigmatized if she was not circumcised. This could mean that her chances for marriage would be jeopardized; a serious issue for a woman's emotional and economic standing in this community. Mosha is deeply concerned about what to do; she feels that no matter what she decides, problems to address will occur.

Questions:

1. If you were Dr. Jones, what would advice would you give to Mosha?

2. In a world of remarkable cultural diversity, how should we decide what is "morally" correct? If a traditional custom is very different from western normative behavior, does that make it wrong? Where do we "draw the line" in our tolerance for practices and beliefs that differ significantly from ours?

3. What do you think about charges of "moral imperialism" made by individuals in developing nations in response to concern expressed by the West over what are labeled as "human rights" abuses (e.g., in India, the selling of kidneys for transplantation; in China, the use of convicted criminals as organ donors; in Korea and some other countries, the use of ultra sound to determine the sex of the fetus so that female fetuses can be aborted)? How would you answer these charges?

Notes

1 Schmich MT. Embryo custody case of a test of law, life. *Chicago Tribune* 1989 Aug. 8:Sec. 1, 1-2.
2 *Ibid*.
3 Schmich MT. Couple in embryo case testify on early hopes. *Chicago Tribune* 1989 Aug. 9:Sec. 1,3.

Chapter 6

What We May Do with Preembryos: A Response to Richard A. McCormick

John A. Robertson

The controversies surrounding *in vitro* fertilization (IVF) arise largely from differing views of the pre-embryo's moral status and of what may appropriately be done with preembryos.

In a recent article the noted Catholic bioethicist, Richard A. McCormick, argues that the genetically unique pre-embryo is not itself a person prior to implantation because it is not yet developmentally individual (1991, pp.8-9). He also argued that key Catholic documents about prenatal life have not considered the biological facts of developmental individuality, and thus have not yet definitively ruled that the pre-embryo is a person.

As a religious matter McCormick's article is an important document. It is a bold and insightful attempt to reconcile Catholic teachings with biological reality, and no doubt will raise controversy within theological circles. As a secular matter, however, McCormick's position is not novel. It reflects the consensus concerning pre-embryo status that has emerged from most official and professional advisory bodies that have examined the issue, such as the Ethics Advisory Board, the Warnock Committe, the American Fertility Society, and others. (Ethics Advisory Board 1979, p. 101; American Fertility Society, 1986, p. 20S; Department of Health and Social Security, Great Britain, 1984, pp. 27, 63).

I am not qualified to comment on the merits of McCormick's theological position, but I do agree with him that the preembryo is not a person. In my view, however, McCormick does not adequately recognize the implications of his position, and may end up taking away with one hand what he gives with the other.

Immediately after concluding that the embryo is not a person and therefore "cannot be the subject of human rights," McCormick sets some rather strict limits on what may be done with preembryos (1991, p.12-13). Because of the preembryo's "intrinsic potential" and uncertainties about the ability to cabin technologies once they are loosed, he proposes a *prima facie* obligation that "the pre-embryo should be treated as a person" (Id.). He also proposes that "any exceptions from the *prima facie* obligation to treat the pre-embryo as a person should be based on criteria established at the national level" (1991, p.10).

If these proposals are strictly applied, it will not be possible to do the things with preembryos -- discard, freeze, research and biopsy -- that are of current interest to clinicians and patients. If we are obligated to treat preembryos as persons (even though they are not), strict limits on actions with preembryos should follow. Only if that *prima facie* obligation permits actions which would not be acceptable if actual persons were involved would McCormick' s position be substantively different.
Even then, it would probably require stricter limits on what may be done with preembryos

---

Source: Reprinted from *Kennedy Institute of Ethics Journal*, Vol. 1, No. 4, pp. 293-305, with permission from The Johns Hopkins University Press © 1991.

than views holding that the preembryo is entitled to a lesser degree of respect.

McCormick's position, though progressive in terms of Catholic doctrine, thus appears to remain restrictive with regard to the questions of immediate interest to scientists, physicians, and patients. Although he does not address these issues directly, his proposal for a *prima facie* obligation to treat preembryos as persons would appear to ban or greatly restrict pre-embryo discard, freezing, research, and biopsy. Yet if preembryos are not persons, such actions would appear to be permissible.

To explore this conflict and identify what we may do with preembryos, I first discuss McCormick's claim that there is a *prima facie* obligation to treat preembryos as if they were persons, showing the implications of this position for four issues at the center of preembryo controversies. I then challenge his claim that policies regarding preembryos must necessarily be set at the national level.

Why Must We Treat Preembyos As If They Were Persons?

Although McCormick argues persuasively that preembryos, because they lack developmental individuality, are not themselves persons, he nonetheless concludes that there is a *prima facie* obligation to treat them as if they were, with any deviation to be established by "national criteria" (1991, p. 9, 10). His reasons for this claim rest on the pre-embryo's potential to develop into an embryo, and the slippery slope consequences of a less rigorous view.

McCormick says that because of the potential of the pre-embryo to implant, develop into a embryo, fetus and eventually a newborn infant, "in viewing the first stage, one cannot afford to blot out subsequent stages" (1991, p.9). Even if the potential of any given embryo to develop into an infant is "significantly reduced," it "remains potential for personhood and as such deserves profound respect" (Id.). Therefore "interference with such a potential future cannot be a light undertaking" (Id.).

Secondly, "uncertainty about the extent to which enthusiasm for human research can be controlled" requires a very rigorous protective stance toward embryos (Id.). A less protective attitude toward embryos will reduce our respect for embryos and fetuses, and "human life in general" (Id.). It will also lead to trivial or frivolous uses of preembryos. Once preembryo manipulation and research begins, the irreversible dynamics of medical technology are not easily stopped.

I question, however, whether the pre-embryo's potential and slippery slope risks, require that preembryos be treated as persons. If preembryos are not persons, then how we treat them is a matter of policy, not moral obligation. The question thus is whether a general policy interest in respect for human life requires that preembryos be treated as strictly as McCormick recommends.

Clearly, preembryos are different from other human tissue. Because they are genetically unique and have the potential to develop into persons, they carry a symbolic meaning not present in other tissue. Their potential to become persons makes their repositories of meaning and value that exist independently of religious views. To express that value, we may accord preembryos respect beyond that accorded other human tissue. However, it must be emphasized that such a judgment is a choice based on utilitarian or constitutive grounds. Because preembryos are too rudimentary in development to have interests, it is not morally obligatory. It may be maintained or relaxed, as other considerations and interests demand.

In each case for decision, the question is whether the symbolic gains of "profound" or "special" respect justify the loss to other legitimate human purposes that restrictions on actions with preembryos would entail. The same point may be posed in utilitarian terms: Is the loss to symbolic respect for human life outweighed by the good from a less respectful stance?

In constitutive terms, do we wish to constitute our stance toward human life as so protective of Preembryos that other goods are foregone?

These questions cannot be answered in the abstract, but must be confronted in the practical situations in which they arise. In examining those situations, we can also see whether treating preembryos as less than persons will yield the slippery slope consequences that McCormick claims.

Preembryo Discard

Given ovarian stimulation regimes that produce multiple eggs in any IVF cycle, couples are often faced with more preembryos than can safely be placed in the uterus. They must either choose either not to fertilize all eggs, which could leave them with too few preembryos to induce pregnancy, or discard the extras. Cryopreservation of extra preembryos does not always alleviate the problem, and may raise independent problems. At some point couples and IVF programs must face the issue of non-transfer or discard of unwanted preembryos.

Although McCormick does not explicitly address this issue, an obligation to treat preembryos as if they were persons would lean very heavily against discard, or at least against egg retrieval practices that make discard likely. After all, if preembryos are to be treated like persons, they should be rescued and implanted, unless implantation poses severe threats to the life or health of the woman.

The reasons for discard, however, seldom rise to that compelling level of justification. Instead, they are reasons based on maximizing the chance of achieving pregnancy and avoiding biologic offspring. For example, suppose the couple undergoing IVF treatment for infertility produces 8 eggs and wants all fertilized in order to have at least 3 or 4 preembryos to place in the uterus. Any preembryos beyond 4 will be discarded, e.g., allowed to divide until they divide no longer.

Although the couple is willing to create 8 embryos to get four, with the excess discarded, their desire to have enough preembryos to implant without unduly risking a multifetal pregnancy (and the need for later selective reduction) should be acceptable. Reasonable persons could find that such action does not greatly diminish respect for human life because discard is occurring for a good reason before developmental individuality has been established.

Cryopreservation would not necessarily alleviate the problem. Suppose the extras were frozen for possible use during a later cycle. For various reasons, ranging from birth of a child, acceptance of childlessness, divorce, age, etc., the couple asks that the preembryos be thawed and not transferred. If creation and non-transfer during a fresh cycle is acceptable, then this action should be as well. Indeed, even if discard of fresh preembryos is not acceptable, discard after freezing might be because there was an attempt to preserve them for later use that did not oocur.

Suppose, however, that extra preembryos (whether fresh or frozen) could be donated anonymously to infertile couples for placement in the woman's uterus, with that couple becoming the rearing parents for all purposes. The couple producing the preembryos, however, still insists on discard, because they do not wish to have biologic offspring reared by others. Again, reasonable persons might agree that it is not callous, frivolous, or highly disrespectful of human life to prefer the destruction of preembryos to having unknown biologic offspring, with all the attendant psychosocial implications for the offspring, and for the social and genetic parents.

In each case the reasons for discard do not appear to be trivial or frivolous, though they reflect a particular view of the importance of preembryos and the competing considerations about which persons reasonably concerned about respect for human life might differ.

Surely one might reasonably believe that a willingness to create but not implant all preembryos does not seriously diminish respect for human life generally, given that discard occurs at a stage before there is developmental individuality.

Yet such reasons do not rise to the level of reasons that would justify discard if preembryos are viewed as persons. If that is the standard, then discard of unwanted or extra preembryos could not in most cases occur. Infertile couples would have to fertilize only those eggs that they would be willing to have placed in the uterus, or accept unwanted donation of preembryos and the possibility of biologic offspring. Thus McCormick's approach would appear to lead to a serious difference with views that do not require that preembryos be regarded as persons.

Cryopreservation of Preembryos

Cryopreservation preserves preembryos that cannot, when created, be safely placed in the uterus for placement in later cycles. It is thought to enhance pregnancy rates from IVF, and saves women from the expense and burdens of later IVF cycles.

Yet cryopreservation may also damage preembryos. As McCormick notes, "thawing of preembryos is not a completely benign process; significant numbers of the preembryos die in the process and injury cannot be excluded" (1991, p.1).

If one accepts that preembryos are not persons, then cryopreservation, if shown to be safe and effective, should be an acceptable alternative for couples undergoing IVF treatment for infertility. Although some preembryos may be damaged in the process, it gives more preembryos a chance to be created and implanted than would otherwise exist. It provides an alternative to discard of preembryos, and minimizes burdens on women and couples undergoing IVF treatment. These are not trivial reasons, and to many persons, would not appear to diminish respect for fetuses, infants, or adult forms of human life.

Yet a *prima facie* obligation to treat the pre-embryo as a person might well require a ban on cryopreservation. Although the procedure allows some preembryos to survive, it does so at the cost of others. Killing some persons to save others, except in dire necessity, is generally not acceptable. Here the dilemma could be avoided by limiting the number of eggs that are fertilized in the first place. Thus McCormick's view of the preembryo may well lead to a ban on freezing, since the need to freeze could be avoided by couples accepting a reduced chance of pregnancy by fertilizing fewer than all retrieved eggs.

Preembryo Research

An important issue of preembryo policy concerns whether and in what circumstances preembryos may be the vehicles or subject of research. On the prevailing view that preembryos deserve some respect but not the respect due persons, preembryo research for legitimate scientific or medical reasons has been found acceptable by most bodies that have examined the subject.

Such research cannot injure the preembryo, which is too rudimentary to have interests that can be injured, and if done for a valid purpose, with institutional review and informed consent, does not substantially diminish respect for human life generally. Indeed, many bodies, such as the Warnock Committee, have found that preembryos could be created for research purposes, even if no placement in the uterus were planned. Because of the preembryo's rudimentary status, use in legitimate research incurs few symbolic costs.

By contrast, McCormick's view of a *prima facie* obligation to treat the preembryo as a person might not permit the same range of preembryo research. Some persons would find that such a standard prohibits all research that is not directly therapeutic to the preembryo. Presumably McCormick would allow at least nontherapeutic research that poses minimal risk to the preembryo. But research posing any risk beyond minimal would most likely be rejected, as might the creation of preembryos solely for research purposes. If one views research leading to preembryo manipulation or discard to be harmful, many kinds of useful research permitted under less restrictive standards would be prohibited.

Preimplantation Genetic Diagnosis of Preembryos

Preimplantation genetic diagnosis involves the removal of one or more cells from the developing *in vitro* preembryo and subjecting its DNA to genetic analysis. Based on the results of the genetic test, the preembryo is either discarded or placed in the uterus. Eventually, such testing may lead to gene insertion or repair at the preembryonic level.

Although still experimental, preimplantation testing offers an alternative to later prenatal diagnosis and abortion for couples at risk for severe genetic disease. Rather than undergo amniocentesis and abortion late in the second trimester of pregnancy, they can screen preembryos for the disease prior to implantation. However, this screening necessarily involves the manipulation and possible destruction of preembryos. Some healthy preembryos will be damaged by biopsy. Others will be discarded on the basis of the genetic test.

If preembryos are not persons, preimplantation genetic testing is acceptable if freely chosen by the couples at risk. Its discard practices are no different from those that occur in many IVF programs. It also has the advantage of moving prenatal diagnosis to an earlier stage, thus avoiding abortion of a more fully developed fetus. Other reservations voiced about the practice go beyond the treatment of preembryos (Robertson, 1992).

However, viewing the preembryo as a person, as McCormick recommends, might also lead to restrictions on this practice. The desire to give birth to offspring without severe genetic disease might not be found to be a sufficient reason to risk damaging healthy preembryos by biopsy. In addition, that desire might not justify discard of preembryos that have the disease in question. The proponents of this view, however, could not consistently argue against preembryo biopsy while permitting prenatal diagnosis and abortion to occur.

Differences

The discussion of preembryo discard, cryopreservation, research, and biopsy shows that there may well be a substantial difference between the actions regarding preembryos permitted under McCormick's *prima facie* obligation test and the less restrictive standards that now generally prevail. In my view, reasonable persons could find that none of these actions, when done for the reasons discussed above, significantly impair respect for human life as either a constitutive or utilitarian matter. In appropriate circumstances, they are the actions that should be permitted with regard to preembryos.

If McCormick's approach would not yield substantially the same conclusions, then he should have to show that the symbolic costs of these actions, despite their benefits, are too great. Of course, reasonable people might differ over these matters, as might the institutions in which they would occur. But reasonable differences of view do not constitute good reasons for prohibiting practices that some find desirable or even necessary. In my view, none of these actions sought with preembryos are so trivial, frivolous, or disrespectful of human life that they should not be permitted.

Are National Criteria Needed for Actions Regarding Preembryos?

Since McCormick does not directly address the four issues just discussed, we do not know whether he would definitively reject them. It may be that he would find some acceptable, though it is certainly plausible under his strong claim of *prima facie* obligation that he would find them all unacceptable.

It may also be that McCormick's acceptance of actions regarding preembryos would turn on the body making the comparison of benefits and risks. In addition to arguing substantively that preembryos should be treated like persons, McCormick (1991, p.13) also makes an important procedural point:

> Because the matter is so important and so controversial, any exceptions from the *prima facie* duty to treat the pre-embryo as a person should be based on criteria established at the national level.

Of course, the morality of a course of action cannot turn on whether a local, state, or national body makes a determination of its acceptability. As a policy matter, however, one may be more willing to accept policies adopted or recommended by a national body than by a local one. In either case, however, the acceptability of the policy is independent of the body recommending it.

With regard to preembryo policy, requiring determinations at a national level, as McCormick suggests, should not be necessary. Many equally important and controversial matters are left to the states and even local units of government, ranging from capital punishment and abortion to pornography and the provision of health care to the poor. Indeed, one beauty of our federal system is that each state may, within constitutional constraints, be a laboratory of social experimentation.

McCormick's recommendation for national criteria also assumes that a national consensus for all actions regarding preembryos is both desirable and possible. Questions of preembryo policy, however, inevitably raise basic value questions for which no national consensus is possible. Nor is it clearly desirable, since people may reasonably disagree about the symbolic value and hence actions taken with preembryos. For example, it may be that some institutions and states will permit preimplantation genetic screening, while others will find it unacceptable.

Finally, as a practical matter setting national preembryo criteria simply may not be politically feasible. At the present time, there is no national consultative body (other than Congress) that could fulfill that role. The Ethics Advisory Board has long been disbanded, and is unlikely to be resurrected. Abortion politics prevented Congress' Bioethics Advisory Board from coming into being. Any similar national body that could set policy on pre-embryo issues is also likely to founder over abortion politics. The exception might be a privately funded board, such as the one proposed by the American College of Obstetrics and Gynecology and the American Fertility Society, but that board might lack the authoritative mandate that presumably McCormick is seeking.

I conclude that there is no need for a national consensus or national body to address these issues before researchers, clinicians, and couples can discard, freeze, research, or biopsy preembryos. While there are important value issues at stake, they are not generically different from the many value conflicts that get resolved at a state or local level. Of course, institutions may require IRB or ethics committee review before permitting them to be done, and applicable state or local law must be observed. If we wait until we have a nationally-announced consensus, however, we may never be able to do anything with preembryos.

Conclusion

McCormick's recognition that the preembryo is not a person because it lacks developmental individuality is an important step forward for Catholics and others trying to come to terms with IVF technology. Taking this claim seriously should permit most of the things that researchers, clinicians and patients now wish to do with preembryos, including discard, cryopreservation, research, and biopsy.

Yet it is not clear that McCormick accepts these implications of his conclusion that the preembryo is not a person. His reasons for claiming a *prima facie* obligation to treat the preembryo as a person can be satisfied by a less restrictive standard that would permit many actions that his *prima facie* obligation would appear to prohibit.

If preembryos are not persons, there is no obligation to treat them as if they were, though we may choose to do so for symbolic or policy reasons. The question in each case involves comparing the harm to symbolic notions of human life versus. the good from the action or manipulation in question. In my view, the purposes generally sought in cryopreservation, discard, research and biopsy are legitimate, and because they occur with an entity that is not yet even developmentally individual, present little risk of diminishing respect for human life. If McCormick disagrees, it may be that he is applying too high a standard to an entity that he acknowledges is not a person and has no human rights.

References

1. American fertility society ethics committe of the ethical considerations of the new reproductive technologies. *Fertility and Sterility* 46;1986:Supplement 1.
2. Report of the committee of inquiry into human fertilization and embryology. In: Warnock M, ed. *Department of Health and Social Security Great Britain*. London: Her Majesty's Stationery Office. 1984.
3. Report conclusions: HEW support of research involving human in vitro fertilization and embryo transfer. *Department of Health, Education and Welfare Ethics Advisory Board.* Washington, DC: U.S. 1976.
4. McCormick RA. Who or what is the pre-embryo? *Kennedy Institute of Ethics Journal* 1991;1:1-11.
5. Robertson JA. Ethical and legal issues in preimplantation genetic diagnosis, *Fertility and Sterility* 1992.
6. Warnock Committee Report. England.

Chapter 7

The Maternal-Fetal Dyad: Exploring the Two-Patient Obstetric Model

Susan S. Mattingly

> *"For ages, medicine has had poor access to the fetus inside the mother's womb. But in relatively recent years, the human body has become transparent. The latest breakthroughs of technology have made it possible, from the very beginning of pregnancy, to consider the fetus as an individual who can be examined and sampled. His or her physician may now establish a diagnosis and prognosis and prescribe a treatment in the same way as in traditional medicine."*[1]

Developments in obstetric medicine during the past ten to twenty years have transformed the clinical status of the fetus.[2] Traditionally physicians have been trained to assess fetal condition by indirect methods: palpating the fetus through the maternal abdominal wall and uterus, measuring hormonal milieu through maternal urine and serum, and estimating statistical risks from parental medical histories. While the skillful use of these methods could produce highly reliable clues to fetal health and development, the fetus itself eluded direct examination. Throughout pregnancy the fetus could not be known, but only inferentially and probabilistically approached. Until recently, suspected fetal anomalies have been treated indirectly, too, by therapeutically managing the maternal environment. Unable to interact with the fetus in clear distinction from its host, physicians conceptualized the maternal-fetal dyad as one complex patient, the gravid female, of which the fetus was an integral part.

High-resolution ultrasonography and techniques for sampling fetal blood, urine, and other tissue have changed this conceptual scheme. These diagnostic tools penetrate the opaque environment and reveal the fetus to clinical observation in all its anatomical, physiological, and biochemical particularity. When anomalies are detected, *in utero* medical and surgical procedures are already beginning to offer alternatives to therapeutic delivery and neonatal treatment. The biological maternal-fetal relationship has not changed, of course, but the medical model of that relationship has a shifted in emphas from unity to duality. Clinicians no longer look to the maternal host for diagnostic data and a therapeutic medium. They look through her to the fetal organism and regard it as a distinct patient in its own right.

What ethical implications flow from the fetus's transformation from inferred to observed entity? Unfortunately, legal developments have tended to preempt ethical exploration of the new two-patient obstetric model. Some physicians, assuming enhanced rights on the part of the fetal patient, have sought and obtained court orders to perform fetal therapies (notably Cesarean deliveries) without maternal consent.[3] Although few in number, these cases raise

---

Source: Reprinted from *Hastings Center Report*, Jan-Feb 1992, pp. 13-18, with permission from © The Hastings Center.

the possibility of a new standard of clinical practice with far-reaching implications for civil and criminal liabilities to physicians and pregnant women. With legal stakes so high, it is not surprising that ethical inquiry has been displaced. Yet in the absence of independent and thorough ethical analysis one cannot judge whether these developments are compatible with fundamental values of medicine and medical care, and so cannot know whether physicians have responsibilities, individually or collectively, to promote or resist them.

Well-grounded in law and ethics or not, cases of court-ordered fetal therapy have set the agenda for debate, focusing attention on the question, *What should the physician do when a pregnant woman refuses medical or surgical treatment recommended for the well being of the newly-individuated fetal patient?* The two-patient problem for the physician is seen to begin at the point of maternal refusal and is framed as a conflict between values of fetal benefit and maternal autonomy. The medical recommendation precipitating refusal is, presumably, unproblematic. But that presumption requires examination. Inherent in any conceptual shift is the potential for equivocation between the old paradigm and the new. If the physician's recommendation of fetal therapy incorporates one-patient thinking about the maternal-fetal relationship, questions about maternal refusal of that recommendation may be spurious, resting on a logically illicit hybrid of one-patient and two-patient conceptual schemes.

We need, I think, to gain a fresh perspective on this issue by stepping back from the legal debate and considering in a systematic way how ethical guidelines for prenatal medical care are altered by transition to the two-patient obstetric model. How do the familiar principles of beneficence, justice, and autonomy operate within the new model in contrast to the old? Fetal rights and fiduciary responsibilities of professionals, parents, and the state may all be affected by the fetus's newly acquired identity as a second individual patient, but to avoid blurring distinctions among these roles my focus will rest on ethical implications for physicians. After all, elevation of the fetus to patient status has occurred not because of any change in the fetus or in the maternal-fetal relationship but because of a change in physicians -- in how they think about and relate to their patients during pregnancy -- so it is in the physician-patient relationship that we should expect the ethical repercussions to begin.

For the Patient's Own Good

The ethical principle guiding initial formulations of medical recommendations is beneficence. It directs physicians to recommend that course of therapy most likely to protect and promote patient health, based on estimates of medical benefits relative to burdens for the various treatment options. In making these complex comparisons, physicians are to ignore their own and third-party interests, responding compassionately to patient medical needs alone. For some purposes it is important to distinguish *positive* duties to offer benefits from *negative* duties not to inflict burdens. "Beneficence" then refers more narrowly to the former duties, "nonmaleficence" to the latter. Nonmaleficence requires that the risks, discomforts, and harms inherent in medical or surgical treatment be offset by proportionate therapeutic gains for the patient. Accordingly, treatment without therapeutic intent is categorically prohibited by the principle of nonmaleficence.

In cases where maternal and fetal burdens associated with fetal therapy are relatively small and prospective benefits to the fetus are substantial, the physician's duty of beneficence on the one-patient obstetric model is clearly to recommend treatment. This is true even if treatment offers *no* medical benefits, only burdens, to the woman in distinction from the fetus. When the maternal-fetal dyad is regarded as an organic whole, what matters is that *combined* maternal-fetal benefits outweigh *combined* maternal-fetal burdens. Distributions of benefits and burdens between fetal and maternal components of the one patient are not ethically relevant.

When fetus and pregnant woman are conceptualized as two individual patients, however, it is no longer appropriate to consider effects of treatment on the two combined. Physicians are to decide what is medically best for each patient considered separately. When fetal benefits outweigh fetal burdens of intervention, beneficence dictates recommending therapy for the fetal patient. But when anomalous fetal conditions pose no threat to maternal health, caring for the fetal patient imposes some degree of discomfort, harm, or risk on the maternal patient with no offsetting therapeutic benefits to her.[4] Maternal medical burdens outweigh maternal medical benefits, such nonmaleficence requires recommending *against* treatment for the maternal patient.

Here is an ethical two-patient problem for the physician that arises well before the point of maternal refusal: Treatment medically indicated for one patient is contraindicated for the other, yet both must be treated (or not treated) alike. It is difficult to see a favorable ratio of fetal gains to maternal losses as a problem and not a solution, of course, for we are accustomed to maternal-fetal balancing on the one-patient model. Also, we know that in most cases pregnant women expect to assume reasonable risks to improve the chances of delivering a healthy baby. Willingness to do so is ideally implicit in the choice of pregnancy, and indeed the argument that the pregnant woman increases her responsibility for the fetus's well-being by choosing not to have an abortion is often cited to support the medical duty to provide fetal therapy.[5] Given persistent economic and social obstacles to abortion, not to mention its precarious legality, the degree to which abortion rights increase maternal responsibilities is, I think, dubious, but that is a side issue. The real question is how maternal duties affect professional duties and exactly which duties are affected. Since beneficence considerations are restricted to medical benefits and burdens, it seems clear that maternal morality must be a factor to be weighed against beneficence at a later stage of ethical analysis.

On the two-patient model of the maternal-fetal dyad, a single treatment recommendation for both patients cannot be justified in terms of the beneficence principle alone, for it includes no provision for balancing burdens to one patient against benefits to another. Indeed, tradeoffs *between* patients are expressly prohibited by the exclusion of third-party interests. Beneficence, applying as it does to patients one by one, is logically unequipped to produce a single recommendation for two linked patients with conflicting medical needs.

Mediating the Conflict

Conflicts between duties of beneficence and nonmaleficence to multiple patients are rare in medicine but they do characteristically occur in two areas in addition to obstetrics: live-donor tissue transplantation and nontherapeutic research.[6] In both fields physicians' unusual divided loyalties -- to patients in need of medical help and to those put at medical risk to provide that help -- have engendered considerable concern and an extensive ethical literature.[7] The resulting codes and practices resist any movement toward a utilitarian ethic whereby imperatives of medical rescue and medical progress would justify imposing relatively small harms and risks on donors and subjects. The rationale for rejecting a balancing approach that trades off benefits against harms between patients hinges on the way medical moral authority is circumscribed. Professional ethical decisions are not generic judgments made from a neutral standpoint preferring always the lesser to the greater harm. They are choices made from the standpoint of the professional as moral agent, hence *causal responsibility* and *motivation* for harm are more significant variables than *quantity* of harm. If physicians *do not* intervene to help a patient in need of a kidney transplant, the patient suffers harm due to progress of the disease condition, the physician's choice being at most a contributing factor; if physicians *do* intervene, the donor suffers harm directly and exclusively from medical intervention. The Hippocratic tradition is shaped by the presumption that moral liability for physician-caused harm to a patient is relieved *only* by therapeutic intent *for that patient,* whereas excusing conditions and motivations for failures-to-benefit are many and varied. Nonmaleficence constrains beneficence and not *vice versa.*

In transplantation and research ethics, nonmaleficence constraints have been cautiously qualified to permit physicians under narrowly specified conditions to treat some patients nontherapeutically in order to benefit others. First, medical burdens inflicted must be smaller in relation to anticipated benefits, than they are when they accrue to one and the same patient. Second, patients treated nontherapeutically must be volunteers. *Recommending* nontherapeutic treatment remains unethical, although *providing* it is permissible at the subject's or donor's request.

On the one-patient model for obstetric care, conflicts between maternal and fetal needs occur within, not between, patients; they are balanced and resolved by physicians under the principle of beneficence in determining the medically indicated course of therapy. On the two-patient model, however, competing maternal and fetal needs must be settled at a different level, by applying standards of justice. According to these standards, physicians are not at liberty to benefit one patient by inflicting medical harms on another, except under stringently qualified conditions. In most cases, pregnant women, continuing to identify fetal needs and interests with their own, will request treatment to promote fetal health, thereby lifting constraints of nonmaleficence and authorizing physicians to proceed with proportionate fetal therapy. For physicians to recommend fetal therapy as if it were medically indicated for both patients, however, would be misleading and unethical.

The question is whether, having removed fetal needs from the calculus of maternal medical interests and having divided one compound professional-patient obligation into two discrete fiduciary commitments, physicians may discount protective duties owed to the woman as an individual patient in her own right. Is this the stage at which professional duties are altered by maternal duties? In other areas of medicine, the injunction against intentional medical harm is not thought to be affected by patient morality or social role: neither moral debts to society nor obligations of family relationship authorize physicians to take a stronger-than-invitational approach in recruiting research subjects or tissue donors. Indeed, incarcerated felons and other institutionalized populations are virtually off-limits to medical researchers, since distinctions between *inviting*, and *advising*, and *requiring* are difficult to maintain in coercive contexts. More to the point, in transplantation ethics, family pressures on the donor are considered a form of moral coercion, increasing rather than decreasing professional obligations to emphasize the optional nature of the transaction. When alternate volunteers or procedures are unavailable or unlikely to yield successful results, this restrained approach on the part of physicians may result in the loss of significant prospective benefits, including lives which might have been saved. That is the price of role-based limits on professional moral agency. But a professional ethics that allow treatment recommendations to be based on moral diagnosis of patients and therapeutic intent for others would also exact a price: It would erode the fiduciary character of the professional-patient relationship, undermining the basis for patient trust.

By separating the maternal-fetal dyad conceptually into two individual patients, the new obstetric model bifurcates the process of formulating medical recommendations: Physicians should recommend beneficial fetal therapy for the fetal patient, but recommending treatment for the maternal patient contrary to her best medical interests is prohibited by standards for the just resolution of duties to multiple patients. In two-patient obstetrics, physicians may at most *invite and encourage* the pregnant woman to submit *voluntarily* to burdensome treatment for the sake of proportionate fetal benefits. Usually the invitation will be readily accepted, so the distinction between *inviting* treatment and *recommending* it will have little practical importance. It is of considerable theoretical importance, however, to the pregnant woman's autonomy.

Honoring the Patient

On the one-patient obstetric model, recommended fetal therapy offers net medical benefits to the pregnant woman, the refusal of which, here as in other medical contexts, should trigger discussion to determine whether her needs and values are in fact incompatible with treatment. Although efforts to encourage consent are appropriate, paternalistic treatment of a competent dissenting patient is unlikely to be justified. In particular, her autonomy cannot be restricted on the grounds that she is causing harm to others, as the pregnant woman on the one-patient model causes harm only to herself.

Rejecting treatment on the two-patient obstetric model is more complicated. The physician's *two* treatment proposals -- the *recommendation* of therapy for the fetus and the *invitation* to nontherapeutic maternal treatment as a means to fetal therapy -- call for two distinct maternal replies, neither of which is a standard exercise of patient autonomy. First, the recommendation of therapy for the fetus requires a *maternal proxy decision* on behalf of the incompetent fetal patient. Maternal responsibility for fetal well-being is certainly relevant at this point, and physicians are morally authorized to challenge proxy decisions that are plainly contrary to the patient's best interests. Yet even if an alternate proxy (the father of the future child, for instance, or a court-appointed legal guardian) consents to therapy on behalf of the fetus, another ethical step remains. The physician's second proposal, the invitation to nontherapeutic maternal treatment, requires a *maternal patient decision*. This second step distinguishes fetal therapy from treatment of an infant or child. Treatment of an infant may impose substantial burdens of financial and personal care on parents, but physicians do not directly cause these harms through nontherapeutic practice of the medical art on parents *qua* patients. New technologies notwithstanding, diagnostic, and therapeutic interventions on behalf of the fetus do entail medical invasion of the mother, and the proxy *for the fetus* has no ethical standing to consent to this invasion. What if the maternal patient declines treatment for herself?

When a proposed course of treatment is in a patient's medical best interests, refusal raises questions about the professional duty of respect for patient autonomy, because the harm caused by not treating her cannot be justified if the patient's refusal was not fully voluntary. When a patient *requests* treatment contrary to her medical best interests, the situation is the same: the request to donate a kidney, for instance, provokes questions about the duty of respect for patient autonomy, because the harm caused by harvesting the kideny cannot be justified if the request was not truly voluntary.

In contrast to both of these cases, *refusal* of treatment *contrary* to a patient's medical best interests prompts no such questions about the duty to honor autonomy. When physicians disregard a patient's refusal of harmful treatment, the violation of patient autonomy is the least of their professional wrongs. Since ethical immunity against medical harm is independent of patient autonomy, it is uncompromised by limits on autonomy -- incompetence, coercion, harm to others -- that sometimes justify paternalism. *Harming* a patient without consent is not medical paternalism but medical maleficence.

A woman's failure to volunteer for fetal therapy may seriously violate her fiduciary responsibilities to the fetus, thus disqualifying her as proxy, but the physician's duties to her as patient remain intact. It is not the woman's *moral obligation to consent* that authorizes physicians to subject her to harm or risk without therapeutic intent; *consent itself* is necessary -- consent that is to the highest degree competent, informed, uncoerced, and harmless to third parties. These exacting standards rule out any attempt to substitute proxy or presumed consent for maternal dissent. As on the one-patient model, physicians would be remiss if they did not make every effort to elicit maternal consent to low-risk, high-gain fetal therapy by providing honest reassurance and encouragement, but in the principles and precedents of medical ethics as applied to the two-patient obstetric model we find no basis for overriding maternal refusals to volunteer for such procedures.

Two-Patient Ethics & the Maternal-Fetal Ecosystem

When the fetus is conceptualized in clinical obstetrics not as an integral part of the pregnant woman (her condition of pregnancy, as it were) but as a second individual patient, the physician's duties to promote fetal well-being are, *prima facie,* increased. Maternal harms no longer weigh against recommendations made for the sake of fetal benefit. Also, the pregnant woman no longer speaks inclusively as maternal-fetal patient; if her decisions are not sufficiently protective of fetal interests an alternate proxy may be sought. But this is only half of the story. The other half is that professional duties to the first patient -- the maternal patient -- are paradoxically increased as well. Detached conceptually from the fetus, the maternal patient suffers medical harms from fetal therapy that are no longer offset by fetal benefits. The physician may not recommend fetal therapy, and the injunction against harming one patient involuntarily to help another is virtually absolute.

Drawing selectively and equivocally from both models -- treating the fetus as an independent patient but continuing to regard the pregnant woman as a compound patient incorporating the fetus -- has, I think, caused the physician's ethical dilemma to be misconstrued as a conflict between the duty to benefit the fetus and the duty to respect the woman's autonomy. If maternal refusal of fetal therapy were a standard exercise of patient autonomy, it would be subject to paternalistic review to guard against harms to others. But fetal therapy is beneficial to the pregnant woman only on the old model, where she *includes* the fetus, while fetal harm is harm to another only on the new model, where the fetus is independent and exclusive of the woman. In fact, maternal autonomy plays a peripheral role on the two-patient model: Maternal autonomy *qua* proxy may be challenged, and maternal autonomy *qua* patient is redundant, a secondary defense against treatment that may not ethically be recommended for her in the first place. From the standpoint of professional ethics, the obstacle to fetal benefit is not maternal autonomy but maternal nonmaleficence. Newly-strengthened duties to help the fetal patient are constrained by stronger duties to do no harm to the individualized maternal patient.

Despite the fetus's new clinical status as a second distinct patient, then, physicians' prerogatives to intervene on its behalf are no greater than before. Whether the maternal-fetal dyad is regarded as one patient or two is less relevant to providing ethical prenatal care than the fact of that dyad's biological unity. Literally, if not conceptually, the pregnant woman incorporates the fetus, so direct medical access to the fetal patient is as remote as ever. Ironically, when the fetus is construed as a second independent patient, physicians' prerogatives to act as fetal advocates are actually diminished. This consequence flows not from any assumed superiority of maternal rights over fetal rights but from differential professional duties to donors and recipients of medical benefits. Two-patient benefit-burden transactions require of physicians a deferential approach to those asked to assume medical risks for others and a readiness to shield reluctant or indecisive patients from involuntary harm. If the example of transplantation ethics is followed in obstetrics, physicians have acquired obligations to neutralize moral pressures on pregnant women arising from family relationships and ensure that any maternal sacrifices to benefit the fetus are strictly voluntary.

But surely our argument has carried us too far. If status as an independent patient affords the fetus relatively *less* protection than its previous state of dependency, instead of revising ethical standards of obstetric care to fit that counterintuitive conclusion one might simply retract the two-patient hypothesis. Perhaps developments in fetal medicine do not require reconceptualizing the obstetric patient after all. Alternatively, since the concept of the fetus as a second patient is already well entrenched in perinatal medical philosophy, one might challenge the orthodox view of the professional-patient relationship, which suppresses dependency relations among patients, and posits them as strangers to one another. Deeply ingrained in the western Hippocratic tradition and the eastern medical traditions as well, the assumption that physicians should treat patients as generic individuals without regard to social role or status reflects an ideal of egalitarian, compassionate, patient-centered medical care.[8] Can professional obligations be made sensitive to relationships of dependency between patients without detriment to that ideal and without simply making an *ad hoc* exception for the case at hand?

Efforts to reinterpret professional ethical principles to accommodate just such relationships are in fact under way in family practice medicine.[9] Family medicine rejects the reductionist model of illness, which focuses narrowly on proximate causes within the patient as a biological organism, espousing instead a biopsychosocial model of health and disease. It looks beyond organic conditions, even beyond the presenting patient, to family relationships and circumstances that affect and are affected by patient health. For diagnostic and therapeutic purposes, the patient is conceptualized in relation to the family ecosystem. This environmental medical model is not entirely compatible with an individualistic patient-centered professional ethic. Responsibilities of family practice physicians to their patients must be understood expansively to include the family context -- guiding patients toward choices that are responsive to their family situations and helping family members fulfill obligations of care to one another.

Adapting the contextual approach of family practice medicine to obstetrics, we might think of the maternal-fetal dyad as an integrated, a two-patient ecosystem whose individual components are not conceptually independent. Caring for one implicates the other and the family context. An environmental medical model would remove the specter of dueling specialists vying for medical control of a complicated pregnancy -- the *reductio ad absurdum* of the two-patient thesis. It would counteract any tendency of physicians to discount the impact of fetal treatment on the pregnant woman now effaced by her clinical transparency, and at the same time it legitimize looking beyond the maternal patient to her protective biological and social role. Helping the pregnant woman fulfill her fiduciary duties to the fetus would again, as on the one-patient model, become a primary professional goal.

Once family roles and circumstances are drawn into the purview of patient care decisions, they may not be selectively considered only when they weigh in favor of treatment. Maternal fiduciary duties, for instance, typically extend beyond the fetus to other family members, and standards of family ethics do not always assign highest priority to fetal needs and claims. If the practice of fetal medicine were informed by an environmental maternal-fetal model, family demands would be acknowledged, not dismessed as irrelevant or even illicit conflicts on interest. By assuming obligations to address a wide range of health-related but nonmedical family problems, physicians may make it possible for the woamn to accept therapy recommended for the fetus, but sometimes physicians must help patients and proxies make tragic choices forced by limited family circumstances, when resources cannot be stretched to meet the basic needs of all.[10] Also, family and medical values will sometimes diverge: increasing the chances for live delivery of a severly damaged fetus, for example, might be a medical value but a family disvalue. A context-sensitive perspective commits physicians to respect a family's well-considered value judgments unless basic family duties are violated.

Not surprisingly, ethical standards evolving in family practice medicine do not sanction doctors enforcing a duty on the part of family members to sacrifice for each other, although reluctance to volunteer might be considered symptomatic of family dysfunction, to be treated through supportive intervention. In family practice, medical authority is exercised by negotiating medical goals and in collaborative decision-making. The physician's last resort in cases of severe and irremediable family problems -- petitioning for the temporary or permanent removal to alternate caregivers of dependents at risk -- is not available for the fetal dependents, of course, although planning for transfer of the neonate might be considered, but then the social meaning of the maternal-fetal relationship is changed. It reverts to the generic relationship of strangers, so the donor protections of two-person ethics apply: physicians should guard the woman from undue pressures to undergo medical harms for someone else's child.

Maternal-fetal conflicts are interesting out of proportion to their incidence in part because they raise in a compelling way questions about the integration of medical and family ethics, an important and underdeveloped topic. Conceptualizing the maternal-fetal dyad as two unrelated patients is bizarre whether the consequence is to tilt the ethical standard toward strongly-weighted professional obligations to protect the maternal donor, as I have argued, or in the opposite direction. Yet the integration of family status into the patient role is not a simple or clearcut matter. Patients who voluntarily present assume *prima facie* duties to act in their own medical best interests, but neither medical ethics nor medical education addresses the task of helping patients combine these duties with the imperatives of their family roles. Family responsibilities are lumped together with patients' idiosyncratic preferences and masked by professional respect for individual patient autonomy. But while exclusion of family concerns from medical attention is often unsatisfactory,[11] to select one familial duty that bolsters the case for medical intervention and graft it onto a medical model that otherwise suppresses family relationships clearly will not do.

To expand the medical gaze to encompass family status is to see that patients as persons in social systems, and this in turn demands a broader view of professional care than is typical of modern scientific medicine. Family practice medicine is an exception, and a biopsychosocial perspective is implicit, as well, in the traditional medical and ethical values of obstetric care. Recent developments in obstetrics, however, particularly the emergence of a subspecialty in fetology, introduce a narrow focus that sees only the fetusas it survives the pathologies of pregnancy.

Constructing a model of the maternal-fetal dyad as a two-patient ecosystem, would restore to medical relevance the relationship of dependence and protection characteristic of the dyad. The effect of such a model would be to join the professional-patient relationships to the two patients almost as closely as if they were a single compound commitment to one compound patient. Protections associated with dependence would be reinstated and the two-patient presumption against maternal medical sacrifice averted. Within a two-patient framework, it is possible, then, to approximate the one-patient standard of obstetric care, but there is no warrant for requiring or permitting physicians to move beyond it toward a stronger posture of fetal protection. One patient or two, independent or dependent, when the various possible models of the maternal-fetal dyad are consistently applied, they converge to reinforce the physician's customary ethical stance -- working cooperatively with the pregnant woman for common, linked goals of infant, maternal, and family well-being.

Notes

1. Daffos F. Access to the other patient, *Seminars in Perinatology* 1989;13(4):252.
2. Manning FA. Reflections on future directions of perinatal medicine, *Seminars in Perinatology* 1989;13(4):342-51. In the introductory paragraphs, I have relied heavily on Manning's excellent account of the way in which technical innovations in perinatal medicine have brought about subtle, but far-reaching changes in underlying philosophy.
3. Veronika E, Kolder G, *et al*. Court-ordered obstetrical interventions, *New England Journal of Medicine* 1987;316(19):1192-96.

4. Harrison MR, *et al.* Management of the fetus with a correctable congenital defect, *Journal of American Medical Association* 1981;246(7):774-77.
5. Engelhardt TH Jr. Current controversies in obstetrics: Wrongful life and forced fetal surgical procedures, *American Journal of Obstetrics and Gynecology* 1985;151:313-18. Engelhardt's argument is cited, for example, by Chervenak FA, McCullough LB. Ethical challenges in perinatal medicine: The intrapartum management of pregnancy complicated by fetal hydrocephalus with macrocephaly, *Seminars in Perinatology* 1987;11(3):232-39.
6. See, for instance, Wolstenholme G, O'Connor M, eds. *Law and Ethics of Transplantation*. London: Churchhill, 1966; Simmons, *et al. Gift of Life: The Social & Psychological Impact of Organ Transplantation*. New York, NY: John Wiley & Sons, 1977; Freund PA, ed. *Experimentation with Human Subjects*. New York, NY: George Braziller, 1970; Levine RJ. *Ethics and Regulation of Clinical Research*. Baltimore, MD: Urban and Schwarzenberg, 1981.
7. Informal practice varies widely, but theoretical medical etihcs assigns no relevance to family responsibilities in arriving at patient care decisions except to the extent that family members are acknowledgded as proxy decision-makers, and then, perversely; they are to ignore responsibilities they or the patient may have aside from their duty to represent the wishes and interests of the patient. For a different view, see Hardwig J. What about the family, *Hastings Center Report* 1990;20(2):5-10.
10. Jonsen A. Do no harm. In: Veatch RM ed., *Cross Cultural Perspectives in Medical Ethics: Readings*. Boston, MA: Jones and Bartlett Publishers, 1989:199-210.
11. See Christie RJ, Hoffmaster CB. *Ethical Issues in Family Medicine.* New York, NY: Oxford University Press, 1986.
10. Physicians and parents have distinct fiduciary responsibilities for the fetal patient, reflecting differences of scope between the professional and parental ethical standpoints. I have developed this point more fully in, Fetal needs. Physicians duties, *Midwest Medical Ethics* 1991;7(1):8-11.
13. Hardwig, *op cit.*

Chapter 8

Selective Termination in Pregnancy and Women's Reproductive Autonomy

Christine Overall

The recent development of a new technological procedure has added additional questions to debates about women's reproductive self-determination. Variously called "selective termination in pregnancy," "selective reduction of multifetal pregnancy," or "selective fetal reduction," the process is performed during the first or second trimester in some instances of multiple pregnancy, either to eliminate a fetus found through prenatal diagnosis to be disabled or at risk of a disability, or simply to reduce the number of fetuses in the uterus. More than two hundred cases of selective termination are known to have been performed around the world (Lipovenko 1989).

There are several methods of selective termination, all of which first involve ultrasound imaging to locate the target fetus or fetuses. One method is the transcervical aspiration of amniotic fluid and fetal tissue (Berkowitz *et al.* 1988). Another is the placing of a needle into the fetal thorax until cardiac motion ceases. In the third method, a lethal dose of potassium chloride is injected into the fetal thorax to stop the heart (Evans *et al.* 1988). In the two latter methods the "terminated" fetus is reabsorbed into the woman's body during the course of pregnancy, and no further surgery is required to remove it from her uterus.

In recent news stories and journal articles some physicians and ethicists have expressed reservations about selective termination, both with respect to its moral justification and with respect to the formation of social policy governing access to and resource allocation for this procedure. Says Abbyann Lynch, former director of the Westminster Institute for Ethics and Human Values in London, Ontario: "It's like saying to a fetus you are good enough to come on the trip but not make the final voyage" (Lipovenko 1989, A4). Margaret Somerville, of the Centre for Medicine, Ethics and Law at McGill University, states:

> With abortion, a woman has the right to control over her own body. Selective reduction is different. Control over the body moves to the right to kill a fetus who is competing with another for space. I have a lot of problems with that (*Kingston Whig-Standard* 1989, 3).

Some commentators are worried that the procedure establishes "precedents for infanticide or euthanasia." They are also concerned that it will be unjustifiably used by women pregnant with twins who wish to reduce their pregnancy to a singleton, and they therefore recommend restricting availability of the process to multiple pregnancies of three or more (Evans *et al.* 1988). In general, according to Walter Hannah, president of the Canadian Society of Obstetricians and Gynecologists, "There's no question there should be

---

Source: Reprinted from *Hastings Center Report*, May-June 1990, pp. 6-11, with permission of © The Hastings Center.

national guidelines [for selective pregnancy termination]" (Lipovenko 1989, A4).

Many discussions of selective termination appear to assume that the procedure is primarily a matter of acting against some fetus(es) on behalf of others. For example, Diana Brahams (1987, 1409) describes the issue as follows: "Is it ethical and legally appropriate to carry out a selective reduction of pregnancy--that is, to destroy one or more fetuses in order to give the remaining fetus or fetuses a better chance?" Richard L. Berkowitz, *et al.* (1988, 1046) poses the problem in the following way: "Is it justifiable to lower the number of fetuses in the uterus in order to reduce an unspecified risk to all the fetuses?" Similarly, in their report on four selective pregnancy terminations, Mark I. Evans *et al.* (1988) discusses the issue as if the primary choice is the killing or the preservation of the fetuses.

However, this construction of the problem is radically incomplete, since it omits attention to the women -- their bodies and their lives -- who should be at the center of any discussion of selective termination. In fact, selective termination vividly instantiates many of the central ethical and policy concerns that must be raised about the technological manipulation of women's reproductive capacities. When Margaret Somerville expresses concern about "the right to kill a fetus who is competing with another for space," what she neglects to mention is that the "space" in question is the pregnant woman's uterus.

According to Evans and colleagues (1988, 293), "the ethical issues [of selective termination] are the same in multiple pregnancies whether the cause is spontaneous conception or infertility treatment." Such a claim is typical of many discussions in contemporary bioethics, which abstract specific moral and social problems from the cultural context that produced them. But the issue of selective termination in pregnancy vividly demonstrates the necessity of examining the social and political environment in which issues in biomedical ethics arise.

Selective termination itself must be understood and evaluated with reference to its own particular context. The apparent need or demand for selective termination in fact is created and elaborated in response to prior technological interventions in women's reproductive processes, themselves the result of prevailing cultural interpretations of infertility.

Hence, it is essential to explore the significance of selective termination for women's reproductive autonomy. The issue acquires added urgency at this point in both Canada and the United States where abortion access and allocation are the focus of renewed controversy. Although not precisely the same as abortion, selective termination is similar in so far as in both cases one or more fetuses are destroyed. The difference is that in abortion pregnancy ends; whereas in selective termination, ideally, the pregnancy continues, with one or more fetuses still present. I will argue that, provided a permissive abortion policy is justified (that is, a policy that allows abortion at least until the end of the second trimester) a concern for women's reproductive autonomy precludes any general policy restricting access to selective termination in pregnancy, as well as clinical practices that discriminate on non-medical grounds as to which women will be permitted to choose the procedure or how many fetuses they must retain.

The "Demand" for Selective Termination

In recent discussions of selective termination, women with multiple pregnancies are often represented as demanding the procedure -- sometimes by threatening to abort the entire pregnancy if they are not allowed selective termination. One television interviewer who talked to me about this issue described women as "forcing" doctors to provide the procedure. Similarly, a case study of selective pregnancy termination (Holder and Henifin, 1988, 21) presents a "Ms. Q" who is pregnant with triplets and asks her doctor to "terminate" two of the fetuses:

> She says she really wants to have a child and "be a good mother," but doesn't feel capable of caring for more than one child at a time. Even though all three fetuses appear healthy, her preference is to abort all rather than have triplets.

The assumption that individual women "demand" selective termination in pregnancy places all moral responsibility for the procedure on the women themselves. However, neither the multiple pregnancies nor the "demands" for selective termination originated *ex nihilo*. An examination of their sources suggests both that moral responsibility for selective termination cannot rest solely on individual women and that the "demand" for selective termination is not just a straightforward exercise of reproductive freedom.

Deliberate societal and medical responses to the perceived problem of female infertility generate much of the need for selective termination, which is but one result of a complex system of values and beliefs concerning fertility and infertility, maternity and children. Infertility is not merely a physical condition; it is both interpreted and evaluated within cultural conditions that help to specify the appropriate beliefs about and responses to the condition of being unable to reproduce. According to the prevailing ideology of pronatalism, women must reproduce, men must acquire offspring, and both parents should be biologically related to their offspring. A climate of acquisition and commodification encourages and reinforces the notion of child as possession. Infertility is seen as a problem for which the solution must be acquiring a child of one's own, biologically related to oneself, at almost any emotional, physical, or economic costs (Overall 1987, Chap. 7).

The recent increase in numbers of multiple pregnancies comes largely from two steps taken in the treatment of infertility. The use of fertility drugs to prod women's bodies into ovulating and producing more than one ovum at a time results in an incidence of multiple gestation ranging from 16 to 39 percent (Hobbins 1988). Gamete intrafallopian transfer (GIFT) using several eggs and *in vitro* fertilization (IVF) with subsequent implantation of several embryos in the woman's uterus to increase the likelihood that the woman will become pregnant may also result in multiple gestation. "Pregnancy rate increments are about 8 percent for each pre-embryo replaced in IVF, giving expected pregnancy rates of 8, 16, 24, and 32 percent for 1, 2, 3, and 4 preembryos, respectively" ("Selective Fetal Reduction" 1988, 774).

A "try anything" mentality is fostered by the fact that prospective IVF patients are often not adequately informed about the very low clinical success rates ("failure rates" would be a more appropriate term) of the procedure (Corea and Ince 1987; Ellis 1989). One physician implants as many as twelve embryos after IVF (Brahams 1987), and a woman who sought selective termination after use of a fertility drug was pregnant with octuplets (Evans *et al.* 1988). Another case reported by Evans and colleagues (1988, 291) dramatically illustrates the potential effects of these treatments: One woman's reproductive history includes three Cesarean sections, a tubal ligation, a tuboplasty (after which she remained infertile), *in vitro* fertilization with subsequent implantation of four embryos, selective termination of two of the fetuses, revelation via ultrasound that one of the remaining twins had "severe oligohydramnios and no evidence of a bladder or kidneys," spontaneous miscarriage of the abnormal twin, and intrauterine death of the remaining fetus.

In a commentary critical of selective termination, Angela Holder (1988, 22) quotes Oscar Wilde's dictum: "In this world, there are only two tragedies. One is not getting what one wants, and the other is getting it." But this begs the question of what is meant by saying that women "want" multiple pregnancy, or "want" selective termination in pregnancy. What factors led these women to take infertility drugs, and/or to participate in an IVF program? How do they evaluate fertility, pregnancy, motherhood, children? How do they perceive themselves as women, as potential mothers, as infertile, and where do children fit into these visions? To what degree were they adequately informed of the likelihood that they would gestate more than one fetus? Were they provided with support systems to enable them to understand their own reasons and goals for seeking reproductive interventions, and to provide assistance throughout the emotionally and physically demanding aspects of the treatment? Barbara Katz Rothman's appraisal of women who abort fetuses with genetic defects has more general applicability (1986, 189):

> They are the victims of a social system that fails to take collective responsibility for the needs of its members, and leaves individual women to make impossible choices. We are spared collective responsibility, because we individualize the problem. We make it the woman's own. She 'chooses', and so we owe her nothing.

Uncritical use of the claim that certain women "demand" selective termination implies that they are just selfish, unable to extend their caring to more than one or two infants, particularly if one has a disability. For example, one physician (O'Reilly 1987, 8558) speaks dismissively of women who are bothered by the "inconvenience" of a multiple pregnancy. But this interpretation is unjustified. In general, participants in IVF programs are extremely eager for a child. They are encouraged to be self-sacrificing, to be acquiescent in the medical system and in the manipulations the medical system requires their bodies to undergo. As John C. Hobbins notes (1988, 1063), these women "have often already volunteered for innovative treatments and may be desperate to try another." The little evidence so far available suggests (Lorber 1988) that, if anything, these women are, by comparison to their male partners, somewhat passive in regard to the making of reproductive decisions. There is no evidence to suggest that most are not willing to assume the challenges of multiple pregnancy.

An additional cause of multiple pregnancy is the conflicting attitudes toward the embryo and fetus manifested in infertility research and clinical practice. One report suggests that multiple pregnancies resulting from IVF are generated not only because clinicians are driven by the motive to succeed -- and implantation of large numbers of embryos appears to offer that prospect -- but also because of "intimidation of medical practitioners by critics and authorities who insist that all fertilized eggs or preembryos be immediately returned to the patient" ("Selective Fetal Reduction" 1988, 774). Such "intimidation" does not, of course, excuse clinicians who may sacrifice their patients' wellbeing. Nevertheless, conservative beliefs in the necessity and inevitability of procreation and the sacredness and "personhood" of the embryo may contribute to the production of multiple pregnancies.

Thus, the technological "solutions" to some forms of female infertility create an additional problem of female hyper-fertility -- to which a further technological "solution" of selective termination is then offered. Women's so-called "demand" for selective termination in pregnancy is not a primordial expression of individual need, but a socially constructed response to prior medical interventions.

The debate over access to selective pregnancy termination exemplifies a classic no-win situation for women, in which medical technology generates a solution to a problem itself generated by medical technology -- yet women are regarded as immoral for seeking that solution. While women have been, in part, victimized through the use of reproductive interventions that fail to respect and facilitate their reproductive autonomy, they are nevertheless unjustifiably held responsible for their attempts to cope with the outcomes of these interventions in the forms that are made available to them. From this perspective, selective termination is not so much an extension of women's reproductive choice as it is the extension of control over women's reproductive capacity -- through the use of fertility drugs,

GIFT, and IVF as "solutions" to infertility that often result, when successful, in multiple gestations; through the provision of a technology, selective termination, to respond to multiple gestation that may create much of the same ambivalence for women as is generated by abortion; and finally through the installation of limitations on women's access to the procedure.

In decisions about selective termination, women are not simply feckless, selfish and irresponsible. Nor are they mere victims of their social conditioning and the machinations of the medical and scientific establishments. But they must make their choices in the face of extensive socialization for maternity, a limited range of options, and sometimes inadequate information about outcomes. When women "demand" selective termination in pregnancy they are attempting to take action in response to a situation not of their own making, in the only way that seems available to them. Hence my argument is not that women are merely helpless victims and therefore must be permitted access to selective termination, but rather that it would be both socially irresponsible and also unjust for a health care system that contributes to the generation of problematic multiple pregnancies to withhold access to a potential, if flawed, response to the situation.

A Grim Option

There is reason to believe that women's attitudes toward selective termination may be similar to their attitudes toward abortion. Although abortion is a solution to the problem of unwanted pregnancy, and the general availability of abortion accords women significant and essential reproductive freedom, it is often an occasion for ambivalence, and remains, as Caroline Whitbeck has pointed out (1984, 251-252), a "grim option" for most women. It is not something women straightforwardly seek, in the way that they may seek a rewarding career, supportive friends, healthy children, or freer sexuality; rather it is wanted "only because of a still greater aversion to the only available alternatives...[Women do not want abortions], although under duress they may resort to them." Women who abort are, after all, undergoing a surgical invasion of their bodies, and some may also experience emotional distress (McDonnell 1984, 33-36). Moreover, for some women the death of the fetus can be a source of grief, particularly when the pregnancy is wanted and the abortion is sought because of severe fetal disabilities (Rothman 1986, Chap. 7).

Comparable factors may contribute to women's reservations about selective termination in pregnancy. Those who resort to this procedure surely do not desire the invasion of their uterus, nor do they make it their aim to kill fetuses. In fact, unlike women who request abortions because their pregnancy is unwanted, most of those who seek selective termination are originally pregnant by choice. Such pregnancies are "not only wanted but achieved at great psychological and economic cost after a lengthy struggle with infertility" (Evans *et al.* 1988, 292).

For such women a procedure that risks the loss of all fetuses, as selective termination does, may be especially troubling. The procedure is still experimental, and its short- and long-term outcomes are largely unknown. Evans *et al.* (1988, 292) state, "Many more cases will have to be observed to appreciate the true risks of the procedure to both the mother and the remaining fetuses," and Berkowitz *et al.* (1988, 1046) say, "Although the risks associated with selective reduction are known, the dearth of experience with the procedure to date makes it impossible to assess their likelihood." Evans *et al.* (1988, 290) add: "[Any attempt to reduce the number of fetuses [is] experimental and [can] result in miscarriage, and...infection, bleeding, and other unknown risks [are] possible. If successful, the attempt could theoretically damage the remaining fetuses."

Note that "success" in the latter case would be seriously limited, assuming that the pregnant woman's goal is to gestate and subsequently deliver one or more healthy infants.

In fact, success in this more plausible sense is fairly low. The success rate for Evans *et al.* was 50%; for Berkowitz *et al.* 66 2/3%. As a consequence, in their study of first trimester selective terminations, Berkowitz *et al.* (1988, 1046) mention the "psychological difficulty of making the decision [to undergo selective termination]," a difficulty partly resulting from "emotional bonding" with the fetuses after repeated ultrasound examinations.

Thus, women undergoing selective termination, like most of those undergoing abortion, are choosing a grim option; they are ending the existence of one or more fetuses because the alternatives -- aborting all the fetuses (and taking the risk that they will never again succeed in becoming pregnant), or attempting to maintain all the fetuses through pregnancy, delivery, and childrearing -- are untenable. Women do not seek selective termination for its own sake, or even simply as a means to an end, but because, as the next section will show, their circumstances and the nature of the pregnancy make any other course of action or inaction unacceptable, morally, medically, or practically.

The Challenge of Multiple Gestation

Why don't women who seek selective termination simply continue their pregnancies? John Woods, a philosopher highly critical of abortion, makes the following claim (1978, 80):

> Pregnancy does not radically impede locomotion, does not necessarily entail a long-term loss of income, does not disrupt a wide range of social and personal relationships, is not a radical and continuous disturbance, is not a socially anomalous condition, and is not an invasion of privacy.

This quotation is extraordinary primarily because of its complete falsity in every clause. As any mother or pregnant woman could explain, pregnancy and its outcome can and do have all of these effects, if not in every case, then in many. Rosalind Hursthouse (1987, 300) remarks, "Most pregnancies and labors call for courage, fortitude and endurance, though most women make light of them -- so why are women not praised and admired for going through them?" No matter how much it is taken for granted, the accomplishment of gestating and birthing even one child is an extraordinary event; perhaps even more credit is owed to the woman who births twins or triplets or quadruplets. Rather than setting policy limits on women who are not able or willing to gestate more than one or two fetuses, we should be recognizing and understanding the extraordinary challenges posed by multiple pregnancies.

There are good consequentialist reasons why a woman might choose to reduce the number of fetuses she carries. For the pregnant woman, continuation of a multiple pregnancy means "almost certain preterm delivery, prefaced by early and lengthy hospitalization, higher risks of pregnancy-induced hypertension, polyhydramnios, severe anemia, preeclampsia, and postpartum blood transfusions" (Evans *et al.* 1988, 292). Another commentator (Hobbins 1988) describes the risks for the pregnant woman as including preeclampsia, serious postpartum hemorrhage, thrombophlebitis, embolic phenomena, and polyhydramnios. The so-called "minor discomforts" of pregnancy are increased in a multiple pregnancy, and women may suffer severe nausea and vomiting (MacLennan 1989), or become depressed or anxious (Scerbo *et al.* 1986). There is also an increased likelihood of Cesarean delivery, entailing more pain and a longer recovery time after the birth (MacLennan 1989).

Infants born of multiple pregnancy risk "premature delivery, low infant birthweight, birth defects, and problems of infant immaturity, including physical and mental retardation" ("Selective Fetal Reduction" 1988, 773). There is a high likelihood that these infants "may be severely impaired or suffer a lengthy, costly process of dying in neonatal intensive care" (Evans et al. 1988, 295). Thus a woman carrying more than one fetus also faces the possibility of becoming a mother to infants who will be seriously physically impaired or will die (MacLennan 1989).

It is also important to count the social costs of bearing several children simultaneously, where the responsibilities, burdens, and lost opportunities occasioned by childrearing fall primarily if not exclusively upon the woman rather than upon her male partner (if any) or more equitably upon the society as a whole -- particularly when the infants are disabled. An article on Canada's first set of "test-tube quintuplets" reported that the babies' mother, Mae Collier, changes diapers fifty times a day, and goes through twelve litres of milk a day and 150 jars of baby food a week. Her husband works full time outside of the home and "spends much of his spare time building the family's new house" (Stevens 1989, A7).

Moreover, while North American culture is strongly pronatalist, it is simultaneously anti-child. One of the most prevalent myths of the West is that North Americans love and spoil their children. In fact, however, a sensitive examination -- perhaps from the perspective of a child or a loving parent -- of the conditions in which many children grow up puts the lie to this myth (Pogrebin 1983). Children are among the most vulnerable victims of poverty and malnutrition. Subjected to physical and sexual abuse, educated in schools that more often aim for custody and confinement than growth and learning, exploited as opportunities for the mass marketing of useless and sometimes dangerous foods and toys, children, the weakest members of our society, are often the least protected. Children are virtually the last social group in North America for whom discrimination and segregation are routinely countenanced. In many residential areas, businesses, restaurants, hotels, and other "public" places, children are not welcome, and except in preschools and nurseries, there is usually little or no accommodation to their physical needs and capacities.

A society that is simultaneously pronatalist but anti-child and only minimally supportive of mothering is unlikely to welcome quintuplets and other multiples -- except for their novelty -- any more than it welcomes single children. The issue, then, is not just how many fetuses a woman can be required to gestate, but also how many children she can be required to raise, and under what sort of societal conditions.

To this argument it is no adequate rejoinder to say that such women should continue their pregnancy and then surrender some but not all of the infants for adoption by eager childless and infertile couples. It is one thing for a woman to have the choice of making this decision after careful thought and with full support throughout the pregnancy and afterward when the infants have been given up. Such a choice may be hard enough. It would be another matter, however, to advocate a policy that would restrict selective termination in such a way that gestating all the fetuses and surrendering some becomes a woman's only option.

First, the presence of each additional fetus places an additional demand on the woman's physical and emotional resources (MacLennan 1989); gestating triplets or quadruplets is not just the same as gestating twins. Second, to compel a woman to continue to gestate fetuses she does not want for the sake of others who do is to treat the woman as a mere breeder, a biological machine for the production of new human beings (Corea 1985; Atwood 1985). Finally, it would be callous indeed to underestimate the emotional turmoil and pain of the woman who must gestate and deliver a baby only to surrender it to others. In the case of a multiple gestation an added distress would arise because of the necessity of somehow choosing which infant(s) to keep and which to give up. For women who seek selective termination, then, it is both the physical stress of large multiple pregnancies and the social conditions for rearing several infants simultaneously that can contribute to making the continued gestation of all their fetuses an untenable possibility.

Reproductive Rights

Within the existing social context, therefore, access to selective termination must be understood as an essential component of women's reproductive rights. But in staking reproductive rights claims it is important to distinguish between the right to reproduce and the right not to reproduce. Entitlement to access to selective termination, like entitlement to access to abortion, falls within the right not to reproduce (Overall, 1987).

Entitlement to choose how many fetuses to gestate, and of what sort, is in this context a limited and negative one. If women are entitled to choose to end their pregnancies altogether, then they are also entitled to choose how many fetuses and of what sort they will carry. If it is unjustified to deny a woman access to an abortion of all fetuses in her uterus, then it is also unjustified to deny her access to the termination of some of those fetuses. Furthermore, if abortion is legally permitted in cases where the fetus is seriously disabled, it is inconsistent to refuse to permit the termination of one disabled fetus in a multiple pregnancy.

One way of understanding abortion as an exercise of the right not to reproduce is to see it as the premature emptying of the uterus, or the deliberate termination of the fetus's occupancy of the womb. If a woman has an entitlement to an abortion, that is, to the emptying of her uterus of all of its occupants, then there is no ground to compel her to maintain all the occupants of her uterus if she chooses to retain only some of them. While the risks of multiple pregnancy for both the fetuses and the pregnant woman increase with the number of fetuses involved (MacLennan 1989), it does not follow that restrictions on selective termination for pregnancies with smaller numbers of fetuses would be justified. Legal or medical policy can not consistently say, "you may choose whether to be pregnant, that is, whether your uterus shall be occupied, but you may not choose how many shall occupy your uterus."

More generally, if abortion of a healthy singleton pregnancy is permitted for any reason, as a matter of the woman's choice, within the first six months or so of pregnancy, it is inconsistent to refuse to permit the termination of one or more healthy fetuses in a multiple pregnancy. To say otherwise is to unjustifiably accord the fetuses a right to occupancy of the woman's uterus. It is to say that two or more human entities, at an extremely immature stage in their development, have the right to use a human person's body. But no embryo or fetus has a right to the use of a pregnant woman's body -- any more than any other human being, at whatever stage of development, has a right to use a person's body (Overall 1987; Thomson 1971). The absence of that right is recognized through state-sanctioned access to abortion. Fetuses do not acquire a right, either collectively or individually, to use a woman's uterus simply because there are several of them present simultaneously. If one fetus alone in a singleton pregnancy does not have such a right, there is no reason to give several fetuses together, either individually or jointly, such a right. Even if a woman is willingly and happily pregnant, she does not surrender her entitlement to bodily self-determination, and she does not, specifically, surrender her entitlement to determine how many human entities may occupy her uterus.

Making Changes

Although I defend a social policy that does not set limits on access to selective termination in pregnancy, there can be no denying that the procedure may raise serious moral problems. For example, as some disabled persons themselves have pointed out, there is a special moral significance to the termination of a fetus with a disability such as Down syndrome (Kaplan 1989; Asch 1989; Saxton 1988). The use of prenatal diagnosis followed by abortion or selective termination may have eugenic overtones (Hubbard 1988), when the presupposition is that we can ensure that only high quality babies are born, and that "defective" fetuses can be eliminated before birth. The fetus is treated as a product for which "quality control" measures are appropriate.

Moreover, since amniocentesis and chorionic villus sampling reveal the sex of offspring, there is also a possibility that selective termination in pregnancy could be used, as abortion already is, to eliminate fetuses of the "wrong" sex -- in most cases, that is, those that are female (Holmes & Hoskins 1987; Kishwar 1987; Steinbacher & Holmes 1987; Rowland 1987).

These possibilities are distressing and potentially dangerous to disabled persons of both sexes and to women generally. But the way to deal with these and other moral reservations about selective termination is not to prohibit selective termination or to limit access to it on such grounds as fetal disability or fetal sex choice. Instead, part of the answer is to change the conditions that generate large numbers of embryos and fetuses. For example, since "many of the currently known instances of grand multiple pregnancies should have never happened" (Evans et al 1988, 296), the administration of fertility drugs to induce ovulation can be carefully monitored (Hobbins 1988), and for IVF and GIFT procedures, more use can be made of the "natural ovulatory cycle" and of cryopreservation of embryos ("Selective Fetal Reduction" 1988, 774). The number of eggs implanted through GIFT and the number of embryos implanted after IVF can be limited -- not by unilateral decision of the physician, but after careful consultation with the woman about the chances of multiple pregnancy and her attitudes toward it (Brahams 1987). To that end, there is a need for further research on predicting the likelihood of multiple pregnancy (Craft *et al.* 1988). And, given the experimental nature of selective termination, genuinely informed choice should be mandatory for prospective patients, who need to know both the short and long-term risks and outcomes of the procedure. Acquiring this information will necessitate the "long-term follow-up of parents and children...to assess the psychological and physical effects of fetal reduction" ("Selective Fetal Reduction" 1988, 775). By these means the numbers of selective terminations can be reduced, and the women who seek selective termination can be protected and empowered.

More generally, however, we should carefully reevaluate both the pronatalist ideology and the system of treatments of infertility that constitute the context in which selective termination in pregnancy comes to seem essential. There is also a need to improve social support for parenting, and to transform the conditions that make it difficult or impossible to be the mother of triplets, quadruplets, etc., or of a baby with a severe disability. Only through the provision of committed care for children and support for women's self-determination will genuine reproductive freedom and responsibility be attained.

Notes

1. Asch A. Reproductive technology and disability, In: Cohen S, Taub N, eds. *Reproductive Laws for the 1990's*. Clifton, NJ: Human Press, 1989.
2. Atwood M. *The Handmaid's Tale*. Toronto: McClelland and Stewart, 1985.
3. Berkowitz RL, Lynch L, Chitkara U, *et al.* Selective reduction of multifetal pregnancies in the first trimester, *The New England Journal of Medicine* 1988;118(16):1043-1047.
4. Brahams D. Assisted reproduction and selective reduction of multifetal pregnancies in the first trimester, *The New England Journal of Medicine* 1988;118(16):1043-1047.
5. Corea G. *The Mother Machine: Reproductive Technologies from Artificial Insemination to Artificial Wombs*. New York, NY: Harper & Row, 1985.
6. Corea G, Ince S. Report of a survey of IVF clinics in the U.S. In: Spallone P, Steinberg LD, eds. *Made to Order: The Myth of Reproductive and Genetic Progress*. Oxford: Pergamon Press, 1987.
7. Craft I, Brinsden P, Lewis P, *et al.*, Multiple pregnancy, selective reduction, and flexible treatment (letter), *The Lancet* 1988;8619:1087.
8. Ellis GB. Trends in medically assisted conception, In: *Hearing before the Subcommittee on Regulation, Business Opportunities, and Energy of the Committee on Small Business*. Washington, DC: House of Representatives, one hundred first Congress. March 9, 1989:246-248.

9. Evans MI, Fletcher JC, Zador EE, *et al*. Selective first-trimester termination in octuplet and quadruplet pregnancies: Clinical and ethical issues, *Obstetrics and Gynecology* 1988;71(3):1:289-96.
10. Hobbins JC. Selective reduction--A perinatal necessity? *The New England Journal of Medicine* 1988;318(16):1062-1063.
11. Holder AR, Henifin MS. Case study: Selective termination of pregnancy. *Hastings Center Report* 1988;18(1):21-22.
12. Holmes HB, Hoskins BB. Prenatal and preconception sex choice technologies: A path to femicide? In: *Man-Made Women: How New Reproductive Technologies Affect Women*. Bloomington, IN: Indiana University Press, 1987.
13. Hubbard R. Eugenics: New tools, old ideas. In: Baruch EL, D'Adamo AF Jr, Seager, J, eds. *Embryos, Ethics, and Women's Rights: Exploring the New Reproductive Technologies*. New York, NY: Haworth Press, 1988.
14. Hursthouse R. *Beginning Lives*. Oxford: Basil Blackwell, 1987.
15. Kaplan D. Disability rights perspectives on reproductive technologies and public policy. In: Cohen S, Taub C, eds. *Reproductive Laws for the 1990's*. Clifton, NJ: Humana Press, 1989.
16. Kishwar M. The continuing deficit of women in India and the impact of amniocentesis. In: *Man-Made Women: How New Reproductive Technologies Affect Women*. Bloomington, IN: Indiana University Press, 1987.
17. Lipovenko D. Infertility technology forces people to make life and death choices. *The Globe and Mail* 1989 Jan. 21:A4.
18. Lorber J. In-vitro fertilization and gender politics, In: Baruch EH, D'Adamo AF Jr, Seager J, eds. *Embryos, Ethics, and Women's Rights: Exploring the New Reproductive Technologies*. New York, NY: Haworth Press, 1988.
19. MacLennan AH. Multiple gestation: Clinical characteristics and management, In: Creasy RK, Resnick R, eds. *Maternal-Fetal Medicine: Principles and Practice*, 2nd edition. Philadelphia, PA: W.B. Saunders, 1989.
20. McDonnell K. *Not An Easy Choice: A Feminist Re-Examines Abortion*. Toronto: Women's Press, 1984.
21. Multiple pregnancies create moral dilemma. *Kingston Whig-Standard* 1989 Jan. 21:3.
22. O'Reilly C. Selective reduction in assisted pregnancies (letter), *Lancet* 1989;8558:575.
23. Overall C. *Ethics and Human Reproduction: A Feminist Analysis*. Boston, MA: Allen & Unwin, 1987.
24. Pogrebin LC. *Family Politics: Love and Power on an Intimate Frontier*. New York, NY: McGraw-Hill, 1986.
25. Rotman BK. *The Tentative Pregnancy: Prenatal Diagnosis and the Future of Motherhood*. New York, NY: Viking, 1986.
26. Rowland R. Motherhood, patriarchal power, alienation and the issue of "choice" in sex preselection, In: *Man-Made Women: How New Reproductive Technologies Affect Women*. Bloomington, IN: Indiana University Press, 1987.
27. Saxton M. Prenatal screening and discriminatory attitudes about disability, In: *Embryos, Ethics, and Women's Rights: Exploring the New Reproductive Technologies*. New York, NY: Haworth Press, 1988.
28. Scerbo JC, Powan R, Drukkar JE. Twins and other multiple gestations, In: Knuppel RA, Drukkar JE, eds. *High-Risk Pregnancy: A Team Approach*. Philadelphia, PA: W.B. Saunders, 1988.
29. Selective fetal reduction (review article), *The Lancet* 1988;8614:773-775.
30. Steinbacher R, Holmes HB. Sex choice: Survival and sisterhood, In: *Man-Made Women: How New Reproductive Technologies Affect Women*. Bloomington, IN: Indiana University Press, 1987.
31. Stevens V. Test-tube quints celebrate first birthday. *The Toronto Star* 1989 Feb. 6:A7.
32. Thomson JJ. A defense of abortion, *Philosophy and Public Affairs* 1971;1:47-66.
33. Whitbeck C. The moral implications of regarding women as people: New Perspectives on pregnancy and personhood, In: Bondeson WB, Engelhardt HT Jr, Spicker SF, *et al*., eds. *Abortion and the Status of the Fetus*. Boston, MA: Reidel, 1988.
34. Woods J. *Engineered Death: Abortion, Suicide, Euthanasia and Senecide*. Ottawa: University of Ottawa Press, 1978.

Chapter 9

Pregnant Woman vs. Fetus: A Dilemma for Hospital Ethics Committees

Martha Swartz

Introduction

Hospital ethics committees are often consulted when competing patient interests blur an otherwise clear course of medical treatment. Nowhere is the potential for competing interests greater than in the field of obstetrics where obstetricians have traditionally viewed themselves as having two patients: The pregnant woman and the fetus.

Legitimate concerns about the health of newborn infants as well as the ever present controversy concerning the legal status of embryos and fetuses make it likely that hospital ethics committees will receive a growing number of referrals in which the ethical dilemma pits the pregnant woman against the fetus she is carrying.

To the extent that ethics committees can articulate the various competing interests and conflicting ethical principles arising in these cases, they can help physicians, patients, and other members of the healthcare team feel more comfortable with treatment decisions.

Because the practical applicability of the outcome of ethics committee deliberations will be influenced by legal considerations, this article will begin with a discussion of the relevant law in the area. Next, a case recently discussed by an ethics committee set in a large urban teaching hospital is described. Finally, specific suggestions are offered about how an ethics committee can be effective when confronted with ethical dilemmas in which a pregnant woman's interests or desires conflict with those of her fetus.

Legal Background

Two types of situations have given rise to the development of law in this area: 1) where the pregnant woman refuses treatment which her physician considers necessary to save the life or enhance the health of her fetus and 2) where the pregnant woman's behavior or lifestyle is believed to interfere with the development of a healthy fetus.

Forced Treatment

Perhaps the most dramatic and most widely reported case involving forced treatment was the case of Angela Carder ("A.C."),[1] a terminally ill woman who was forced to undergo a Caesarian section to attempt to save the life of her 26 1/2week-old fetus, notwithstanding pleas by the woman herself, her husband, her parents, and her physicians that she not be put through such an ordeal. In the face of these refusals of surgery, the hospital administration petitioned the court for an order which would compel treatment to save the life of the fetus. In granting the hospital's petition, the judge weighed the value of the woman's necessarily

---

Source: Reprinted from *Cambridge Quaterly of Healthcare Ethics*, Vol. 1, pp. 51-62, with permission of Cambridge University Press © 1992.

truncated remaining life against the fetus's potential life. Both the woman and the premature child died shortly after delivery.

In re A.C. was subsequently overturned by the District of Columbia Court of Appeals,[2] which held that in virtually all cases the question of what is to be done is to be decided by the patient -- the pregnant woman -- on behalf of herself and the fetus. If the patient is incompetent or otherwise unable to give an informed consent to a proposed course of medical treatment, then her decision must be ascertained through the procedure known as "substituted judgment", not through the balancing test applied by the lower court.[3]

However, the decision of the District of Columbia Court of Appeals is controlling only in Washington, D.C.; elsewhere, the overwhelming trend has been to override the pregnant woman's objections to treatment. In a study published in the New England Journal of Medicine in May, 1987, Kolder, *et al.*[4] reported that fifteen court orders were sought in 11 states and obtained in all except one case.

The same article reports that court orders have been obtained in several other types of cases in which competent women have refused treatment that physicians have recommended to save the life or enhance the health of the fetus. These treatments include court-ordered blood transfusions, forced detention, and administration of medication to diabetic women, and forced intrauterine blood transfusions in cases involving Rh sensitization.[5] Moreover, it is likely that many pregnant women who initially refuse treatment are coerced to comply through threats that a court order will be obtained.

This propensity toward overriding the objections of pregnant women to treatment can be attributed to a number of factors. Prime among them is a consideration of the societal cost of rearing children with handicaps that might have been avoided through prenatal intervention.[6] Other factors include:

1. The growing emergence of the anti-abortion movement, which imbues the fetus with legal personhood, the logical extension of which, in the minds of some people, is the fetal right to medical treatment;[7]

2. The theory that a woman's voluntary decision to continue a pregnancy creates in her special obligations to optimize the fetus's chances for good health;[8]

3. The continued difficulty of physicians to feel comfortable when a patient's decision concerning her medical care conflicts with what the physician believes is in her "best interest" and a corresponding lack of understanding about patients' rights to refuse recommended treatment ("physician paternalism;")

4. A societal minimalization of the value of women apart from their child-bearing roles;[9] and,

5. A lack of appreciation for economic, cultural, educational or philosophical differences in the patient that account for her decision. Significantly, Kolder *et al.*[10] report that among the patients ordered to undergo treatment in their survey, 80% were Black, Asian, or Hispanic, 44% were unmarried, and 24% did not speak English as their primary language. Also, several of the reported cases[11] involving forced Caesarian sections or forced transfusions involved women who refused treatment based on their religious beliefs.

An anecdote from my personal experience illustrates the effect these last three factors often play in physician decision-making. A group of physicians specializing in maternal-fetal medicine, most of whom were male and all of whom were more educated and more financially secure than the patient, were presented with a hypothetical case involving a 20-year-old woman suffering from premature contractions at 26 weeks gestation. At first, she agreed to stay in the hospital to receive intravenous medication to stop the contractions; but after 2 days on intravenous therapy, she indicated that she needed to go home to take care of her 2-year-old child. She had neither the finances nor the social support to make alternative child care arrangements.

The majority of physicians present advocated petitioning the court for an order compelling the patient to stay in the hospital to avoid a premature delivery. They viewed the patient as "hysterical" and were unsympathetic to her child care needs. Few had any compunctions about physically restraining the patient should she refuse to voluntarily abide by the court order; they saw no distinction between this competent pregnant woman's refusal of treatment and an incompetent patient's noncooperation with treatment, which is routinely handled by physical restraints.

Given this apparent comfort level with overriding the objections of pregnant women to undergo medical treatment,[12] there are many future possibilities for court orders to force pregnant women to receive treatment to enhance the health of the fetus. Increased conflicts between physicians and their pregnant patients are likely with the advent of new technological developments in the areas of prenatal diagnostic testing and intrauterine surgery.

Court Orders to Force Lifestyle Change

The national epidemic of drug abuse (of which pregnant women are a part) has led some judges to issue orders aimed at preventing pregnant women from taking drugs during their pregnancies. For example, a court in Washington, D.C. recently ordered a pregnant woman who pleaded guilty to forging checks but who tested positive for cocaine imprisoned until her baby was due.[13] (It is unclear why her urine was tested for cocaine if the charge against her were forgery!)

In Florida, New York, California, and Illinois, criminal charges have been brought against women whose children were born addicted to cocaine.[13,14] The charges have ranged from delivery of a controlled substance to a "minor," to criminal "child" abuse and neglect to involuntary manslaughter.

The most widely publicized case of this type was *In re* Pamela Stewart,[15] a situation involving a woman who ignored her physician's advice to abstain from drugs and sexual intercourse during pregnancy and gave birth to a severely brain damaged child who subsequently died. She was charged with criminal failure to provide help to a "child" under California law and briefly jailed. The court later ruled that the law did not apply to fetuses.

Several state legislatures have also attempted to address the problem of drug abuse among pregnant woman. Bills have been introduced in both the Illinois and Minnesota state legislatures[16] to require drug screening of newborns and the reporting of positive results to the local welfare agencies. Counties in other states have established policies that have the same effect.[17]

Commentators have suggested[18] that the present trend toward regulating pregnant women's behavior might lead to extension of child abuse and neglect charges against women who drink alcohol, smoke, fail to exercise, or fail to follow prescribed diets during pregnancy. In Massachusetts, a woman was recently charged[19] with motor vehicle homicide in the death of her 8 1/2-month-old fetus who was stillborn after an accident in which the woman was allegedly intoxicated.

Rights of Pregnant Women

Courts facing situations in which a pregnant woman is viewed as endangering the health of her fetus are often forced to make decisions on an emergency basis, often without hearing directly from the woman herself. This is especially true in cases where physicians have applied to the court for an order to proceed with treatment. As a result, courts are often not conversant with the applicable law. Uncomfortable with what they may view as life/death decisions, courts may prefer to "err on the side of life," i.e., issue a decision that protects the fetus at the expense of the pregnant woman's rights.

From what body of law are courts deriving their decisions? The common-law right to bodily integrity and the Constitutional rights to liberty and privacy protect a competent woman's right to direct the course of her medical treatment. Under the common-law right to bodily integrity, every competent adult has the right to determine what shall be done with his or her body.[20] A physician who touches a patient without the patient's consent is liable for battery[21]. When a patient is incapable of participating in medical decision-making by virtue of mental incompetence, most courts apply the "substituted judgment" doctrine, which mandates that efforts be made to ascertain through oral or written evidence what the patient would have wanted under the circumstances if she were competent.[22]

One manifestation of this right that is often discussed in the context of forced treatment is the reluctance of courts to order competent adults to submit to bone marrow or organ donation to save the life of another.[23] In fact, the District of Columbia Court of Appeals in *In re* A.C.[24] cites these cases in support of its position that the "substituted judgment" doctrine rather than a balancing test should be applied to incompetent pregnant patients where physicians are recommending treatment to benefit the fetus.

The Constitutional rights to privacy and liberty were first applied in a reproductive rights context in Griswold v. Connecticut,[25] the case in which the right of married people to use birth control was held to be a Constitutionally protected privacy right. The right was further developed in Roe v. Wade[26] in which the U.S. Supreme Court held that a women's right to abortion was a protected privacy right. Although the Webster Court[27] suggested that the right to abortion was a liberty interest rather than a privacy right, thus less deserving of the strictest protection, it did not directly overrule Roe.

The Roe Court[28] secured the right of pregnant women to obtain abortions throughout their pregnancies to protect[29] their lives or their health. However, several states have attempted to narrow that right. For example, in Pennsylvania, the legislature passed a law[30] which prohibits abortions after 24 weeks gestation except in very limited circumstances. Under this law, a court could order that a woman continue a pregnancy that would be detrimental to her health as long as it would not "substantially and irreversibly impair a major bodily function."

In a well-known New York case, *In re* Nancy Klein[31], abortion opponents appealed a lower court's order granting the request of the husband of a comatose pregnant woman that the woman have an abortion because physicians testified that a continued pregnancy would have deleterious effects on the woman's chance for recovery. The case went all the way up to the U.S. Supreme Court which rejected the group's request. The woman had the abortion and subsequently emerged from the coma.

Some commentators take the position that abortion law should not be discussed in the context of refusal of treatment cases because the right to refuse medical treatment involves the right to be free from unwanted bodily intrusion; whereas, the right to an abortion involves an affirmative right to direct that a medical procedure be performed. However, abortion law is included in this discussion because both types of cases involve a pregnant woman's right to direct the course of her medical treatment.

Moreover, because of the apparent conflict posed by each situation between the pregnant woman and the fetus, it appears that courts and physicians will continue to blur the distinctions.

Fetal Rights

If pregnant women were treated the same as nonpregnant women and men, their rights to refuse treatment would be relatively clear. However, courts, like obstetricians, often view the pregnant woman as a "container" holding another living person, the fetus. Thus, many courts, like the lower court in, *In re* A.C., feel compelled to engage in a balancing test, weighing the privacy/bodily integrity rights of the pregnant woman against the fetus's "right to life."

Historically, fetuses have not been viewed as persons with legal rights; their rights have not been viewed as vested unless and until they are born alive. For example, in estate law, a fetus can be named as an heir, but property is vested only after a live birth. In personal injury law, in many states, the parents of a stillborn viable fetus may sue a negligent third party for wrongful death; however, some states still require that a live birth take place before the parents may recover damages. In criminal law, the states are split as to whether a fetus can be victim of criminal or vehicular homicide.[32,33]

Most courts distinguish between previable and viable fetuses,[32] affording more legal rights to the latter than to the former. However, some courts[34] have gone so far as to allow recovery for any injury suffered after the point of conception.

Notably, all of the statutes and case law have had as their goal a means for parents to have some redress against a third party who has negligently or intentionally destroyed a fetus; none of them was intended to be a means for a fetus to obtain redress against a pregnant woman. Nevertheless, some state courts are allowing children to sue their mothers for injuries they suffered while in the womb. For example,[35] in Michigan, a court allowed a son to sue his mother for negligently taking tetracycline, causing his teeth to be discolored.

The other area of the law that is being used to protect fetuses is child abuse and neglect law. Traditionally, these laws prohibit parents from abusing or neglecting their children. Generally, the penalty for violating the laws is the removal of the children from the home or, in especially egregious circumstances, incarceration or other criminal sanctions. To cover fetuses under these acts, the definition of "child" is being broadened in some states.[36]

The controversy about expanding the applicability of child abuse laws to cover fetuses was succinctly illustrated in conflicting opinions issued by two New York county judges in the fall of 1988. Both were confronted with pregnant women who had used cocaine during pregnancy and were charged with child neglect. The Nassau County judge held that the woman's use of cocaine and failure to obtain prenatal care were acts of neglect, writing, "There is no reason to treat a child in utero any differently from a child ex utero where the mother has decided not to destroy the fetus or where the time allowed for such destruction is past."[13,37] Conversely, the Bronx court concluded, "I see no authority for the state to regulate women's bodies merely because they are pregnant."[13,38]

Society's Interests

Perhaps the strongest argument in favor of compelled medical treatment or forced detention of pregnant women to enhance the health of their fetuses arises not from fetal rights *per se*, but from society's interest in avoiding the financial and social burdens created by children born with handicaps that might have been avoided through appropriate prenatal care. Even the most protected of Constitutional rights can be restricted where a compelling state interest necessitates the overriding of these rights.

For example, in those cases where a competent adult has refused life-saving medical treatment, even courts that acknowledge that such a right is a Constitutionally protected privacy right will engage in a balancing test which weighs the individual's right against various state interests.[39]

The problem is that even where society's interest is viewed as sufficiently compelling to justify the restriction of a pregnant woman's liberty, the implementation of that interest is problematic. Notwithstanding, the previously described anecdote about physicians practicing maternal-fetal medicine, many physicians will feel uncomfortable physically restraining a competent pregnant woman in order to administer court-ordered treatment. Also, in cases involving drug or alcohol abuse, imprisonment and fines are likely to have an equally deleterious effect on the fetus and other children in the home as on the pregnant woman.

Certainly, the more reasonable approach would provide pregnant women with the social services, financial resources, and education which would encourage them to voluntarily act in a manner which is consistent with the fetus's health. Although it may be morally and ethically appropriate in most cases in which: 1) a woman's own health would not be adversely affected and 2) the fetus is viable for the woman to make decisions that would enhance the fetus's chance for good health, legislating morality in these cases raises more questions than it would answers.

The Role of Ethics Committees

As the law in this area develops and as fetal medical technology increases, it is likely that ethics committees will see an increasing number of referrals involving pregnant women and their fetuses. Thus, the ethics committee's educational and policymaking roles in this area can be expected to increase. This article focuses, however, on the ethics committee's consultative role.

In their consultative role, ethics committees generally must ask as one of their threshold questions: "Whose interests are we obligated to protect? The patient's? The family's? The physician's? The institution's? Society's?" In cases which involve a pregnant woman, ethics committees must first confront another problem: "Who is the patient? The pregnant woman? The fetus? Both? At what point, if ever, in gestational development does the fetus have health interests that require or deserve protection?"

Any model that relies on fetal viability as a threshold point for defining fetal rights must acknowledge that developing technology may significantly reduce the gestational age at which fetuses are generally considered to be viable. However, for lack of a more just alternative, and considering current legal precedent, fetal viability seems to be an appropriate starting point for considering fetal interests in ethics committee deliberations. By no means, however, should fetal viability be the endpoint of any analysis; many people would contend that a woman's autonomy interests should prevail no matter what the gestational age of the fetus.

One useful way to analyze these dilemmas is based on the autonomy/beneficence model.[40] This model acknowledges the physician's dual obligations to respect the autonomy of the pregnant woman in decision-making, while offering his or her professional advice about what would be in the best interest of the woman and her fetus. The model also acknowledges the pregnant woman's ethical obligations to preserve/enhance the health of her fetus on the one hand (at least when the fetus is viable) and her sometimes conflicting right to personal autonomy.

In applying this model to conflicts between pregnant women and their physicians, Frank Chernevak and Laurence McCullough[40] describe four kinds of common areas of dispute:

1. Conflicts between the maternal autonomy-based obligations of the physician and the maternal beneficence-based obligations of the physician, e.g., the Jehovah's witness refusing blood or the woman refusing a Caesarian section because she fears scarring. In these cases, they advocate weighing the potential goods against the potential harms, concluding that in some cases, autonomy takes precedence and in others, beneficence predominates.

2. Conflicts between the fetal beneficence obligations of the pregnant woman and the

fetal beneficence obligations of the physician, e.g., where physicians recommend the surgical placement of an intrauterine shunt into the fetus's head to alleviate hydrocephaly, but the woman believes that the procedure is too risky for the fetus. Here, they conclude that because there is no clear medical answer, the woman's decision should be respected.

3. Conflicts between maternal autonomy-based obligations of the physician and fetal beneficence-based obligations of the physician, e.g., where a physician recommends intrauterine blood transfusions or Caesarian section in the event of fetal distress, and the woman refuses treatment because she believes that the procedure will be painful. Here, Chernevak and McCullough engage in a balancing test between the woman's right to autonomy and the benefits to the fetus offered by treatment. They conclude that if fetal risks are minimal and the benefit sought is substantial and the risk to the woman is "one she should reasonably accept," then intervention should take place.

4. Conflicts between maternal beneficence-based obligations of the physician and fetal beneficence-based obligations of the physician, e.g. a maternal malignancy that requires drugs toxic to the fetus. Chernevak and McCullough conclude that because there is "no clearly convincing moral argument that the woman's life is more important than that of the fetus," the woman's decision should be accepted.

This model provides some helpful guidance for analysis; however, the authors' applications of the model, at least in some of the examples, seem to devalue autonomy considerations while promoting fetal beneficence considerations. Their conclusion in example 3 suggests that they may be allowing their own beliefs about what they think would be "reasonable" to confuse the weighing process. Similarly, their reasoning in example 4, that a woman's life is not necessarily more important than that of the fetus, fails to recognize that many patients and their families would strongly reject that position, based on their own moral or religious beliefs. However, notwithstanding the flaws in their reasoning, they rightly conclude that the woman's decision should prevail.

Case Discussion

Of all the examples discussed by Chernevak and McCullough, the most problematic is example 3, where the pregnant woman rejects a treatment which might have some detrimental effect on her, but that would likely benefit the viable fetus. The following case was discussed some time ago at a large urban hospital ethics committee.

A 17-year-old woman in her first pregnancy came to the hospital clinic for a checkup when she was 32 weeks pregnant, having had no previous prenatal care. An ultrasound showed that the fetus had hydrocephaly. Physicians recommended that the woman have a Caesarian section because the fetus's head would be too large for a vaginal delivery. Both the woman's and the fetus's life might be endangered if a vaginal delivery were attempted.

The woman refused consent to a C-section. This was an unwanted pregnancy and she did not want to undertake the additional risk entailed by a C-section nor did she want the scarring associated with the operation. There was no suggestion that the woman was incapable of participating in medical decision-making.

One physician had told the patient about the option of cephalocentesis, a procedure in which the fluid would be removed from the fetus's head while still in her uterus, thus allowing for a vaginal delivery, but in all likelihood resulting in the death of the fetus. The woman chose this option; however, the consulting neonatologist vehemently opposed the idea.

An ad hoc group of five ethics committee members met with the obstetrician and the neonatologist. Journal articles describing the alternative treatments and the ethical ramifications of the options were discussed. Questions posed by the ad hoc ethics consultative committee motivated the physicians to perform additional diagnostic tests on the fetus. The physicians were encouraged to discuss the case with their colleagues at neighboring academic medical centers.

The risks and benefits of a C-section versus cephalocentesis were laid out as they applied both to the pregnant woman and to the fetus. A C-section would be more risky to the woman than a normal vaginal delivery. However, it would be far less risky than attempting a vaginal delivery of a hydrocephalic infant.

Obviously, a C-section was much more likely to result in a live baby than was cephalocentesis. Also, the medical and legal risks of producing an even more severely handicapped baby as a result of the cephalocentesis were discussed.

The possibility of petitioning the court for an order to perform the C-section was discussed. In view of judicial approaches in other jurisdictions, it was considered likely that the court would grant such an order. Thus, going to court would operate only to provide legal protection for the physicians and institution; it was unlikely to offer any insights that would make physicians more comfortable with their decisions from an ethical standpoint.

The pregnant woman's rights to autonomy in medical decision-making were discussed. However, the gestational age of the fetus led some members of the committee to advocate that the fetus had its own independent right to medical treatment.

Most of the discussion centered around the prognosis of the fetus if it were delivered by C-section. With additional information provided as a result of the ethics committee questions, physicians diagnosed an additional fetal anomaly that doomed the fetus to death within a few days after birth. This fact seemed to be pivotal in enabling both the obstetrician and the neonatologist to feel comfortable respecting the woman's decision.

The ad hoc ethics consultative committee performed a number of valuable functions in this case:

1. Presenting the case allowed physicians to ventilate their feelings and frustrations about a very tragic dilemma.

2. Playing out the scenarios that would follow from different approaches illustrated the limited helpfulness of judicial intervention in these cases.

3. In presenting the case to the ad hoc committee, the physicians were helped to articulate the issues they found confusing. Crystalizing the issues led them to a sense of empowerment and control.

4. In responding to questions from committee members, physicians were motivated to obtain additional medical and social facts that eventually influenced their ultimate approach.

5. Questioning by the ad hoc committee also helped to highlight the "hidden agendas," i.e., the personal values, religious beliefs, social biases, professional styles, and personality characteristics that were secretly influencing the physicians' judgment in the case.

Whether these functions could be performed as easily in a larger group as they were in the smaller ad hoc consultative group setting depends on the interpersonal dynamics of any particular ethics committee. Clearly, smaller groups tend to be more flexible and thus more available to deal with emergencies.

It is unclear whether some special format is needed for ethics committees confronted with these type of conflicts because of the existence of two potential patients. In the preceding example, the two interests emerged naturally: the obstetrician represented the woman's interest (with some ambivalence toward the fetus), and the neonatologist represented the interest of the fetus. However, this may not always be the case. One advocate might be assigned to the pregnant woman and another advocate to the fetus to insure that their respective interests will be represented. However, this adversarial approach to ethical problem solving presupposes a solution that benefits one party to the exclusion of the other. In many situations, a compromise solution is possible. In any case, deliberations that try to apply an autonomy-beneficence model will generally explore the risks and benefits of various alternatives to both the pregnant woman and the fetus, without resorting to the adversarial approach.

Finally, special attention should be paid to the particularly high potential for personal, cultural and religious biases that may influence physician decisions and committee deliberations in this area. A significant effort should be spent in helping physicians and committee members to articulate their biases and understand how such biases might be affecting their judgment.[41]

Notes

1. *In re* AC. No. 87-609 (DC 16 Jun 1987).
2. *In re* AC. No. 87-609 (DC Cir. 26 Apr 1990).
3. See note 2. *In re* A.C. 1990:3-4.
4. Kolder VEB, Gallagher J, Parsons MT. Court-ordered obstetrical interventions, *New England Journal of Medicine* 1987;316(19):1192-6.
5. See note 4. Kolder *et al*. 1987;316(19):1195. See also: In the Matter of Madyun Fetus. 114 *Daily Wash L Rep*. 2233 (D.C. 26 Jul 1986). A court ordered a Caesarian section to avert the development of a fatal infection in the fetus over the objection of a woman who wanted natural childbirth. Jefferson versus Griffin Spalding County Hospital Authority. 274 S.E. 2d 457 (Ca. 1981). A court ordered a Caesarian section over the religion-based objection of a woman suffering from placenta previa to save both the woman and the fetus. The woman left the hospital before the order was implemented and later delivered a healthy newborn via a vaginal delivery. *In re* Unborn Baby Wilson. No. 81-108 AV (Mich. Ct. App. 9 Mar 1981). The administration of insulin to a diabetic woman was ordered over her religion-based objections. *Raleigh Fitkin-Paul Morgan Memorial Hosp. versus Anderson*. 42 N.J. 421, 201 A.2d 537 (1964), Cert. Denied, 377 US 985 (1964). Blood transfusions were ordered performed on a pregnant woman not withstanding the fact that the fetus was previable. Kolder *et al.* (see note 4, p. 1193) also described court orders having been obtained in Colorado for two women with diabetes, 31-33 weeks gestation, who refused treatment. *Taft versus Taft*. 388 Mass. 331, 446 N.E. 2d 395 (1983). A pregnant woman refused an operation to dose her cervix to avoid miscarriage of her previable fetus, her husband sought a court order to override her objections, and the court refused to restrict the woman's constitutional rights. See generally: Rhoden NK. Caesareans and Samaritans, *Law Med Health Care* 1987;15(3):118-25. Rhoden NK. The judge in the delivery room: The emergence of court-ordered cesareans, *Calif Law Rev* 1986;74:1951-2029. Nelson L, Milliken N. Compelled medical treatment of pregnant women -- life, liberty, and law in conflict, *J Am Med Assoc*. 1988;259(7):1060-6. Annas G. Protecting the liberty of pregnant patients, *New England Journal of Medicine* 1987;316(19):1213-4. Jurrow R, Paul R. Caesarean delivery for fetal distress without maternal consent, *Obstet Gynecol* 1984;63(4):596-9. Annas G. Forced Caesareans: The most unkindest cut of all, *Hastings Center Report* 1982;12(3):16-17; Bowes W, Selgestad B. Fetal versus maternal rights: Medical and legal perspectives, *Obstetrics and Gynecology* 1981;58(2):209-14.

6. Johnson DE. The creation of fetal rights: Conflicts with women's constitutional rights to liberty, privacy and equal protection, *Yale Law Journal* 1986;95:599-625.
7. See note 5. Rhoden. 1986;74:1965.
8. See note 5. Rhoden. 1986;74:1979. Referring to Robertson J. The right to procreate and in utero therapy, *Journal of Legal Medicine* 1982;3(3):333-66.
9. Even the fact that some programs that train obstetricians identify themselves as "maternal-fetal" fellowships reveal a bias toward viewing pregnant women as "mothers" primarily and as patients with independent medical interests only secondarily. This "pronatalist" bias is also apparent in discussions concerning the selective termination of multiple fetuses induced by hormonal therapy. Se, e.g., Overall C. Selective termination of pregnancy and women's reproductive autonomy, *Hastings Cent Rep*ort 1990;20(3):6-11. Significantly, the tendency of courts to override women's objections to medical treatment extends beyond pregnant women. The New York Times recently reported that in a study of right-to-die decisions in which courts were faced with situations in which a patient had no advance directive so that the courts were forced to "construe" the patients' wishes, courts said that they could not construe female patients' preferences in 12 of 14 cases. In contrast, in cases involving men, the courts were unable to construe male patients' preferences in only 2 of 8 cases. The author of the study noted that in court opinions in these cases, "women are referred to by their first names and construed as emotional, immature, unreflective and vulnerable to medical neglect, while men are called by their last names, and construes as rational, mature, decisive, and assaulted by medical technology." From: [Anonymous]. Courts, wills and women, *The New York Times* 1990 Jul 23:sect A:2.
10. See note 4. Kolder *et al.* 1987;316(19):1193.
11. See not 5. *In re* Unborn Baby Wilson. Jefferson versus Griffin Spalding County Hospital Authority.
12. Robertson J. Legal issues in prenatal therapy, *Clin Obstet Gynecol* 1985;29(3):603-11. Holder A. Maternal-fetal conflicts and the law, *Female Patient* 1985;10:80-90. Lenow J. The fetus as a patient: Emerging rights as a person? *Am J Law Med* 1983;9(1):1-29.
13. [Anonymous]. When the courts take charge of the unborn. *The New York Times* 1989 Jan 9;sect A:1.
14. [Anonymous]. *Philadelphia Inquirer* 1988 Dec 17;sect A:3. The New York Times Magazine has reported that prosecutors in Florida, Georgia, South Carolina, Massachusetts, California, and Michigan have charged pregnant women whose infants were born addicted to cocaine or whose urine tested positive for cocaine use with delivering a controlled substance to a minor. [Anonymous]. *The New York Time Magazine* 1990 Aug 8:33. Although courts have dismissed charges against most of the women, a Florida Court of Appeals recently upheld the conviction of a woman charged with delivering cocaine to her newborn. [Anonymous]. Appeals court in Florida backs guilt for drug delivery by umbilical cord, *The New York Times* 1991 Apr 20;sect A:5. Also, in Illinois, a court recently ordered a pregnant cocaine addict who was near the end of her term confined to a drug treatment center in an effort to protect her fetus. [Anonymous]. Court orders pregnant woman held in drug treatment center, *The New York Times* 1991 Apr 13;sect A:3.
15. *People versus Stewart*. No. M50819, slip op., at 7-8, 10 (San Diego County, Cal., 26 Feb 1987).
16. [Anonymous]. Crime and pregnancy, *Am Bar Assoc Journal* 1989;Aug:14.
17. See note 13 describing policies in Nassau County, New York, and Los Angeles County, California, requiting drug tests for newborns and possible removal of the child from the home by the Department of Social Services.
18. Field M. Controlling the woman to protect the fetus, *Law Med Health Care* 1989;17(2):11429. [Anonymous]. Maternal rights and fetal wrongs: The case against criminalization of `fetal abuse', *Harvard Law Rev*iew 1988;101:994. [Anonymous]. Maternal substance abuse: The need to provide legal protection for the fetus, *South Calif Law Review* 1987;60:1209-41. Robertson J, Schulman J. Pregnancy and prenatal harm to offspring: the case of mothers with PKU, *Hastings Cent Report* 1987;17(4):23-40, which describes maternal phenylketonuria, a condition that causes mental retardation to offspring unless the pregnant woman's diet is controlled.
19. [Anonymous]. [Photograph]. *Philadelphia Inquirer* 1989 Sep 29;sect A:8.

20. *Scholendorf versus Society of New York Hospitals*, 211 N.Y. 125, 129-30, 105 N.E. 72, 93 (1913). The court held: "Every human being of adult years and sound mind has a right to determine what shall be done with his own body: And a surgeon who performs an operation without his patient's consent commits an assault for which he is liable in damages."
21. Swartz M. The patient who refuses medical treatment: A dilemma for hospitals and physicians, *Am J Law Medicine* 1985;11(2):147-94.
22. *In re* Spring. 380 Mass. 629, 405 N.E. 2d 115 (1980). In re Jobes. 108 N.J. 394, 529 A.2d 434 (1987).
23. *McFall versus Shimp*. 10 Pa.D&C 3d 90, 91 (Allegheny County Ct. 1978). The court refused to order Shimp to donate bone marrow that was necessary to save the life of his cousin, McFall, holding "for our law to compel defendant to submit to an intrusion of his body would change every concept and principle upon which our society is founded. To do so would defeat the sanctity of the individual, and would impose a rule which would know no limits, and one could not imagine where the line would be drawn." See also the case of the Curran twins, in which the father of a leukemia-stricken boy sought the appointment of a guardian by the Illinois Supreme Court to consent to the testing of the bone marrow of the boy's twin half-brothers over the objections of the twins' mother; a lower court had refused to order the tests saying it would be an invasion of the twins' privacy. [Anonymous]. Guardians named for children in marrow suit, *The New York Times* 1990 Aug 18;sect A:26.
24. See note 2. *In re* A. C 1990:31.
25. *Griswold versus Connecticut*. 380 US 479, 485-6 (1965).
26. *Roe versus Wade*. 410 US 113, 153 (1973).
27. *Webster versus Reproductive Health Services et al.* No. 88-605, slip op. (US 3 Jul 1989).
28. See note 26. *Roe versus Wade*. 1973:164-5.
29. After Overriding the governor's veto, the Louisiana state legislature passed a law prohibiting all abortions except those performed to save the life of the mother or in cases of rape or incest that is reported within 7 days. The law is presently being appealed to the Fifth Circuit Court of Appeals. *Sojourner T. versus Roemer*, No. 91-2247 (DC La. Aug. 7, 1991). Guam has also passed a law severely restricting abortions. The Pennsylvania, Louisiana, and Guam laws are unlikely to be presented to the U.S. Supreme Court in the near future.
30. 18 Pa. C.S.A. Section 3211 (1989).
31. [Anonymous]. With court's OK, abortion done on comatose woman, *Philadelphia Inquirer* 1989 Feb 12;sect A:8.
32. See Notes 12. Lenow. 1983;9(1):3-15.
33. See note 6. Johnson. 1986;95:600-13.
32. See note 12. Lenow. 1983;9(1):3-15.
34. *Hornbuckle versus Plantation Pipe Line*, 212 Ga. 504, 93 S.E. 2d 727 (1956). *Bennett versus Hymers*, 101 N.H. 483, 485, 147 A.2d 108, 110 (1958).
35. See note 16. [Anonymous]. 1989;Aug:16.
36. N.J. Stat. Ann. Section 30:4C-11 (West 1981) authorizes the Bureau of Children's Services to petition to care for an "unborn child" when it appears that the "child" is of such circumstances that his welfare will be endangered unless proper care or custody is provided.
37. *In re* Ruiz. 27 Ohio Misc. 2d 31, 500 N.E. 2d 935 (1986). The trial court ruled that a viable fetus is a child and that the mother's prenatal use of heroin constituted child neglect. *In re* Baby X. 97 Mich. App. 111, 293 N.W. 2d 36 (1980). The court held that evidence about a woman's prenatal "abuse" or "neglect" could be considered in proceedings to determine whether she should be deprived of the custody of her newborn.
38. *In re* Steven S. 126 Cal. App. 3d 23 (Cal. App. 1987). *In re* Dittrick Infant. 263 N.W. 2d 37 (Mich. App. 1977). The courts ruled that fetuses were not "children" under child neglect laws.
39. *Cruzan versus Director*, Missouri Department of Health. 58 U.S.L.W. 4916, 4918 (US 25 Jun 1990). *Citing Superintendent of Belchertown State School versus Saikewicz*. 373 Mass. 728, 370 N.E. 2d 417 (1977). The U.S. Supreme Court upheld the decision of the Missouri Supreme Court to consider the state's interest in preserving life in deciding whether to allow the guardians of a patient in a persistent vegetative state to withdraw her artificial nutrition and hydration.

40. Chernevak F, McCullough L. A practical method of analysis of the physician's ethical obligations to the fetus and pregnant woman in obstetric care, *Resid Staff Physician* 1989;35(1):79-87.
41. That a woman's decision should prevail in the vast majority of cases is now the official policy of George Washington University Medical Center, the site of the *In re* A.C. case. As the result of an out-of-court medical malpractice settlement with Angela Carder's parents, the hospital issued a policy that states, "When a fully informed and competent pregnant patient persists in a decision which may disserve her own or fetal welfare, this hospital's policy is to accede to the pregnant patient's preference whenever possible." [Anonymous]. *The New York Times* 1990 Nov 29;sect B:14.

SECTION 2

PEDIATRIC ISSUES

Chapter 10

Cases 2.0

Case 2.1: **BILLIE "B"**

An 8-year-old Down's syndrome child was swimming in his family's backyard pool when he jumped head-first into the water. He broke his neck at the C2 portion of the spine, but was immediately rescued by his parents, who called the emergency service. The boy could not talk, but was alert.

Seven months later, after several moves from outlying to more progressively intensive hospitals, Billie was still in a pediatric intensive care unit, completely paralyzed, with significant brain damage. He required a succession of shunts to relieve pressure on his brain; he was ventilator dependent, was fed through a gastrostomy, and could not communicate in any way with caregivers or family.

A plan was proposed to the parents for yet another shunt operation. They now refused, stating that Billie's progress was nothing of the sort. He had been the recipient of fine care, but this was as far as they were willing to go. They wanted him to remain on the respirator and to be fed, but they wanted him to be DNR and to have no new interventions.

The managing physician, a pediatric neurologist, actually refused to meet with the parents or the rest of the staff (who supported the parents) because his own convictions about preserving the life of this child were at risk. He was afraid they might talk him out of his own values.

When a family conference was finally arranged with caregivers, an ethicist, social workers, and staff, the physician and the ethicist (who had gotten some legal advice before the meeting) argued that not to shunt Billie was to abandon and "abuse" him. It would be akin to murder one. The Department of Children and Family Services would be notified by someone, they feared, and a charge of child-abuse would be brought against the physician for neglecting his patient. For the patient would most surely die if he did not get the shunt.

The mother tearfully spoke of her child's values. Although he was retarded, after years of working with him, he had learned to eat by himself and learned to swim in a rudimentary way. She said, "All Billie lived for was to eat and swim. Now he cannot even do that."

Can potentially life-saving therapy be avoided and the child allowed to die?

Case 2.2: **REFUSAL OF MEDICAL TREATMENT FOR RELIGIOUS REASONS**

Sharon R. is a thirteen-year-old girl who was initially admitted to a Community Hospital nearly two years ago with a three-week history of chest pain and progressive shortness of breath on exertion. She tired easily according to her mother. It was noted on admission that she appeared thin and undernourished. Height and weight were more than two standard deviations below the mean for her age group. A chest x-ray revealed opacification of the right chest and a mediastinal shift to the left. After one liter of serosanguinous fluid was removed from her chest, a large anterior mediastinal mass became evident by x-ray.

The fluid drawn from her chest contained lymphoblasts and lymphocytes. After further studies, the following diagnoses were made:

1. Malignant lymphoma, lymphoblastic type, involving the mediastinum, right pleural cavity, and right supraclavicular nodes.
2. Undernutrition.
3. Idiopathic seizure disorder.

Sharon was given chemotherapy and radiotherapy at the Children's Research Cancer Center. There was a rapid and complete regression of the tumor. During the next four months, Sharon suffered moderate toxic side-effects -- including anemia, weight loss, oral ulceration, and radiation pneumonitis, requiring a hospitalization and adjustment of the chemotherapeutic dosage.

The management of these problems was complicated by the patients's refusal to permit blood transfusions on religious grounds. Sharon and her family were Jehovah's Witnesses. Their wishes in the matter were honored--especially since it was not thought that blood transfusions were absolutely essential for effective management of Sharon's problems to this date. Her red blood cell count had never dropped dangerously.

Sharon had remained in initial complete remission for sixteen months, and she had been treated on an outpatient basis for fourteen of these months. There was a good chance that Sharon had successfully fought off the lymphoma. Her last bone marrow confirmed this assumption.

One week ago she was again admitted to the Children's Research Cancer Center for treatment of a cough , fever, and fatigue. She was found to have diffuse pneumonia of the left lung, for which she was given antibiotics and supportive measures. The pneumonia is due to pneumocystis carinii, an organism that often affects persons with lowered immunological resistance. Her admission hemoglobin of 7.3GM% progressively declined to 4.4GM%, and her condition rapidly deteriorated. In addition her white blood cell count plummeted to dangerously low levels. The postulated mechanisms for her anemia and low white blood count were effects of chemotherapy and/or infection; bone marrow showed no residual tumor. The questions of whether she had lymphoma outside the bone marrow, whether the lymphoma could ever recur, and whether the marrow aplasia would recover, were judged to be undecidable.

The physicians treating Sharon now judge that a blood transfusion is essential if there is to be any hope of saving her life. Both parents refused, although the father spent most of his time denying the disease as he sits in front of the television in the parent's lounge. Sharon was asked directly if she wanted the blood transfusion when her mother was out of the room. She was very sick. She did say, however, "I do not want to die and go to hell." She and her mother spend time with their Bibles every day, even though Sharon can hardly speak.

Sharon's social history is very important and is well-known to the physicians. Her natural father calls each day to check on her progress. He and Lily, Sharon's mother, were divorced when Sharon was only 1 year old. He did not contest the divorce and custody of the child went to Lily. He now lives in another state. He repeatedly demands that the physicians, "Take that crazy woman out of the room and save my daughter." It is not clear whether her natural father followed any particular religion. Lily reported that Sharon's natural father had never visited her. His child-support payments had come erratically through his sister who still lived in town.

Lily married again when Sharon was three. This marriage also ended in divorce 7 months later. At the divorce proceedings, Lily accused this husband of physical and emotional abuse. It was, like the first marriage, stormy. In fact, Lily accused this husband of sexual abuse of Sharon. Nonetheless, the judge pointedly noted in the divorce decree that no evidence was introduced to support this charge. Nothing is known of this husband, except that he was a Baptist and that Lilly and Sharon had become Baptists with him.

Between marriages, Lily supplemented the meager and sporadic child support payments by working as a waitress at the sandwich counter of a local drugstore. She reported that the income was insufficient to provide for her needs and those of Sharon. "I made just too much to draw welfare, and too little to pay all the bills," she said.

Lily married Bill R.F., two years before Sharon became sick. Bill did not abuse her and Sharon like her other husbands, Lily reported. They both became Jehovah's Witnesses because he was a lifelong member of the church. The doctors treating Sharon all thought that Lily was manipulative, domineering, and probably unstable. A social worker evaluated Sharon, however, and found that her cognitive, emotional, and personality development were all normal. Since the marriage to Bill, a person Sharon admires, both she and her mother have been very active in the church.

According to the social worker, neither Sharon nor her mother seem to understand the rationale behind the Jehovah's Witness objection to blood transfusion. One gets the strong impression that the primary interest of both is honoring Bill's deep, lifelong convictions. Lily wants to preserve her marriage after two previous "disasters." Sharon responds to the affection and kindness Bill displayed in the past. Both think they will go to hell if they accept blood.

The hospital attorney, Littman Bowers, is consulted about the possibility of turning to the courts to get approval for treatment. The attorney counsels against trying to obtain court approval. He notes that the judge in this jurisdiction always rules in favor of the right of the free expression of religion. The attorney has argued before the judge on a number of cases and in one, the judge protected a family who appealed to what the attorney thought were outlandish beliefs in order to justify child abuse.

The reporters would sensationalize the case if it became a matter of public record. The hospital would be portrayed as interfering with the internal workings of a family and defaming these honest, hard-working people, by charging them with child-neglect (the formal, legal charge that must be brought as part of the request for a court order for the transfusion). There would be an onslaught of negative publicity. Though, if pressed by the physicians, the attorney would have to pursue court action for them.

Sharon's natural father phones again, this time saying, "Lily is entitled to adopt some cockeyed religious beliefs if she chooses, but I will be damned if she is going to sacrifice my child's life to save her marriage to that jerk!" He announces that he is flying into town immediately and getting a lawyer who will try to transfer guardianship to him. He slams the phone with the statement: "If you delay in getting an authorization for a transfusion, and she dies before I get to town, I will slap you with a murder charge!"

Consider the following questions: Should Sharon have input in deciding whether to receive a blood transfusion? How do we incorporate, protect, and respect a child's values? Does the natural father have a right to influence the decision? What is the significance of a patient's and family's religious beliefs in deciding a course of medical treatment?

We are indebted to Glenn C. Graber, Ph.D., University of Tennessee, Department of Philosophy, for developing parts of this case.

Case 2.3: "**CHRIS**"

Chris was born at 28 weeks AGA to a 23-year-old single black female college student with pre-eclampsia and premature rupture of membranes. He had significant asphyxia at birth (apgars 4 & 8) and was intubated in the delivery room. He was hypoglycemic and had difficulty regulating his core body temperature. Within the first 24 hours, Chris also manifested severe hypotension which required pressors in order to keep him alive. He experienced a drop in blood count (hematocrit) from 56 to 38 which required transfusion with packed red blood cells through an umbilical vein catheter. He was transfused several times over the next 5 days for decreasing hematocrit; and on day 4 of life, he had multiple tonic-clonic seizures for which he was started on phenobarbital and dilantin.

On day 6, ultrasound of the head showed a Grade IV intraventricular hemorrhage (IVH). On day 8, a heart murmur was heard at the left upper sternal border, and Chris' ventilator requirements increased. This was consistent with Patent Ductus Arteriosus, a condition in which the connection between the pulmonary artery and the aorta re-opens; thus diverting blood flow from the systemic circulation back to the lungs. This is usually treated with Indocin, a drug which closes the ductus; and if Indocin is unsuccessful, surgery is performed to ligate the ductus. Indocin was successful in Chris.

Throughout this time, Chris was still in respiratory distress requiring continued ventilator support. In the beginning, it was unclear whether Chris' problem was caused by Hyaline Membrane Disease (HMD) or pneumonia. As time passed, it was clearer that HMD was the likely cause of Chris' problem. His respiratory illness was further complicated by the Patent Ductus and the grade IV IVH. Chris also experienced hyperbilirubinemia for the first 2-3 weeks of his life; contributed to by IVH, bruising at birth, and the side effects of Indocin. The major complication of this is kernicterus; a condition in which the brain can be damaged by the high levels of bilirubin (which is a breakdown product of hemoglobin in blood). At approximately 3 weeks of age, Chris' head size began to increase an he became more irritable with handling. Ultrasound showed increased size of the lateral ventricles of the brain, consistent with hydrocephalus; but there was no extension of the hemorrhage. This was treated successfully with the placement of an intraventricular shunt. (A device which is inserted into the ventricle to drain off the excess cerebral spinal fluid that collects in there and can cause eventual mental deterioration and death.)

At 4 weeks, Chris has stabilized. He is still on the ventilator at moderate settings with no sign of the side effects of prolonged ventilator use at this point. Feedings are through a feeding tube placed through his nose into his stomach as Chris has not shown an ability to suck yet. Chris' weight at birth was ll90mg and is not lll0mg (about 2.5 pounds).

Social Background

Chris' parents are both 23-years-old, unmarried, but they live together. They are college students at a local college in Chicago, and the father works part time. The pregnancy was unplanned, but the parents wanted Chris and were concerned and involved in his care. Their reactions to Chris' illness were different in many ways. The mother seemed more devastated and was unable to stay in the unit for long periods of time especially at the beginning. As time wore on, she visited every day, and her visits grew longer. But, it was clear that she was emotionally distraught with Chris' illness and with the surroundings in which he was placed.

When caregivers explained Chris' condition to both parents, it was not always clear that she understood or wanted to take part in the more technical aspects of the decision-making (Although she was clearly intelligent enough to do so). The father, on the other hand, seemed to thrive on the technical aspects of Chris' condition. For example, he was a full explanation of Chris' hemorrhage down to the anatomy affected. He asked pointed and concerned questions; and in the beginning seemed to be the one making most of the decisions. Chris' parents seemed a close couple. They spoke in private about his condition and comforted each other. They visited often, but didn't stay for long periods. They were easily accessible at home.

Medical Facts

Intraventricular Hemorrhage is a condition in which the immature blood vessels in the area of the brain surrounding the ventricles break and bleed into the substance of the brain. They can also break into the ventricles themselves causing a clinical picture of hydrocephalus. Hydrocephalus is a condition in which too much fluid in these ventricles can cause compression of the tissue around them, thus causing damage. The sequelae from this range from death due to hemorrhage to mental and motor deficit. It is usually classified into 4 grades. Recent literature suggests that the prognosis is not as uniformly poor for all grades as was once thought. Infants with grades I and II hemorrhage have between an 80-90% chance of remaining normal or with minor deficit, (i.e, They don't have spastic hemiplegia or mental deficits, but there is an increased incidence of learning disability and fine motor deficit.) Grades III and IV hemorrhage have a poorer prognosis with anywhere from 40-70% of patients experiencing major deficit (i.e. spastic hemiplegia and mental retardation) especially when associated with clinically overt hydrocephalus. Still it is extremely difficult to predict the prognosis of infants with grades III and IV hemorrhage; partly due to lack of numbers and partly because it's difficult to use the above statistics on an individual basis. Certainly mortality rates are higher for those with a more severe bleed; but not significantly higher. This is complicated by the fact that these infants often die of other causes. Thus, grades III and IV hemorrhage can not be considered terminal lesions.

Their ethical impact centers more on the difficulty of predicting mental and physical handicap: some of which is so severe, that many have questioned whether an all out effort should be made to save these patients. Is their life, such as it is, preferable to death?

Hyaline Membrane Disease is a form of respiratory distress found at an especially increased incidence in premature infants. The etiology is still in doubt, but most clinicians today believe that a decrease in surfactant and a decrease number of mature alveoli cause a picture in which individual alveoli collapse. (Alveoli are the tiny sacs at the terminal branchings of the lung that carry on the lung's basic function of O2 and CO2 exchange). If respiratory function can be maintained on a ventilator until the lungs mature, this disease presents minimal long-term problems. There are two situations where this is not the case. The first is when HMD is so severe that the ventilator requirements are increased to the point of causing side effects.

One of these side effects is Broncho-Pulmonary Dysplasia which is a fibrous inflammatory change in the lung tissue with variable severity and consequences which range from minimal Chronic Obstructive Pulmonary Disease to death. The other side effect is pneumothorax which is a more acute problem that requires chest tube placement as a life-saving measure. The second situation is the one in which the HMD is so severe that it never resolves and the infant goes on to die.

Problem

Chris' mother now requests that "nothing further" be done to save her son, since he is "suffering so much." The father seems to concur. Both begin to talk more about Chris' suffering and letting him go. The couple, while respectful, note that they have little money and cannot foresee caring for their son at home should he develop and grow up retarded. They emphasize, tearfully, that they are the ones who will have to live with the consequences of your decisions about intervening further in Chris' beginning-of-life crisis.

Case 2.4: **DO MULTIPLE FAILURES ADD UP TO DYING?**

K.A. is an 8-year-old girl of Greek descent who was admitted to a children's hospital on January 5 with complaints of abdominal pain and fever for one month. She had been seen by her local physician during the month and found to have enlarged spleen and liver with a left ear infection which resisted treatment with two different antibiotic regimens. At four months, K.A. was diagnosed as having B thalassemia major, a difficult genetic disorder, for which she has been receiving transfusions every three to four weeks since. She has also been receiving chelation therapy for the past five years in order to rectify overloads of iron which appears in this disease.

The initial physical examination upon this admission showed a thin white female with "thalassemic" facies, marked hepatomegaly (liver enlargement) and moderate splenomegaly (spleen enlargement). The left ear was draining purulent material.

During the last six months, this child has had a stormy hospital course caused by multi-system illnesses. A brief summary of her past and present problems includes:

1. *Fluids/Nutrition:* She is currently maintained on a central H-A because she cannot tolerate food orally due to severe diarrhea. Thus, all of her food is in liquid form. There can be no "pleasure" in eating.

2. *Respiratory*: After an episode of sepsis (a systemic infection) several months ago, she was placed on a respirator. She has now become ventilator-dependent, which means that she can only tolerate short periods of time off the respirator without become asphyxiated. Currently she has been weaned off the respirator at night. When she is awake, she begins voluntary ventilation through a tracheotomy (a hole in her throat) by using 25-30% pure oxygen.

3. *Cardiovascular*: Her LV function is markedly impaired. As a result she receives serious cardiac drugs such as Digoxin, Lasix and Aldactone. This defect is not reversible, but can be controlled with the drugs.

4. *Gastrointestinal Tract*: She suffers from two problems:
   a. Chronic diarrhea, whose cause is most likely an infection.
   b. Hepatosplenomegaly, whose cause is most likely an iron overload, but could also be attributed to an infection.

5. *Infectious Diseases*:
   a. Systemic histoplasmosis which persists even after a six week course of Amphotericin B, a potent antibiotic, and daily administration of ketaconozola, another potent antibiotic.
   b. Pseudomonas sepsis and colonization, also persisting to date.
   c. Herpes simplex persisting even after treatment with Acyclovir. The persistence of the infections means that her immunological system is severely impaired.

6. *Neurological*: She suffers from dementia and aphasia (lack of oxygen), both of which show slight improvement lately. However, she still has an encephalopathy of unknown etiology.

7. *Immune Dysfunction*: An initial CBC, blood test, showed severe lymphopenia (ALC

110), a reduction in white lymph cells; T4/T8 ratio was also markedly decreased. HTLV III screen was positive; and antibody liters were markedly elevated (1:35000), confirmed by CDC and NCI. In other words, the child has also contracted AIDS.

8. *Social*: The mother has not left the hospital since this admission. The patient is the second of two children. The father owns a restaurant in the far suburbs, about 50 miles away from the hospital. The first child stays with the father and goes to school. Now and then they are both able to visit. When they do, they all insist upon doing everything for their daughter/sister.

9. *Economic*: The estimated hospital bill, not counting physician and specialist fees, after 7 months, is greater than $250,000.

Among the many questions this case poses are: Is the girl to be considered to be dying? If not, what obligations persist should new problems develop? If she is considered to be dying, even though no single current problem can be said to be terminal at this time, what obligations do we have to keep her alive? Could we simply terminate the life-support system one morning, for example? Also, the economic questions must also be raised. Is it proper for our society to keep a marginal patient like this alive at such great cost, when so many others are not able even to see a doctor? Finally, what impact will her continued hospitalization have on the family and caregivers? Physicians are currently divided about recommending any course of treatment in addition to current care, even though the mother and father want everything done to preserve their daughter's life.

In short, the girl continues to suffer and there is no clearly definable treatment plan. What should be done and why?

Case 2.5: **PAMELA HAMILTON**

> *Is any among you afflicted? Let him pray. Is any merry? Let him sing psalms. Is any sick among you? Let him call the elders of the church: and let them pray over him. Anointing him with oil in the name of the Lord. And the prayer of faith shall save the sick; and the Lord shall raise him up; and if he have committed sins, they shall be forgiven him.*
>
> James 5:13-15 (King James Version)

This passage forms the cornerstone of doctrine of the Church of God of the Union Assembly. The organizing tenet of the church appears to be members' opposition to medical treatment. A typical church service includes testimonies by those present of episodes of divine healing. All members are forbidden to use "medication, shots, or injections of any kind," including pain medications. They will accept chiropractic treatments and repairs of cut flesh and broken bones, however, believing that these treatments merely prepare the way for God's healing action.

Other rules of the church include bans on the use of "any adornment" (including makeup, fingernail polish, or jewelry), shaving legs, or cutting of their hair by women. (This last one makes it especially difficult for a female member to accept the prospect of the chemotherapy side effect of hair loss.) Women are not permitted to teach or take any leadership role in services in the church.

The church also prohibits tobacco smoking and alcohol, mixed swimming, attendance at movies or ball games, and chewing gum in church.

Pamela Hamilton is the 12-year-old daughter of an ordained minister in this sect. Her father, Larry Hamilton, is pastor of a 38-member congregation near LaFollette, Tennessee.

Pamela has three brothers, ranging in age from 3 to 14. Their mother was killed in 1981 in an auto-train wreck. Their father remarried within a few months, and he and his new wife are expecting a child in the Fall of 1983.

In July 1983, Pamela's parents took her to a chiropractor in response to her persistent complaints of a pain in her left leg. He referred her to an orthopedic surgeon, who discovered a tumor as well as a fracture. Biopsy confirmed the diagnosis of Ewing's sarcoma.

Apparently, the Hamiltons did not register any objection to any aspect of the treatment of the broken leg. Installing the pin involved the use of anesthesia and pain medications, and the child was also given sedatives and other medications during her hospitalization. The hospital staff say they were unaware of any religious objections to these medications on the part of the family.

Initial Refusal of Treatment

Nor, apparently, was anything said about an intention not to bring the child back for the recommended work-up and treatment of the tumor. They merely failed to return for the scheduled follow-up appointment. When the appointment was not kept, the Oncologist sent the usual letter of reminder urging the Hamiltons to re-schedule the appointment; and, when no response was received to this, he followed up further with a telephone call to Mr. Hamilton.

DHS Involvement

It was not until sometime in early August that the Oncologist became convinced that his efforts to persuade the father to authorize treatment were not going to succeed. At this point, he contacted officials of the state Department of Human Services (DHS) to notify them of the Hamiltons' intention to refrain from medical treatment for Pamela's tumor.

The state, acting under the ancient legal doctrine of *parens patriae*, assumes final responsibility for the welfare of dependents within its jurisdiction. For example, any child whose "parent, guardian, or custodian neglects or refuses to provide necessary medical...care" may be declared a "Dependent and neglected child" and the state may intervene to protect the child's welfare [*Tenn Code Annotated*, Section 37-202(6.iv)].

Court Actions

On August 26, the local Juvenile Court issued an order requiring the Hamiltons to take Pamela to St. Jude Children's Research Hospital in Memphis, Tennessee for evaluation and treatment. On September 13, after attempts by the family to resist this order, Pamela was taken to St. Jude Hospital by a court-appointed guardian and admitted for a work-up. Rev. Hamilton refused, however, to permit the use of pain medications during any of the diagnostic tests. Pamela voiced agreement with her father's position on this matter. So all of the tests -- including a bone marrow aspiration -- were performed without anesthesia or painkillers.

Juvenile Court Hearing

In depositions read at the subsequent court hearing on September 17, St. Jude physicians reported that their medical evaluation confirmed the diagnosis of Ewing's sarcoma. No metastases were detected. They expressed the judgment that, without treatment, Pamela would die within six to nine months, but that there was a chance of "50% or better" for a long-term remission with a combination treatment of chemotherapy and radiation therapy. Just under fifty percent of the Ewing's sarcoma patients treated at St. Jude since the early 1960s are still alive; and, the protocol currently being employed appears to have an even higher success rate.

Mr. Hamilton's attorneys argued against treatment, citing the sanctity of the family and the right to religious freedom.

Pamela's Wishes
Pamela herself shyly told observers in the crowded judge's chambers that she believed God was more powerful than doctors. "I believe in God, and I believe God can heal me without taking medicine and all that stuff."

Pamela told her court-appointed guardian that she did not believe doctors' prognosis that she would die within six months from the cancer if she did not receive medical treatment. "Do you want to die?" she was asked. "When the Lord gets ready for me," she replied.

The Court Decision
Juvenile Court Judge Charles Herman issued his decision immediately following the 14-hour hearings. Before reading his decision, Judge Herman addressed Pamela directly: "The court is aware of what you have gone through and you have gone through it courageously. You are one of the most courageous people I have ever come in contact with in my life."

Saying that this was "the most difficult decision I have faced on the bench," Judge Herman ruled in favor of treatment. "To allow her to die would constitute a grave public wrong," he stated. Thus, he placed Pamela into custody of the state DHS and ordered medical treatment for the cancer.

Hospitalization
An ambulance was called to the courthouse, and television cameras recorded the scene as Pamela -- tearful, reaching out to her father, and making a feeble attempt to resist being parted from him -- was strapped to a stretcher for transport to East Tennessee Children's Hospital.

Further Court Action
However, the Hamiltons' attorneys immediately sought, and received, a stay order from the state Court of Appeals pending their review of the decision; and thus treatment was delayed for four days.

However, after hearing the case, they upheld the lower court ruling, as did the Tennessee Supreme Court.

Sequelae
After six months of treatment by chemotherapy and radiation therapy, an evaluation revealed no signs of tumor cells present. However, nine months later, new tumors were discovered.

What should be done now?

Used with permission of Glenn C. Graber and David C. Thomasma, co-authors, *Euthanasia: Toward an Ethical Social Policy*.

Case 2.6: SPINAL STABILIZATION?

N. is a 12-year-old girl with severe athetoid cerebral palsy. She has no purposeful use of her arms and has no effective expressive language. Because of the severity of her disabilities, no IQ or other measure of intellectual function is known.

She is seen at a University hospital because of her difficulty sitting. On examination she has a severe scoliosis measuring 135 degrees with the 11th and 12th rib inside the pelvis. Multiple attempts at devising wheelchair supports have been attempted and are not effective.

The definitive treatment is spinal stabilization, which would require anterior fusion, halo femoral traction and finally a posterior fusion. This implies about one month of hospitalization and two major surgeries. She has been seen at a Community hospital where the parents were told by the orthopedic surgeon there that she was "not worth my time."

The goal of surgery would be improved sitting. Is this worth the expenditure of time and resources? Her parents are willing to listen to your advice, but are also concerned, not only for her own well-being, but also about escalating health care costs. Their primary value seems to be that she not suffer unduly. Since she cannot understand what will be happening to her, they are worried that the operation will cause undue pain and suffering, with significant risk, and only a minor improvement, given her status.

Nonetheless, it does not seem right to discriminate against her just because she is so retarded and disabled. Indeed, laws protecting defective newborns demonstrate the commitment of society to the disabled.

What will be your recommendation?

Case 2.7: THE CONJOINED TWINS

The Lakeberg twins were born at Loyola University Chicago Medical Center on June 29, 1993, joined at the chest, from the sternum down. Their plight became the focus of national media attention during July and August 1993, and again in June 1994. For this reason their real names can be used in this case.

The ethical problem associated with conjoined twins are perplexing and complicated. This is because they involve questions of social justice and clinical uncertainty. Medical technology has given us so many choices that we lack the wisdom to select the best from among them. Ultimately, the physicians, other members of the health care team, and the parents must evaluate the risks and benefits of a course of action based on medical evidence and ethical considerations. Since these births are extremely uncommon, medical and ethical discussion about the care of conjoined twins rarely takes place. The opportunity to explore this issue in depth occurred for medical staff and ethicists at Loyola University of Chicago Medical Center in June 1993. To this discussion was added the newer concerns of a nation on the brink of developing a National Health Care Plan.

The Lakeberg twins were born on June 29, 1993, conjoined at the heart, from the sternum down: a physical metaphor for the conjoining of cherished values in society -- the value of human life, the energy and cost of medical intervention, the problems of social justice and allocation of health care, and the role of parenting itself. Discussion about their care, their survival, their parents, and the nature of civil society all began when the Lakebergs themselves approached the media. Their plight and that of the twins became the focus of national media attention during July and August 1993,[1,2] and again in June 1994, when the surviving twin, Angela died on June 9, just over two weeks shy of her first birthday.[3] She became the longest living survivor after surgery on this type of conjoined twining. But the questions persist: It is a good opportunity, then, to examine what we learned from the Lakeberg twins.

Mr. and Mrs. Lakeberg lived in rural Indiana. They had a five-year-old healthy daughter, who was born in 1987 without anomalies. Some problems existed in their lives already. They had been ejected from the trailer park where they lived for failure to pay rent, and Mr. Lakeberg was on probation for assaulting a family member. Later the father's escapades added a sad, carnival atmosphere to tragedy as it unfolded.

Amy and Angela Lakeberg

Mrs. Lakeberg, 24-years-old, was 16 weeks into her second pregnancy when an ultrasound examination revealed conjoined twins of the thoracopagus type. She was referred to Loyola University Medical Center after initial care in Indiana. There was good prenatal care, with the ultrasound on February 9, 1993 consistent with 17.8 weeks. There was no family history of congenital anomalies. However the mother does have a history of mitral valve prolapse. The mother denied use of drugs, alcohol, or tobacco.

The ultrasound evaluation demonstrated a sharing of a common heart and liver with a single umbilical cord with four vessels. Separate GI tracts and stomachs existed for each twin. No other obvious anomalies of either of the twin's heads or extremities was noted. A fetal ECHO on May 5 demonstrated markedly abnormal cardiac anatomy with three atrioventricular values, two well formed and one hypoplastic. There were two aortic and two pulmonic values.

At least two well-formed ventricles each gave origin to two great vessels. There was also a least one large basal inlet ventricular septal defect identified at this time. At 17 weeks, the medical staff at Loyola met with the Lakebergs to discuss the situation. They were told that if the pregnancy was brought to term, there was an overwhelming chance that one of the twins would die, and a very significant chance that both twins would die.[4] The Lakebergs decided to carry the pregnancy to term, following an aborted visit to an abortion clinic.

Amniocentesis performed one day prior to delivery revealed a mature lung profile. The babies, Amy and Angela, were born at 37 weeks gestation by Caesarean-section. As expected, physical examination was remarkable for thoracopagus conjoined twins. There was a six vessel cord that had four arteries and two veins. Initial combined weight of the twins was 4.2 kg (small for gestation). Initial heart rate was approximate 100 beats a minute with spontaneous respirations. The Apgar scores for both twins were 7, 8, and 8 at one, five, and ten minutes.

Initial testing showed that the twins shared one common complex six-chamber heart and one common liver; there were separate lungs, kidneys and GI tracts. Ultrasound indicated normal brains. The babies became ventilator dependent by six hours of life.

Hospital Course

The following is a summary of their hospital course relative to major organ systems. It shows a number of problems experienced by the twins:

1. *Respiratory*: Pulmonary function secondary to the non-compliant joined chest wall was always marginal. This raised the first and, as it turned out, the final question of whether individual lung function was possible. As respiratory failure ensued the medical team hurriedly wrestled with the question of whether to intervene with mechanical ventilation or not. The twins were intubated after 6 hours of life for progressive carbon dioxide retention after failing nasal oxygen, under the assumption that improvement of a transient postnatal respiratory condition would enable later extubation. They remained dependent on synchronous servo volume ventilation. All attempts at extubation were unsuccessful because of a thoracic-like dystrophy due to the way they were joined. Pulmonary function testing on each twin suggested that independent respiratory function would be unlikely for either child. This was the first major ethical issue to be faced after the twins were born. What should the goals of mechanical ventilation be if the respiratory failure did not improve. In that case, should mechanical ventilation be withdrawn?

2. *Cardiovascular*: The twins remained hemodynamically stable on Digoxin and Lasix.

Evaluation of cardiac catherization revealed that Angela had a left double-outlet right ventricle with the aorta and pulmonary artery in a transposed position. There was a supracardiac total anomalous pulmonary venous return (TAPVR). The pulmonary artery was small and a VSD was present and moderate in size. The Inferior Vena Cava appeared to be single and coursed from Angela to Amy. Amy had a right double-outlet right ventricle with mild valvular pulmonary stenosis and more significant subvalvular aortic stenosis. There was a partial anomalous supracardiac pulmonary venous drainage.

3. *Infectious Disease*. During the course of their hospitalization at Loyola the twins experienced two life-threatening infections. These were both treated successfully. At both points no ethical discussion occurred about continued treatment of the infections with antibiotics because the infections were nosocomial. The parents spoke proudly to the media about how Dr. Muraskas saved the lives of their babies.

4. *Neurological.* Ultrasound revealed normal anatomy and a neurological examination revealed no major deficits.

Initial Medical and Ethical Discussions

As noted, the first ethical dilemma came at six hours of life when the twins had to be put on the respirator. The question then was what the goal of treatment would be? Would either or both ever live off the respirator once it had been started? Should the intubation be seen as an intervention for an acute emergency, with later withdrawal? Why start it if the twins were not going to be separated? Should it be used if the likelihood of living off of it would be almost zero? JM decided to put them on it despite these questions from TM on the grounds that he needed more time to conduct further tests. Many said later that at this point we sentenced Angela to life.

Early in their treatment, on July 9, a meeting was held at Loyola to discuss the medical and ethical issues involved in the case. Participants at this interdisciplinary care conference included the Director of the Neonatal Intensive Care Unit (TM), the attending physician (JM), the managing physicians, other neonatology attendings and residents, a pediatric radiologist, other pediatric specialists, including a pediatric cardiovascular surgeon, medical students, nurses, social workers, the unit chaplain, and members of the ethics consult service (DCT) (PM).

Three possible courses of action outlined were:

1. Do nothing, in which case the babies would inevitably die; a subset of this course of action was to withdraw the respirator and allow the children to die;

2. Attempt to separate the twins at Loyola after medical testing was completed; and,

3. Send the twins to another site (e.g., Children's Hospital of Philadelphia -- CHOP) with greater experience in separating conjoined twins.[5,6]

During the course of one year, the ethical issues focused on three major areas: First, is it ever moral to kill one to save another? Second, how far can parents push doctors and hospitals to provide extraordinary (some would say futile) care? Third, in a National Health Plan should the public support such extremely controversial care?[7] Yet the case was far more complex than these ethical precipitates, more complex ethically, emotionally, professionally, and socially.

The ethics consult note said, in part, that this case demonstrated a problematic application of the "best interests" principle. Whose best interests are being served if the twins are separated? The baby who lives? The baby who dies? Medical science, because of the opportunity to scientifically document and evaluate another case of conjoined twins, or no one, since the probable outcome is death for both infants?

Historically, there is legal and ethical support for reasonable attempts to separate twins with conjoined hearts. The underlying moral argument suggests that it is better to try and save one life than to passively allow two deaths to occur. The situation, however, is replete with ethical dilemmas. Is it right to sacrifice one baby so that the other can live?[8] Can the rule against killing be suspended if the outcome is very poor, or very little likelihood exists that the one surviving twin would eventually survive?[9] If that rule can be suspended, on what grounds would the action be justified? Are the physicians obligated to two babies or only one? Is it ever justified to expend social resources on what is essentially medically futile treatment, even if the possibility of pursuing that treatment is available? Given the slim chance of success and the scarcity of medical resources, is it appropriate to attempt separation? If separation is attempted, it is certain one baby will die; the chances of the other baby living outside the hospital have never been documented. As noted, there was further evidence in this case that independent respiratory function was extremely unlikely. Should medicine always push every envelope of possibility so it can continue to advance? Most surgeons consulted and commenting in the media noted that all such surgery is experimental because, in the words of Louis Keith, M.D., "surgeons generally have no benchmarks of prior experience to guide them. Each operation must be devised as it proceeds in order to deal with the anatomic problems that present themselves."[10]

The ethical situation of saving one twin rather than letting both die is less ambiguous when there are objective medical criteria which indicate that one of the twins has a better chance of survival. In the present case, the evidence suggested just such a scenario -- one twin was more likely to survive separation. The parents, along with the some of the medical team, were committed to doing everything possible to save the life of at least one of the twins. Kenneth Lakeberg articulated this commitment as a form of "winning the lottery," realizing nonetheless that the chances were extremely small.[11] We think at this point in the case, the family essentially became addicted to the media. No matter what JM or Dr. O'Neill said, the family, enjoying the national spotlight, would insist that everything be done. Growing up in the rural farmlands of Indiana and now to be seen throughout the world turned out to be a critical factor in the family's decisions about the twins.

After further medical review, however, the physicians at Loyola again decided against recommending the separation surgery. The husband was willing to accept this considered judgment, but the wife thought that "she could not live with herself if she did not at least try to save one life." The physicians at Children's Hospital of Philadelphia agreed all along with the Loyola physicians that the chances of survival of one twin were remote, but they agreed to consider the possibility of surgery after further tests. The babies were transferred there for additional testing and consideration.

Philadelphia

Amy could not survive because she did not have necessary structures. Transplantation was not an option. Though the outcome for the surviving twin was regarded very slim, nevertheless the physicians agreed to the surgery.

They were wary of trying to "sell" the family on such a surgery, so they asked the family to reconsider for another day.

When they still pressed forward with their request, the surgery was planned for August 20, 1993. At 0700, the twins were brought to the operating room, after a tearful good-bye from assembled family and friends. Dr. James O'Neill, Jr. performed the initial component of the surgery by separating the liver. This portion of the operation went smoothly. After this, Dr. William Norwood took over the direction of surgery. Angela came off bypass uneventfully, with excellent cardiac function, something that could not have been predicted completely before the surgery.

As known in advance that she would, Amy died during the surgery. The surgery took much less time than thought. When asked by the media about the ethics of killing one child to save the other, as it was put, Dr. O'Neill remarked that there was widespread support for the action. This is probably not the case. O'Neill said that when the blood vessels connecting Amy with Angela were severed, cutting off the blood flow and causing her death, "nothing was said, but I know everybody felt it."[12]

Almost twelve months later Angela continued to be dependent on mechanical ventilation, and was taken off for short periods from the negative pressure respirator (like an iron lung that created a vacuum atmosphere), but was still in serious condition. Angela experienced thoracic wall instability and chronic lung changes. She remained on a significant amount of oxygen. She tolerated her feedings well and was gaining weight. Angela faced many critical steps toward continued survival, or even eventual discharge from the hospital. During her brief life, her mother was able to visit her only three times; a milestone was passed in December when she was held by her mother for the first time. At the time of her death, another visit was being planned for her first birthday. She smiled at caregivers who said they were surprised by her death from cardiorespiratory insufficiency, since she had been stable for some time. Yet this is how we knew she would die. The caregivers in Philadelphia said it was worth it, and so did the family members before her funeral.[13] We think these statements reflect the bond created by family love and by health care providers, but also may entail a metaphysics that would argue that it is better to live than not to have lived at all. The problem is: what kind of life was it for Angela?

Ethical Questions

These are just a few of the ethical questions that linger from the case:

1. Should we ever ration healthcare at the bedside, or should we ignore the needs of the community and the scarcity of medical resources, pursuing instead health care of the individual(s) at hand?

2. Other families argued that, because they had never brought their cases to the media, their children who needed expensive health care never got it, and died. Is this just?

3. Are there reasons beyond medical ones for doing what many consider to be medically futile therapy? Do family values trump medical ones?

4. What is the role of parenting and protecting the vulnerable from harm in this case? Is it a form of denial to "want everything possible done," or may it instead stem from a desire to "accept what God has given us?"

5. Do the "Baby Doe" Regulations apply to this case? Were the Loyola physicians and support staff, along with the ethicists, discriminating against the infants on the basis of handicap by deciding not to separate them?

Case 2.8: **DENIAL AND A HYDROCEPHALIC INFANT**

Baby M is a 25-day-old infant with severe hydrocephalus born at 23 weeks gestation. It was a twin gestation, but the other twin died after two weeks of age in the Newborn Intensive Care Unit. The mother was a 32-year-old single WF who had used cocaine during her pregnancy, but otherwise had no known health problems. She visited Baby M every day, asking each time whether her baby would get better.

Baby M had no ability to move her extremities. A CT of her head showed severely dilated ventricles with a thin rim of cortex surrounding them (about 5MM thick). The brainstem appeared intact, but the infant would not be able to breathe on her own. The physicians had tried to explain the poor prognosis for this infant, and suggested terminating life-support, but the mother continued to ask whether her baby would get better as she got older. She was repeatedly told that the infant would remain paralyzed, would have no cognitive function, and would always require life-support. She had, in fact, already coded once and had been resuscitated by the resident on-call, since no DNR orders had been agreed upon.

After all the struggles to keep the baby alive, the mother was having an even harder time deciding whether the infant should be disconnected from the respirator. After one week of deliberation following the doctor's recommendation, she did decide that the respirator should be disconnected. She refused to sign any papers, however, because she said she needed time to say good-bye. She visited her baby every day for the next 2 weeks, each time saying she would agree to disconnect the respirator next time she was visiting.

At 45-days-old, Baby M finally was disconnected from the respirator. The mother watched tearfully, but quietly. After a few minutes, the nurse turned the baby over and reported to the physician, "The heart is still beating." The mother cried out, "Please resuscitate her then." The physician replied, "I'm sorry Mrs. M., we cannot resuscitate her now. We have already discussed this, and we have decided that she should not be kept alive any longer."

The mother objected and said they she could not stand by and let her baby die this way. What should now be done?

Based on a case presented by Andrea Poirier,
Class of 1993 medical student

Notes

1. Toufexis A. The ultimate choice, *Time Magazine* 1993 Aug 30:43-44.
2. Siegel B. Two babies, one heart--and a dilemma, *L.A. Times* 1993 Nov 7:1.
3. Brandon K, Cawley J. Lakeberg baby dies; medical debate lingers. *Chicago Tribune* 1994 June 10:Sec.1,1,24.
4. Barth RA, Fily RA, Goldberg JD, *et al.* Conjoined twins: Prenatal diagnosis and assessment of associated malformations. *Radiology* 1990;177:201-207.
5. O'Neil JA, *et al.* Surgical experience with thirteen conjoined twins, *Annals of Surgery* 1988;208(3):299-312.
6. Albert MC, Drummond DS, O'Neil J, *et al.* The orthopedic management of conjoined twins: A review of 13 cases and report of 4 cases, *J Ped Ortho* 1992;2:300-307.
7. Editorial. *Chicago Tribune* 1994 June 9:Sec.1, 23.
8. Annas GJ. Siamese twins: Killing one to save the other, *Hastings Center Report* 1987 April 17:27-29.
9. O'Neill JA, *et al.* Surgical experience with thirteen conjoined twins, *Annals of Surgery* 1992 Sep. 2;8(3):229-312.

10. McNamee T, Wisby G. Modern medicine unable to save win: Angela's short life strained faith, ethics, *Chicago Sun-Times* 1994 June 10:6.
11. McNamee W:6.
12. Brandon K. For survivor, What are we really creating? *Chicago Tribune* 1994 Feb 21:Sec.1, 1,6.
13. McNamee W:6.

Chapter 11

Caring for Life in the First of It: Moral Paradigms for Perinatal and Neonatal Ethics

Warren T. Reich

It is the contention of this paper that the ethics of caring for life in the first of it -- examining our responsibilities to the fetus and the newborn infant in a medical setting -- has been too narrowly conceived, and that its basis should be broadened.

Until now, writings on the ethics of perinatology and neonatology have placed too much emphasis on rights and duties, making use of the language of ethical principles that require major philosophical theories as their starting-points. I will point to some limitations in those approaches and will make an appeal for another approach that takes more unabashedly as its starting-point the moral experiences of patients, parents, physicians, nurses and other agents in these human dramas. For I believe that if some neglected methodologies in ethics that pay closer attention to moral experience as their starting-point -- in particular, the ethics of value and virtue -- could be brought to bear on the ethics of caring for the infant and fetus, ethical discussions in our country might show a richer and more appealing moral fabric.

Furthermore, were such an approach to be taken, international and intercultural dialogue on these ethical questions would become a more profitable undertaking, for our methodology would then allow us to take more seriously the moral experiences, the moral perceptions, and the moral sentiments of people, without having to assume that all must learn the Anglo-American language of ethical principles and duties.[1]

Thus, when we come to the final debate on the ranking of values that are experienced in various ways in the human perinatal situation, we could negotiate those differences by making use of principles that have evolved from centuries of experience in making moral judgments. But that would reduce principles to their appropriate role, for we would then have a greater assurance that we are aware of and involved in a sufficiently broad and deep range of values and commitments that in fact make up the stuff of the morality of perinatology and neonatology.

I start my appeal with a narrative.

The Case of the White Oaks Boy

I was alone, waiting for the start of an ethics case conference in an all-purpose room of the Child Development Center. I remember that the cement block walls of the 1960s vintage building were painted with a stark yellow (they must have wanted it to look like sunshine, to cheer up the handicapped, I said to myself). Feeling very much the displaced, developed adult consultant, I was in the grip of wondering whether the gray molded plastic chair would

Source: Reprinted from *Seminars in Perinatology*, Vol. 11, No. 3, pp. 279-287, with permission of W.B. Saunders Company © July, 1987.

really continue to support me, when the pediatric resident, who would be presenting the case -- and whom I will call Dr. McDonough -- arrived and started telling me the following story while we waited for the other committee members.

"The patient is 21-years-old," he said, "is the size of a seven-year-old, and has the mental age of a two- to two-and-a-half-year-old.

"We have two questions about this patient: First, what decisions should we make about his care right now? And second, at some point I'd like to discuss how the decisions we are faced with now trace their origins back to decisions that were made about him when he was a neonate. Currently, in our department, we are starting an interdisciplinary inquiry into quality of life in pediatric decision-making; and we want to find out how the patient's present situation -- and our responsibilities to him -- relate to the promise he held at birth and the decisions that were made about him then. So far we have not been able to do a history on him as a neonate; but I can tell you something about him as a survivor of what was apparently a fairly intense neonatal treatment. Let me describe his present situation and see what you think of his quality of life and our responsibilities."

"Michael, the patient, has had a history of lung infections and malnutrition. He was admitted to the hospital this time for an appendectomy; but then he experienced post-operative aspiration pneumonia, and because of this and his history of chronic lung disease, he was then admitted to Pediatric Intensive Care."

"No crises arose that created a moral quandary, but there was a discussion among the staff on the ethical aspects of his care, especially on what may lie in his future."

"Here was a patient who was recovering from pneumonia, and the question arose: What if the antibiotics don't work? He has a persistent problem of lung infections. If he needed a respirator, should we use it? Some of the staff -- in particular, the chief resident, Dr. Stafford -- were saying: 'There's so little there; so little quality of life; so little human life. He is not ambulatory; he doesn't have any intellectual life; he has no companionship and seems incapable of it; his parents never visit him at White Oaks and they've never visited him here. He's just one of our White Oaks patients, like so many others, and each time we get him better, he just goes back to White Oaks, and that's no life.'

"He requires a lot of attention," Dr. McDonough continued. "Right now he can eat by mouth, but with difficulty. It takes an awful long time to feed him. Dr. Stafford drew his own conclusions in that brief conversation when he said: 'This is all a waste. Why are we doing this?'

"I recall," Dr. McDonough continued, "that the nurses disagreed with him. One of them said very bluntly: 'You can't withhold treatment from these patients. They have the same rights as anyone else. They have the right to be treated!' The chief resident (Dr. Stafford) did his job: during this episode he treated the boy aggressively, but he rather resented the reason for such aggressiveness. You may still see some resentment in him when the conference starts.

"There was a saying around the hospital: If this is a White Oaks patient, we have to go all out. White Oaks has expressed its policy to the hospital: Always treat the residents of our home aggressively -- full code -- don't ask questions.

"Besides," Dr. McDonough continued, "this was during the time of the federal Baby Doe regulations, which had the effect of hardening attitudes in the Pediatric Intensive Care Unit. I might also add that there was additional pressure on the chief resident because attendings rotated every month, and there was no Director of the PICU -- it was just then being organized as a formal, separate unit."

Itchy to shift attention elsewhere, I asked my conversation partner: "Dr. McDonough, what was this patient like? How did he strike you? What did you think of him?" McDonough, his face now transformed by curiosity and amazement, told me what I (as a non-physician) regard as the "real story" inside the case history.

He said: "Michael is a very strange individual. He shows unusual behavior. I'll never forget him -- how he seems to be capable of just three things.

"First, if you call out his name very loudly he turns to you and bestows on you a wonderful smile. It is the smile of a saint. I've never seen anything like it before: beautiful but eery -- and he keeps smiling at you for a while.

"Second, he has a toy tractor in his bed. He holds it in front of his face and spins the two back wheels for several hours at a time, but with a look of great concentration.

"The third thing about him I'll never forget: he does what I would call finger ballets. He touches his fingers together, then closes his hands, opens them again as though he were playing 'Here's the church and here's the steeple,' and then, well, he does a kind of ballet with his fingers. Again, he has a look of concentration on his face like Vladimir Horowitz performing on piano."

"How do you feel about him?" I asked Dr. McDonough.

"...I will confess to feeling fear and a bit of fright when I'm in his presence. I haven't had much experience at this." Then, under his breath, Dr. McDonough added quietly: "He's like an alien to me. I don't know his world."

Then, abruptly changing his mood, this amazingly candid young clinician added soberly: "I suspect that, in the end, I would interpret all his behavior as learned behavior. I must confess to having some of the reservations of the chief resident: I wonder if it will be worth it to offer maximum treatment next time around. But I'm sure we will. I suppose it's our duty. Just like I suppose it was the duty of the hospital staff to treat him when he was a newborn."

Then I did something very spontaneously. Attracted to the story of this boy-man Michael, I asked Dr. McDonough if he would take me to see him. McDonough said he would be glad to; he had to examine Michael anyhow.

By the time Dr. McDonough had raised his stethoscope to Michael's chest and touched him with it, I had already attempted to enter into Michael's mentality. I could sense something like a feeling of gratitude in Michael, reflected on his face as he stared at the device that was connected with McDonough's head: "Thank you, Dr. McDonough, for this beautiful tube of yours." Michael reached out and softly gripped the stethoscope as though it were part of his doctor-friend's body.

I stood there a long time, never taking my eyes off Michael as long as he held that life-giving tube and stared at it with restful, smiling eyes.

A Choice of Moral Paradigms

The foregoing narrative is complete in itself, without any ethical show-down on whether Michael will continue to be treated aggressively. It sets the stage for our discussion, for my primary goal in this paper is to focus a strong spotlight on the perspectives that influence our choice of approaches to the ethics of neonatology and perinatology.

There are three paradigms for approaching ethical issues; and it may be instructive to use those paradigms for evaluating the state of the field of perinatal and neonatal ethics.[2] Those three paradigms correspond to the various types of normative judgments that are basic to all of ethics: judgments of duty, of values, and of character (or virtue).

The Duty-Based (Principle-Based) Paradigm

Judgments of duty -- which determine which actions are morally obligatory -- respond to the question: What morally ought to be done? The paradigm of an ethic of duty could also be called the paradigm of ethical principles, for duties or obligations are usually expressed and measured by principles that articulate moral demands. A principle-based ethic of duty dominates the contemporary ethics of neonatology and perinatology,[3] as it does bioethics more generally.[4]

This dominant approach frequently takes the form of "quandary ethics," meaning that the author takes as a starting-point a sharply defined moral dilemma as epitomized in a severely truncated case characterized by contrasts of claims and interests. After defining the issues, the author then usually moves toward a resolution of the dilemma by arguing for an overriding duty through application of tested ethical principles that are known *a priori* and that are applicable to all people in such situations. Clarity and consistency of expression and cogency of discursive moral reasoning are emphasized in a principle-based ethics of duty.

In the White Oaks case, what appears to be the only serious allusions to ethics are suggestive of an ethic of duty. Some of the hospital staff suggested that, judged in terms of a quality-of-life criterion, persistent treatment of Michael (should he need a respirator) would be a "waste" and hence there would be no obligation to offer that treatment. Similarly, those inclined to more aggressive treatment were inclined to a duty rooted in the rights of the retarded patient. One of the shortcomings of a principle-based ethic is that it focuses so exclusively on a single quandary and the general ethical principles that are applicable to it, that it creates a mentality prone to overlooking other important moral issues. Those other considerations are often highlighted in the other two paradigms.

The Value-Based Paradigm

A second paradigm of ethics entails an approach in which judgments of value are its starting-point. Value judgments examine in what sense and to what degree particular states of affairs or goals are good or bad. When one takes this approach, one begins not by asking what must I do, but rather: What is going on around me, and how should my behavior fit into that?[5] This approach is more fundamental than that of an ethic of duty, for it invites one to perceive a full range of values and disvalues, and allows room for the intuitive dimensions of perceiving and appreciating values, and in determining what behavior is fitting in the context of those values,[6] before deciding whether and to what degree principles are needed for moral judgments.

The story of Michael, the White Oaks boy, seems to open the door to a broad range of value's related to the staff, and in particular, the patient. Just as other stories and lyric writings bring within range of our moral vision the inferiority of the retarded and comparably disabled individuals,[7] this brief narrative invites the reader into the inner world of this still-infant-like man and the values -- however singular and non-standard -- that it represents. The wonder of Michael's smile, his concentration on his tractor, and his finger ballets suggest that there may be far more of a self -- and self-related values -- in this individual than our systematic ethic has previously invited us to consider.

A narrative has the power of engaging us in the value content and the moral force of characters' points of view; and the point of view of the retarded, especially the retarded child, is a world that, by and large, has not been taken seriously in the ethics of perinatology and neonatology. Nor have there been many scientific inquiries into our communication with the inner world of the retarded child,[8] and those that exist are generally not familiar to the average clinician-specialist who is active in the care of infants. A serious inquiry into the inner world, aims and journey of the mentally retarded infant -- examined perhaps in patients like Michael who remain infants mentally -- might well lead to new perceptions of value that would be important, even crucial, to an ethics of neonatology and perinatology.

The Character-Based (Virtue-Based) Paradigm

A third paradigm for bioethics is the ethics of character or virtue. This approach begins with the question: What dispositions or characteristics of individuals or societies, for which they could be accountable, are commendable or reprehensible? In this context, the question is not simply what should be done for a patient but what sort of moral agent should the care-giver be. The character-based approach begins with a consideration of the values and expectations involved in the roles of family members, professionals, and others; the commitments that are entailed in those roles; and the virtues that should characterize individuals and groups that are in a position to care for the patient.

In the White Oaks story one is struck by the absence of any person who has a truly personal commitment to Michael's welfare -- for neither parents nor his institutional custodians nor even the hospital staff seem to have more than a narrowly-based concern for the tasks they must perform for Michael. Arguments regarding obligations created by Michael's rights are somewhat ill-fated, since there is doubt as to whether there is anyone with Michael's best interests at heart who would be attentive to his true needs. Michael's best interests require, at a fundamental ethical level, one or more individuals whose attitude toward him is characterized by virtues such as benevolence, compassion, and fidelity.

The three paradigms of ethics provide a framework for illustrating what the ethics of perinatology and neonatology can be and in what ways it may have been incomplete up to this point. Now I want to offer a more sustained argument and explanation of my central thesis: that the language of rights and duties, while it has been highly instrumental in advancing the welfare of the retarded generally and of retarded children in particular, is inadequate as a foundation for an ethic of the care of human life in the first of it; and that a language of values and virtues would provide a more appropriate starting-point for this sort of ethic.

The Shortcomings of Rights Language

Through international declarations of rights, national and international law, court decisions, and federal and state regulations, the language of rights has provided an essential component in advancing an awareness of and in providing for many of the needs of the retarded and of handicapped infants and children. Yet the care of these populations is not satisfactorily addressed in rights language, for several reasons.

Identifying the Duty-Bearers

The first objection to rights language in this context pertains to the welfare rights of the retarded, such as the rights to proper medical care, physical therapy, education, training, guidance, etc., that have been articulated by the United Nations.[9] If these human rights are to be taken seriously, they should be seen as consisting of ethical claims of the right-holder to be provided with specific goods or services by some duty-bearer, i.e., by some party or parties who have corresponding obligations. But there is often an ambiguity in identifying the second party who has the obligation to satisfy the rights of retarded persons: Is it the family (parents, the whole family), the local political community, the nation, the world community, national, or international organizations? And when the duty-bearer is identified, the right often fails the test of practicability, for the resources frequently are not available to satisfy the claims of every right-bearer. And since no one can be obliged to do the impossible, many of the rights of the retarded cannot be taken at their face value.

For example, in its attempt to create a policy regarding treatment of handicapped infants -- the so-called Baby Doe problem -- the U.S. federal government, in the early 1980s, claimed that pediatric units had the duty to fulfill the handicapped infant's right to treatment and held hospitals and hospital units responsible for withholding treatment. Yet those institutions clearly did not have the resources for fulfilling that obligation, even if the obligation had in other respects been rationally sustainable.

Consequently, human rights of the retarded and of handicapped infants, though by no means useless or unreasonable, are inadequate to serve as the core of an ethic of caring for these individuals. Those interested in ethical issues in perinatology and neonatology would more profitably begin by examining the components of the character-based ethic of social benevolence, for even the doctrine of human rights of the retarded is fundamentally expressive of an ethic of character. The real value of that sort of rights language is its manifesto value: It proclaims a vision of what the world of the retarded and non-retarded should be and the kind of benevolent social character that should distinguish the human community if it is to be the sort of moral community that embraces disadvantaged individuals in a worth manner.

Rights as Adversarial

A second objection is that rights language is too adversarial in the case of positive rights (rights to goods and services) that affect the child as a family member.

Some bills of rights for children include demands that are clearly addressed to parents: "the right to grow up nurtured by affectionate parents" and "the right to be supported, maintained and educated to the best of parental ability." Commenting on these special rights, one philosopher has pointed out that they place the parent in the role of a potential adversary, for these are rights which a child or child's representative may claim against his or her own parents.[10]

A likely effect of pressing for the recognition and enforcement of these rights is that calling into question the good will of the parents would undermine the natural affection and sympathy that most parents feel for their children. This would be an unfortunate consequence, inasmuch as the need for adult love and affection are so crucial to the development of the child.

Ultimately, the shortcoming of urging rights language for gaining positive services for infants and children is the assumption that rights convincingly capture the core meaning of the moral status of retarded children. But that is deceptive, for their moral status resides in and is fostered by family relationships -- as well as professional health-care relationships -- that are characterized by acceptance, trust, affection, and care.

Excessive Abstractness in Rights Approaches

A third objection against rights language in the neonatal and perinatal settings deals with a third kind of rights: the philosophically-argued, autonomy-based rights that are a keystone in much of the contemporary ethics literature that addresses the question of saving or not saving the life of a handicapped, mentally deficient infant.[11] The objection is that this sort of rights language is excessively abstract, for it arises from conceptual constructs that are isolated from the particular experience of the retarded and of our relationships with the retarded and the handicapped infant.

This problematic approach is found in a dominant, duty-paradigm school of thought in contemporary moral philosophy, generally traceable to Immanuel Kant, that grounds rights and duties in the need to respect the dignity of persons. A major distinction is drawn between those who are merely human and those humans who are persons. Individuals are not valued for being human; it is persons who are respected, and only persons are subjects of rights. Persons are respected and have rights because they are free, autonomous agents. Accordingly, our most fundamental obligations to others are grounded in the autonomy of the persons to whom we have obligations. Autonomous individuals are those who are (or are capable of being) conscious, self-reflecting individuals who can make rational decisions on their own behalf. Therefore, the existence of rights and duties, as well as serious obligations in beneficence, depend upon our assessing the prerequisites for rationality in each individual human being.

To make an autonomy test the requirement for having a fundamental moral claim to respect for one's life is objectionable partly because it discriminates in a fundamental way against the mentally retarded as a group (even when the author argues for a safety-net principle for meeting the needs of this group). But there is a more radical, philosophical objection: This rights-based approach is based on the assumption that the moral status of human beings should be assessed in an isolationist manner; and it places autonomy above all other morally significant values in assessing moral status. Thus, the neonatal ethic of autonomy-based rights, due to the single-concept abstractness of the philosophical theory which shapes it, loses sight of the moral relevance of the primary relations in which we care for one another, particularly friendships and family.[12] An alternative starting-point for an ethic of perinatology and neonatology would be grounded in the moral experiences encountered in those settings. Some elements of that approach will be outlined in the final section of this paper.

Experiential Ethics and the Retarded Infant

To expand our vision of the ethics of the care of the retarded infant or child to include, for example, the view of the retarded infant as one's child or friend rather than simply as the potential holder of rights is to radically alter the possible basis of an ethic of perinatology and neonatology. This expansion involves a shift from a principle-based ethic to an experiential ethic. A principle-based ethic is the more deductive, norm-based ethic in which standards of moral behavior -- whether articulated in the form of ethical rules or even virtues -- are simply applied to a variety of moral problems. The other, being advocated here, is what I would call experiential ethics, in which a more inductive process is used. In this perspective, the starting-point for ethics (though surely not its entire scope) is the study of *particular sets* of moral values and behavior; only secondarily does ethics entail the development and analysis of a *general* conceptual construct, secular or religious, that can then be applied to dilemmas of moral choice.

An experiential ethic begins with a perception and interpretation of values related to moral experience -- persons, relationships, roles, attitudes, behaviors -- which are conveyed through life experiences, narratives, images, models known from behavioral sciences, etc.[13] By taking this experiential approach we make sure that we are addressing the right sorts of questions and not just those that best illustrate some already established ethical principles; we become aware of values that we may have overlooked; we become alert to the force of values that we may have minimized; and we become aware of the sort of moral agents we might become and the sort of moral community we would want to build, whether in hospitals, families, communities, nations, or world.

The experiential starting-point requires that we first ask ourselves the question, "What is going on in the world of the care of the mentally retarded infant?" To understand and interpret this world requires a phenomenology of human moral behavior. An important gateway to this fuller experiential moral world can be found in the work of the philosopher Emmanuel Levinas, which is dominated by the image of responsiveness to the stranger.

The Image of Stranger

Levinas presents an ethic of responsibility that is based on the human encounter and communication with the other. He contends that prior to and presupposed by all systematic philosophical ways of thinking about our relations with other is the basic experience of encountering strangers. Thus, the starting-point for knowing what we owe morally to others is "the existing individual and his ethical choice to welcome the stranger and to share his world by speaking to him."[14]

Now both the mentally retarded and the handicapped infant are pre-eminently strangers, for our society has shown an inability to face them and to relate to them with equanimity. For ages we have placed them in the social and moral categories where we relegate what is threateningly strange. Indeed, the very strangeness of the mentally retarded and of the handicapped infant may account for the struggle between the contrasting ethical approaches that are described in this article. For, simply in asking some of the usual questions in neonatal ethics we seem to be asking ourselves: Why should we do for these strangers what we have grown accustomed to doing for others who are familiar to us? Furthermore, our penchant for having recourse to rights language may also be accounted for by our conviction that the mentally retarded and the handicapped child are strangers, for rights (conveniently) transcend the question of whether the rights-holder is familiar or strange. Thus, by acknowledging the rights of mentally retarded infants we can continue to regard them as strangers, for if "people generally" must fulfill those rights, that preserves and reinforces the distance between each of us and these strangers.

Yet, in the ethic of responsibility that I am proposing, it is appropriate to acknowledge that the mentally retarded and handicapped infants are strangers. For in this theory they are on the same basic plane with all other individuals, precisely because our moral relations with others begin with the radical phenomenon that all Others are strangers. Thus, *the impression that the mentally retarded and the handicapped infant are strangers basically does not differ from the radical experience between the self and the Other, in which all Others are initially strangers.* The initial experience that handicapped neonatal patients are strangers to parents or other care-givers is simply a more intensified experience, but ultimately not essentially different from the initial strangeness of our relations with all Others.

The experience of the stranger leads to the experience of responsibility. An experiential ethic would eventually come to know how we ought to act socially by first asking: How do we become social? In the "I-Other" encounter, when I meet with the other person who is stranger to me, I may either decide to assimilate the Other to my categories and make use of the Other, or I may take the risk of taking the Other seriously, of responding to him or her.

There is a strong inclination in human individuals and groups to maintain an egocentric attitude and to think of other individuals either as extensions of the self or as alien objects to be manipulated for the advantage of the individual or social self. According to Levinas, neither of these egocentric views does justice to our original or fundamental experience of the other person, which is one of communicating with the Other, speaking to the Other.

Even the questioning glance of the Other is seeking for a meaningful response. I may, of course, choose to give only a casual answer; but if I give a real response, I put something of my world into words. Thus, a free interchange involves giving, it entails an initial act of generosity, for I give something of my world, even if it is a limited word with dubious assumptions. A response is radically a choice for generosity and communication, i.e., for the social. And in responding to the Other who inhabits a strange world, I become aware of what it means to become responsible, i.e., what it means to be able to respond.

Furthermore, it is in responding to the Other that I become aware of the arbitrary attitudes and actions into which my uncriticized freedom can lead me, and see the need of doing justice to the Other. In perceiving the negative and positive values in my response (and in the response of others), I am then in a position to think in terms of conceptual constructions that might best articulate these moral experiences.

Our task in ethics is to develop the implications of this ethic of responsiveness to the handicapped infant seen as stranger. The thrust of an ethic based on this metaphor would be to break the preoccupation of ethics with reasonings stemming from the ethical analyst's point of view -- assimilating the "problem" of the mentally retarded into the conceptual world of the bioethics policy-molder -- and re-center ethics on the stranger, by allowing his or her story to refocus our vision and expose the relativity of our own orientation to what is meaningful.[15] Quite possibly, the story of Michael in "The Case of the White Oaks Boy" suggests a moral re-centering of this sort. Another example is the following study.

Parenting and Bonding With Handicapped Infants

An example of an ethic of responsiveness to the mentally retarded infant, viewed initially as stranger, has been presented by William F. May in an article on the values inherent in parenting and bonding with mentally retarded children.[16] In his description of the process of bonding -- which is difficult to summarize in a way that retains the empirical richness of the original description -- May shows how the process honors and values the other who is retarded and generates loyalty and trust between those who are bonded. May's detailed analysis of bonding focuses on the changes the birth of a retarded child calls for in parents' lives under three headings: detachment from the past, transition, and attachment.

The birth of a retarded baby causes more than detachment from past assumptions and priorities: parents suddenly feel isolated, burdened, guilty, and a failure. To become loyal to this child requires a reconsideration of many other relations. Parents of the retarded child need a period of transition and assimilation, to sever themselves from their former expectations and enter a new world. The process of attachment normally includes experiences of reciprocal interaction such as touching and eye-to-eye contact with the baby. This can be more difficult with the retarded child who, more than other infants, often appears as a stranger. Yet bonding does take place, May points out, and of an order and depth that sometimes suggests a powerful transformation of life.

May's portrayal of parenting and bonding conveys a sense of values and virtues. It portrays the human context in which the act of bonding reaffirms the world and the worth of the retarded child, provides the matrix for the moral status of the child, and engenders loyalty between him or her and the parents. It also conveys the value of the parent's life whose worth has at least been questioned initially by the arrival of a child that is not the dream child who had been anticipated. The parents' response is not inherently altruistic: parents are challenged to be one or the other or a combination of both; but there is no way that they can remain what they were before.

An ethic of responsibility shows what values are possible in an unavoidable situation of response. The moral response that we observe in the bonding of parents with their retarded children does not constitute, of itself, a universal norm that is binding on all others in similar situations. Rather, such parents manifest one model of benevolence in parenting; and that model presents an image of valued moral behavior that carries moral force, making possible a spirited rejection or spirited emulation on the part of others.

Conclusions: Clinical Implications

The thrust of this paper has been to make an appeal for a new approach to the ethics of perinatology and neonatology. The implications of this appeal are diverse and will be seen in a variety of perspectives by the various disciplines and professions that have an interest in this field of ethical inquiry and action. Although detailed clinical implications of this appeal require further studies of the sort advocated in this paper, some general clinical implications can be indicated, for the clinician participates more directly in the context of experiential ethics than any ethical scholar.

At the very least, an experiential ethic of neonatology and perinatology requires that attention be given to more complete case histories. Descriptions of attitudes, perceived values, commitments, and roles should not be denigrated as elements that are too "subjective," for they provide the objective matrix of many of the ethical dimensions of ethics in a clinical setting. Attention should also be paid to literature touching on the experiential aspects of cases: publications as diverse as behavioral medical studies[17] and literature on the images and metaphors that shape the perinatal world[18] can provide insights into the care of the mentally retarded or otherwise handicapped infant and child.

Clinicians should be aware that an experiential ethic introduces to the ethical agenda the moral commitments, attitudes, and character traits (or virtues) of the parties involved. This is of considerable importance, for it is often the conflicting commitments of the professionals and parents that gives rise to the ethical conflicts. These commitments must be submitted to critical evaluation, for they could range anywhere from heroic service to blatant neglect; and a principle-based, duty-based ethic (e.g., regarding the rights of infants and other parties) will be instrumental in negotiating the priorities among various parties' commitments. Complementing the principle-based approach, however, and more fundamental than it, is the experiential approach that I have described. The importance of this experiential approach on the clinical level can be seen in the fact that clinicians are often in a position to foster commitments such as the bonding of parents and often do so routinely. This is entirely appropriate from an ethical perspective, for the self-conscious fostering of appropriate attitudes and commitments is integral to a character-based ethic.

In addition, deliberate exposure of oneself to a rich range of values, disvalues, and commitments -- which an experiential ethic entails -- requires that the clinician deal with uncertainties. At the same time it may become apparent to the physician that moral principles can, at times, mask that uncertainty.

Finally, the underlying appeal of this paper is that clinicians and other parties to the ethics of neonatology and perinatology will see themselves as more than the objects of ethics -- those who are "part of the problem" and who then receive the solution "from outside." The experiential paradigm, emphasizing values and virtues prior to principles, enhances the moral agency of clinicians, for it offers a vision of ethics in which the decision maker -- whether patient, clinician, or other -- is the active subject of ethics.

Notes

1. An earlier version of this paper appeared as: Reich WT. Mas Alla de los Derechos: Hacia una Etica del Cuidado del Niño Mentalmente Retardado. In: *Retardo Mental XXII Anniversario de Avepane*. Caracas: Avepane, 1985:406-416.
2. See Reich WT. Bioethics in the 1980's: Challenges and paradigms. In: Sondheimer H, ed. *Biomedical Ethics: A Community Forum*. Syracuse, New York, NY: SUNY Upstate Medical Center, 1985:1-35. Reich WT. Paradigmen fuer die bioethik: Lagebericht und lagebeurteilung, *Mensch, Medizin, Gesellschaft* 1986;11:231-236.
3. See Reich WT, Ost DE. Infants: Ethical perspectives on the care of infants. In: Reich W, ed. *Encyclopedia of Bioethics*. New York, NY:Macmillan Free Press, 1978:724-735. McCormick RA. *How Brave a New World*? Garden City, NY: Doubleday, 1981. Tooley M. *Abortion and Infanticide*. New York, NY: Oxford University Press, 1983. Weir RF. *Selective Nontreatment of Handicapped Newborns: Moral Dilemmas in Neonatal Medicine*. New York, NY: Oxford University Press, 1984. Engelhardt HT. *The Foundations of Bioethics*. New York, NY: Oxford University Press, 1986. Shelp E. New York, NY: Macmillan Free Press, 1986.
4. See, for example, Beauchamp TL, Childress JF. *Principles of Biomedical Ethics* 2nd Edition. New York, NY: Oxford University Press, 1983. Veatch RM. *A Theory of Medical Ethics*. New York, NY: Basic Books, 1981.
5. See Niebuhr HR. *The Responsible Self: An Essay in Christian Moral Philosophy*. New York, NY: Harper & Row, 1963.
6. Mieth D. *Moral und Erfahrung: Beitraege zur theologisch-ethischen Hermeneutik*. Freiburg, West Germany: Herder, 1977.
7. See, for example, Rilke RM. The idiot's song, In: Mitchell S, ed. and trans. *The Selected Poetry of Rainer Maria Rilke*. New York, NY: Random House, 1984. Faulkner W. *The Sound and the Fury*. New York, NY: Random House, 1946.
8. See, for example, Fraser WI, Grieve R, eds. *Communicating with Normal and Retarded Children*. Bristol, England: John Wright & Sons, 1981.

9. United Nations General Assembly. *Declaration of the Rights of Mentally Retarded Persons*. G.A. Res. 2856, 26:U.N. GAOR Supp. 3, at 73, U.N. Doc. A/8588, 1971.
10. Schrag F. Children: Their rights and needs, In: Aiken W, LaFolette H, eds. *Whose Child? Children's Rights, Parental Authority, and State Power.* Totowa, NJ: Rowman and Littlefield, 1980: 237-253.
11. See Engelhardt. *The Foundations of Bioethics*. Shelp. *Born to Die*? and Murphy JG. Rights and borderline cases, In: Kopelman L, Moskop JC, eds. *Ethics and Mental Retardation*. Boston, MA: Reidel, 1984:3-17.
12. Hauerwas S. *A Community of Character: Toward a Constructive Christian Social Ethic*. Notre Dame, IN: University of Notre Dame Press, 1981.
13. Mieth D. *Moral und Erfahrung*.
14. Levinas E. *Totality and Infinity: An Essay on Exteriority*. Lingis A. trans. Pittsburgh, PA: Duquene University Press, 1969. Burggraeve R. The ethical basis for a humane society according to emmanuel levinas, *Ephemerides Theologicae Lovaniensis* 1981;57:5-57.
15. Ogletree TW. *Hospitality to the Stranger: Dimensions of Moral Understanding*. Philadelphia, PA: Fortress, 1985:2-3.
16. May WF. Parenting, bonding, and valuing the retarded. In: Kopelman L, Moskop JC, eds. *Ethics and Mental Retardation*. Boston, MA: Reidel, 1984:141-160. Further work on values and virtues can be found in, Hauerwas S. *Responsibility for Devalued Persons: Ethical Interactions Between Society, the Family, and the Retarded*. Springfield, IL: Charles C Thomas, 1982.
17. Guillemin JH, Holmstrom LL. *Mixed Blessings: Intensive Care for Newborns*. New York, NY: Oxford University Press, 1986.
18. Fiedler LA. The tyranny of the normal. In: Murray TH, Caplan, AL, eds. *Which Babies Shall Live*? Clifton, NJ: Humana, 1985:151-159.

Chapter 12

Siamese Twins: Killing One to Save the Other

George J. Annas

Early this year, physicians at Philadelphia Children's Hospital sought permission to separate infant Siamese twins with conjoined hearts. A decade earlier, the same hospital sought similar permission in a case in which Surgeon General C. Everett Koop was attending physician. Both cases reveal our ambivalent attitudes toward treating such children: Can one twin be sacrificed so that the other may be made "human?" Do physicians have responsibilities to two patients, or only to the twin who may have some chance of surviving?

The separation of Siamese twins with conjoined hearts, while a rare event, has received some ethical and legal discussion. Most of it, unfortunately, has been characterized by fuzzy thinking and flawed analogies. Perhaps this is inevitable. Siamese twins have always been seen as bizarre. Their very name comes from history's most famous such twins, Eng and Chang Bunker. Born in Siam in 1811, they were exhibited around the world by P.T. Barnum. They lived until 1874 and died within three hours of each other. The second most famous are Amos and Eddie Smith, fictional Siamese twins who appear in Judith Rossner's challenging novel, *Attachments*; they also spent time with Ringling Brothers Barnum & Bailey.

Siamese twins continued to be referred to in freakish, sideshow terms ("double-headed monster," thoracopagus monster, monstruo doble, an les monstres á deux têtes) in the medical literature well into the twentieth century. Conjoined twins are the product of a single ovum; they have the same chromosomal composition and sex. Approximately three-quarters are joined at the chest (thoracopagus twins) and have a conjoined heart. It is believed that surgical separation is "hopeless" in the vast majority of these cases; and even where success is theoretically possible by sacrificing; one of the twins, no twin with a conjoined heart has survived for more than a few months.[1] On the other hand, unlike the Bunkers and the Smiths, no thoracopagus twins with conjoined hearts have survived longer than nine months remaining attached, apparently because their heart mass is not strong enough to maintain adequate circulation to both bodies.

Straining for Analogies

The case that has received the most commentary occurred in October 1977 at Children's Hospital in Philadelphia. Survival of both twins following separation was impossible, and survival of one very unlikely. Could one twin be "sacrificed" so that the other might have a chance to live? Because the parents were deeply religious Jews, they would not consent to separation without rabbinical support. The nurses were mostly Catholic, and would not be involved unless a priest assured them it was morally acceptable.

Source: Reprinted from *Hastings Center Report*, April 1987, pp. 27-29, with permission of

Dr. Koop, among other things, feared potential homicide charges, and would not perform the separation unless a court granted him prospective legal immunity from criminal prosecution.

Unlike cases involving an anencephalic baby, a Tay-Sachs baby, or a trisomy-13 baby, the suggested justification for letting one child die is not because it is dying anyway. Rather, there is a possible (albeit highly experimental and so far unsuccessful) intervention that has the potential to permit one of the two children to live. The case is more analogous to attempted selective feticide, when amniocentesis discloses that one of two fetuses is affected with a severely handicapping condition and the mother would abort both if she did not have the option to abort only the affected twin. But while the current abortion laws permit the woman to make this decision prior to viability, after birth selective infanticide is not an option. But should it be if the twins are physically connected and can be regarded as literally, although innocently, killing each other?

The rabbinical scholars involved in the 1977 case reportedly relied primarily on two analogies.[2] In the first, two men jump from a burning airplane. The parachute of the second man does not open, and as he falls past the first man, he grabs his legs. If the parachute cannot support them both, is the first man morally justified in kicking the second man away to save himself? Yes, said the rabbis, since the man whose parachute didn't open was "designated for death."

The second analogy involves a caravan surrounded by bandits. The bandits demand a particular member of the caravan be turned over for execution; the rest will go free. Assuming that the named individual has been "designated for death," the rabbis concluded it was acceptable to surrender him to save everyone else. Accordingly, they concluded that if twin A was "designated for death," and could not survive in any event, but twin B could, surgery that would kill twin A to help improve the chance of twin B was acceptable.

The Catholic logic, which employed the principle of the double effect, was even more strained. That principle states generally that if an action has two effects, one good and one bad, it can still be acceptable, provided the good effect does not come about because of the bad effect, and there is a proportionate reason for permitting the bad effect. Here the bad effect is the death of twin A, the good effect the possibility of preserving the life of twin B. When the carotid artery feeding blood to the brain of twin A is tied off, this causes the death of twin A. It was argued that this action, however, was done not to terminate twin A's life, but to preserve the life of twin B by protecting it from the poisons that would build up in twin A's blood after its death.[3]

The application of the principle of the double effect, however, seems to fail because it is precisely the bad effect that permits the good effect: killing twin A permits twin B to have a chance to live (twin A's blood becomes poisoned and threatens twin B only after it is dead). One might respond that it is better that twin B have a chance to live than that both twins die, but this does not address the fact that twin A has been killed to try to save twin B. In other words, the good end has been used to justify the evil means, unless one argues further that twin A threatens twin B merely because its body requires more support than their shared hearts can provide. Then one is relieving the pressure on twin B's heart by tying off the carotid artery, and twin A's death becomes an inevitable but unintended result of a good act.

A three-judge panel of the Family Court heard the hospital lawyers make two additional arguments on behalf of Dr. Koop. The first was that because the two twins had only one heart between them, there was only one person. This argument was rejected because the concept of brain death was already well established. (Nevertheless, they might have concluded that a child with one body and two heads is just one child, and that removing one of the heads would be similar to removing an extra arm or leg.)

Their second argument was an analogy similar to the rabbinical one. Two mountain climbers are attached to each other by a rope. One falls from his perch, but is saved from instant death by the rope attached to his partner. His partner has a more secure hold, but not so secure that he can hold both of them. In this circumstance, (like the parachute case) the lawyers argued that it was acceptable for the mountain climber with the more secure hold to cut the rope to save himself.

After deliberating for a few minutes the court authorized Dr. Koop to perform the surgery. It was done the next day. The separation was successful, but the surviving twin died three months later.

Three things should be noted about the 1977 case: (1) The analogies are weak. In all of them adults are consciously and voluntarily engaged in known, risky behaviors; and one adult always puts the other's life in peril by his own actions. Neither voluntary assumption of the risk nor any personal act on the part of the twins can justify treating them like mountain climbers or parachuters. (2) There was great consternation and ethical and legal debate about this case, which was seen as problematic by almost everyone involved. (3) Homicide charges were considered such a real possibility that the surgeon demanded a court order before he would proceed.

In a similar case in Little Rock, Arkansas, that same month, surgery was not performed until both the State Attorney General and the County Prosecutor agreed that no criminal prosecution would be pursued. The Arkansas case was described by the physicians involved as an "amputation" (of the right twin from the left twin). Even though the surgical result was recognized as very suboptimal, the physicians thought "it seemed unwise in view of the prolonged survivals of some dicephalus twins not to attempt separation.!"[4]

Ten years later, in early 1987, physicians at Philadelphia Children's Hospital confronted almost the same situation. In the interim, there had been debate on Baby Doe regulations, which mandated treatment for most seriously ill newborns, and the first (and still the only) attempted criminal prosecution of a physician for nontreatment of a newborn--the Danville, Illinois, Siamese twins case. Nonetheless, the legal aspects of the case seem to have been handled more calmly. The surgeon, James A. O'Neill, Jr., did not demand or expect prospective legal immunity from a court. The hospital's lawyers, however, did ask the District Attorney's office to sign a letter saying the surgeons would not be prosecuted for homicide. The D.A.'s office complied but thought the exercise unnecessary.

Instead of going to court, the surgeon sought concurrence from a group not available in 1977: the hospital ethics committee. The committee talked the matter over for an hour and a half, and agreed with the surgeon's plan. He was pleased with both the process and the outcome. The surgery was performed, but neither twin survived.

The Potential to Survive

This can be seen as an easy case in two ways. First, we can assume that there are "objective medical criteria," which can determine which one of the twins has a significantly better chance to survive. Then the decision is not which twin will survive (their own condition has determined this), but whether the separation should be carried out at all. Also, since the separation procedure remains experimental and survival is unprecedented, the parents unquestionably have a right to refuse the surgery.

Second, we can take the "monster" approach, concluding that the twins are so grotesque that they are not really human. Therefore, we are justified in doing anything medically reasonable to make at least one of them "human," even if it will very likely result in both of their deaths.

But suppose there is no significant difference in the survival potential of the two twins. Then neither is "designated for death," but one must be chosen to die for the sake of the other. How is this decision to be made? The more apt (though equally unlikely) analogy is now clear. A man jumps from a burning plane with two infant children in his arms. His parachute opens. As he descends, he begins to lose his grip on both of them. Assuming he is justified in dropping one, which one does he drop to save the other?

If this is the case with Siamese twins, the fairest way to determine which would potentially survive is random, by the flip of a coin. Besides eliminating human prejudice, this has a potential advantage for the surviving twin (assuming that someday one will survive), who doesn't have to live with the knowledge that his life was paid for by a conscious decision to kill his identical twin. A decision to kill one to save the other in this circumstance would be homicide (as Dr. Koop knew), but the relevant legal issue is whether it would be justifiable homicide.

The closest legal cases deal with necessity, actions taken in response to natural disasters or acts of God. In a lifeboat, for example, casting lots to see which individuals get thrown overboard has been thought to be acceptable if some must die so that the others can keep the boat afloat. But having the stronger simply throw the weaker overboard is not justified by the circumstances. What seems to be at issue in the case of Siamese twins is the more modern notion of the "choice of evils" defense, which now serves to exculpate justified conduct no matter what the source of the threat.[5]

Restated, does society regard it as "justified" to kill one twin to attempt to save the other? As long as the "rescue" attempt is medically reasonable and the choice of which twin to kill is made fairly, the answer is almost unquestionably yes. But, although flipping coins would be fairest, society would likely find it too callous and arbitrary. That is why we continue to look for "objective medical criteria" to decide, for example, who gets the next heart for a transplant. In this instance we would probably let the physician decide which twin is most likely to survive, to maintain the fiction that the decision is an "act of God." Likewise, our parachutist with his two infants would probably instinctively drop the one he held in the weakest grasp, to try to hold onto at least one child.

A more formal best interests analysis "works" only if we make some strained assumptions. Having twin A separated from twin B is in twin B's best interests if it enhances his chances to survive. It cannot, however, be said to be in twin A's best interests objectively, since twin A is experiencing life and is not suffering, and its life will be cut short by the procedure. On the other hand, we could accept the "monster" analysis and conclude that the life of such a twin is so degrading that it is better off dead.

If we want to fantasize a substituted judgment scenario, we can ask twin A if he will consent to being killed, since he will die soon in any event and, unless he undergoes this sacrifice, his twin brother will also die. Since his twin brother carries his identical genes, the only way his genes have any chance to survive is if he makes the supreme sacrifice. Using this wildly speculative sociobiological scenario, one might conclude that twin A might consent to die for his twin--or at least that the parents of twins A and B should be permitted to make this terribly difficult decision under these unique and tragic circumstances.

We can complicate the matter further by unequivocally declaring that there are two patients here, not just one. Thus separate representation in some form should be considered. Prior cases have all assumed that one child must die for the other to have a chance to live, and this may indeed be true. But unless each child has its own advocate, alternatives that might permit them both to have some chance at survival might not be vigorously pursued. In future, for example, the twin who will not have its circulation maintained may possibly be a candidate for a heart transplant. Although this may present a logistical nightmare, an attempt might be made to put the "doomed" twin on a heart transplant list, and if a heart becomes available before separation surgery must be performed (and it cannot be used by a more "medically suitable" candidate), to try to preserve the lives of both children.

This approach "solves" the problem of choosing between the two twins, but brings us back to a question that underlies our entire discussion: When is it reasonable to perform an experimental intervention on a human being that has little chance of success? In terms of separating Siamese twins with conjoined hearts, most people would agree with the fictional physician in Attachments who concluded, "The condition is enough reason to attempt the cure."

Stated somewhat differently, it is better to intervene to try to save one life than to passively observe two lives end. Both law and ethics support reasonable medical attempts to separate Siamese twins with conjoined hearts. Nonetheless, defining a rationale better than human instinct is perplexing, as is developing a fair and useful procedure to apply it.

Notes

1. Marin-Padilla M, Chin AJ, Marin-Padilla TM. Cardiovascular abnormalities in thoracopagus twins, *Teratology* 1981;23:101-13.
2. Drake DC. The twins decision: One must die so one can live, *Philadelphia Inquirer* Oct. 16, 1977.
3. Meehan FX. The siamese twin operation and contemporary catholic medical ethics, *Linacre Quarterly* 1978;45:157-62.
4. Golladay ES, Williams GD, Seibert JJ, *et al.* Dicephalus dipus conjoined twins: A surgical separation and review of previously reported cases, *Journal of Pediatric Surgery* 1982;17:259-64.
5. Robinson PH. Criminal law defense: A systematic analysis, *Columbia Law Review* 1982;82:199, 234-35.

Chapter 13

A New Understanding of Consent in Pediatric Practice: Consent, Parental Permission, and Child Assent

William G. Bartholome

The meaning and importance of the concept of the informed consent of the patient has evolved in dramatic and important ways over the past two decades. Although its roots relate largely to the legal aspects of medical practice, the concept has emerged as a fundamental aspect of the ethical practice of medicine.[1] It is felt to be expressive of the core ethical values of knowledge and freedom. Informed consent rests primarily on the ethical principle of respect: respect for the patient as a person with basic rights to know or to be informed and to exercise the right of autonomy or self-determination.

Although pediatricians have recognized the importance of this concept to the ethical practice of medicine,[2] they have also realized that it had limited direct application in pediatrics since most of their patients lacked the capacity and legal power to give informed consent to their medical care. Clearly the concept can be incorporated into the care of many adolescents and most young adults; this has been acknowledged by the American Academy of Pediatrics in a variety of publications and policy statements.[3,4]

One practice widely adopted by pediatricians was to attempt to adapt the concept of informed consent by granting the parent the power to give consent by proxy. This seemed appropriate since parents are the legal guardians of the child. However, serious limitations of proxy consent have now been acknowledged.[5,6] One of the more obvious limitations is that the right of consent also encompasses the right to refuse consent. This right has been interpreted as including even the right to refuse a life-sustaining treatment. Allowing a proxy to exercise the right to refuse consent would confer on a parent a right to refuse any medical care their child might need, including life-sustaining medical treatments. Recognition of such a right would mean that a parent would have a right to endanger or even neglect the child. Clearly such a right is incompatible with the most basic understanding of child abuse and neglect, especially the concept of medical neglect.

Another serious objection to parental proxy consent is that pediatric health care providers have a wide range of ethical and legal duties and obligations that are owed to pediatric patients independently of parental desires or "consentings." The Committee on Bioethics of the American Academy of Pediatrics acknowledged that "the most basic ethical principle" in the context of care of critically ill newborns is that "the pediatrician's primary obligation is to the child."[7] Such an understanding of the role of the pediatrician and the nature of the basic ethical relationship in pediatric practice is obviously in serious tension with any concept of a parental right to decide.[8]

Source: Reprinted from *Pediatric Annals*, Vol. 18, No. 41, pp. 262-265, with permission of Pediatric Annals © April, 1989.

Parental Permission

Although it might be possible to formulate a complex concept of proxy consent with built-in exceptions and limitations, another approach would be to use the concept of consent to refer exclusively to the autonomous authorizations provided by those with the capacity and legal power to make such authorizations. This approach was first proposed by the President's Commission for the Protection of Human Subjects of Biomedical and Behavioral Research in its recommendations regarding research involving children:

> The Commission uses the term parental or guardian "permission," rather than "consent," in order to distinguish what a person may do autonomously (consent) from what one may do on behalf of another (grant permission.)[9]

Clearly in this context it was inappropriate to conceive of a parent as having the "right to volunteer" the child to be a research subject, particularly in situations in which a child was asked to participate in a project not intended to be of direct benefit to himself or herself.

This proposal has now been generalized to include the entire range of decision-making involving the health care of infants and young children. It is based on the idea that parents and health care providers have a shared responsibility for the health and welfare of the child. The provider has the legal and ethical obligation to obtain the informed permission of the parents prior to any medical intervention (except in emergency situations when the parent could not be reached.) However, such permission would *not* be treated as a sufficient basis in and of itself to justify medical intervention into the life of a child. In that sense the parent does not have a right of consent (a right and power to authorize the intervention) nor a right the refuse consent (a right and power to "block" the intervention.) The ethical principles that justify medical interventions into the life of a child are that they are undertaken in response to demonstrable health needs of the child and are intended to protect and serve the child's interests.

Another very important aspect of this change from the language of consent to that of permission is that clearly parental refusal to grant permission does *not* relieve the physician of duties and obligations to the child. In any such situation a pediatrician would have the duty of working with the parents to help them reassess the situation and, if necessary, to seek permission through involvement of appropriate agencies or the legal system. This is most obvious in cases in which the parent refuses to grant permission and the physician believes that the failure to provide care would be a significant risk to the child's health, i.e., would endanger the child's health or welfare.

The Concept of Child Assent

A much more challenging and fundamental aspect of this proposal to replace proxy consent with parental permission is that pediatricians have long recognized that decision making involving the care of children and adolescents must include the perspective and "voice" of the child. Individual advocacy for children assumes that the voice and interests of the child are of paramount concern to pediatricians. Instead of trying to select an arbitrary threshold beyond which children would be considered competent to make their own decisions and to provide consent, pediatricians have attempted to involve children in their medical care to the extent of their capacity.

Child assent allows for the explicit acknowledgement of this important set of ethical issues. Children are respected as persons with a developing capacity for participation in decision-making. The concept of assent asks that pediatricians involve children to the extent of their capacity; that children participate in making decisions about their health and health care to the extent that they are able.

Since assent is a relatively new concept, it is important that pediatricians understand the basic "building blocks" or elements. Assent has been defined to include at least three basic elements. The first is an ethical duty which most contemporary pediatricians have recognized and attempted to discharge: the duty to assist the child or adolescent in developing an age or developmentally appropriate awareness of the nature of the illness. It has been assumed that the care of the child is facilitated by this awareness. From an ethical perspective it can also be argued that respect for the child as both *the* patient and a developing person obligates the physician to play this important role.

The second element of assent is the ethical duty to disclose to the child or adolescent the nature of the proposed treatment and what he or she is likely to experience. Again, many contemporary pediatricians routinely disclose information regrading proposed diagnostic or therapeutic interventions to their patients. It is assumed that children are much more likely to cooperate in undergoing a particular procedure if they are told in advance what to expect. Also, the negative psychological consequences of procedures can be significantly reduced by allowing children to anticipate and to prepare themselves for the intervention.[10] From an ethical perspective it could be argued that this duty of disclosure is based on the broader duty of truth-telling, or that the child is entitled to this information.

The third element is the most challenging, and again it is one that many pediatricians have attempted to honor.[10] It is the obligation to solicit the child's or adolescent's expression of willingness to undertake the proposed treatment. The child's, and particularly the adolescent's, willingness to undergo or undertake a particular treatment is a critical determinant of the ultimate success or failure of that treatment. The ethical aspects of this element call attention to the principle of respect for the emerging autonomy and developing capacities of children to make decisions and to serve as the guardians and caretakers of their health.

Proxy consent is replaced by a model of decision-making that involves a sharing of decision-making authority and responsibility. In the care of an infant, toddler or pre-school child this sharing includes primarily the health care providers and the parents or guardian of the child. It involves the ethical and legal obligations of the health care provider to the child and, the legal and ethical obligation of the provider to seek the informed permission of the parent or guardian. In the case of the school-aged child or adolescent the new model includes the additional ethical requirement of the assent of the child as outlined above.

Dissent of the Child

What is to be done if the child refuses to assent, or "dissents?" Clearly there are many situations in which children may withhold or temporarily refuse to assent to a proposed treatment in an effort to gain some control. Often they are attempting to understand what is happening to them or trying to deal with fear or the anticipation of a painful experience. The obligation to solicit assent in such a situation functions by asking that we be willing to hear, to respect, to respond to these needs even if it might temporarily delay intervention. Manipulation, coercion, or force are to be avoided. However, they may be required in unusual emergency situations or as a last resort when all attempts to gain assent have failed. But even in this context the ethics of assent require an explanation of the need for the treatment and, often, an apology to the child who was asked to undergo the procedure against his or her will.

In some situations, child's dissent may be ethically binding. Obviously dissent in non-therapeutic research is one example. However, the persistent objection of a child might also demand respect in a wide range of clinical situations in which the intervention was not considered essential or could be deferred to a later date.

Conflicting Ethical Judgments

One of the major objections to the model of shared decision-making proposed here is the inevitability of conflicting judgments and decisions if provider, parent and child or adolescent are all to share in this process. One of the most attractive aspects of proxy consent is that it seemingly placed ultimate decision-making authority and responsibility in the hands of the parent or guardian. Just as obviously, this was the most dangerous and ethically inappropriate aspect of the concept. However, the proposed model does demand that mechanisms be created and be available to providers, parents, and pediatric patients for addressing ethical conflict. A wide range of such mechanisms should be considered, including medical consultations or "second-opinion" provisions; liaison psychiatric, psychological or social service consultation; "case management" or multi-disciplinary conferences; pastoral care consultation; consultation with a clinical ethicist or hospital-based ethics committee; and others. In rare cases of refractory conflict formal legal adjudication may be appropriate.

Conclusion

This brief ethical analysis of informed consent proposes that the concept has a limited direct application in pediatric practice; i.e., that it can only be directly used in cases involving emancipated or mature minors, adolescents, and young adults who have the capacity and legal power to provide this kind of autonomous authorization. In the care of infants, children and younger adolescents, the concept should be understood and applied by pediatricians as the combination of two related concepts: the legal and ethical requirement to obtain parental permission to proposed medical interventions; and the ethical requirement to solicit the assent of the child patient whenever feasible. This new model for decision-making allows for a sharing of ethical responsibility among health care providers, parents, and pediatric patients and respects the important ethical duties, obligations and rights of each.[11]

Notes

1. Faden R, Beauchamp TL. *History and Theory of Informed Consent*. New York, NY: Oxford University Press, 1986.
2. American Academy of Pediatrics, Task Force on Pediatric Research, Informed Consent, and Medical Ethics. Consent, *Pediatrics* 1976;57:414-16.
3. American Academy of Pediatrics: Conference on Consent and Confidentiality in Adolescent Health Care. Elk Grove Village, IL: American Academy of Pediatrics, 1982.
4. American Academy of Pediatrics, Committee on Adolescence. Counselling the adolescent about pregnancy options, *Pediatrics* 1989;83:135-7.
5. Langham P. Parental consent: Its justification and limitations. *Clinical Research* 1979;27:1-18.
6. Gaylin W, Macklin R. *Who Speaks for the Child: The Problems of Proxy Consent*. New York, NY: Plenum Press, 1982.
7. American Academy of Pediatrics. Committee on Bioethics Treatment of critically ill newborns, *Pediatrics* 1983;72:565-6.
8. Bartholome WG. The child-patient: Do parents have the right to decide? In: Spicker SF, Healey JM, Engelhardt HT, eds. *The Law-Medicine Relation: A Philosophical Exploration*. Boston, MA: D. Reidel Publishing, 1981.
9. National Commission for the Protection of Human Subjects of Biomedical and Behavioral Research. *Report and Recommendations: Research Involving Children*. Washington, DC: DHEW Publ. No. (OS) 77-0004, 1977.
10. Kavanagh C. Psychological intervention with the severely burned child: Report of an experimental comparison of two approaches and their effects on psychological sequelae, *Journal of the American Acadamy of Child Psycholgy* 1983;22(2):145-156.
11. Leiken SL. Minors assent or dissent to medical treatment, *Jounal of Pediatrics* 1983;102:169-76.

Chapter 14

The Anatomy of Clinical-Ethical Judgments in Perinatology and Neonatology: A Substantive and Procedural Framework

Edmund D. Pellegrino

Clinical ethics is distinguished by the fact that it must focus on practical decisions. In the "moment of clinical truth," a decision must be made, often under pressures of time, and when the facts are incomplete or uncertain. Retreat into the back-and-forth debates of the classroom is neither possible nor ethically responsible. Despite the difficulties, every clinician must make decisions that are morally defensible. He or she must knowledgeably and skillfully confront the central moral question: "What is the right and good thing to do for this patient?"

Answering that question today is more difficult than ever. The issues are more complex than ever, the range of choices wider. There are more parties to the decision: the patient, the family, the institution, the law, public policy, and economics. All must be decided without the benefit of consensus on the most sensitive and fundamental moral questions.

For the perinatologist and the neonatologist, clinical-ethical decisions are further complicated by the vulnerability of their patients, who include the pregnant woman, the fetus, and the newborn infant. The skills of ethical analysis are as essential as the knowledge of pathology and physiology.

The objective of this report is to examine the anatomy of clinical-ethical judgments, and to offer a substantive and a procedural schema -- a framework of issues and questions that should help in answering the practical question: "What shall I do in this case?"

Three Ethical Obligations

The framework that will be described here is essential to fulfilling three ethical obligations that bind every clinician, no matter what his specialty may be. First is the obligation to understand and know the structure of one's own values, i.e., to understand the foundation on which one builds moral choices in response to a concrete clinical dilemma. Second is the obligation to have some working knowledge of the formal discipline of ethics. In my own teaching, I often encounter clinicians who do not appreciate that ethics is a discipline, that like the basic and clinical sciences, it can be learned, and that it can provide an orderly, systematic, and rational approach to clinical ethical decisions. Third is the obligation to carry out the process of ethical decision-making itself, and the decision reached thereby in a morally defensible way. A right decision derived or implemented unethically is as faulty as a morally wrong decision.

These three obligations are not spelled out in the Hippocratic Oath, the ethical

---

Source: Reprinted from *Seminars in Perinatology*, Vol. 11, No. 3, pp. 202-209, with permission of W.B. Saunders Co. © July, 1987.

guidelines of the American Medical Association, or any of the several codes that have emerged since the Nuremburg trials.[1] They may be implied in some of these codes, but they must be made explicit. This is especially true for the neo- and perinatologist, who faces ethical dilemmas that could scarcely be imagined by the authors of our traditional ethical codes, even a decade ago, to say nothing of 2,500 years ago.

To fulfill his or her ethical obligations, the clinician needs two analytical structures: one substantive and one procedural. Both converge on the central question of what is the right thing to do in a particular case. The substantive structure consists of four conceptual questions that shape all our moral choices and the procedural structure consists of five steps that enable us to make the actual concrete decision.

The Substantive Structure

Four questions, or levels of consideration, comprise the skeleton on which all moral choices ultimately hang. Each question and its subquestions shape our moral philosophy, our understanding of morality, what it requires, how we ought to behave in our professional lives, and why we do so. Each probes the levels of belief or concern on which we base our choices, but do not make explicit. Each is connected with the other in actual practice.

The four substantive issues are these: (1) the philosophy of the physician-patient relationship to which we subscribe; (2) the interpretation we: place on the principles of ethics common to clinical ethical-decisions; (3) the theory of ethics we favor; and (4) the ultimate source of our morality. Implicit assumptions in all these issues are buried in every clinical decision. They reveal themselves in any careful analysis of clinical-ethical judgment.

Ethical Models of the Physician-Patient Relationship

The first question concerns the nature of the physician patient relationship. It is central to all clinical-ethical decisions. What we think is right and wrong in professional ethics depends on what we think is the proper moral role for the physician in meeting the patient's needs. This is true whether the patient is an adult or an infant. The infant is, of course, vastly more dependent on the physician than a competent patient. Decisions are made with surrogates who act on behalf of the infant. But the patient is in the final analysis, the infant.

A series of analogical models are used in defining the physician-patient; relationship, that is to say, we usually like a relationship from outside medicine and apply it to the medical relationship. These models overlap somewhat but the question is which model is the primary one, the one we turn to resolve conflicts in our obligation.

Some of the most frequently used models follow; each has fundamentally different ethical implications. The first is the physician-patient relationship as applied biology. This is a dominant view for many academicians. Here the physician's major responsibility is technical and scientific competence. Competence is his primary obligation. The nonscientific elements in the relationship are not denied, but they are not intrinsically part of medicine. They can, and should, be left to others -- social workers, nurses, psychologists -- as the patient's needs may dictate. The prime good is the medical good of the patient and what is medically indicated is what should always be done.

The second model is the relationship as a contract for services, usually analogous to a legal contract.[2] Here, the physician's obligations are defined by negotiation and are not fixed. The physician is expected to perform as agreed, and failure to do so constitutes a breach of contract.

With this model, ethics is usually given a legalistic caste and the relationship between physician and patient is based less on trust than on mutual agreement of specific performance criteria.

The third model is the covenant.[3] This suggests a quasi-religious relationship, a binding promise like that between the Lord and his people in the Old Testament. Here the physician's obligation to help and heal transcends a contract or scientific relationship. Physician and patient are bound to each other in a trust relationship essential to healing. In this view, the obligations of a biological contract "and most other models are morally sparse."

The fourth model is the commodity transaction.[4] Here medical care is likened to the purchase of another commodity in the marketplace. The physician is a businessman, or entrepreneur, seeking his own interests, which presumably will eventually redound to the benefit of all, the patient included. The ethical obligations are those of the businessman, tempered somewhat by the nature of the kind of activity involved in healing, but nonetheless essentially the same as the merchant's. Medical knowledge is simply another form of proprietary knowledge to be used for the physician's profit.

The fifth model is the social functionary,[5] in which the physician is seen as essential to maintenance of a properly functioning and productive society. He serves the patient because it is good for society to do so. Within this model he may be a bureaucrat, or a proletarian, a worker in a corporate endeavor. In either case, he serves not solely as the patient's advocate, but also as the advocate for an institution. Conflicts of obligations, as gatekeeper or guardian of the public health and as patient advocate, are built into this model.

The sixth model is the one I favor.[6] In contrast with the others, it is not analogical. It is derived from the nature of medicine as a special kind of human activity. It depends on the internal morality of medicine itself. This morality -- the obligations imposed on the physician -- arises in the vulnerability of the sick person, the nature of the physician's promise to help in the face of that vulnerability, and the nature of healing as the immediate aim of the relationship. I have developed this model in detail elsewhere. The model focuses on the nature of illness, the inequality in knowledge and power between physician and patient, and the obligations that arise out of that fact and the existential state of the patient. My view emphasizes beneficence in trust, fidelity to promises, and effacement of the physician's self-interest. These obligations are built into the very nature of healing.

Although medicine and the physician-patient relationship are some of all of these things, the important question is: Which model do you choose when these several facets of the relationship conflict, as they often do, in concrete decisions? The answer to this question is the most pressing and fundamental problem in professional ethics today.

A question which, in a sense, precedes these is: Who is the patient? To whom is the physician primarily responsible? In the case of the competent adult, it is clearly the patient himself, not the family, society, or the institution. Each has some interest that deserves consideration, but the values and choices of the competent adult predominate.

In the case of infants, the answer is more difficult. Some would argue that the "patient" is the family and that their values and needs should predominate. Others, because of the economic impact of decisions with neonates, would place social concerns first. Still others insist that the interests of the infant are primary and that his or her benefit must dominate when there are conflicts of interest. The complexity and reality of these conflicts are evident in the well-publicized controversies surrounding the cases of Baby Fae, Baby Doe, Baby Jane Doe, and the role of government in how such decisions are made.

Interpretation of Ethical Principles

Whatever model we choose must be fitted to the three major ethical principles that figure in most clinical-ethical decisions. These are beneficence, autonomy, and justice. Secondary principles that derive from these are confidentiality, truth-telling, and promise-keeping. While most physicians will accept these principles, the way they are interpreted varies considerably. As a result, there may be wide variations in our moral judgment about what is the right and good thing to do in a particular case.

The Principle of Beneficence

Beneficence, acting in the best interest of the patient, is historically the first principle of medicine. It is central to every code of medical ethics since the Hippocratic Oath. But beneficence may be interpreted in different ways and with different degrees of stringency. Thus, some limit beneficence to non-maleficence, the negative ethical obligation that forbids harming the patient. However, others accept a positive ethical obligation to do good. But what level of doing good do we mean -- only if it means no inconvenience to ourselves, at some small or great inconvenience, or even danger. Or is sacrifice of an even higher degree required? Defining the level of beneficence to which we feel bound is one of the most debated questions today.

In addition to the obligation of beneficence, there are questions about what in fact is in the patient's best interests. In the case of competent adults, we have some idea of the patient's value system and wishes to guide us. But in the case of the infant, we cannot know what he or she would wish. Some argue that the safest course under these circumstances is medical indication; if there is medical benefit to be obtained then a treatment should be used. Others would interject the projected "quality of life" of the infant with severe congenital defects. Others would consider the "burden of life" in their decision. If that burden is too great, they hold that beneficence dictates nontreatment.

The definition one uses of beneficence will often depend on answers to the deeper levels of questioning, the ethical theory one espouses, or the ultimate sources of one's morality. It is essential to clarify what we mean by beneficence to make rational decisions in particular cases.

The Principle of Autonomy

The principle of autonomy, respect for the patient's moral right to decide for himself and the physician's obligation to respect and enhance that decision, has come to challenge beneficence as the primary principle in medical ethics. This is perhaps the most fundamental change in physician-patient relationships in the history of medical ethics. Previously, beneficence was exclusively interpreted in terms of what the doctor thought best for the patient. Indeed, the patient's opinion was rarely sought. The whole thrust of Hippocratic ethics is toward the physician as a benign authoritarian or father figure.

A number of questions must be asked about the interpretation of autonomy. Is it unrealistic to expect someone who is ill, in pain, and anxious to be able to make objective choices? Or to understand enough about the medical decision to judge wisely? Can the parents of a really sick child make the difficult decision about what is best for that child? That is the view of the strong paternalists, those who think the physician always knows what is in the patient's best interests and is obligated, therefore, to do what is medically indicated?[7]

Others on the other hand hold a "weaker" view, namely that there are times when the physician should override the patient's autonomy, i.e., when the patient is very ill, when the choice is between certain death and an effective treatment, or in the case of infants or incompetent adults, when the patient's surrogates have opted against beneficial medical treatment.

Should autonomy become an absolute principle to be abrogated only when it ends in direct harm to innocent parties as Engelhardt holds?[8] Or should you balance beneficence and autonomy as McCullough and Beauchamp suggest?[9] Or should a different concept of the relationship be examined, such as Thomasma and I suggest in a forthcoming book that focuses on the idea of beneficence in trust?[10]

The Principle of Justice
Justice is another of those words we all use to bolster our arguments. Yet, as Plato showed in the first book of his Republic, we do not always understand what we mean when we use this powerful and complex word.[11] Is it enough to say that justice is to render to others what is owed them? Do we render good for good and harm for harm? Do we temper justice with charity as the Christian Gospels teach? What kind of justice does the model of the physician-patient relationship we choose dictate? Can we justly reject or refuse to treat patients who are the victims of their own self-abuse, i.e., some AIDS victims, the smokers, drinkers, drug addicts, sociopaths, and criminals?

What rule do we use to translate our concept of justice into a concrete decision? Is it equity of access to health care, need, merit, social worth, ability to pay, first come first served, citizens of your own country over others? Do we use the rule of similar treatment for similar people in similar situations?

These are all fundamental questions in peri- and neonatology, where we must deal with infants who cannot defend their own rights against the rights of others. Does justice permit letting an uncomplicated Down's syndrome infant die because his or her parents feel they cannot cope emotionally or economically with a retarded child? Is it just for the parents of a badly handicapped infant with a terminal disease to demand treatment to the bitter end when they are using up society's resources in money, facilities, or personnel?

Do the sick have any claim in justice on the rest of society? Do those more fortunate have an obligation to the less fortunate? Which of the two current theories of justice is the more pertinent to the care of neonates, Nozick's[12] or Rawl's?[13] Manifestly answering the question, What is justice?, is as difficult and as inescapable as Plate's question, What is truth?

Yet, if we are to make rational clinical-ethical judgments, we must arrive at some position on the way we interpret not only justice, but beneficence and autonomy, and how to resolve conflicts between them. But what we think of these three principles will have deeper groundings in the last two levels of the structure of ethical decisions: ethical theory and the ultimate source of morality we espouse.

Grounding of Ethical Principles
Clinical-ethical judgment and decision-making cannot be rational processes if we do not understand the grounding of the principles we use, for it is from that grounding that we draw their interpretation.

There are a variety of ethical theories, most of which cannot be discussed here.[14] They all depend on some theory of the good. Only the two major theories, consequentialism and deontology, can be examined in this brief report.

Consequentialism
Consequentialist theories of ethics hold that the right and good action is determined by its consequences, by the amount of good versus harm pain versus pleasure, cost versus benefit. Is the center of the good your own egotistical self-interest or the good of everybody? Are you a utilitarian who seeks to maximize utility or good for the greatest number? Beneficence and justice are often justified on consequentialist foundations.

Deontology
The deontological theories of ethics hold that the goodness of an act is inherent in the act itself. In this view, some acts are always right or wrong in respect of the consequences they produce. Should the truth always be told, promises always kept, confidentiality always protected? Some answer yes, some no. The principle of autonomy is often based in a deontological foundation. Justice and beneficence can also be interpreted deontologically.

Deontological viewpoints are apt to be nonnegotiable, creating conflict when the participants in a clinical-ethical decision do not all share this theory of ethics. Even if they do, they might differ on whether the act in question is morally licit, or not. Consequentialism. has its problems too, since the "calculus" of harms and benefits is often difficult to carry out and frequently debatable in its conclusion.

The simple definition of consequentialism and deontology do not exhaust the differences or similarities between them. Also, there is considerable overlap in actual practice. Usually, a blending of both theories occurs in concrete decisions. For the neonatologist and perinatologist, the question is where to place his own primary emphasis.

Ultimate Sources of Morality

This is the most fundamental level of ethical concern and often the most firmly held. It represents the set of moral beliefs most closely identified with the person, the rules by which he orders his own life, the beliefs he gives up last, if ever.

When is said and done, what do you believe validates your moral values? The existentialists hold that morality is self-generated. Each person makes his own values as part of his own life project. Others bold morality to be whatever society, culture, or custom dictates. The right and good, therefore, change with geography, history, and society. Another view is that what is right is what we can make the strongest and most coherent argument for. Still others use ultimate criteria like moral sentiment, and biological or economic utility. Finally, a large number of people find the ultimate source of morality in religion, in beliefs revealed or commanded by a personal God, the cosmos, or a worldly spirit.

These sources can only be enumerated without evaluating them, which requires a full course in the philosophy of religion. What is important for the clinician is to recognize the source of his own and his patient's morality. In the case of neonatology and perinatology, these will be the values of parents, society, or institutions. These must be understood if conflicts are to be resolved in morally defensible ways.

In a morally pluralistic society, one in which ultimate sources of morality may differ sharply, it may be preferable to turn to the internal morality of medicine itself as suggested in the previous discussion of the sixth model of patient care. This is a common ground for all health professionals, and patients as well. This does not mean that the deeper sources of morality are to be ignored, but only that we must seek some ground for possible consensus in the practical world of clinical-ethical decision-making.

The Purpose of Ethics

One question that under lies the whole idea of a schema for ethical decisions is what purpose ethics itself fulfills. The modern view is largely that the purpose is conceptual clarification and analysis, understanding the terms and logic of ethical judgments and the assumptions on which they are based. This contrasts with the view that ethics has normative content that can tell us what we ought to do and how we should live. The latter is the classical understanding of ethics as found from its beginnings in Plato and Aristotle and in the moral teachings of most of the world's religious and philosophical systems.

Many clinicians, with their scientific and pragmatic training, judge ethics to be useless and frustrating. It seems that ethics cannot arrive at proven conclusions that will convince everyone. There seem to be no "right" answers. Therefore, one view is as good as another. This is the road to moral relativism and ultimately moral chaos. It destroys the possibility of rational clinical-ethical judgments. It also defeats itself, since the view that ethics is useless is itself also no more than an opinion.

Most of the discussion in this report has tried to show that the resolution of ethical conflict and dilemma is possible, that an orderly and systematic approach can contribute to the quality of the decision. There may well be more than one well-argued case for resolution of some ethical issues, but this does not mean that all arguments are equally coherent. Some arguments are better than others. Some are patently indefensible.

There is no real alternative to ethics so long as we are rational creatures and wish to respect each other's moral values without submitting to them without examination. A democratic society is based finally on a continuing dialogue among its citizens on the moral values that make for a good society. Medicine and medical ethics are two of the most significant arenas for this dialogue today. A pluralism of well-founded and rigorously argued judgments is preferable to moral privatism in which each person retreats into the redoubt of his own beliefs and refuses to examine them critically.

All humans make moral judgments. Ethics provides the skills whereby those judgments can be understood, assimilated, and transmitted to others. It is indispensable to a liberal education and a free society.

The Ethical Work-up: A Procedural Schema

Thus far I have emphasized the substantive framework for clinical-ethical judgment. This is essential to fulfill two of the three ethical obligations of the clinician outlined at the beginning, namely, understanding one's own value system on four major levels, and possessing some knowledge of ethics as a formal discipline. The third obligation, making the actual clinical decision and implementing it in a morally defensible way, requires a procedural schema. This schema is a set of steps to be used in making the decision itself. This is the ethical work-up. It consists of five steps.

Establish the Facts

The first step in an ethical analysis, as in a clinical analysis, is to establish the technical facts as securely as possible. Confusion in the ethical decision is as much the result of uncertainty about the facts as about the ethical issues. Indeed, the issues are in large part defined by the particular features of the case in hand.

Clinicians are inclined to make authoritative statements, some that do not bear up under careful scrutiny. Clinical judgments about diagnosis and especially prognosis and treatment are probability statements. The clinician should be clear about the degree of certitude and uncertainty in the facts upon which he bases his ethical judgments.

The patient, or the surrogate decision-maker in the case of infants, should be helped to understand the essential facts and the uncertainties as well. The clinician must communicate the diagnosis, the prognosis treated and untreated, and the potential benefits and side effects of treatment.

He must be certain as well about whether the patient is "brain dead," in a permanent vegetative state, or is terminally ill, and what he means by these terms. These judgments and judgments about the patient's competence figure importantly in most ethical decisions.

Determine What is in the Patient's Best Interests

While it is easy to assert that beneficence is crucial to medical ethics, it is much more difficult to say precisely what will be in the patient's best interests, since this is a value-laden judgment. Such things as the balance of harm and benefit, effectiveness, and relationship to the patient's concept of quality of life must be figured into the decision. The patient's best interests are not fully assumed in what is medically indicated. The patient's perception of what is good in terms of his own life plan, the values he wishes to protect, and his spiritual goals are even more important than medical benefit. Indeed, medical benefit ought to serve those other values.

The patient is a moral agent, and in the case of infants, the patients have moral agents who are responsible for what they decide. Their judgment of the infant's best interests may not always coincide with the physician's. Therefore, it is incumbent that the physician be as careful as possible not to interject his own values in determining what is "best" for the infant. Indeed, when we do not know the values of the patient, as in the case of an infant, best interest should be as close to medical indication as possible. Quality of life determinations of best interest are particularly dangerous.

Define the Ethical Issues and Principles

This step depends on the various levels of substantive ethics discussed earlier. It is essential to recognize where there are conflicts, how they might be resolved, and what principles, theories of ethics, and sources of morality and philosophy of physician-patient relationships are being used. This is the heart of the ethical analysis.

Dealing with ethical principles such as respect for autonomy and beneficence, it is often necessary to decide which carries greater moral weight in a particular case. The arguments we use reveal what we think are our ethical obligations to the patient. Indeed, we must appreciate that usually the ethical judgment involves not absolute right and wrong, but a conflict between competing good things. This is the "tragic choice" that makes ethical analysis so painful at times.

State Your Decision in Concrete Terms

The essential feature of clinical ethics that distinguishes it from a classroom exercise is that, at some point, the discussion must come to an end, and a position must be taken. A moral choice cannot be avoided. This is painful, but inescapable. Ethics does not require that one be perfect. We must make the best decisions we can given the complexity and uncertainties of the case. Clinical ethics like clinical diagnosis ends in action. It is a moral responsibility to choose that action as intelligently as we can. Our decision must be clearly cited. Ambiguity is acceptable in discussion, but dangerous when action is finally taken.

Justify the Decision

The decision is truly ethical only if it is justified in rational terms. Ethics is a formal discipline, a systematic, orderly, critical examination of the rightness and wrongness of a particular act with a view to determining out ethical obligations. It examines the meaning of the terms we use, the logic of our argument, and the assumptions from which we start.

This means we must also examine the arguments for and against our decision. In this way we can check our own logic and reexamine our own values and beliefs against those of others who may have good arguments to the contrary. The purpose of an ethical analysis is not to. prove that we are right, but to arrive at the best defensible judgment in the interests of the patient.

As any clinician recognizes, these processes are fully analogous to the way we analyze clinical problems, conduct a differential diagnosis and arrive at a treatment regimen. The capacities to make clinical-ethical judgments and other clinical judgments are really the same, and the two are in, separable in clinical practice.

Carrying Out the Ethical Decision

Assuming that we have, through the two schemata described above, arrived at an ethically defensible clinical-ethical decision, we must conduct the process of decision-making itself in a morally defensible way. We must deal ethically with all the participants in the decision. This usually centers on the question, "Who decides?"

When the patient is competent he or she decides. The limitations on a competent patient's autonomy are two: asking the physician to do something that violates the physician's moral beliefs, or something that produces direct and serious harm to a third party. Under these circumstances, the physician cannot presume to override the patient's wishes. But he must withdraw from the case, respectfully giving his reasons and avoiding recrimination.

In neonatal and perinatal medicine, these situations are not uncommon. Catholic physicians, for example, cannot be asked to perform abortions or to withhold treatments of benefit to the child simply because the parents think the child's quality of life or the economic or psychological burdens of raising the child are too much to bear. Another example would be the refusal of transfusions by Jehovah's Witnesses when such a treatment would be life-saying for an infant. In many clinical situations, the fundamental values of parents, or pregnant women, can conflict with those of the physician. These conflicts can be handled in a way that protects the infant and, if possible, respects the values of the parents.

In dealing with incompetent patients, there is a moral obligation to transfer the moral rights of the patient to a valid surrogate, someone who acts for, and presumably protects the interests of, the incompetent person. With once-competent adults or older children, we seek a "substituted" judgment, a decision, based on knowledge of the patient's values, and as close as possible to what the patient would have chosen were he or she able to make the choice.

In perinatology and neonatology, we can have no idea what the fetus' or infant's values might be or what he or she would consider a quality life. The principle of respect for autonomy simply does not apply. We must depend on the family or guardian for a surrogate decision. But we cannot assume that they will automatically share the same view as the physician about the best interests of the infant.

The situation may become a difficult one, because biologic relationship does not automatically confer moral competence or morally correct motivations. One of the unsettled questions of great importance in peri- and neonatal medicine is whether parents and physicians should be entrusted with final decision-making authority, or whether concerned third parties or government may intervene if they think an injustice is being done.

The physician, who should be the advocate of the patient, has a serious responsibility to make some judgment about the moral validity of a surrogate decision-maker. He has a bond, or covenant, with the patient that compels him to act in the patient's behalf. He must be the patient's advocate when he perceives that these surrogates may not be acting in the patient's best interest because of some conflict of interest or a mistaken notion about what is best. The difficult fact is that, to some extent, the physician must make a judgment about the moral competence of the parents--an extremely vexatious matter as the cases of Baby Doe, Baby Jane Doe, and Baby Fae amply illustrate.

This is not to depreciate the interest and the importance of the parents, rather it is to question whether their authority is absolute or can be questioned. That is the question behind the recent debates about the so-called Baby Doe regulations of the DHHS. Much more discussion on this issue is needed.

It is crucial to remember always that the fetus and the infant are peculiarly vulnerable. We cannot tell what their future values will be. We do not know what each will consider a life worth living. One can argue back and forth about the Baby Doe case and whether or not those parents acted in the best interest of the infant. Whatever one's substantive view may be, one ought to try to discern the motives behind the decision. Sometimes there is a serious conflict of interest. Also there can be a conflict among the surrogates, e.g., when father and mother differ between themselves whether a seriously ill infant should be treated. In such cases, a determination must be made about who best represents the interest of the infant. A few states are now beginning to develop a hierarchy for moral decision-making.

But that is a legal hierarchy. It does not necessarily correspond with the moral competence of the surrogates.

The special moral status of the fetus and the infant make the substantive and the procedural issues in neo- and perinatology more complex than in adult medicine. Perinatologists and neonatologists have the same moral obligations as other physicians, complicated by the special vulnerability of their patients. They have the obligations of all physicians to understand the deeper structures in the anatomy of clinical-ethical judgments, to use an orderly approach to making the actual decision and to carry out the decision-making process itself in a morally defensible manner. The purpose of this report has been to suggest substantive and procedural schemata that can make clinical-ethical judgments more orderly and more explicit.

No matter what schema is proposed or used, the final determinant of the patient's best interests is the character of the physician, his disposition to act in a morally responsible way. Given the complexity of ethical decisions in pert- and neonatology, the type of person the physician is, is even more important than the way he structures his decisions. The best safeguard for the vulnerable patient is always a combination of a virtuous physician dedicated to the patient's welfare and an explicit and orderly system of ethical analysis.[15,16]

Notes

1. Seldin D. *The Boundaries of Medicine*. Presidential Address, Transactions of the Association of American Physicians, 1981;494:75-86.
2. Veatch RM. *A Theory of Medical Ethics*. New York, NY: Basic Books. 1981.
3. May WF. *The Physician's Covenant*. Philadelphia, PA: Westminster, 1983.
4. Sade R. Medical care as a right: A refutation, *New England Journal of Medicine* 1971;285:1288-1292.
5. Parsons T. *The Social System*. London, England: Frex Press, 1954.
6. Pellegrino ED. Toward a reconstruction of medical morals: The primacy of the act of profession and the fact of illness, *Journal of Medicine and Philosophy* 1979;4:32-56.
7. Childress JF. *Who Shall Decide?* New York, NY: Oxford, 1982.
8. Engelhardt HT. *The Foundations of Bioethics*. New York, NY: Oxford, 1986.
9. Beauchamp TL, McCullough LB. *Medical Ethics: The Moral Responsibilities of Physicians*. Eaglewood Cliffs, NJ: Prentice-Hall, 1984.
10. Pellegrino ED, Thomasma DT. *For the Patient's Good: The Restoration of Beneficence in Health Care*. New York, NY: Oxford, 1988.
11. *The Republic of Plato*, trans. Bloom A. New York, NY: Basic Books, 1968.
12. Nozick R. *Anarchy. State, and Utopia*. New York, NY: Basic Books, 1974.
13. Rawls J. *A Theory of Justice*. Cambridge, MA: Harvard, 1971.
14. Frankena W. *Ethics*. Englewood Cliffs, NJ: Prentice Hall, 1973.
15. Meilander GC. *The Theory and Practice of Virtue*. Notre Dame, IN: University of Notre Dame, 1984.
16. Pellegrino ED. The virtuous physician and the ethics of medicine, In: Shelp E, ed. *Virtue and Medicine: Explanations in the Character of Medicine, Philosophy and Medicine*, Vol. 17. Holland, Netherlands: Reidel, 1985.

Chapter 15

Abating Treatment in the NICU

Robert F. Weir

As with any case analysis, the first task in commenting on the case described by Robert J. Echenberg, "Permanently Locked-In Syndrome," is to be clear on the diagnosis. Clarity in diagnosis is especially important in cases involving medical conditions with a variety of symptoms and a range of severity, as in the three types of infantile spinal muscular atrophy (SMA). SMA type I, commonly known as Werdnig-Hoffmann disease, has an early onset, either *in utero* or within the first three to six months after birth. An infant with Werdnig-Hoffmann disease exhibits profound hypotonia, absent tendon reflexes, inability to sit unsupported or to roll over, poor head control, motor and respiratory paralysis, and impaired sucking and swallowing. Life expectancy is very short, with many of these children dying in the first year of life and virtually all others dying in their second or third year, even with aggressive medical management.[1]

The second, or intermediate, type of SMA among children begins to manifest itself in an affected child after the first six months of life. The child, having achieved the ability to sit unsupported, never achieves the ability to stand or walk unaided. Children with this form of the disease are prone to respiratory infections, contractures, and scoliosis, but usually survive into adolescence or early adulthood. Medical management is directed at maintaining optimal function, with spinal surgery, mechanical ventilation, and electric wheelchairs being commonly used.[2]

SMA type III, or Kugelberg-Welander disease, appears in late childhood. Children with this mild form of SMA are able to stand and walk with a waddling gait. They continue to have the ability to ambulate until they are approximately thirty years of age. They have normal or only slightly depressed reflexes and a normal life expectancy.

The infant in this case had the most severe of the three types of SMA. As illustrated by the case description, cases of Werdnig-Hoffmann disease pose difficult ethical problems and painful emotional issues for parents, physicians, nurses, and other health professionals. Unlike children with some other neuromuscular conditions (such as Canavan's disease), children with Werdnig-Hoffmann disease are mentally normal and remain alert and attentive to their environment despite progressive paralysis. Their lives can be sustained for a limited period of time by chronic mechanical ventilation and gastrostomy placement, if their parents and physicians decide on aggressive medical management. However, such an approach is both medically and morally problematic because it dooms these infants to a state of complete immobility with respiratory infections posing an ongoing threat to life.

The dilemma posed by the case is clear. On the one hand, the infant in this case was described as "mentally intact" and "well developed and bright-eyed," with the apparent abilities

---

Source: Reprinted from *Journal of Clinical Ethics*, Vol. 3, No. 3, pp. 211-213, with permission from Journal of Clinical Ethics.©

to "see, hear, taste, smell, and feel." On the other hand, she was, with the exception of slight facial movements, totally paralyzed, dependent on a ventilator, and sustained by technological feedings. Her disease was described as "progressive, relentless, and totally irreversible."

Given these contrasting facts, the adults who deliberated about initiating, continuing, or abating different forms of life-sustaining treatment were pulled in opposite directions. Most of the physicians thought the best course of action was to withhold medical interventions (such as CPR or gastrostomy placement), given the perceived futility of such interventions. Some of the neonatal intensive care unit nurses and a few of the physicians seem to have favored such interventions, given the infant's mental alertness and their own emotional attachment to her. Other nurses were clearly troubled by the pain and suffering they seemed to be inflicting on the patient, although the only clinical sign of this perceived suffering given in the case description was the cardiac instability that appeared at each tube feeding. Unfortunately, the young, unmarried parents did not or could not participate in these deliberations because of their overriding interpersonal concerns.

Three comments about this case may be helpful. First, the major concern expressed by Echenberg is procedural in nature. He asks, "Who should speak for these tiny patients if the family, either by choice or incompetence, abdicates its responsibility?" He indicates that one option, a court-appointed guardian, was not chosen because a *guardian ad litem* would not be involved in the "patient's direct care" and therefore would have difficulty making "an empathetic decision."

The option actually chosen represents a hybrid of existing models of collective decision-making in pediatric contexts. On the one hand, the procedural question was answered in a fairly straightforward manner by having a perinatal ethics committee discuss the case. This model, convening a meeting of a multidisciplinary pediatric ethics committee to give collective advice on a case, has been used in many hospitals since the early 1980s.[3] The advantages of this model are several, especially when compared with leaving selective nontreatment decisions entirely to the discretion of parents or individual physicians: It provides an institutional mechanism for securing knowledge and information (both medical and nonmedical) relevant to a case, and it increases the likelihood that a difficult decision will be made with impartiality, emotional stability, and consistency from case to case.[4]

On the other hand, the comments in the case description about the committee's deliberations are suggestive of a second model for collective decision-making, used in many hospitals as a supplemental alternative to an ethics committee, and as a substitute for an ethics committee in other hospitals or pediatric services not having such a committee. This model, often taking the form of a care conference, does not emphasize the importance of multidisciplinary perspectives on a difficult case as much as the personal participation of the attending physician, a few nurses, and perhaps another health professional or two who have actually been involved in a case. In this model, personal experience with a case and the personal capacities for empathy, emotional bonding, and caring (for the patient, for the parents) tend to be valued more than the abilities to be impartial and consistent from case to case.

In this case, the pediatric ethics committee seems to have moved in the direction of a care conference. The actual decision to abate life-sustaining treatment, following a discussion of some of the relevant medical, ethical, and social factors in the case, seems not to have been a thoughtful, deliberative decision that reflected the consensus and advice of the ethics committee. Rather, floundering in the midst of medical and moral uncertainty, the committee began "weighing the intuitive assertions of those most closely involved with the patient's moment-to-moment care."

The result was a group process dominated by shared intuitions, an anecdotal story, personal feelings regarding the patient and her parents, subjective concerns about her suffering and quality of life, an emphasis on caring, and a celebration of "community."

Second, the committee seems to have been remiss in failing to discuss some important substantive matters. Faced with the case of a two-and-one-half-month-old child with a severe, progressive neurologic impairment but undiminished mental alertness, the committee found itself "treading in unfamiliar waters." According to Echenberg's account, the committee could no longer "make rational recommendations based on factual, medically understood data, nor could we rely on traditional moral and ethical principles of autonomy, beneficence, non-maleficence, or justice." Again he says that "traditional ethical theory . . . , logical rules, predetermined principles, and commonly trusted beliefs... were not of great help."

A case involving a child with Werdnig-Hoffmann disease is undeniably difficult for all persons involved. For physicians and nurses to be moved by perceptions or the suffering of a young patient is commendable. For committee members to express a collective desire for nurses to participate more in patient-centered decision-making is long overdue. For the committee to acknowledge the medical and moral uncertainty it faced is laudable. For anyone to participate in a decision to abate life-sustaining treatment in the case of a mentally alert, brighteyed young patient, knowing that her death will soon follow, is certainly emotionally taxing.

Yet the psychological and emotional aspects of the case do mean that the members of a pediatric ethics committee are excused in forgoing substantive matters. Simply mentioning the difficulty of applying some of the principles of biomedical ethics to the case does not mean that the principles were incapable of providing any insight or guidance for decision-makers. The principles are not, after all, a mantra that merely has to be recited for ethical guidance?[5]

Likewise, simply stating that some physicians at the ethics committee meeting thought the available treatment possibilities were futile in this case does not automatically mean that the physicians were correct, or that the committee might not have benefited from a discussion of the, concept of futility. Given the different meanings of futility and the recent literature on the subject, the committee members could have discussed what they meant when they said treatment would be "futile," or whether they actually thought that mechanical ventilation (already being used) and a gastrostomy tube (being considered as an option) were both futile in this case, or why one but not both of these technologies was futile, or why CPR was futile, or how the use of these technologies in this case was different from their use in other cases.[6]

In addition, the repeated vague references to the patient's suffering could have been used as the basis for a helpful, rational discussion of suffering in neonatal and other young pediatric patients. For instance, physicians and nurses involved in the patient's care could have been asked for empirical signs of her suffering that could have supplemented and validated the nurses' ability to "read" the baby's facial expressions.

The committee could also have discussed the concepts of benefit and harm and their applicability to the case. In this and other cases of Werdnig-Hoffmann disease, for instance, would the provision of mechanical ventilation and technological feeding be "beneficial" to the patient in the sense of corrective therapy, or would the use of these technologies be '"beneficial" only to the medical and nursing staff in the sense of making the medical management of the patient easier? Could the use of these technologies in this case be judged as harmful to the patient, either in the sense of interfering with her future interests, impairing her psychological welfare, or as aimless cruelty?[7]

Third, the committee seems to have had no substantive standard, much less a policy, that could be used in arriving at a decision to withhold life-sustaining treatment from this patient. Of the several possible substantive standards, the patient's-best-interest (PBI) standard is the most widely accepted. The case description uses the language of "best interest" several times, yet the committee does not seem to have discussed what the PBI standard means, the variables that can be used in determining whether treatment is or is not in a patient's best interest, or how the PBI standard applies to the Werdnig-Hoffmann case under consideration.

As described elsewhere, the PBI standard has several variables that can be used in making decisions to abate treatment in pediatric cases. The variables are as follows: (1) the severity of the patient's medical condition, (2) the availability of curative or corrective treatment, (3) the achievability of important medical goals, (4) the presence of serious neurological impairments, (5) the extent of the patient's suffering, (6) the multiplicity of other serious medical problems, (7) the life expectancy of the child, and (8) the proportionality of treatment-related benefits and burdens to the child?[8]

If the ethics committee had discussed these variables at its meeting the outcome for the child with Werdnig-Hoffmann disease would not have changed: the child would still have been allowed to die without any effort at CPR being made. However, the committee meeting would have been different, with more emphasis on reason and less on the emotional aspects of the case (as important as they are). In addition, if the committee had earlier used the PBI standard to formulate an institutional policy on selective nontreatment decisions, the policy to abate life-sustaining treatment in Werdnig-Hoffmann cases might have led to an earlier decision. Depending on when the child's condition was diagnosed, the child might never have been placed on a ventilator.

Notes

1. V. Dubowitz. *Muscle Disorders in Childhood.* Philadelphia, PA: Saunders, 1978:146-57.
2. Gilgoff IS, Kahlstrom E, MacLaughlin E, Keens TG. Long term ventilatory support in spinal muscular atrophy, *Journal of Pediatrics* 1989;115:904-9.
3. Weir RF. Pediatric ethics committees: Ethical advisers or legal watchdogs? *Law, Medicine & Health Care* 1987;15:99-108.
4. Weir RF. *Selective Nontreatment of Handicapped Newborns.* New York, NY: Oxford University Press, 1984:253-74.
5. Beauchamp TL, Childress JF. *Principles of Biomedical Ethics*, 3rd Edition. New York, NY: Oxford University Press, 1989.
6. Schneiderman LJ, Jecker NS, Jonsen AR. Medical futility: Its meaning and ethical implications, *Annals of lnterna Medicine* 1990;112:949-54; Tomlinson T, Brody H. Futility and the ethics of resusitation, *Journal of the American Medical Association* 1990;264:1276-80.
7. Weir RF. *Abating Treatment with Critically Ill Patients.* New York, NY: Oxford University Press, 1989:340-54.
8. Weir RF, Bale Jr JF. Selective nontreatment of neurologically impaired neonares, *Neurologic Clinics* 1989;7:807-21.

Chapter 16

A Paradigm for Making Difficult Choices in the Intensive Care Nursery

William E. Benitz

Putting Theory into Practice

In the 10 years since the birth of "Baby Doe," the decisions confronted daily by neonatologists and parents of sick or premature infants have been the focus of a great deal of attention. Issues raised by these decisions have been vigorously debated and discussed in the popular media in political and governmental forums, and in the professional literatures of a variety of academic disciplines. These discourses have illuminated a number of moral and ethical principles that may govern these decisions and have contributed to the development of regulatory and procedural constraints upon this process, including requirements for establishment of infant care review committees at all hospitals that provide neonatal intensive care services. However, the philosophical concepts espoused by theoreticians, although often helpful as abstractions, are rarely invoked at the bedside as decisions are sought for individual patients. No clear consensus has emerged on how these ideas should be incorporated into clinical practice or on the role of mandated ethics committees or discretionary ethics consultants. Consequently, there are wide disparities in decision-making processes both within and among institutions. Failures of these systems to protect neonatal patients or their families remain distressingly common and have attracted considerable attention in the lay press. Although there can be no universal decision tree that can dictate the course of this complex process in all cases, a clearly articulated operative paradigm that defines essential features of an effective and equitable decision-making process is essential to identify the causes of failures and conflicts that arise when the process is dysfunctional and to prevent such problems by providing a framework for training practitioners to deal with these issues.

The following discussion describes an approach that has been applied and refined over the past 10 years in my own practice of neonatology in a busy tertiary care nursery. The purpose of this description is not to suggest that this approach provides the definitive answer to the ethical questions raised by neonatal intensive care but rather to suggest a starting point from which practical strategies for dealing with difficult choices in neonatal medicine can be developed, evaluated, and refined.

Acknowledge Procedural Paradigms

The observation that the particulars of each case require individualized consideration has led, in part, to the argument that a framework for approaching ethical decisions is neither necessary nor desirable. As Loewy pointed out, this avoidance of a framework in itself

---

Source: Reprinted from *Cambridge Quaterly of Healthcare Ethics*, Vol. 2, 1993, pp. 281-294, with permission of Cambridge University Press © 1993.

constitutes a framework that denies any requirement for disciplined reasoning.[1] Decisions based entirely upon subjective impressions of what "seems to be the right course" are intrinsically idiosyncratic and thus cannot be impugned or defended through rational discourse. As a consequence, it is impossible to dissect this process in retrospect to identify potential errors or their antecedents when the decisions reached are not satisfactory.

Therefore, this paradigm presupposes that nothing learned from present or past instances can be of any value as difficult choices are contemplated in subsequent cases. In this circumstance, there can be no expectation that discussion of ethical issues by prospective participants in ethical decision-making will be of any benefit. The vast energy devoted to ethical controversies, as reflected in part by the very existence of journals such as CQ, provides prodigious evidence of a deeply shared belief that these discussions are not futile. To those who have participated in many such decisions, it is obvious that experienced practitioners (whether physicians, ethicists, or others), who could not be more skilled than novices if no learning or generalization were possible, do bring skill and insight to the process. Whether by design or default, experience in dealing with ethical issues leads to adoption of ideas or behaviors that guide subsequent considerations. In addition, even naive participants (such as students or parents who unexpectedly find themselves in these circumstances) come with tacit assumptions about the nature of the decision-making process. Denial of the utility or necessity of these conceptual frameworks cannot negate their existence but can only obscure their influence. Acknowledgment of the existence of procedural paradigms, whether explicitly articulated or tacitly assumed, is a prerequisite to clear thinking and accurate communication as ethical decisions are deliberated.

Although paradigms for approaching ethical dilemmas necessarily must evolve from a collective experience with similar cases, there can be no guarantee that the resulting "self-generated" paradigm will ensure optimal outcomes from the process it directs. If an opportunity to improve performance is not to be missed, it is incumbent upon those who can anticipate their need to participate in such decisions to clearly articulate and continually refine the paradigm(s) they utilize. Construction of conceptual paradigms to guide the process by which decisions are made on behalf of sick infants must be undertaken carefully, with a clear understanding that the chosen paradigm has a powerful potential to dictate not only the process, but the outcome. This potential is obviously true of some determinate paradigms, such as those that dictate that no resuscitation will be attempted for infants below a specified birth weight or that maximum intensive care will be applied without wavering until the patient expires. The potential may be less apparent for more flexible paradigms, which may superficially appear to provide for substantial adaptation of solutions to a patient's individual circumstance but are nonetheless covertly or inadvertently restrictive. Example 1 provides an example of such a circumstance, in which a tacit assumption that an infant could not be permitted to die without referral for intensive care could have led to an unnecessary separation of a dying infant from her family.

Example 1

Baby girl A, an infant with anencephaly, was delivered at Community Hospital by nonelective Caesarean section because of fetal distress. Neonatal intensive care services were not available at this hospital. Although resuscitation was not required at birth, respiratory and cardiovascular vital signs were unstable, and prolonged survival was not expected. Because within memory all other infants whose life had been in jeopardy at Community Hospital had been immediately transferred to an intensive care nursery, the attending pediatrician assumed that this newborn could not receive care at that hospital and recommended transfer to the intensive care nursery of a distant referral center. Her mother, having undergone Caesarean section, could not have visited her at that nursery for at least several days. After consultation with the neonatologist at the referral center and further discussions with family members and nursing staff, it was decided that the infant should remain at Community Hospital. Care appropriate for a healthy infant was provided, a "Do-not-resuscitate" order was entered, and the baby expired within a few days.

When different parties to this process assume different paradigms, an especially pernicious set of problems may arise. Accommodation of different approaches to decision-making is possible (although often difficult) when these differences are recognized and specifically addressed by at least one of the parties involved. Accommodation is impossible if none of the parties are aware of the assumptions upon which their behavior is based. In this situation, the choices of paradigms may not dictate the solution to the ethical dilemma, but instead may preclude realization of any resolution, foreordaining a failure of the process to effectively address the needs of the infant patient. Example 2 describes such a quandary. Here, the tacit expectation of the hospital staff that the parents could comply with their recommendations came into conflict with the parents' expectation that their wishes would be paramount.

Example 2

Three months after birth at 25 weeks gestation and a weight of 750 grams, Baby G had massive obstructive hydrocephalus due to a large intracranial hemorrhage and severe respiratory failure due to bronchopulmonary dysplasia. Both of these problems were progressive in spite of aggressive therapy, and it was the judgment of the medical staff that the problems were refractory to treatment. Because further treatment was considered futile, discontinuation of intensive care was recommended to the family. Based upon their belief in a miraculous recovery promised by a religious advisor, the family refused to consider any limitation of care. Frustrated by the family's refusal to accept their recommendations and feeling coerced into providing care contrary to good medical judgment, the medical staff became increasingly angry. Simultaneously, the family was angered by their perception that the medical staff did not respect their right to determine the course of their child's care. Sensing hostility toward their demands, they stopped visiting the infant and became difficult to contact by telephone. Because no dialogue about the infant's care could take place, she remained intubated and on mechanical ventilation and continued to have regular ventricular punctures for control of her hydrocephalus.

Without recognition of the processes and assumptions invoked by different participants, such conflicts are extraordinarily difficult to resolve. Adoption of a consistent and rational approach by the medical staff (and ethics committee, when one is involved) not only ensures that these participants have an awareness of the postulates and procedures underlying their behavior but greatly simplifies identification, integration, accommodation, and/or modification of the assumptions brought to the problem by uninitiated participants (parents, in particular).

Establish a Therapeutic Alliance

Formation of a therapeutic alliance on behalf of the sick infant is a prerequisite to effective selection and implementation of care options. This therapeutic alliance must have an inclusive constituency and demands mutual respect and trust among all participants. The idea of a therapeutic alliance on behalf of a patient is neither new nor limited to neonatal medicine. The often-overlooked second sentence of Hippocrates' first aphorism states "It is the duty of the physician not only to do that which belongs to him, but likewise to secure the cooperation of the sick, of those in attendance, and of all external agents."[2] After more than three millennia, the force of this duty has not diminished.

The parents and primary physician are obviously key members of this alliance, but it should include all other healthcare professionals who have contributed to the patient's care and any family members or others (such as a priest or pastor) whom the parents may wish to involve. The alliance may fail if any interested person feels excluded from the process. A nurse whose opinions are not solicited or grandparent who is not informed of the infant's condition, for example, may subsequently undermine efforts to achieve consensus. In some instances, the respect and trust underlying the collective decision-making of this assemblage will carry over from established relationships, but often respect and trust must be established de novo. In all cases, each individual must be able to expect that his or her opinions will be heard and that he or she will be fully and honestly informed. In particular, it is imperative that the parents are well informed of the medical realities. However, the importance of ensuring that other participants (including the medical staff) are informed of the parents' (and each other's) expectations and anxieties should not be overlooked.

To a large extent, the responsibility falls to the primary physician to ensure that these relationships are established and nurtured. Much can be achieved as the physician provides medical information to the infant's family. This information should be presented concisely and in language understandable to the audience, but it must be complete and accurate. If parents have any reason to suspect that medical information is being withheld or misrepresented, trust cannot be established and an effective therapeutic alliance cannot be sustained. Although empathy with parents confronted with difficult choices is often appropriate for health care professionals, it must be conveyed with considerable circumspection. Telling parents that "I know how you feel" is likely to be perceived as presumptuous and will compromise the credibility of the speaker (unless he or she actually has also lost a child or had a child with a life-threatening disease).

Finally, it must be evident that all parties seek to act in the best interests of the child, even if they do not immediately agree upon what those "best interests" are. This necessity may seem obvious, but in my experience perception or suspicion that at least one party is motivated by other factors is very common. For example, a parent may seem to be motivated by worries about the costs of hospitalization, or a family may suspect that a physician is trying to prevent malpractice litigation (either against himself or another party). If overt, such issues may have to be addressed explicitly before attention can be focused upon the decisions to be made on behalf of the infant. However, latent or diffuse doubts can often be assuaged by the simple (and sincere) statement that "I am very concerned about your baby" or "I know that you are very concerned about your baby." Such statements not only redirect attention to the infant but reinforce the coalition formed on his or her behalf.

Example 3 illustrates a failure to develop and maintain a therapeutic alliance between the medical staff and Baby G's parents. Reestablishment of this relationship was a prerequisite to resolution of the situation.

Example 3

At nearly 5 months of age, responsibility for Baby G was transferred to a physician who had not previously participated in her care. She continued to require daily ventricular punctures for control of severe hydrocephalus and had markedly elevated carbon dioxide tensions in spite of continued mechanical ventilation at high ventilator settings. When not obtunded by the effects of her hydrocephalus and apparent carbon dioxide narcosis, she was often agitated and required frequent administration of sedative drugs. Following an acute exacerbation of her respiratory insufficiency (during which her arterial CO2 tension exceeded 130 mmHg), her parents were contacted to arrange an urgent meeting to discuss her deteriorating condition. On arrival for that meeting, the parents appeared to be angry and alienated. Beginning the meeting with an apology for the hostility they had perceived towards their previous requests, the physician promised that they would be listened to and that their values would be respected in present and future interactions. Baby G's condition was reviewed in detail, including the apparent medical futility of continued intensive care. Her parents continued to express their belief in an imminent miraculous recovery and would not contemplate any reduction in the aggressiveness of care provided for her. Apparently feeling less threatened by the medical personnel, they agreed to resume regular visits and to communicate with the physician directly several times each week.

Understand the Nature of Decisions

Widespread and profound misunderstanding of the nature of the decisions that parents and medical professionals are called upon to make on behalf of desperately ill infants is a major cause of confusion and mischief in this process. The popular perception that unitary and irrevocable choices about continuation or withdrawal of care determine life or death does not reflect the realities of these situations. Contrary to a nearly universal misconception, these decisions rarely determine whether an infant lives or dies. Life and death are not (and should not be) in the hands of parents or physicians. When it is evident that intensive care cannot result in long-term survival (i.e., is futile), the "decision" that the child will die has already been made and cannot be revoked, no matter how willfully the participants in this process may wish to do so. Inability to reverse the progression of life-threatening disease and avert death is confronted sufficiently frequently to ensure humility in this regard for most of us who work in neonatal intensive care. Conversely, we are often surprised by infants who appear to be dependent upon life-sustaining technologies but survive (sometimes for a very long time) after application of these technologies is discontinued, reminding us that cessation of intensive care is not tantamount to a decision to permit an infant to die. Although death may appear likely and imminent upon implementation of a decision to limit or discontinue specific medical interventions, this outcome is rarely a certainty, and it is not wise to suggest to parents that death will occur within any preconceived interval.

Understanding that "life or death" is not the prerogative of the interested parties, then, forces recognition that decisions can be made only about matters over which these parties are able to exercise control. The question at hand then becomes one of how best to care for an infant under difficult circumstances, because autonomy can be exercised in the selection of the medical and social measures that will be invoked on behalf of the infant. These choices can and do influence the time of death in many instances, because continuation or discontinuation of truly life-sustaining therapy may delay or hasten death, but prospective articulation of these decisions as "how to care" issues ensures that interventions affecting the quality of survival or the process of dying are not neglected, as may happen if the decision is perceived as a simple "life-or-death" dichotomy.

In spite of another seemingly ubiquitous presumption, implicitly reinforced in many discussions of these issues in the popular and professional literatures, "withdrawal of care" is never an option. No matter what the circumstance, every infant is entitled to basic humane care and comfort and never more so than when death appears imminent. Ensuring that the infant is not cold, wet, hungry, in pain, or alone is obligatory, and the abandonment entailed in an implicitly global "withdrawal of care" would be reprehensible at best. Just as the parents should be encouraged to remain involved with their baby no matter what course of treatment is selected or outcome is expected, they also must be assured that the medical personnel will not abandon their professional obligations to the infant, even if aggressive application of technological interventions is no longer deemed appropriate. Decisions to "limit" treatment may be appropriate, but this phrasing also may lend itself to misinterpretation. If care is limited, it should not be because of agreement that some arbitrary global level of intensity should not be surpassed but rather because specific aggressive interventions (e.g., mechanical ventilation or cardiotonic drugs) are deemed inappropriate under the circumstances at hand. Because this process ultimately reduces to selection of the interventions to be implemented for the infant, the process is not fundamentally different from one by which decisions are made for sick infants under more ordinary circumstances.

Assuming the existence of a single "correct" choice for each case leads to two misapprehensions. First, it must be understood that what is "right" for one family and their infant may not be so for another under similar conditions, so that judgmental interactions must be avoided as the decision-making dialogue evolves. Second, there is no mandate that decisions cannot or should not be reconsidered or changed. Change may be appropriate when new information comes to light, as might be the case when an infant is clearly not responding to intensive care or when an untreatable metabolic disease is diagnosed. A change in perception of the infant's condition or in the values ascribed to various features of this condition may also lead to reconsideration of a previous choice. Because availability of new information and changes in perceptions and values are virtually universal in the course of caring for sick babies, frequent reevaluation of the choices made in their interests is not only permissible but essential. All participants in this process should understand its dynamic nature and know that a change of mind implies neither error nor weakness but may be the natural consequence of conscientious attention to the problem as it unfurls.

Agree upon an Objective

Much of the confusion and conflict that has bedeviled those responsible for sick infants in various capacities has arisen from failure to articulate and agree upon a realistic primary objective. Medical care can be provided for an infant in pursuit of three different goals: 1) salvage of a long-term survivor; 2) prolongation of life (while accepting that long-term survival is not achievable); and 3) minimization of suffering (or, equivalently, maximization of comfort).

In our nursery, we assume that salvage will be the objective of care until sufficient information is available to permit or compel adoption of another objective. Thus, premature or distressed infants are aggressively resuscitated in the delivery room and intensive care is initiated and continued until it becomes apparent that the infant is not able to respond to such interventions. When survival of a functional individual is likely to result from care that does not qualify as heroic, we are compelled by societal constraints to apply that care, even if parents ask that it not be given. Circumstances in which long-term survival of a functional individual is not a realistic expectation or can be achieved only at the expense of heroic therapy or inordinate suffering, then, both permit and compel identification of prolongation of life or minimization of suffering as the specific objective. As a practical distinction, the objective of continued intensive care must be prolongation of life if recovery sufficient to permit survival after discontinuation of intensive care cannot be anticipated, but salvage may be pursued if intensive care is not expected to be necessary indefinitely. Articulation of one of these objectives may significantly simplify consideration of other issues, but those involved in the choices must also recognize that achievement of the chosen objective is not always within their control, so that it may be necessary to change objectives or accept that the desired outcome is not attainable.

In many instances, the circumstances make selection of an objective of care easy. For most sick infants, survival and achievement of a state of good health are the expected results of medical interventions, and there is no need to consider objectives other than salvage. Other conditions, such as profound congenital malformations or multiple organ failure due to asphyxial or septic shock, are so clearly incompatible with recovery that salvage is obviously not a realistic objective. The challenging cases are those for which this choice is not immediately apparent; in these instances, it may be difficult to determine or agree upon either the objective criteria for or the subjective values ascribed to survival as a "functional individual," the meaning of "likely" as it applies to the probability of favorable responses to interventions, or what constitutes "heroic" therapy or "inordinate" suffering. Considerable judgment, wisdom, and compassion must be exercised as the medical staff helps the family elucidate the specifics of these issues in their individual case and to balance them as they select an objective for continuing care of their infant.

Agreement on one of these objectives has immediate practical implications for the infant's care, both with respect to selection and application of medical technologies and in the assessment of and responses to the infant's suffering. If salvage is the objective, intensive care should be applied with a vengeance, limited only by the magnitude of the patient's needs and respect for the hazards of the interventions themselves. In this instance, suffering incurred as a consequence of aggressive care or invasive procedures may be quite acceptable, because it is readily justified by the rewards to be gained from survival long beyond the period for which hospitalization and intensive care are required. Because good medical practice dictates that unnecessary suffering must be avoided, the medical staff is nonetheless obligated to ascertain that suffering occurs only as a consequence of medical necessity in the pursuit of stabilization, recovery, and healing.

When prolongation of life is the objective, technological interventions may be applied more or less aggressively than would be the case for a patient for whom salvage is pursued. Prolongation of life by technological means can be rational only if the aggregate benefits that accrue from longer survival outweigh the negative consequences. It might therefore be appropriate to reduce suffering by performing laboratory studies (and the associated arterial punctures, heel sticks, and phlebotomies) less frequently than would be the usual practice for monitoring infants for whom salvage is the objective. Conversely, concern about long-term toxicities that might constrain interventions when long-term survival is sought and expected should not restrain application of technologies when the objective of care is limited to prolongation of life. For example, administration of high concentrations of oxygen might be avoided in infants who are expected to survive, so that the risk or severity of bronchopulmonary dysplasia due to pulmonary oxygen toxicity could be minimized. This long-term concern would not justify restriction of oxygen supplementation for an infant who is not expected to survive beyond hospitalization, especially if high inspired oxygen concentrations improve the baby's comfort level by reducing air hunger. During pursuit of this objective, suffering (and other burdens imposed by continued intensive care) must be regularly evaluated by the family and the medical staff to ascertain that it is warranted by the benefits of the interventions required.

If the objective is to minimize suffering, medical interventions can be justified only to the extent that they alleviate suffering. Interventions that prolong life may be undesirable, even if they impose no burden of suffering in themselves, because they will increase the duration of suffering from other causes, including that of the terminal disease process. For example, antibiotic treatment of bacterial pneumonia may not be appropriate for an infant with multiple organ failure following severe intrapartum asphyxia. However, fear that their application may shorten the duration of survival should not prevent use of treatments (such as opiates for patients in pain) that increase patient comfort, but measures intended to reduce suffering simply by hastening death (i.e., euthanasia) are not acceptable (in my opinion). It is apparent that these objectives are not entirely mutually exclusive. Salvage necessarily entails prolongation of life and attention to issues of comfort or suffering, and efforts to prolong life may be tempered to a greater or lesser extent by the desire to minimize suffering.

It is neither appropriate nor helpful for medical professionals to acquiesce to a request for pursuit of salvage when this objective is not realistic. Continued application of intensive care with the apparent objective of salvage after presentation of an opinion that salvage is not achievable is likely to be interpreted by the family as behavioral evidence that the medical staff does not believe their own prognosis. This apparent inconsistency between word and action quickly undermines trust and impedes communication. Tacit assumption of different objectives by different parties inevitably leads to conflict and confusion. Parents who are committed to salvage may be infuriated if they perceive that the medical staff is not applying medical interventions with maximum intensity or is not attempting to wean their infant from intensive care, as might be appropriate if the primary objective is simply prolongation of life.

These problems can be circumvented only if the objectives of the medical staff are clearly articulated for the family's benefit and are in accordance with their expectations. When parents are unable or unwilling to accept limitation of intensive care based upon a hopeless prognosis, it is often helpful if their implicit choice of objectives is explicitly articulated as prolongation of life, with the understanding that one benefit of this will be to provide time for them to understand and accept the medical futility of continued intensive care.

Example 4

At the next meeting with Baby G's parents, the physician reiterated that her progressive respiratory failure would inevitably lead to death in spite of continued mechanical ventilation. Indicating that he would feel dishonest if he suggested that salvage was even a remote possibility, he indicated that their request for continued intensive care would be taken to be a request for continued prolongation of life and would be honored as such. Because prolongation of her life could make sense only if the quality of her existence justified the suffering engendered by intensive care, her parents help in optimizing the quality of her daily experience was solicited. They agreed to increase their participation in her care, especially to hold and soothe her when she appeared unhappy or agitated. Subsequently, they began to spend several hours daily at her bedside. About 10 days later, they expressed the opinion that the suffering they observed during these daily visits could not be justified by the minimal apparent benefits derived from continued intensive care. They requested that assisted ventilation be discontinued, and the infant died shortly after this request was implemented.

Identify Medically Viable Options

The options for medical care presented to the infant's family, from which a course of action may be constructed by members of the therapeutic alliance, must be selected carefully. These options must be medically viable, in the sense that they are both technically available and can be expected to promote achievement of the identified primary objective of care. Identification of potential therapies with these characteristics requires medical expertise and thus is both the right and obligation of the responsible physician. Although it is quite appropriate to ask the family to participate in selection of a specific therapeutic plan if two or more alternatives are equally sound in the opinion of the physician, implicitly or explicitly to ask or permit family members to identify other therapeutic measures they might wish to employ is a breach of the implied contractual obligation of the physician to provide the expertise for which the family has engaged his or her consultation. Thus, although the parents should have a major role in selection of the primary therapeutic objective, most decisions regarding the implementation of care in pursuit of this objective should be made by the medical personnel. These choices must be considered very carefully, however, and should always be fully explained to parents and other parties in the therapeutic alliance.

Treatments that do not contribute to the desired outcome should not be implemented merely because of the technological imperative of their availability.

Although this concept may seem obvious, its practical implementation is often less than straightforward. Caretakers tend to focus upon the beneficial effects of medical interventions and discount or overlook adverse consequences, which frequently become more serious threats to the infant than the original disease itself. For example, bronchopulmonary dysplasia as a consequence of mechanical ventilation and oxygen supplementation may be perpetuated and exacerbated by continued use of these causative agents in its management. I have participated in the care of many infants whose survival was both longer and of better quality after apparently life-sustaining measures (e.g., mechanical ventilation or vasoactive drug infusions) were discontinued. One such situation is described in Example 5. Several babies whose survival was not expected after cessation of mechanical ventilation are now rather healthy schoolchildren. This potential for medical interventions to worsen rather than ameliorate a patient's condition must be respected, but half-measures should also be assiduously avoided. If a therapeutic intervention is to be applied, it should be performed to the best ability of the care providers. For example, use of mechanical ventilation for the purpose of prolonging life requires periodic measurement of blood gases and adjustment of ventilator settings to ensure that the level of support provided is sufficient to spare the patient from distress due to inadequate ventilation. (However, these evaluations and adjustments may be significantly less frequent than might be the case when attempting to wean a patient from assisted ventilation.)

Great care may be required to ensure that the recommended therapeutic plan does not make a bad situation worse. This concern often arises when the objective is to minimize suffering for an infant who requires a level of intensive care that may not be truly life sustaining. Such a situation might exist for an infant with severe neurologic limitations who requires assisted ventilation because of a short-term or self-limited pulmonary condition. If the infant would likely die without any intervention, institution of ventilation may not be appropriate because the suffering incurred by doing so may not be justified by the benefits of survival. If nonintervention is expected to result in an immediate period of unmanaged respiratory distress that does not lead to death and poses the hazard of incremental hypoxic-ischemic neurological injury, this course of action will result in greater suffering both immediately and in the long term. Because this outcome is not consistent with the objective of minimizing suffering, this course should be avoided. Even the mention of treatments that are not actually available or practical, such as suggestion of a spinal cord transplant for an infant with spina bifida, should be avoided because these spurious comments raise false hopes and create expectations that cannot be met.

Example 5

A 3-month-old premature infant with severe chronic lung disease remained on mechanical ventilation at high pressures, rates, and oxygen concentrations. Attempts to gradually wean the ventilator rate consistently resulted in unacceptable respiratory acidosis, and he required progressively increasing ventilator support. The medical staff expected that his survival would not exceed 2 weeks. His father insisted that he would not permit the medical staff to "let his baby die." After a painstaking discussion of the hazards of this treatment, he agreed to a trial of rapid weaning from ventilation, with the understanding that an exacerbation of respiratory failure would result in resumption of the current level of ventilator support. The ventilator rate was reduced to zero in three large steps, each of which resulted in improvement in ventilation and oxygen saturations, and he was extubated within 2 days. His chronic pulmonary disease remained difficult to manage, but it was apparent that positive pressure ventilation offered neither immediate nor long-term benefits. He remained off the ventilator but died suddenly 3 months later, shortly after discharge from the hospital.

Respect the Values of the Patient's Family

Accurate medical information, including the prognosis for both duration and quality of survival and the impact of possible interventions on the infant and family, provides much of the necessary factual information, but the values of the family (as expressed by the parents) are the essential determinants of the importance attached to each of these facts. Although the physician's medical expertise generally takes precedence in selection and implementation of specific therapeutic plans, these family values should be paramount in choosing among medical options that are similarly efficacious. For example, it may be appropriate for the family to decide whether a problem (such as pyloric stenosis) is better managed by medical or surgical interventions if the expected long-term benefits are comparable because families may place different values on the short-term consequences of the alternatives (e.g., avoidance of surgery and anesthesia may be preferred to more rapid resolution of vomiting).

Family values may be even more important in selecting the primary therapeutic objective. Unless the family's choice is in conflict with generally accepted societal values (such as requesting only pain medication for an infant whose disease could be cured by a routine medical intervention) or is inconsistent with medical realities (such as insistence on attempted salvage of an infant with irreversible multiple organ failure), the values that the family brings to these decisions should be the principal determinants of the chosen course of action. In making these choices, it is often appropriate for the family not only to take into account the consequences of the decision for the baby but also to weigh the effects of their decision on the family in its entirety. For example, a decision to proceed with heart transplantation for an infant with a hypoplastic left heart will have ramifications for every member of the family, including a significantly increased burden of daily infant care and a long-term, intensive involvement with medical care institutions for the parents and reduced parental energy for and attention to siblings. Although purists might maintain that only the costs and benefits that accrue directly to the infant should be considered as decisions are reached on his or her behalf, failure to consider the effects of these choices on the rest of the family is a major reason for the all too frequent statements by parents that they would not have agreed to aggressive medical intervention for their baby if they could have foreseen the outcome.

A parent's reluctance or fear of inability to undertake the long-term care of a handicapped infant should not be sufficient in itself to justify changing the objective of care for the infant during an acute perinatal illness nor should parental guilt or grief compel indefinite prolongation of life, but these family-focused matters do deserve consideration in context with other issues. Discussions with medical professionals, including nurses and social workers as well as physicians, or with other families who have confronted similar choices may help parents integrate the relevant medical information with their value systems. As the situation permits, taking time for these conversations may be quite useful to parents as an objective for care of the infant is chosen, and the values that they use to reach their conclusions may become evident to other participants in this process. The family's values may be different from those of the medical personnel involved in both content and application, and this difference should be accepted throughout these discussions, which should not be used as a vehicle for challenging, criticizing, or attempting to change a family's value system.

When a family elects to pursue prolongation of life or attempted salvage of an infant against difficult odds, other participants in the child's care or external observers may express distaste for the expenditure of resources entailed in this endeavor. Clearly, instances occur about which most observers would agree that massive utilization of precious medical and financial resources have been made without any expectation that the patient could return to a state of health, cognition, or independence from intensive care. It is arguable that these resources have been "wasted" with respect to benefit to the patient, but our society has placed a very high value on empowerment of families to make decisions of this sort, and these expenditures must be viewed as part of the cost of this reverence for individual (family) autonomy. Health care professionals may quite properly ask whether this societal choice is appropriate when many have little or no access to health care and health care costs consume a rapidly escalating share of the gross domestic product,[3] but this concern for distributive justice has no place at the bedside of a sick infant. Until we reach a societal consensus that defines how expensive care with limited expectations for long-term benefit is to be allocated, cases such as those of Baby L[4] and Mrs. Wanglie,[5] in which the family's requests for continuation of expensive intensive care come into conflict with a care giver's perceptions of social justice, will continue to demand that medical professionals choose between their specific responsibility to their patient (and his or her family) and their more generic responsibilities to society. In the meantime, medical professionals who provide such care will remain obligated to respect the mandate that society has given the patient's family to make these choices on his or her behalf.

Role of the Ethics Committee

I provide the following counsel for physicians responsible for helping families make difficult choices on behalf of their infants.

1. Be aware of the nature of the decisions that parents and medical personnel are called upon to make and the processes that are used to make them.

2. Take advantage of the time spent informing the family of the medical facts to establish a therapeutic relationship that includes other interested parties.

3. Establish a consensus regarding the objective to be pursued.

4. Respect the values of the family whenever these are paramount in making choices, but apply your medical expertise carefully and wisely.

When these strategies are followed, it will seldom be necessary to consult an ethicist or ethics committee to resolve conflicts or dilemmas.

On the rare occasions when an adversarial relationship develops between a family and medical professionals or when conflicts arise that cannot be resolved within the healthcare team, the ethics committee may serve as a valuable external referee. By examining the process that resulted in the impasse, the committee may be able to determine which essential steps in the decision-making paradigm have not been successfully completed and then recommend ways to correct these procedural errors. Rectification of the process should allow the primary participants to proceed to resolution without explicit direction of the outcome from the committee.

The examples described above provide instances in which such intervention could have been effective. In Example 1, the committee would be able quickly and simply to articulate the tacit objective (minimizing suffering) and validate the decision to provide basic comfort-directed care at the community hospital. In the case of Baby G (Examples 2-4), committee intervention could have been helpful at each point described in these examples. At the point described in Example 2, recognition by the committee that divergent operative paradigms were in use by the medical staff and parents might have helped the medical staff to acknowledge the extent to which their behavior attempted to limit parental autonomy and thus facilitated consideration of the question of whether this limitation was appropriate. In addition, the committee could have requested clarification of the physician's opinion regarding the intractability of Baby G's condition, both from the attending staff and outside consultants, if necessary. If recovery sufficient to permit survival without intensive care was even remotely possible, the committee could have suggested that the medical staff accept the parent's request for pursuit of salvage, even if they perceived the likelihood of success to be small. If this outcome was clearly not a realistic possibility, the committee could recommend adoption of prolongation of life as the operative objective. However, to elicit the parents' concurrence in implementation of this objective demanded reestablishment of a therapeutic alliance between the medical professionals and the patient's family. An experienced committee, familiar with clinical strategies, such as those recently presented by the group at the Massachusetts General Hospital,[6] may be able to counsel the medical staff regarding restoration of such a relationship. In some cases, the committee may recognize that the relationship is hopelessly fractured and may recommend transfer of responsibility for the infant's care to a new, previously uninvolved physician (which happened fortuitously in this case at the point described in Example 3). The committee's task in these circumstances is to ensure that all parties understand the nature of the decisions they are undertaking and are actively engaged in both the care of the infant and the ongoing reassessment of his or her care needs, daily experience, and long-term prognosis. As indicated in Example 4, this process can lead to resolution, as all parties begin to pursue a mutually agreed-upon objective.

Committee review may also be useful on occasion to evaluate potential interventions for which ethical propriety is not obvious to the care providers. In Example 5, for instance, the committee could have been called upon to decide whether an attempt to rapidly wean the baby from high ventilator settings was ethically appropriate and could therefore be presented to the parents as a legitimate medical option, because this maneuver might be expected *a priori* to result in significant worsening of respiratory failure as well as elimination of a major source of continuing lung injury. In such instances, the role of the committee is to identify management plans that are ethically acceptable and to exclude any that are not while clearly articulating the basis for these selections or rearticulating controversial decisions in terms that are more conducive to achievement of consensus. In the cases of Baby L[7] and Mrs. Wanglie,[8] for instance, the committee might appropriately have identified continued care with the objective of prolonging life as an ethically reasonable choice, while supporting sustained efforts to help the family to understand the likelihood of the possible outcomes and to integrate this information with their own values[9] and indicating that intensive care with the expectation of recovery to a state of health was neither medically realistic nor ethically supportable. In most cases, there will be several ethically and medically appropriate options, and the committee should not attempt to direct which of these viable options should be chosen for implementation by the parents and medical staff.

No matter how well conceived and carefully implemented, any system for approaching these difficult and emotionally charged decisions will fail on occasion. The ethics committee may not succeed in the interventions outlined above, and the parties may reach an impasse. Cases in which parents refuse permission for performance of life-saving interventions (as in the case of Baby Doe) or insist upon interventions that have no therapeutic value or frankly endanger the child may come to this juncture. A final function of the committee in these situations may be to ensure that there is no recourse other than litigation. As several recent cases have demonstrated, the courts may be the final forum in our society where resolution of these issues can be sought, even though the results of invoking the legal system often are not satisfactory to all participants.[10,11,12]

As the committee struggles with these challenging responsibilities, it should continually assess and refine the local paradigm with which difficult choices in neonatal medicine are approached. If this procedural paradigm is to be effectively applied, the committee must also ensure that members of the healthcare team are well educated in both its theory and practice. The true measure of the success of these efforts will then be how rarely the committee must provide consultation to seek resolution of problems in the care of individual babies.

Notes

1. Loewy EH. Suffering as a consideration in ethical decision-making, *Cambridge Quarterly of Healthcare Ethics* 1992;1:135-42.
2. Hippocrates. *The Aphorisms of Hippocrates*. Birmingham, AL: Gryphon Editions, 1982.
3. Garfunkel JM. Priorities for the use of finite resources: Now may be the time to choose, *Journal of Pediatrics* 1989;115:410-11.
4. Paris JJ, Crone RK, Reardon F. Physicians' refusal of requested treatment -- the case of Baby L, *New England Journal of Medicine* 1990;322:1012-5.
5. Miles SH. Informed demand for "non-beneficial" medical treatment, *New England Journal of Medicine* 1991;325:512-5.
6. Jellinek MS, Catlin EA, Todres ID, Cassem EH. Facing tragic decisions with parents in the neonatal intensive care unit: Clinical perspectives, *Pediatrics* 1992;89:119-22.
7. Paris JJ, Crone RK, Reardon F. Physicians' refusal of requested treatment -- the case of Baby L. *New England Journal of Medicine* 1990;322:1012-5.
8. Miles SH. Informed demand for "non-beneficial" medical treatment. *New England Journal of Medicine* 1991;325:512-5.
9. Troug RD, Brett AS, Frader J. The problem with futility, *New England Journal of Medicine* 1992;326:1560-4.
10. Paris JJ, Crone RK, Reardon F. Physicians' refusal of requested treatment -- the case of Baby L, *New England Journal of Medicine* 1990;322:1012-5.
11. Miles SH. Informed demand for "non-beneficial" medical treatment. *New England Journal of Medicine* 1991;325:512-5.
12. Stevenson DK, Ariagno RL, Kutner JS, Raffin TA, Young EWD. The `baby doe' rule, *Journal of American Medical Association* 1986;255:1909-12.

SECTION 3

ISSUES IN PRACTICE

Chapter 17

Cases 3.0

Case 3.1: **"MOMMA"**

Momma was a 68-year-old woman and mother of 8. She spent most of her married life in the kitchen. She came from Italy when she was a little girl, and married young. She could still not speak English very well.

Her husband never involved her in major decisions in the family, nor did the children. She was just "Momma." They all loved her.

Momma started having black stools. She was admitted to the hospital and had a sigmoidoscopy which showed a mass. The biopsy report came back indicating adenocarcinoma. Her liver function tests were abnormal, raising the strong likelihood of metastases to the liver.

The surgeon visited Momma with a translator, hoping to discuss her medical problems and a proposed treatment plan. Momma referred him directly to her husband, saying, "He'll know what to do. He makes the decisions in this family." In this discussion the surgeon did not mention to the patient that she had cancer.

When the surgeon talked with Momma's husband (who could speak English) and children about her condition, he said, "She must have been feeling weak and tired for a long time and did not complain." He stressed the need to talk with Momma so that decisions could be made in regard to surgery and chemotherapy. There was an emotional outburst in the family, with much wailing and carrying on. The family requested that he not tell her of her diagnosis or prognosis.

The surgeon, sensitive to their grief, suggested that they go home and think about their approach for a day. Meanwhile, he would honor their request for 24 hours, after which he planned to get her involved in decisions in her care.

The husband immediately shouted at the surgeon that he would sue him if he so much as gave a minor hint to his wife about her illness.

When he calmed down, the husband explained that his wife had never been "bothered" by the rest of the family in decisions they had made over the years. He also stressed the importance of their Italian heritage saying that it was their tradition to protect loved ones from the knowledge of a disease like cancer -- a disease that could result in death.

The surgeon was committed to the modern notion in healthcare of the autonomy of the patient. The standard care in this type of cancer is surgery to remove the colon cancer in order to prevent bleeding, obstruction or perforation. The liver metastases are incurable even with chemotherapy. Options for treatment are:

1. Palliative supportive care only;
2. Chemotherapy with the expectation of a 35% chance of a temporary tumor size reduction and possible prolongation of life. However, the chemotherapy may be associated with significant side effects.

The surgeon needed to discuss with her the potential benefits and side effects of the various treatment options in order that she can make an informed decision.

What should the surgeon do?

Case 3.2: **THE ETHICS OF ACCEPTING MEDICAID PATIENTS**

Harvey Mitchell, MD, is an internist in solo practice in a small city in the Northeast. One day he receives a message to call an old classmate, Linda Cohen, MD, who practices in an academic medical center at the other end of the state. The message indicates that Dr. Cohen would like to refer a patient named Bernadine Johnson, who is moving to Dr. Mitchell's area. Dr. Mitchell returns the call the following day, only to discover that Dr. Cohen is out of town. He tells Dr. Cohen's secretary that he would be happy to see Ms. Johnson, and to ask the patient to authorize the transfer of records. Dr. Mitchell tells his receptionist to schedule Ms. Johnson if she calls, and also mentions it to his nurse, who often screens new patients over the phone to assess their needs.

A few days later, Dr. Mitchell's nurse buzzes his office. She says, "Your remember that referral from Dr. Cohen you mentioned? Well, she just called for an appointment, and I said I'd get back to her. She has Medicaid, and it took me 20 minutes just to review all of her problems on the phone. In case you didn't know...she has poorly controlled diabetes with congestive heart failure, a chronic, non-healing foot ulcer, peripheral neuropathy, retinopathy and recurrent UTIs. She wants us to coordinate all her care and make appointments with the subspecialists she needs. What do you want me to do?" Dr. Mitchell sighs and says, "Tell her that we're not taking any new patients, and give her Dr. Perry's number."

The following day, Dr. Cohen calls Dr. Mitchell. "Harvey, I just heard from Bernadine Johnson, who said she couldn't get an appointment at your office. Did your receptionist just make a mistake, or what?" Dr. Mitchell hedges. "Well, it's been really busy here, and besides, it sounds like she would be better off with Dr. Perry, who works in the community health center."

"But Harvey, I referred her to you because her care is complex and I trust your judgment as a physician. Do you only see a certain kind of patient? Why are you turning her away?" Dr. Cohen asks, her anger rising. "How can you justify discrimination?"

Commentary

> "In truth, one ought always to ask oneself what would happen if everyone did as one is doing..." Jean-Paul Sartre

The initiation of the patient-physician relationship is based on mutual agreement regarding medical care for the patient. A physician may not discriminate against a class or category of patients who fall within his or her specialty; however, in the absence of an existing relationship, a physician is not ethically obligated to provide care to an individual except in specific situations, such as an emergency, under a contract, or when no other physician is available. So says the ACP "Ethics Manual."[1] So what applies here?

If Dr. Mitchell refused to care for all patients of a particular race, the case would be a clear one of unethical discrimination against a class. If he refused to care for a patient of that race because he knew from another physician, for example, of that patient's history of prescription drug fraud activities, the case would also be clear -- no ethical obligation. But Dr. Mitchell says he cannot accept Ms. Johnson as a patient because she has Medicaid.

Clearly, Dr. Mitchell is not ethically obligated to accept all Medicaid patients into his practice. The context for deciding to accept any individual patient, i.e., the current composition of a practice, is an important factor. Dr. Mitchell might already have many Medicaid patients, or might be a regular volunteer at the free clinic. Also important is the selection process. Is it ethical for a physician to regularly use criteria other than clinical expertise and factors intrinsic to the patient/physician relationship in choosing patients? Would Dr. Mitchell be on the same moral footing when he reuses new patients because their illness is not within his area of competence, because he does not speak their language, or because the patients do not have private insurance?

The ACP "Ethics Manual" states unequivocally that the welfare of the patient must take primacy over the physician's fiscal considerations; it is less clear, however, on the role of fiscal considerations in the physician's acceptance of a new patient.

In 1990, Medicaid reimbursement levels averaged 69% of Medicare prevailing charges,[2] and an even lesser percentage of private insurance payments. It is conceivable that a private practice could not be sustained on Medicaid reimbursement alone. Dr. Mitchell's decision is certainly ethical if accepting Medicaid threatens the viability of his practice (in which case, all his patients will suffer). Ethics does not require that he accept all people who have Medicaid any more than he is required to work 18 hours a day in order to meet the needs of all potential patients. But does that mean he is ethically justified if he does not accept any Medicaid patients?

When Dr. Mitchell says, "I lose money on every Medicaid patient," he probably means that Medicaid reimbursement does not cover his overhead costs, averaged out for each patient. But general internists see an average of 117 patients per week[3] and the vast majority of those patients do not have Medicaid. If Dr. Mitchell's practice is typical, the marginal cost of a few Medicaid patients would not threaten his practice nor dramatically lower his overall income level. The key lies in a fair and equitable distribution of Medicaid patients throughout medical practices. Physicians can satisfy both ethical and financial requirements by a commitment to this fair-share principle.

However, a 1992 report by the AMA Council on Ethical and Judicial Affairs stated that as many as one-third of physicians provided little or no free or reduced-pay care, and that "a disproportionate share of uncompensated care was provided by those practices which already had relatively high levels of Medicaid patients."[4] Some physicians are not seeing their fair share of the less-profitable patients. If other physicians in the community are willing to accept Medicaid patients, are the physicians who do not accept them relieved of their obligation? How many physicians are referring to Dr. Perry at the community health center? Is it fair to their colleagues for some physicians to avoid the less financially appealing patients, especially those needing complex care? Is it fair to the patients who get left out? Does this satisfy the collective obligation of the medical profession to society?

Some physicians might avoid this obligation in the belief that Medicaid patients are more likely to sue or for fear their presence in the waiting room will cause non-Medicaid patients to leave the practice.[5,6] But recent studies comparing medical malpractice claims by Medicaid versus non-Medicaid recipients do not support the belief that Medicaid patients are more litigious.[6,7] And one physician whose practice includes a large number of Medicaid patients had this to say about his mix of patients: "Although many colleagues tell me, `off the record,' that they shun Medicaid chiefly out of fear of losing private patients, I've found such defections to be largely a myth. Currently, about half my patients are Medicaid recipients, yet I've heard no complaints from the non-Medicaid segment."[5]

Although they are a fact of life, financial considerations should not interfere with the physician's primary commitment to patients. Reform that replaces out current patchwork approach to health care with a cohesive and coherent system that provides adequate access to care for all Americans is much needed. Reimbursement is most properly dealt with as a policy matter at the system level -- not at the level of physician and patient.

As a practical matter, any given patient will probably ultimately receive care, albeit perhaps after being shuffled from physician to physician or to a clinic. Or the patient might end up in the emergency room. But delaying care can hurt patients and be inefficient. To enter the medical profession is to recognize the obligation to participate in medicine's collective responsibility to all who are sick, and to ensure that resources are used wisely. Otherwise the profession has a collective duty that no one physician is obligated to fulfill. Where once the profession taught its students and young physicians the "ancient message that a physician is bound by `professing' humane kindness (humanitas) and compassion (misericordia) to those in need," one physician has noted that any sense of obligation to care for the poor is diminishing and that, as a consequence, the cynicism of both physicians and patients is fueled when young physicians are taught that they may put their own financial interests ahead of patient needs.[8]

This cynicism is fueled further by the reluctance on the part of some physicians to be honest about their reasons for refusing patients. As in this case, if a "wrong" answer is given to an appointment secretary's inquiry about insurance or ability to pay, there can suddenly be no room in the doctor's schedule for a new patient. This phenomenon has been written about as it applies to Medicare patients.[9] Obviously, lying to a prospective patient or the referring physician about the reason for not accepting the individual cannot be condoned. Truth-telling is a basic tenet of the medical profession; it is essential to relationships with colleagues and patients, and the social contract within which medicine is practiced.[10]

Case 3.3: **NON-COMPLIANT DIABETIC**

DS, a 52-year-old male, first visited the clinic in January of 1988. He had a 12 year history of insulin dependent diabetes, hypertension, and renal disease. DS had not checked fingersticks at home and he ate an irregular diet. He occasionally forgot to take insulin. He was not compliant with medication and took his medicines only when he felt "bad". DS smoked one pack of cigarettes per day but he denied alcohol or drug use. DS was unmarried and unemployed. DS lived with his mother who was demented. He had not seen a physician in years. His initial BUN and creatinine were 35 and 2.2, respectively (normal .7 - 22 BUN, 0.7 - 1.5 creatinine); his hemoglobin A1C was 12.4 (normal 5.5 - 8.5). He was continued on insulin and started on nifedipine because his blood pressure was 185/105. DS was offered diet counselling but declined. He failed to keep his appointments after two visits and was lost to follow up.

In September, 1988, DS presented to the emergency room complaining of headache, nausea and vomiting. His blood pressure was 200/110. Glucose was above 600. BUN and creatinine were 40 and 3.1 respectively. He was admitted and treated with insulin and antihypertensives. On the second day of his hospitalization, DS left against medical advice. Two days later, he presented again to the emergency room with similar symptoms and was admitted. DS signed out against medical advice after two days, saying he felt better. He did not take insulin and medication with him. DS failed to keep his follow-up visits.

In March, 1989, paramedics were called to his home. DS had fallen and was unable to get up. He was admitted with a diagnosis of renal failure and was immedicately dialyzed. DS left against medical advice on hospital day five with a quintan catheter in place.

Three weeks later DS presented to the emergency room complaining of swelling and fever. There was pus at the catheter site. Blood cultures were positive for S. epidermidis. Echocardiogram revealed a small vegetation on the mitral valve. He was treated with vancomycin. Home therapy was arranged. A new catheter was placed. Eventually, a right brachial AV shunt was placed for permanent vascular access. Discharge planning and social services assisted DS.

Over the next two years the patient had two admissions for infections and left against medical advice both times. He was often non-compliant with dialysis. He was seen by psychiatrists who judged him to have a mixed personality disorder, but they believed he was competent to make his own decisions.

DS was found comatose in his home in May, 1991. He was dialyzed in the emergency room. He left against medical advice after three weeks saying he had had enough of doctors. The patient was subsequently lost to follow up.

Consider the following questions:

1. Is the physician obligated to continue to treat DS?

2. What ethical dilemmas do noncompliant patients pose for health care providers?

3. What about financial considerations and the scarcity of medical resources? Is this a factor in your analysis concerning whether DS's physician is obligated to treat him? What about the issue of patient autonomy?

Used with permission of Christine Rosanze, M.D., University of California, Davis, Medical Center.

READINGS

1. Holm S. Words: What is wrong with compliance? *Journal of Clinical Ethics* 1993;19(2):108-110.
2. Warren JJ. Ethical concerns about noncompliance in the chronically ill patient, *Progress Cardiovascular Nursing* 1992;7(4):10-15.
3. The Diabetic Control and Complications Trial Research Group. The effect of intensive treatment of diabetes on the development and progression of long-term complications in insulin-dependent diabetes mellitus, *New England Journal of Medicine* 1993;329(14):977-986.
4. Guathier CC. Philosophical foundations of respect for autonomy, *Kennedy Institute of Ethics Journal* 1993;3(1):21-37.
5. Veatch RM. Voluntary risks to health, *Journal of the American Medical Association* 1980;243(1):50-55.
6. Reichard P, Nilsson B, Rosenquist U. The effect of long-term intensified insulin treatment on the development of microvascular complications of diabetes mellitus, *New England Journal of Medicine* 1993;329(5):304-309.

Case 3.4: TRUTHTELLING: REVEALING GENETIC INFORMATION

Mr. Carson, a 43-year-old Atlanta man, is diagnosed as having amyotrophic lateral sclerosis, or ALS, a motor neuron disease. A careful history reveals that Mr. Carson's father and two uncles also developed the disease in their early forties. There appears to be additional evidence that the man's grandfather died of ALS as well. The neurologist concludes that the patient is suffering from a form of ALS that is transmitted as a autosomal dominant with nearly complete penetration. The patient reveals that, about 20 years before, he lived in California, was married, and had one child, Dave, by that union. Since then he has had little contact with the family. However, he knows that Dave is now 21 and a premed student in the process of applying for medical school.

The neurologist believes that the son should be informed that he has a fifty-fifty chance of developing ALS, most likely by the time he is in his late forties. Mr. Carson insists that his son not be informed until Dave has been accepted to medical school. He does not want Dave to make reference to this possible difficulty in his application form. In addition, he believes that the stress will affect his son's attitude and therefore his chance to be accepted to medical school. Dave plans to be married within six months.

1. Discuss some of the major signs and symptoms of ALS. Why is this genetic disease so devastating in the lives of those afflicted and their families? In what ways are their minds affected?

2. Do you agree with Mrs. Carson's insistence that his son not be informed of his flawed genetic heritage, at least until he is accepted to medical school? From an ethical standpoint, would this decision be fair to the school that matriculates Dave?

3. Describe the dilemma faced by the neurologist. Mr. Carson is his patient, not the son. What struggles might be going through his mind with respect to patient autonomy versus physician authority. What right does Mr. Carson have to confidentiality? What right does Dave have to disclosure of information?

4. Do you think that Dave should get married? If he does marry, should the couple attempt to have children or should they consider sterilization? What kind of fact does Dave need on hand to be open and honest with his future wife?

5. Whatever the doctor decides (either to inform Dave or to keep quiet), are there legal ramifications in this case? For example, what kind of court suits might be initiated by Dave or his father?

6. In what ways might the voluntary waiving of rights be helpful or hurtful in family relationships in this case?

Used with permission of Charles Webber, Ph.D.

Case 3.5 **LETTER TO HOSPITAL ADMINISTRATOR**

Dear Administrator:

This letter is a plea for easement from what I believe to be most unreasonable demands from your organization.

On December 29, 1992, I was taken to your emergency room. I was seeking relief from persistent and severe sinus headaches and was referred to the hospital by your Physician Referral Service. It was there that I was diagnosed as having suffered a right frontal parietal hemorrhagic infarct and was admitted to the hospital. I repeatedly told all pertinent staff and physicians that I had no insurance and no means to cover extensive medical bills. In fact, I tried to remove myself from the hospital on the first day only to be confronted by a cadre of medical and security personnel to prevent my exit.

I consented to stay only after my wife became hysterical upon being told by a doctor that if I did leave the hospital, I would be back before the night was over on a steel table with him performing an autopsy on me.

During my eight-day stay I requested release daily only to be subjected to more medical tests and examinations. *Everyone was continuously reminded that I had no insurance and no means to pay for that elaborate treatment. My requests as to what each test was for, what was hoped to be learned from the test, and how much money each test cost were never satisfactorily answered -- especially about costs. I made every effort to minimize costs by suggesting that certain tests not be made and even refusing to take a CATscan one week after my release after consulting with medical personnel and learning that it was too soon for a CATscan to be informative. I refused nearly $600.00 worth of out-patient tests because I could not pay for them and I did not fill several prescriptions for the same reason. While I was trying to do everything possible to minimize my costs, it seemed that the staff was doing everything possible to maximize the charges -- such as keeping me in intensive care for my entire stay.* That was not needed according to the medical professionals that I have since questioned. The only medication that I requested was something to ease my headaches. Most of my meals were purchased separately from the cafeteria or brought in from the outside.

What was learned after accumulating $15,759.00 in hospital charges and $3,980.00 in doctors's charges? *Nothing except that I am in good health which I knew before ever going to your institution.* The staff had many theories of what may have caused my condition, but no definite answers. I could have accomplished the same ends by spending a week at home in bed. It certainly would have been less menacing, less intrusive, and most assuredly less expensive. *Actually a suite in a luxury hotel would have been less expensive and they would have let me check out when I wanted to*!

I am well aware of the high fatality rate and frequent incidence of permanent brain damage from parietal hemorrhagic infarct. However, the early physical motor and mental tests clearly demonstrated that the damage to my brain was quite minimal -- if present at all. *I could have been released then and sent home to bed or transferred to a veteran's or county hospital.* All of the subsequent high-tech and costly tests were performed to confirm the various doctors' and interns' theories that the bleed was caused by some particulate matter in the blood stream lodging in the brain.

Everything in my body was CATscanned except for my hands and feet. Many other elaborate and more dangerous tests were performed. Nothing was learned. True, they did discover a very small leakage between the chambers in my heart. But that is not uncommon. Few hearts are perfectly sealed. For their theories to be true, a piece of particulate matter -- which did not appear in tests -- would have to break loose in the blood stream, pass through the tiny leakage in my heart, and then be routed to the brain. The probability of all these things occurring at once is exceedingly small. Much more could have been learned from a short old-fashioned conference with me rather than the heavy reliance on the high technologies that are very impersonal and most costly. All that these aggressive treatment techniques did were to build an exceptionally high medical bill and learn nothing. Furthermore, they were conducted with all staff being repeatedly advised that I did not have the means to pay for them.

I do not question the doctors' good intentions nor their integrities. But a most fundamental fact was overlooked by all. The best source of information is from the patient himself. *Far too often this type of modern medical care may save the patient -- if indeed it does -- while simultaneously destroying him financially -- thus ruining the rest of his life.* To paraphrase Norman Cousins -- Modern medicine seems too intent to treat the disease and not the patient. The only part of my disease that was treatable was to employ drugs to assist the body to absorb the additional blood in the brain. This the doctors refused to consider.

If any of the medical personnel would have taken just a little time to explain to me my condition, I would have quickly figured out its cause. It was only after I researched the subject in my local library and reflected on it that I can provide the answer. It is very much related to my original complaint. My allergies caused me to have sneezing spells. Ten to fifteen sneezes in a row in rapid succession were not uncommon. After these bouts I would have to lay down due to dizziness or headaches or both. I did not sneeze properly. I tended to sneeze with my mouth closed. This caused tremendous pressures in my head. I frequently felt a sharp pain behind my right eye after sneezing. I have since retrained myself to keep my mouth open when I sneeze and taken steps to filter the air in my household. The results? Greatly reduced sneezing in both frequency and severity, and no headaches. Not one! No dizziness. *And I learned that myself for free.*

But you are not interested in my health, so I'll get on with the finances. I was an executive with International Harvester in their Engineering and Research organization. Since their demise, I have been self-employed as a speaker and entertainer. Though not getting rich, I was at least surviving and had earned a national reputation as a quality attraction. Additionally, I believed it to be an activity that I could carry on regardless of my age. However, several things have occurred to radically change my comfortable existence. I was working nation-wide in the university and college market during the school year, state and county fairs during the summer, and for business and professional organizations' conventions year round. All three of those markets have been decimated by the current economic conditions. Most states have slashed their education spending to the point where many public universities and colleges have severely restricted enrollment as well as their course and curriculum offerings. Budgets for state and county fairs have been likewise pared. The recession has greatly reduced attendance and participation in conventions as well limiting their expenditures as well.

Most states attribute their need to reduce all non medical expenses due to the *imposed and uncontrolled explosive growth of Medicaid and Medicare costs.* This is not what I say. *This is what they say - repeatedly.* My earnings for 1992 were *net loss* of $6,294.95. My wife's earnings for that period were $9,783.75. All these financial records have been sent to the hospital's patient financial services department.

1993 is no better. The various budgets have been restricted even further. An additional hardship has been inflicted on my self-employment status lately due to the death of my father. As a result, my mother -- who is in her 90's and nearly blind -- had to be moved from Florida to here so that she could be cared for. Thus, I am not free to travel as freely as before. I have tried to seek conventional, temporary and contract employment with little success. Despite having a college background in the sciences, extensive experience, an excellent work history, a willingness and eagerness to work and a high degree of computer expertise, no one will consider hiring me at 62 years of age. I have been told -- unofficially and very much off the record, of course -- *that this is due to the high employer medical insurance risks and costs of my age group.* My personal good health seems to be of no interest to the insurance companies. It's simply a matter of my falling into a particular group. In an effort to circumvent these difficulties, my wife and I have started a small computer consulting service called L-A Computer Sciences. But not enough time has elapsed for it to produce significant revenue.

I have applied for hardship relief with the hospital and the Medical Practice Plan. The hospital is still considering the application. The Practice Plan's offer was to pay one-half of the bill in $50.00-a-month payments. It was given as a take-it-or-leave-it proposition. He was not concerned that his offer, however generous, was well beyond my current means. I suggested to both the hospital and to the Medical Practice Plan of using my services to work off some of the bill. *That offer was spurned by both.* Their only interest was money.

Now you can continue to press me for payment. It doesn't matter if your demands are for $1,900.00, $19,000.00, $190,000.00. All are well beyond anything I have. *I cannot give you what I do not have.* The only dependable income I have is a small disability check from the Veteran's Administration. My savings are exhausted. There are no stocks, bonds, CD's, trusts, IRA's or other financial investments whatsoever. Right now I am living on odd jobs if and when they are available. You can try to ruin my credit rating, though medical source complaints are so common now that they carry little weight. You cannot overcome my life span of responsible credit management by a one-time medical charge. However, you can force me into bankruptcy. All that will do is diminish whatever earning ability that I now have. My assets are quite modest and would not be appreciably effected.

Don't stop reading now, there is still more.

On February 15, 1993, my wife took me to the same University Medical Center for an Ears, Nose, and Throat examination that was scheduled during my stay in the hospital. After my examination was started, she felt faint and asked for a place to lay down. Instead of providing that, she was taken by ambulance next door to the hospital emergency room. This was done without my knowledge. There she was diagnosed as being dehydrated -- she wasn't and said so; and as having the flu -- she did and had contracted it while continuously staying with me during my confinement in the hospital. The doctor ordered a series of tests and a saline intravenous feeding. *Instead of saline solution she was mistakenly given a high-glucose solution at an unrestricted flow rate*. Yes, there were many apologies. After I learned where she was I retrieved her. But the fact of the matter is that my wife was much more ill when I picked her up than what she was a short time before. She still shows symptoms from the mistreatment. (Perhaps there are grounds for litigation.) So what did she get for her $675.65 hospital bill and $52.00 doctor's bill?

You damn near killed her! That's what.

The pancreas was not made to cope with such high sugar doses in such a short time. *I can only speculate what your charges would be had you killed her.*

Yours is the only industry where you solely determine what services and goods are needed, when, how, and where these will be dispensed and what the charges for these will be without any regard for the user's ability to evaluate, compare or pay for them. You have no competition. You would certainly not hire anyone on those conditions. Yet you impose this on those in need of your services. Though you cloak yourselves in the noblest of terms, your actions are much more predatory in nature. At least it seems so in my case.

I feel as though I have been mugged. I realize that this comparison will be offensive to you, but the similarities are striking. I was steered to a strange place, my life was threatened, followed by demands for money. I would have preferred the mugging. My losses would be limited to the cash on my person at the time. In many ways the mugger is much more honorable. At least there is no pretense as to what he is nor what he wants.

My professional contracts all contain an unconditional 100%-Money-Back-Guarantee of my clients' complete and total satisfaction in every way. (That option has never been exercised by any of my customers.) Just imagine what would happen if the health care industry operated under that kind of discipline. I am sure you would immediately conjure up endless reasons of why that would be impossible and forecast a picture of complete doom and gloom if that standard was imposed. It is not impossible. I can tell you from personal experience that you would pay much closer attention to your patient's expectations, feelings, and general welfare. *You would not be now facing an irate nation demanding the health care reform.*

Very truly yours,

John and Mary Doe

Patient Numbers - 780008 & 788115 (not the real numbers)

cc:Mrs. Hillary Rodham Clinton, The White House, Washington D.C. 20500

Joint Commission of Accreditation of Health Care Organizations, 1 Renaissance Blvd., Oakbrook Terrace, IL 6018

Illinois Department of Public Health, Central Complaint Registry,
525 W. Jefferson, Springfield, Illinois 62761
Illinois State Medical Society, 20 N Michigan Ave, Chicago, Il. 60602
Supervisor, Patient Financial Services, University Hospital
Manager, Patient & Information Services, University Hospital
Van Ru Credit Corp., P.O.Box 46249, Lincolnwood, Il. 60646-0249
Allied Medical Acc'ts Control, Assoc'd Bureaus Bldg., 260 E. 260 E Wentworth Ave., St. Paul, MN 55118

Modified and used with the permission of the original patient.

Case 3.6: **WHEN FINANCES MAY INFLUENCE PHYSICIAN'S DECISION**

The following case history presents an example of the potential influence of financial incentives on physicians' clinical decision-making. A common medical scenario is presented in which there is potential influence from the organizational setting and the contractual arrangements under which the care is provided.

Case History

Ted and Ned are 46-year-old, asymptomatic, sedentary identical twins. Both are executives in local corporations. Former smokers—both smoked about one-half pack per day from their late teens to their early 30s, when they quit as a New Year's resolution—they have been generally healthy except for mild obesity, secondary to many executive lunches. As a New Year's resolution for 1990, Ted and Ned agree to join a local gym to "tone up" and get back in shape (both had been college athletes). The gym required a note from the men's doctors before they could start the exercise program, but no specific tests were mandated.

Ted had enrolled in GreatCare, an IPA-model HMO, because he liked the "comprehensive care" concept, including an emphasis on prevention and wellness. He also valued the idea of no out-of-pocket health care costs other than the premium deducted from his paycheck. Because it is an IPA-model HMO, in which the HMO contracts with independent providers in private practice, Ted was able to select a local physician about whom he had heard good things.

Unbeknownst to Ted, his physician had agreed to certain contractual arrangements with the HMO. Among them were a 15% discount in his usual fees and an additional 15% withholding. The HMO would return the 15% withholding to the physician only if his referral account for specialist services and laboratory tests had a surplus at the end of the year. If the referral account had a surplus, the physician would get his withheld funds and a bonus equal to half of his share of any surplus in the referral pool. The HMO, which had grouped Ted's physician with four others in his community as a risk pool, provided him with the names, addresses, and telephone numbers of these other physicians and encouraged him to contact the group to "discuss the use of referral funds from their aggregate pool."

Ned had elected traditional indemnity fee-for-service health care insurance, in which his premiums and out-of-pocket payments were higher than Ted's. He felt that it was important to retain complete freedom of choice with respect to doctors, despite the somewhat higher overall costs. As is usual in traditional fee-for-service health care, Ned's doctor is paid for each patient visit and every service performed.

Ted and Ned met at the gym for their first joint workout. Ned explained that his physician would not write a note for him to start the program without first performing an

ECG and exercise tolerance test (results of both were normal). Ned takes some pride in what he considers to be his doctor's comprehensive approach to his health care, and the extra attention he got for clearance for the exercise program. Ted wants to know why his doctor hadn't ordered the tests also. After some thought, Ned begins to wonder if the expensive and time-consuming tests he received really were needed. Both brothers are confused.

Commentary

The physician's primary obligations should be to the patient, not to the system under which he or she provides care, and certainly not to the physician's own pocketbook. It is obviously easiest to follow the ethical course under medically clear circumstances: An exercise tolerance test would be medically unnecessary for a 20-year-old female college athlete, about to join a gym, who has no risk factors.

Many situations require physician judgment as to whether an intervention or test is appropriate given the individual patient. The objectivity of physician discretion should not be allowed to be affected by external forces.

Says the ACP Ethics Manual: "The welfare of the patient must at all times be paramount, and the physician must insist that the medically appropriate level of care takes primacy over fiscal considerations...The guiding principle should always be care consistent with humanistic, scientific and efficient medicine...In the final analysis, no external factors should interfere with the dedication of the physician to provide optimal care for his or her patient."

Used with permission of *ACP Observer*[11]

Case 3.7: **MR. C.'S WIFE**

Mr. C. has had diabetes since age 8. Both legs have been amputated below the knee. Mr. C. has diabetic complications including nephropathy and retinopathy. He has been unemployed for twenty years and he receives a social security check each month. His hobby is collecting and showing farm equipment. During the last year he has been hospitalized 6 times.

At this time, further surgery is planned for his right knee. A consult was called on Monday, January 22, because his wife expressed concern about the use of life saving therapies following surgery.

A patient-staff meeting was held at 3:00 pm, January 22. Present at the meeting were: The managing endocrinologist, her resident, a Risk Management member, a social worker, Mrs. C., her daughter, a son, and later the patient himself, and the ethics consultant. At 4:00 pm, Mr. C. joined the meeting.

Mrs. C. appeared to be both anxious and defensive. She said that under no circumstances would she allow any life support procedures to be used on her husband. She also insisted that she should be present when he signed "papers" (presumably informed consent papers, or advance directives). She repeatedly said that she did not think her husband was capable of making decisions for himself in regard to his treatment. She indicated that on several occasions in the last week he has been uncommunicative and confused. She said that one day, when asked if he remembered her visiting the previous day, he did not.

Mrs. C. appeared to be deeply concerned that life saving measures would be used in her husband's care and she wants to insure that she has the right to make decisions regarding his treatment. She said that her husband agrees with her about the use of life support measures such as respirators and that he wants her to be the one to make decisions for him.

The managing physician said that, at this time, Mr. C. appeared to be depressed but that his depression did not interfere with his ability to make decisions for himself. It was explained to the family that sometimes life support measures are taken during surgery that are temporary in nature and not used to prolong life indefinitely. Mrs. C. seemed to have trouble understanding this and, at one point, became somewhat threatening, saying "My attorney said the minute (you) put them (life machines) on, we'd be in court!" Mrs. C. made reference to her lawyer numerous times throughout the meeting.

Mr. C.'s wife also expressed anger and frustration with her husband's behavior. She said, "I put my foot down (about medicines, etc.)...he does what he wants to do. No one is there. He cheats (with his insulin)." She was referring to what Mr. C. does when he is at home alone and she is at work or away. She also said, "He doesn't always tell me the truth and he doesn't always tell the doctors all they need to know (about symptoms he has)." Mrs. C. was distressed because she said her husband is reluctant to accept his limitations. She seemed to be very concerned about prolonged hospitalizations and "extraordinary" care. She talked about a previous experience with her father who died slowly and she said she did not want her children to undergo what she went through with her father. She also expressed concern about her finances. She said that her health insurance stopped in November when her office shut down.

Mrs. C. had contacted a lawyer, "Joe," before coming to the meeting. She appeared to be determined to make it clear to those present that she has sought legal advice regarding her husband's care.

When Mr. C. joined the meeting at 4:00 pm he appeared to be lucid and alert. He spoke clearly and he was able to answer questions without confusion. Mrs. C. asked him if he remembered the visit from the previous day. She seemed to want to prove her point that he did not remember well. He said, "Yes." She asked, "Do you remember who was there?" and he said, "Of course I do, my mother and you..." His mother had been to visit at that time. So at this time, at least, his memory was fine.

Mr. and Mrs. C. seem to have a distrustful relationship. For example, several times Mrs. C. made reference to "her house" even though they live together. This mistrust seemed to extend to the problem of live saving therapy, about which they disagreed over details. Nonetheless, Mr. and Mrs. C seemed in the final analysis to be in agreement concerning the use of live saving therapies. Mr. C. said he did not want to be kept alive for an indefinite period of time on life support machines and that he would refuse dialysis for an extensive period of time. He agreed that Mrs. C. could make decisions for him if he were unable to do so, and intended to draft a durable power of attorney to that effect. Mrs. C. said that she was opposed to organ donation. By contrast, Mr. C. said he wanted to donate his organs for research purposes if they could be helpful. Mrs. C. did not totally agree to respect his wishes in this regard.

The endocrinologist asked Mr. C. if he knew the lawyer who was advising his wife. He said that he did not but indicated that her choice of a lawyer was her business; he had more important concerns on his mind. When asked further if this lawyer had ever represented her in legal action against her husband, Mrs. C. hedged. She said that "that was all in the past." "Let's not talk about this now." Mr. C. shook his head, indicating "no," to this question, although he seemed to have heard the question properly.

The meeting ended at approximately 4:30 pm.

Respect for patient autonomy is an important principle in making ethically responsible decisions about medical treatment for patients. Decision-making normally occurs within the context of a shared dialogue between the patient and the physician. Family members often participate in this dialogue, especially when the patient is incompetent or comatose. In this case, the patient's wife has expressed concern about her husband's ability to make decisions regarding his care. She is advocating herself as the person who would be the most effective at expressing his wishes. Yet, at this time, Mr. C. does not seem to need anyone to make decisions for him. In regard to future developments, both Mr. and Mrs. C. appear to be in agreement about long-term use of live-prolonging therapy, but disagree about details sufficiently that troubles will lie ahead. Regardless of what their underlying motives might be, each of them wants to be able to refuse medical treatment that would continue life indefinitely through artificial means (e.g., respirator, dialysis). Mr. C. seemed willing to allow his wife to make decisions for him when he is unable.

On Wednesday, January 24, at 3:30 pm, the ethics consultant visited Mr. C. in his room. His wife was also there. The consultant spent about one hour talking with them. Mr. C. appeared tired, but alert and communicative. At the beginning of the conversation, Mrs. C. said she was, "very upset" because she had brought in a Living Will for her husband to sign and she could not get the nurse to act as a witness. The consultant explained that it was hospital policy -- employees are not supposed to act as witnesses for Living Wills. The consultant talked with both of them about the Living Will, and the more helpful Durable Power of Attorney, and asked Mr. C. directly what he thought about signing the document at hand. He said he wanted to. She also asked again about the lawyer who was helping Mrs. C., since a concern of the team was that there was some underlying tension between the couple. Mr. C. said he had no problems with her choice of a lawyer, "since she'll do whatever she wants anyway."

During the talk on Wednesday, both Mr. and Mrs. C. appeared to be confused about the tests that were being performed and the treatments that might follow. Several times Mr. C. indicated his frustration with is knee, asking, "Why can't they just treat my knee?...why are we talking about all of these other things?" Jane F., a 4th year medical student, stopped by to check on Mr. C. and was able to alleviate many of the concerns by answering questions about tests and procedures.

After the meeting with the family on Wednesday, the ethics consultant believed the couple shared the same values regarding the use of artificial life support, despite the many unanswered concerns in this case. She also believed that Mr. C. wanted to sign a Living Will and that he was willing to allow his wife to assume decision-making powers if he became not competent.

Nonetheless, the situation about advance directives is less than ideal, particularly when being honest about the tensions between husband and wife. They tended to answer questions immediately, but on both sides of the issue, one saying "yes" and the other "no." This is worrisome, not so much in the long term, but about the specific details of treatment.

What should be done? Should the advance directives be followed?

Case 3.8: OVERRIDING A PATIENT'S LIVING WILL

J.B. was an 8l-year-old active and alert man who was actively engaged in his business and the development of a recreational camp for the physically disabled, this later interest stemming from his elder son's disability from polio which left him unable to walk. On routine physical examination, he was found to have a prostatic nodule, for which a transperineal needle biopsy was performed. During the next several hours, the patient became febrile and hypotensive. A leukocytosis an thrombocytopenia develop with peritoneal signs. A diagnosis of septic shock and an acute abdomen secondary to ischemic bowel was made. The relative risks of operating versus not operating in a case of presumed small bowel infarction were discussed with the patient and family, and an operation was readily agreed upon.

A celiotomy, a dusky left colon was discovered which extended below the peritoneal reflection. The mesenteric arteries were pulsatile and venous thrombi were not noted. The decision was made not to resect the ischemic colon, a colostomy thus being avoided, and the patient was closed and treated with vasodilators post-operatively. During the next few days, he had rectal bleeding and mucosal sloughing requiring transfusion, confirming the diagnosis of ischemic colitis. By the fourth postoperative day, the patient was off cardiac support and vasodilators and tolerating a clear liquid diet.

On the fifth postoperative day, he began to experience more respiratory depression associated with poor expectoration. A chest x-ray demonstrated bilateral pneumonia and pulmonary edema. Systemic antibiotics were begun. His respiratory rate continued to increase throughout the day, and by evening was 40-50/minute. Arterial blood gases at that time revealed a pH of 7.38, p02 42 torr, and pC02 54 torr. He was electively intubated at this time. The patient was extubated eight days later with normal arterial blood gases and ventilatory capabilities.

After extubation, the patient stated that he had a living will, and he now requested that no further heroics be done to save his life, including reintubation should that become necessary. He had been alert and oriented for the last eight days since surgery. During that day, he became increasingly unable to handle his secretions, became febrile again, increased his respiratory rate to 40/minute and became hypercarbic and hypoxic. Re-intubation was recommended, and the patient refused. His family was divided regarding whether to re-intubate their father, and two family members who believed he should be intubated contacted the patient's lawyer. The lawyer insisted that the patient be ventilated, and informed the family that this was the only responsible course of action.

Case 3.9: GRANDMA OR THE HOUSE

A 76-year-old woman was admitted to the hospital on 1/8/85 with a diagnosis of respiratory failure believed to be related to congestive heart failure and pneumonia. Her medical history was significant for congestive heart failure, atrial fibrillation, and a stroke in the past. Despite these problems, up until a couple of days prior to admission, she had almost normal function. She was mentally alert and had largely recovered from the stroke. The patient's admitting physician diagnosed rapidly progressing respiratory insufficiency, evidence of pneumonia by history, exam, chest x-ray, white cell count, and renal failure due to dehydration. The patient was intubated and admitted to the ICU. Antibiotics were begun. The following day the attending physician found the patient in the intensive care unit much more stable, awake, alert, and apparently oriented, responding appropriately to questions. Over the next few days, the patient became slowly more obtunded, and remained ventilator dependent, despite efforts of the pulmonary service to wean her.

By two weeks after admission, no real progress had been made. In the evening of 1/22/85, the patient extubated herself and suffered a cardiopulmonary arrest. She was resuscitated and placed back on the ventilator. There was an initial marked worsening in her neurologic status following this arrest, and her course was further complicated by worsening gastrointestinal bleeding, requiring transfusions. However, over the next few days she gradually became more alert mentally and she was seen in consultation by cardiology because of persistent heart problems. The cardiology consultant felt that the patient had mild to moderate aortic stenosis and possible mitral stenosis, and suggested that a cardiac catheterization might be appropriate if her mental status improved. Over the next few days her mental status did improve, and on 1/29/85 a cardiac catheterization was done. This revealed significant three vessel CAD, and mild to moderate mitral stenosis. However the mitral stenosis was not felt to be severe enough to explain her persistent respiratory insufficiency. It was also felt that the patient may well have a hypertrophic cardiomyopathy.

About this time, the patient's husband began to question the extent of our care. He did not want to abandon his wife, but did not want her to suffer needlessly, either. We told him that, in our opinion, it was too early to abandon intensive care efforts. The patient began to become more agitated and required some sedation. On 2/6/85, a family conference was held with the patient's husband and son. We agreed that the patient would not be resuscitated in the event of a cardiac arrest.

A tracheostomy was scheduled, although the husband objected to this because he did not feel that his wife would want to go on living on a ventilator. The medical ethics department was consulted.

The ethicists spoke with the patient concerning her present condition, and asked her if she agreed with discontinuing the ventilator as her husband desired. She shook her head "yes." However, she was apparently unable to shake her head "no" and she was also sedated with Haldol and Ativan, so it was difficult to know exactly what her degree of mental awareness was.

On 2/8/85, the attending physician had a long discussion with the family. By this time, the husband was adamant about discontinuing the ventilator. He could not understand why he would not be allowed to make that decision. He felt his wife was clearly suffering unnecessarily, and that this is not what she would want. He was not a man of means, and continuing this hopeless but expensive care would likely cost him his half of the worth of their house. He loved his wife deeply and could not bear to see her suffer. However, he thought it was very cruel and inappropriate to discuss things with his wife in her present condition. He became extremely agitated when the attending physician asked the patient, in the presence of the himself and other family members, if she wanted the ventilator discontinued, and if she understood that discontinuing the ventilator might result in her death.

The patient was transferred out to a private room, and the ventilator was continued. The patient's husband and son became more agitated daily. They stated that they felt betrayed by the patient's attending physician because he had won their confidence early but now would not discontinue the ventilator. Slow progress was made in continuing efforts to try and wean the patient. On 2/22/85, although the patient did not meet criteria for long term survival off the ventilator, she was extubated. She showed evidence again of persisting respiratory failure. By that time her mental status had slowly deteriorated to the point where she was able to do little more than nod her head. The attending physician must now decide whether to re-intubate.

Consider the following questions:

1. What factors are important to consider in your decision regarding re-intubation (e.g., family's wishes, medical indications, societal values)?

2. How do we balance our desire to prolong life against our need to refrain from providing what some might consider to be futile medical care?

3. Does the issue of resource allocation figure into your decision?

4. What about quality-of-life considerations?

5. Does the patient's age influence your decision?

Case 3.10: **HIGH COST OF MEDICAL CARE**

The patient is a 5-year-old child who was sitting in the front seat of an automobile when struck by a passing car and thrown into the street. The poverty stricken family was from out of state. Since they were not on the State's welfare system they were not eligible for Medicaid. The patient was stabilized initially at a primary care institution and then transferred for tertiary care. The extensive list of injuries included a severed spinal column, fracture of the cervical vertebrae, skull fracture, and other multiple injuries. She was therefore attended by different surgical teams with appropriate medical support. Following several intermediate operations to stabilize the neck, to evacuate hematoma, and to treat bleeding in the GI system, appropriate ICU care was instituted with the concomitant high ratio of personnel to patient. Serial evaluations of her neurologic status were performed with little indications of high cortical functioning, and her neurologic assessment at the end of two months was one of apparent irreparable CNS damage along with complete severing of the spinal cord. She did not meet the criteria for brain death since the EEG, while grossly abnormal, did show some activity. At that time a staff conference was held with all involved parties, including the family. Assessment of the neurosurgical and neurology services was that she had received severe and likely permanent damage to the CNS. The family agreed with the general consensus that a status of "Do-Not-Resuscitate" should be instituted, but requested that no active intervention to discontinue life support systems be undertaken.

She survived in this state for several months with supportive care, hyperalimentation, etc. Suddenly she began responding and, to truncate the clinical history, she is, at 14 months post injury, a normally sentient 5-year-old with no neurologic function below the level of C-5.

Plans were made for home support with the parents becoming conversant in ventilator care. The girl used a wheelchair with a portable ventilator attached. She learned to "grunt" with exhalation on the respirator to communicate "yes" or "no."

It is perhaps relevant to note that her family is an extended family living together. They were under rather severe social and interpersonal stress prior to the patient's illness. One member of the family was psychotically depressed and no members were at work. After the initial contacts with the family, and in conversations with the agencies who had been helping this family earlier, it had been felt there was no possibility for this patient ever to return to that home in anything other than a completely recovered state. However, either coincident with this illness, or secondary to the challenge of this illness, the family rallied. New housing arrangements were made, members of the family began working and the potential for home care was clearly present given the family resources at the time the girl was discharged.

Another relevant feature of this case was the cost of the treatment: total charges without physician component were $260,000 for the first 14 months. Breakdown of these charges include $15,000 for x-rays, $16,000 for medical supplies, $60,000 for respiratory support, $46,000 for intensive care, and $82,000 for intermediate care following the intensive care period. Most of this cost is borne by the taxpayer.

After the girl was brought home in the care of the family, arrangements were made to provide a van for her transportation to and from the hospital. This van was provided, like all of her care, through a special fund for uninsured patients in the State. Fortunately, the State in which this case occurred was reasonably wealthy. The van was stolen. Stolen twice, in fact. Some health professionals suspected the family was getting a kickback from the thief, since they had learned how to manipulate the system. Their suspicion was part of a larger feeling that began to grow in this "Million-dollar" case, that saving a life had consequences down the road that were difficult for the child, the family, and society itself.

Questions raised in this case included:

1. Should this much energy and time, not to speak of health care resources, be spent

on a single life? The issue of allocation of financial resources, which, while remote from the mind of the treating physicians, may be addressed in your discussion.

2. Is it right to make quality of life judgments in constructing a treatment plan? If so, is life permanently attached to a respirator and permanently paralyzed and completely dependent on others, worth living?

3. Should the initial resuscitation have been abandoned in light of the probable severely compromised neurologic outcome?

4. Would not these health care dollars be better spent providing for primary care to save many lives, a hospital-based hypertension program in the inner city, for example?

5. Since over 30 million Americans are underinsured, and cannot get care, is it just to expend so much for so little?

Case 3.11: NOT "LETTING GO"

Mrs. L.B., 76-years-old, has multiple medical problems including an idiopathic intestinal pseudo obstruction which produces a situation of megacolon. This condition meant that her daughter, a nurse, had to help each week in reaming out the colon, since she was unable to eliminate in the normal manner. She has very poor nutritional uptake and is on a central IV line. In the past she has undergone angioplasty, she has had multiple strokes, renal problems, decubi, and compressive lung changes. She lived in a nursing home, but her daughter mentioned above, helped out a great deal. Mrs. L.B. is a widow. Her daughter, an only child, never married.

She was transferred to the hospital for surgery on the colon, so that her care might become a little easier. She was scheduled for surgery to remove the colon, but on the operating table, suffered a heart attach and another stroke. The surgery was never performed. These events left her in a comatose state, unable to communicate, and respirator-dependent for her continued existence.

After a stormy course complicated by all the conditions mentioned above, she remained in the Surgical Intensive Care Unit. Her Medicare and Medicaid DRG's ran out, and her care is now, in essence, provided by the hospital and its personnel.

The managing physician, her surgeon, recommended to the daughter that a DNR order placed on her mother. The daughter refused. The daughter requested that a tracheostomy be done instead, so that her mother might do better on the respirator and avoid infection as far as possible. This procedure was instituted. L.B. was returned to the surgical intensive care unit following this surgery.

At that time a chart note indicated that future problems might involve not only the DNR status, but also questions concerning removing the respirator and/or nutrition.

The surgeon, residents, ethicists, and medical students met two weeks later to discuss again the medical ethical principles regarding L.B. Delores, her daughter, is perceived as not willing to "let go." Yet L.B., after suffering a heart attack and severe stroke, will not recover any meaningful life. Since the last discussion, L.B. Has successfully been weaned off the respirator, much to the astonishment of the surgical and nursing team.

On the bases of the patient's best interests, the team agreed on the following treatment plan:

1. No new intervention should be used if L.B. suffers an arrest;
2. Current care will continue, with an effort to drop oxygen content (at 50% now);
3. If she continues to improve respiratory function, the tracheostomy tube will be removed.

She will be transferred to the regular floor, where the care is not as intensive and expensive.

The ethicist present argued that since no new intervention could possibly improve her status, this plan was justified. Her condition will progressively decline. However, everyone present at this discussion noted that they had not expected her to survive this long, and not only has she survived, she has been weaned off the respirator. The senior attending dared the question: "Are we not actually trying to cut off this lady's care because her care has become an expensive burden on the hospital?" And a resident asked: "Can we go ahead and institute the DNR order on grounds that it is useless treatment, even though her daughter will not let us"?

Notes

1. American College of Physicians Ethics Manual. *Ann Int Med* 1992;117:947-60.
2. Physician Payment Review Commission. Annual report to Congress. Washington, DC: 1991.
3. American Medical Association. Physician Marketplace Statistics. Chicago, IL: 1991.
4. The Council on Ethical and Judicial Affairs of the American Medical Association. AMA Council Report C: Caring for the Poor. Chicago, IL: 1992.
5. Attwood C. It's unfair -- and unwise -- to shun Medicaid patients. *Medical Economics* 1991;22-28.
6. MxcNulty M. Questions and answers: Are poor patients likely to sue for malpractice? *JAMA* 1989;262:1391-2.
7. Mussman MG, Zawistowich L, Weisman CS, Malitz FE, Murlock LL. Medical malpractice claims filed by Medicaid and non-Medicaid recipients in Maryland. *JAMA* 1991;265;2992-4.
8. Miles SH. What are we teaching about indigent patients? *JAMA* 1992;268:2562-3.
9. Butler RN. Doctors are refusing to treat Medicare patients. *The Washington Post* 1992;May 12.
10. Every physician should participate in implementing the fair-share principle. This can be done by providing care to the poor in the office setting at no cost or at reduced cost, by serving at clinics that treat the poor or shelters for the homeless or abused women, by accepting Medicaid patients in sufficient numbers, or by participating in programs developed by medical societies to care for the poor. (American College of Physicians)
11. *ACP Observer* Oct. 1990;10(9):1,8-9,12. In the Introduction to the case, Edwin P. Maynard, MACP and Chair of the American College of Physicians Ethics Committee noted: "This is the first in an occasional series of case studies on ethics with commentaries developed by the College's Ethics Committee. This series will elaborate on controversial and subtle aspects of issues not previously addressed in detail in the ACP Ethics Manual or other College position statements, and to make our policies more relevant to daily practice by discussing their application in specific situations. The most relevant issues and concerns of all, however, are those that are identified by our members. We hope this series will prove valuable."

Chapter 18

Communication About Advance Directives: Are Patients Sharing Information with Physicians?

Suzanne B. Yellen, Laurel A. Burton, and Ellen Elpern

Introduction

Historically, patients have deferred to physicians' judgments about appropriate medical care, thereby limiting patient participation in treatment decisions. In this model of medical decision making, physicians typically decided upon the treatment plan. Communication with patients focused on securing their cooperation in accepting a treatment decision that essentially had already been made.

In recent decades, however, this approach has been challenged and largely replaced with a model that emphasizes patient autonomy and the right of individuals to participate in or even direct decisions related to their medical treatment. In the patient autonomy model of medical decision making, the physician is viewed as an expert consultant who delineates the risks and benefits of all reasonable treatments. After a presumed thorough review of possibilities, the "informed" patient, in collaboration with the physician, selects the treatment most consistent with his or her values and individual treatment goals.

The concept of patient autonomy has been applied to the full spectrum of illness ranging from time-limited treatments to end-of-life decisions. Advance directives (ADs), such as the living will (LW) and durable power of attorney for healthcare (DPAHC), have emerged as a means of promoting patient autonomy, especially in end-of-life decisions.

The Patient Self-Determination Act (PSDA) of 1990 has made patient autonomy in end-of-life decisions a key standard. According to this act, institutions receiving federal funds for patient care are required to ask all adult patients whether or not they have some form of AD (e.g., LW or DPAHC). Institutions also must provide written information about ADs, although the specifics of how this information is communicated has, to a large extent, been left in the hands of individual institutions in accordance with state law.

The PSDA has tremendous implications for the field of patient-healthcare provider communication. Despite the emergence of ADs with the Quinlan case in 1976 and considerable attention given to life-support issues in both popular and professional publications, communication about ADs between patient and physician has been limited, [1,2,3] although reasons for communication difficulties have not been specified in the literature. One possible explanation for these difficulties is an extension of communication problems noted in the "do-not-resuscitate" (DNR) literature. Specifically, physicians are uncomfortable discussing resuscitation with terminally ill patients[4] for fear of taking away hope, unleashing an emotional reaction, or causing a depressive reaction.[5] A consequence of this discomfort

Source: Reprinted from *Cambridge Quaterly of Healthcare Ethics*, 1992, Vol. 4, pp. 377-387, with permission of Cambridge University Press © 1992.

is that resuscitation discussions are delayed until, on the average, 3-9 days before the patient dies,[6] when the patient is not competent to be involved in the discussion. Consequently, resuscitation discussions are more often held with family members (in up to 86% of cases) than with patients directly (22-26% of cases).[7]

Research in communication about resuscitation and ADs has generally focused on the physician as the initiator and provider of information. Less attention has been paid to the role or desire of patients to initiate end-of-life discussions.

As part of a larger investigation of patient opinions and behaviors about ADs, the present study examined patient communication patterns and preferences and sought to determine the extent to which patients direct communication towards physicians about end-of-life treatment decisions and ADs. Patients and potential patients were interviewed to answer the following questions. How many patients discuss treatment preferences about end-of-life decisions directly with physicians? Does communication directed to physicians differ as a function of whether or not patients have a written advance directive? Does communication differ as a function of patient category (e.g., inpatient, outpatient, or nonpatient setting) or health status? Are patients who have advance directives making their physicians aware of them? Do patients feel that the responsibility for initiating discussions about advance directives rests with physicians? What is the preferred method of communication of information about advance directives, in keeping with federal mandate (PSDA)?

Hypotheses

Although many of the above questions were exploratory in nature, several specific hypotheses were tested. First, we predicted that execution of an AD would be a function of perceived health, such that people who believed their health was "poor" would be more likely to have completed an AD than those who felt their health was either good or fair. Second, it was hypothesized that people with perceived poor health status would be more likely than those in good or fair health to have specifically discussed treatment preferences with their family and/or physicians. Finally, the data were explored to assess the degree to which execution of an AD and communication about treatment preferences were related to patient category (e.g., inpatient, outpatient, or nonpatient setting).

Method

Subjects

Subjects were 131 persons (50 males, 81 females) who volunteered to participate in the study. Participants included hospital inpatients, outpatients, and healthy nonpatients. The inpatient sample included 42 adults utilizing the medical and surgical services at Rush-Presbyterian-St. Luke's Medical Center, a 900-bed tertiary care academic facility serving the Chicago metropolitan area. Fifty outpatients were recruited from persons with appointments at the offices of a cardiologist and an oncology group. Nonpatients were 39 adults who were not in active treatment for a medical problem. All patients were recruited on the basis of their availability to the interviewers on the days of data collection. The refusal rate was 4%.

Procedure

An interview format was used to administer the questionnaire. Potential study subjects were approached by one of the data collectors who explained the purposes of the study and requirements for participation. People who were unable to speak or understand English were excluded from consideration. Written informed consent was obtained for those who agreed to participate after the purpose of the interview was explained. The study was approved by the Human Investigations Committee of Rush-Presbyterian-St. Luke's Medical Center.

Questionnaire

A structured questionnaire developed specifically for this project used a forced choice format to assess attitudes, behaviors, and communication patterns related to ADs. (In Illinois, the LW and the DPAHC are the ADs recognized under state law.) The questionnaire consisted of several sections: 1) demographic information; 2) communication about treatment preferences and ADs with physicians; 3) beliefs about ADs; and 4) preferred communication format for receiving information about ADs. Interview questions were pilot tested on a limited number of patients and nonpatients, after which items that caused confusion were identified and revised. Interview procedures were standardized across interviewers, and a standardized definition of an AD was provided to those subjects who did not understand this term.

Analyses

A software package[8] was used for statistical analyses. Frequency data were tabulated, and percentages were calculated. Planned comparisons between categorical variables (e.g., group of patient, perceived health status, having executed an AD, communication patterns) were analyzed using chi-square analyses in accordance with a priori hypotheses. Percentages for dichotomous responses were converted to proportions and tested with a Test for Significance of Proportion.[9] A p-value of .05 was considered to be statistically significant. No adjustments were made for multiple comparisons.[10]

Results

Demographics

The subjects ranged in age from 18 to 88 years. Age was normally distributed, with the mean age of 52.8 years. Mean age for male and female participants did not differ significantly: mean age for males was 53.9 years; mean age for females was 52.1 years. The subjects were predominantly Caucasian, Christian, and well educated, and over half had some form of education beyond high school graduation (Table 1). Chi-square analyses revealed no significant differences among inpatients, outpatients, and nonpatients with respect to communication patterns and preferences; therefore, data were collapsed across patient category and analyzed as a single sample.

Communication of Treatment Preferences

In 88 of the 131 cases (68%), respondents reported that discussions about treatment preferences in the event of illness and patient incompetence had been held (the "communicators"). However, the majority of these discussions were not held with respondents' physicians. Of the 88 respondents who had communicated about treatment preferences with someone, only 13 (14.8%) reported discussing treatment preferences directly with their physician. Considering the entire sample, less than 10% reported speaking with their physicians about treatment preferences (See original article for Figure 1). Most often, these discussions were held with family members and/or close friends.

Data were further examined to determine the percentage of subject agreement with a statement that physicians should initiate discussions with patients about ADs and to explore whether there were differences between respondents who had discussed treatment preferences with their physicians versus those who had not. Neither the communicators nor noncommunicators seemed to believe that the burden of initiating AD discussions rested with the physician. Only 6 of the 13 communicators (46%) and 27 of the noncommunicators (37.0%) believed that physicians should initiate these discussions.

Table 1. Demographics of Subjects in a Study of Patient-Doctor Communication Concerning Advance Directives

Characteristic	% of Sample
Sex	
Male	38
Female	62
Race	
Caucasian	80
African-American	14
Latino	2
Asian	4
Martial Status	
Single	23
Married	56
Separated/divorced	13
Widowed	8
Religious preference	
Jewish	7
Catholic	35
Protestant	44
Other	10
None	4
Education	
Grade School	10
High School	39
Trade/Vocational School	7
College(undergraduate)	24
Postgraduate	19
Recent hospitalization (past 2 years)	
None	38
Twice	28
>2	14
Recent intensive care stay	
Yes	23
No	76
Health status	
Good	61
Fair	25
Poor	13

Communication Patterns among Patients with or without an Advance Directive

Thirty-one (23.7%) of the 131 patients in the study had completed an advance directive at the time of interview. Of this sample of "completers," however, only 15 (48%) had informed their physician of the existence of their AD. Further, a significant proportion of completers (19.4%; z = -3.44, p < .01) failed to discuss the terms of the AD or treatment preferences with their physicians, and a small minority (9.7%) of patients with an AD failed to notify physicians, family members, or friends of the fact that they had an AD. Having an AD does not necessarily mean that this information will be transmitted to attending physicians.

The pattern of data for the group of "noncompleters" was similar to that of the completers. Ninety-nine patients (76.3%) had not completed an AD at the time of the interview. Of this group of respondents, 60 (61%) had discussed treatment preferences with someone; however, only 8 (8%; z = -8.4, p < .01) had discussed preferences directly with a physician.

Data were also examined to determine if perceived health status influenced the likelihood of executing a LW, discussing treatment preferences with someone, or discussing them specifically with a physician. We hypothesized that people who perceived their health status as "poor" (as opposed to "good" or "fair") would be more likely to have an AD and to have discussed treatment preferences with their loved ones as well as their physicians. A chi-square analysis indicated only an effect for health status on execution of an AD; X^2 (df = 2) = 8.62, P = .013. People who believed their health was poor were more likely to have completed an AD than were people whose health was believed to be good or fair. Perceived health had no effect on either discussion of treatment preferences (P = .78, ns) or the likelihood of discussing treatment preferences with a physician (P = .82, ns).

Comfort in Discussion of Advance Directives with Various Hospital Personnel

Most patients anticipated either some or a great deal of comfort in discussing ADs with their physicians, and overall comfort level with physicians was markedly higher than that with other healthcare or hospital personnel (Table 2). Of the 131 participants, 91 (69.5%) anticipated that they would be very comfortable discussing ADs with physicians and 32 (24.59/0) felt that they would be somewhat comfortable.

Patient Beliefs about Advance Directives

Study participants indicated agreement or disagreement with statements designed to evoke attitudes about ADs. Several attitudinal statements were presumed related to known communication difficulties that physicians have in discussions of foregoing life-sustaining treatments (e.g., discussion of CPR in terminally ill patients). The percentage of subjects that agreed with a statement "Patients want their physician to bring up the issue of ADs first" was only 43%, and 44% believed that discussion of ADs was depressing and related to thoughts about dying. However, some (21%) agreed that ADs were primarily necessary for those who were old or sick. With the exception of responses to the statement that ADs were for those who were old or sick (21%, z = -7.25, P < .01), the probability agreement with these statements did not differ significantly from chance.

Communication of Advance Directives

Each subject's first choice of various methods in which information about ADs could be communicated was recorded, and percentages were calculated for each class of response. Choices were written information, videotaped information, face to-face discussion, or a combination of the above (Table 3). The most preferred method of communication involved face-to-face discussion (39%).

Table 2. Comfort Levels of Potential Patients Discussing Advance Directives

Treatment team member	Very comfortable	Somewhat comfortable	Not at all comfortable
Attending physician	91 (69.47%)	32 (24.43%)	8 (6.11%)
Psychologist	48 (36.64%)	45 (34.35%)	38 (29.01%)
Nurse	59 (45.04%)	46 (35.11%)	26 (19.85%)
Chaplain	72 (54.96%)	22 (16.79%)	37 (28.24%)
Admit clerk	15 (11.45%)	40 (30.53%)	75 (57.25%)
Social worker	48 (36.64%)	49 (37.40%)	34 (25.95%)
Lawyer	36 (27.48%)	34 (25.95%)	61 (46.56%)

Table 3. Preferences for Communication about Advance Directives

Manner of delivery	% of sample
Written information	31.8
Video presentation	0.7
Face-to-face discussion	39.3
Combination	17.8
Do not want information	2.9
No Preference	6.1

The provision of written information was selected by 32% of the sample, and a combination of written information with face-to-face discussion was selected by 18% of subjects.Over half of our sample preferred that some form of face-to-face communication be a part of the process of delivery of information about ADs.

Discussion

Our data have implications for both patient-doctor communication and the Patient Self-Determination Act (1990). Physicians have difficulty initiating discussions about various end-of-life issues, often delaying these discussions until the probability of dialogue with the patient becomes a moot point.[11] Traditionally, the responsibility for communication failures has rested on the shoulders of the physician. Our data show communication difficulties but suggest that they may be bi-directional. Patients may not see themselves as active participants in the medical decision-making process and therefore may fail to either discuss end-of-life treatment options with physicians or to notify physicians of the existence and content of their ADs. Our study indicated that: 1) patients are communicating treatment preferences and wishes to limit treatment but are not discussing them with their physicians; 2) patients who have considered treatment limits and have formalized them in an AD do not necessarily share this information with their physicians; and 3) having an AD or communication about treatment preferences is not a function of patient or nonpatient settings. Our data also suggest that communication failures usually do not stem from either anticipated discomfort in discussing ADs with physicians or from the belief that it is the physician's responsibility to initiate the discussion.

The relatively few empirical studies focusing on the extent to which physicians and patients directly discuss life-sustaining treatment[12,13] and DNR orders[14,15] report competing findings. Lo *et al.*,[16] who examined patient attitudes toward discussing life-sustaining treatments in a chronic illness patient population (e.g., cancer, angina, chronic obstructive pulmonary disease (COPD), chronic renal failure), found that 70% of patients discussed treatment preferences with either family or friends, but only 6% of patients had discussed life-sustaining treatments directly with physicians. The limited number of doctor-patient discussions of resuscitation preferences (3-16% of respondents[17,18,19]) has also been found in other studies. Further, Lo *et al.* found that 68% of respondents wanted to have discussions about life-sustaining treatments with their physicians, but only 53% of this group preferred that their physician bring up the matter of life-sustaining treatment first, a finding that is supported in the present study. In contrast, Stolman *et al.*[20] found that 51% of their sample recalled discussing resuscitation directly with a physician. The failure to obtain consistent results among these studies may be explained by methodological differences in the way the subject population was defined. Stolman and her colleagues derived their sample from a pool of terminally ill patients, 73% of whom had already been designated as DNR following discussion with their doctors. The present study, as others, derived its sample from populations in which death was not imminent and resuscitation status had not necessarily been addressed. [Frankle *et al.*[21] found that neither communication nor desire for communication about life support was related to terminal or nonterminal illness status. However, terminal illness was defined by specific diagnosis (e.g., cancer, AIDS, end-stage liver disease) rather than by the expectation that death would occur within 6 months.] The relatively high percentage of doctor-patient communication about resuscitation found by Stolman *et al.* might thus be limited to illness contexts in which death is imminent, and future research should examine communication patterns across various levels of illness severity. In nonterminally ill patient populations, however, it is obvious that despite increased public awareness about ADs within the past 5 years (in our sample, 75% had heard of either LW or DPAHC and 71% had a relatively accurate understanding of their purpose), there has not been a concomitant increase in the likelihood of patients and physicians talking about ADs.

A potential limitation of the generalizability of these communication-specific findings involves the demographics of our sample, which was predominantly white and well-educated. A well-educated sample may result in an over- rather than underestimation of the probability that physicians and patients are talking to one another. However, level of education and verbal ability may be irrelevant when it comes to discussing topics related to death and end-of-life decisions. Irrespective of the direction of the bias, these findings warrant replication using a sample more representative of the Chicago metropolitan area.

Our data did not address specific reasons for communication failures. One possible reason is that time restrictions of office visits with physicians do not permit exploration of future treatment (or lack of treatment) possibilities. Another possibility is that patients may share information about ADs with their primary physician but not with a medical specialist. A more plausible explanation, however, involves role ambiguity on the part of both patient and physician that occurs as the focus of treatment changes from curative to palliative care. Stewart and Roter[22] offered a model of doctor-patient relationships that varies as a function of both physician control and patient control, such that relationships can be described as paternalistic (high physician control-low patient control), mutual (high physician and patient control), consumerist (low physician control-high patient control), or default (low physician and patient control). Assuming their model is dynamic, the actual expression of the doctor-patient relationship changes as a function of illness stage and needs of the patient.[23] Thus, a shift in physician-patient control may accompany the transition from curative to palliative treatment, and previously well-defined roles may become ambiguous. Role ambiguity and associated discomfort caused by this shift have important implications for communication, particularly in sensitive end-of-life issues. Because roles are ambiguous, each member in the doctor-patient dyad may look to the other for clues as to how to proceed in communication about ADs, CPR, and other decisions to actively limit agressive treatment, with the result that no communication occurs.

Better understanding of the shift in doctor-patient roles when treatment changes from curative to palliative care could reduce discomfort associated with role shifts and foster better communication in the doctor-patient relationship. Attempts cited in the literature have focused on clarifying both the role of the physician and the manner of delivery of information in palliative care.[24] Attention is also being devoted to changing the patient role. Research is beginning to address the question of doctor-patient communication from a patient perspective by determining patient communication style as either active or passive and then teaching the patient to be more direct with his or her healthcare provider in the medical interview.[25] This method, along with other forms of "assertiveness training" could give patients increased role flexibility and encourage more participation in the communication process. However, all patients may not desire a high degree of communication, and physicians should direct initial inquiries into determining the extent to which patients want to be involved in the medical decision-making process. For example, our results indicate that only a small percentage (3%) of people do not want to receive information about ADs, whereas others[26] have found higher proportions (30-41%) of patients who do not want to talk to their doctors about life-support preferences.

The PSDA specifies that procedures must be established to provide information to patients about ADs, but the extent and manner in which this information is disseminated may differ widely among institutions. Although the spirit of the act encourages timely discussion of ADs, literal adherence to the law will more likely involve routine questions asked by admitting clerks (e.g., "Do you have a living will? Would you like to receive in (oration about it?") than establishment of a process to increase doctor-patient discussion. Our results suggest that simply providing written information to patients about ADs and expecting them to actively pursue discussion of this topic with physicians will be inadequate. Over 50% of our sample preferred either face-to-face communication about ADs or discussion along with written information. The lack of an opportunity for physician or medical center-initiated communication may likely result in failure on the part of patients to review materials about ADs received in the admitting department. Research in New York State at Memorial-Sloan Kettering Cancer Center has indicated that legislation can have virtually no impact on patients being admitted with an appropriate resuscitation status.[27] Without active communication about ADs between patients and their physicians, it is likely that the impact of the PSDA on the number of ADs executed will be minimal.

Remediation of communication difficulties should be directed to both physicians and patients, particularly because physicians cannot reliably predict resuscitation preferences of patients.[28,29] Physicians may not ask patients about whether or not they have completed ADs, and patients who have completed them may not inform their physicians,[30] as indicated in the present study. If physicians are aware that patients do not necessarily communicate about their ADs, then physicians may become more vigilant in making requests for this type of information a standard in medical practice.

Assessing physician beliefs about the impact of AD discussions with patients might help identify and challenge inappropriate assumptions regarding the anticipated reactions of patients. Findings of Emmanuel *et al.*[31] suggest a prevalent belief among both patients and physicians that planning for ADs is primarily for older and sicker people. This belief was cited as a barrier to planning for 24% of their sample; however, the manner in which these data were generated did not allow for determination of whether or not 76% actually disagreed with the belief. Further, their results indicated that the younger, healthier people in their sample were actually more interested in discussing and planning ADs than were the older, sicker people. In the present study, this specific belief was assessed systematically and revealed a low percentage of agreement. This finding, which was statistically significant, provides additional support to the findings of Emmanuel *et al.* and suggests that physicians who believe that they should not initiate discussions about ADs with younger and healthier patients may be operating under a false assumption.

Physicians may be reluctant to discuss life-sustaining treatments due to misperceptions about the consequences of initiating these discussions.[32] However, the assumed vulnerability of patients to discussions of ADs has not received empirical support either in past research[33] or in the present study. Although almost half of our sample (44%) believed that discussion of ADs could be depressing and related to thoughts of dying, only a very small percentage (3%) stated that they would not want to receive this information, suggesting that although these discussions may be distressing, patients are still willing to engage in dialogue about ADs with physicians and other hospital personnel. The anticipation of patient distress on the part of the physician should not be used as an excuse for failing to discuss this important topic. Our study and others[34] indicate that beliefs about the impact of AD discussions are indeed important; however, further systematic investigation is needed to precisely determine those beliefs of patients and physicians that interfere with initiation of discussions.

Efforts to improve communication should be directed towards patients as well as physicians. Preliminary findings of experiments conducted by Degner[35] suggest that increasing patient participation results in increased hope, "fighting spirit," and improved quality of life. Most importantly, there was no evidence of harm by increasing patient involvement in the decision-making process.

As the PSDA is implemented, there is a moral necessity to train and empower patients and physicians alike to engage each other in on-going, prospective discussions about treatment and care preferences. Neither physicians nor patients need fear such communications. Indeed, for both groups, this mutual enhancement of patient autonomy carries the potential for mutual benefit to the doctor-patient dyad.

Notes

1. Emmanuel L, Barry M, Stoeckle J, *et al.* Advance directives for medical care--a case for greater use, *New England Journal of Medicine* 1991;324:889-895.
2. Gamble E, McDonald P, Lichstein P. Knowledge, attitudes, and behavior of elderly persons with living wills, *Archives of Internal Medicine* 1991;151:277-80.
3. LaPuma J, Orentlicher D, Moss R. Advance directives on admission: Clinical implications and analysis of the Patient Self-Determination Act of 1990, *Journal of the American Medical Association* 1991;266:402-5.
4. Stolman C, Gregory, J, Dunn D, *et al.* Evaluation of patient, physician, nurse, and family attitudes toward do-not-resuscitate orders, *Archives of Internal Medicine* 1990;150:653-8.
5. Holland J. Clinical course of cancer, In: Holland J, Rowland J, eds. *Handbook of Psychooncology*. New York, NY: Oxford University Press, 1989:75-100.
6. Bedell S, Pelle D, Maher P, *et al.* Do-not-resuscitate orders for critically ill patients in the hospital: How are they used and what is their impact, *Journal of the American Medical Association* 1986; 256:233-7.

7. See note 6. Bedel, *et al.* 1986:233-7.
8. Wilkinson L. *SYSTAT: The system for Statistics*. Evanston, IL: SYSTAT, Inc., 1987.
9. Bruning J, Kintz B. *Computational Handbook of Statistics*. Glenview, IL: Scott, Foresman and Co., 1977
10. Rothman KJ. No adjustments are needed for multiple comparisons, *Epidemiology* 1990;1:43-6.
11. See note 6. Bedell, *et al.* 1986:233-7
12. Lo B, McLeod G, Saika G. Patient attitudes to discussing life-sustaining treatment, *Archives of Internal Medicine* 1986;146:1613-5.
13. Frankl D, Oye R, Bellamy P. Attitudes of hospitalized patients toward life support: A survey of 200 medical inpatients, *American Journal of Medicine* 1989;86;645-8.
14. Seckler A, Meier D, Mulvihill M, *et al.* Substituted judgment: How accurate are proxy predictions? *Annals of Internal Medicine* 1991;115:92-8.
15. Schmerling R, Bedell S, Lilienfeld A, *et al.* Discussing cardiopulmonary resuscitation: A study of elderly outpatients, *Journal of General Internal Medicine* 1988;3:317-21.
16. See note 12. Lo, *et al.* 1986:1613-5.
17. See note 13. Frankl, *et al.* 1989:645-8.
18. See note 14. Seckler, *et al.* 1991:92-98.
19. See note 15. Schmerling, *et al.* 1988:317-21.
20. See note 4. Stolman, *et al.* 1990:653-8.
21. See note 13. Frankl, *et al.* 1989:654-8.
22. Stewart M, Roter D. *Communication with Medical Patients*(Introduction). Newbury Park, CA: Sage Publications, 1989.
23. See note 22, Stewart, Roter 1989.
24. Kinzel T. Relief of emotional symptoms in elderly patients with terminal cancer, *Geriatrics* 1988:43:61-68.
25. Degner L. *Fostering Patient Participation in Treatment Decision-making*, Paper presented at the 1991 International Consensus Conference on Doctor-Patient Communication. Toronto, Canada: Nov. 1991.
26. See note 13. Frankl, *et al.* 1989:645-8.
27. O'Hare D. *DNR orders in New York State*, Paper presented at Controversies in the Care of the Dying Patient Conference. Lake Buena Vista, FL, Feb. 1991.
28. See note 14. Seckler, *et al.* 1991:92-8.
29. Uhlmann R, Peralman R, Cain K. Physicians' and Spouses' predictions of elderly patients resuscitation preferences, *Journal of Gerontology: Medical Sciences* 1988;43:M115-121.
30. See note 3. LaPuma, *et al.* 1991:402-5.
31. See note 1. Emmanuel, *et al.* 1991:889-895.
32. See note 3. LaPuma, *et al.* 1991:402-5.
33. See note 1. Emmanuel, *et al.* 1991:889-895.
34. See note 1. Emmanuel, *et al.* 1991:889-895.
35. See note 25. Degner. 1991.

Chapter 19

Advance Directives and Surrogate Laws: Ethical Instruments or Moral Cop-Out?

Erich H. Loewy

The Patient Self-Determination Act has spawned a great deal of activity by states as well as by hospitals. Advance directives have become firmly established by law, and statutes establishing hierarchies of surrogates have proliferated. Such activities are intended to foster informed patient choice when it comes to end-of-life matters.

Whether, ultimately, they will do this or whether they will, in fact, reduce ethical medical decision-making will depend on the why these instruments and laws are used. In this article, I caution against the almost unbridled enthusiasm with which these steps have been greeted. Whether health care professionals will use these instruments to enhance dialogue and to see choice as being made not only by and for individuals, but by and for individuals who are meshed in community remains to be seen.

The federal Patient Self-Determination Act (PSDA), which became effective in December 1991, has spawned a rash of legislation in the several states. In an effort to comply with the PSDA as well as with the state acts, hospitals have rather hurriedly begun to assess ways and means of implementing these acts. Legislation at the state level has been aimed not only at supporting the PSDA, but also at extending it, as when states such as Illinois passed a surrogate act that determines the general hierarchy of surrogates for patients who become incompetent or unconscious and who have not executed an advance directive for themselves. The fear of being at the mercy of either crass medical or crass legal paternalism stimulated the PSDA and its offspring. It was aimed at giving patients legitimate choices when it comes to their own end-of life decisions.[1]

There would seem to be few reasons to quibble with such an attempt: All of us want to exercise control over our own destiny and want to have a chance to finish our own "work of art" in our own way. Our particular way of living, of valuing and of envisioning our destiny and, therefore, our own style, is unique to us. We are, as Cassell[2] pointed out some time ago, the artists of our own life.[2] As good a composer as Mahler may have been, he would have found it difficult to complete Schubert's "Unfinished Symphony" in Schubert's own way, just as Van Gogh would have had difficulty completing a Rembrandt self-portrait in a way that would have pleased Rembrandt. The passage of the PSDA and the attempts in several states to bolster and extend it should therefore be expected to be embraced with open arms.

I do not want to downplay the importance of these various attempts to give patients more control over their own destiny. Such a move is a long-overdue acknowledgment of the fact that there are other than what the profession generally sees as "strictly medical"

Source: Reprinted from *Archives of Internal Medicine*, Vol. 152, Oct. 92, pp. 1973-1976, with permission from American Medical Association © 1992.

considerations that must enter into making choices at the bedside. The fact that such considerations are of great importance to medical practice has been acknowledged by compassionate and thoughtful physicians since medicine first began to be practiced, but it frequently has not been acted on, especially in this century. And yet, I want to introduce a word of caution. I fear that the generally enthusiastic reception that the PSDA (and the whole notion of advance directives), as well as other laws establishing a hierarchy of surrogates, has been given may be motivated less by a genuine respect for actual informed patient choice than by the feeling that physicians and hospitals now need not trouble themselves in making truly critical and sometimes agonizing decisions. On the whole, advance directives and acts such as the Illinois Surrogate Act, by producing some order in a legally chaotic situation, give some legal protection to physicians and hospitals. Giving such protection, if the shield of protection is used wisely and responsibly, may be an ethically good thing. It may, on the one hand, encourage physician communication and enable patient choice; but, on the other hand, the protection given by this law may be used by institutions and physicians to distance themselves all too easily from a particular patient's particular situation by taking refuge in a generic rule. Medicine does not want to throw out the baby of genuine and ethical caring with the bathwater of physician paternalism.[3]

The way physicians, as well as society, have seen medical obligations has changed over time. In ancient times, and up to the time of Newton and Bacon, the obligation to save life was not conceived to be a medical obligation. Rather, the threefold obligations of ameliorating suffering, of helping nature restore function or health, and of refraining from treating those "hopelessly overcome by illness" were accepted.[4] Despite Hippocrates' personal feeling that love for medicine is not possible without love for patients, medical ethics during Hippocratic times was an "ethic of outward performance" in which the concern of medicine was not primarily to help patients for the sake of helping others, but to help patients so that the reputation and standing of medicine could be kept high?[5] It was only later, and only briefly, when Scribonius Largus, in the first work on professional ethics that we would today recognize as patient-centered ethics, spoke of and accepted an "ethic of inward intention," one in which physicians performed "a good act of healing in the face of illness"[6] primarily to benefit patients themselves.[5,7,8] During those times and up to the very present, however, medicine continued to be a predominantly paternalistic profession in which pursuing as well as defining the patient's good was accepted by all as the profession' s task. Even when, after Newton and Bacon, medicine progressively concerned itself with treating those "who were overcome with illness" (at first mainly to learn from them, later to benefit them), and as it became a more and more "scientific" enterprise, paternalism remained the order of the day.[4] Physicians defined what was proper and chose what to do; patients "complied."

In this century, and stimulated by a capitalist philosophy in which autonomy is the highest good and beneficence only a very questionable general obligation, physicians have more and more been seen as entrepreneurs. Patients have been transformed into consumers; and physicians, into "bureaucrats of health."[9,10] Indeed, the physician as entrepreneur and the "medical-industrial complex" (a term coined, but a concept hardly thought appropriate, by Relman[11]) interested in pursuing profit have been touted as the proper basis of medical morality.[10] Market forces and competition would see to it that the best possible care at the lowest possible cost would be supplied to alert and freely contracting consumers. Such an ethic, of course, returns us once again to one of "outward performance." Physicians perform "a good act of healing in the face of illness" (and at the lowest possible cost) not as much to benefit patients as to attract more customers to themselves.[3] Such a philosophy must, of course, rest on the assumption that patients and physicians are truly "equal contractors." If patients and physicians are, indeed, equal contractors and patients employ their physicians for a specific self-chosen act of healing, then adhering blindly and in lockstep fashion to advance directives makes sense.

I want to be clearly understood: I do not want to return the profession to a time when crass paternalism was the order of the day. There is still too much of this abroad. But neither do I want to see the profession surrendering (and surrendering gladly) its basic and ultimate responsibility: a responsibility that we have come to accept as transcending the technical. The concept of physicians as "bureaucrats of health" who (no matter how well) perform a technical task does not foster true autonomy; true autonomy, which implies freedom of choice, is possible only when patients and physicians act jointly. Advance directives can help bring about situations in which a dialogue between physician and patient is improved, or they can bring about a situation in which physicians and health care institutions abrogate their responsibility and justify this abrogation by a mere obeisance to the concept of autonomy.

Advance directives, properly used to foster true patient autonomy, have much to recommend them. Among other things, they can: (1) stimulate patients to think about such issues; (2) allow patients to speak about their preferences with their physician, their relatives, and their friends; (3) permit patients either to express their wishes or to select a trusted other who can make choices for them; and (4) help resolve some of the fears of entrapment by the medical system. All of these advantages, however, imply leadership by health care professionals who must carefully inform, discuss, listen to, and ultimately counsel and advise patients and their families. When done properly, this should (at first, but perhaps not ultimately) take more, rather than less, time.

I fear that advance directives are often not quite used in this way. Ideally, advance directives stimulate dialogue between health care givers and their patients so that patients can truly become more (even if not completely) equal partners (I deplore the word contractor: physicians are, after all, not plumbers!). When patients execute advance directives without extensive discussion with trusted health care providers, they often make choices that are motivated by unrealistic fears. These fears are often created and played on by the media, which have exaggerated and distorted reality.

A patient's understanding of what is to be done (What is cardiopulmonary resuscitation? Why are ventilators used?, is often quite meager when he or she signs such directives and it is properly the physician's task to see that this is not the case. When, for example, patients insist that they "would never want to be on a ventilator," it is the physicians task to explain what a ventilator entails. Ventilators, after all, can be used temporarily (as in anesthesia or to tide a patient over a bout of severe pneumonia) or permanently (as when a patient with chronic lung disease finally becomes entirely and permanently ventilator dependent), or they can, and quit, properly so, be used as a comfort measure. When patients decline cardiopulmonary resuscitation or intubation, similar careful explanations are in order. Such explanations must delve into some of the details of what is proposed; they must address the patients' understanding or misunderstanding of what is involved; and they must deal with the patients' impressions and fears. Patients often believe (and, regrettably, so do physicians) that once a procedure or a course of therapy is started it cannot be stopped. It is frequently not so much their opposition to being on a ventilator, to being intubated, or to undergoing cardiopulmonary resuscitation as their fear that if the outcome is not what is hoped for, therapy must come what may, be continued. Patients do, not, as they understand it, want to commit themselves to being permanently ventilator bound or to living on in a severely mentally reduced fashion, and, given the alternatives as they see them, they are simply not willing to "give it a shot." Alleviating such fears, and often helping patients to clarify such conditions in an advance directive, may help to clarify the situation. A blanket statement that "I would never want a ventilator used" (or to be resuscitated or intubated) is hardly one that ought to be accepted without careful and repeated explanation.

The patients' fears and their frequent misunderstanding of medical facts point out the fallacy in the doctrine of "equal contractors": When one party to a bargain is fearful and when his or her technical information and understanding is sketchy or distorted, while the other party has no fear and has information and understanding that are more accurate equality does not truly exist. This calls into question the very basis of equality on which entrepeneurialism is founded the claim that physician and patient meet as equal contractors to make and carry out choices. Looking at patients as "equal partners" gives rise to the danger of inequality being exaggerated owing to the circumvention of explanation and dialogue. Instead of fostering autonomy, it very well may do the opposite: patients will be free to make choices but will not truly understand the implication of the choices they make. The inequality of patient and physician, while it cannot be entirely eliminated, can be attenuated and individually addressed. Physicians who truly subscribe to meaningful patient autonomy (as I do) will be ethically compelled to do all they can to lessen this difference and to restore their patients autonomy.[12]

The fallacy of equal contractors likewise explains why stimulating competition and relying on the market to decrease medical costs and increase medical quality have simply not worked. For the reasons given, and others as well, patients cannot truly and freely select the type of health care they want the same way they select pear, shoes, or automobiles. Not only is it much easier to know what kind of pear, shoe, or automobile I want, and at what price, but if I make a wrong choice my life is not threatened. I do not, so to speak, make such choices "under the gun." Since the theory of equal contractors is a fallacy when it comes to selecting medical care, the market, as we have, to our regret, come to find out, neither reduces costs nor improves quality.

Patients have become increasingly more distrustful of the entire medical establishment, albeit somewhat less so of their own particular physician. (This is somewhat akin to polls that how that citizens mistrust Congress but tend to trust their own representative.) Advance directives are, in part, an expression and outcome of such distrust. This distrust is not entirely unjustified. When physicians see themselves as entrepreneurs whose chief interest (and whose chief legitimate interest according to some) is in accumulating as much material gain as possible, when they own and are known to own laboratories and free-standing surgical or x-ray clinics, and when they are, known to derive excessive profit from a practice whose conditions only they themselves can control, trust is not apt to be greatly enhanced. This is especially true since layman: (1) know perfectly well that they have little chance of truly understanding what is and what is not needed and (2) suspect (and often with good reason) that physicians are apt to profit greatly from the suggestions made. Patients fear not unreasonably if entrepeneurialism is indeed a proper basis for medical morality exploitation by an establishment for its own financial purposes. Furthermore, in our system of medical care, in which insurance is often either nonexistent or totally inadequate when it is needed most, patients fear pauperization by a basically entrepreneurial system that is only to eager to treat them until their last, or their family's last, penny is gone.

In some states (Illinois is an example), a new act prescribes a hierarchy of surrogates to be used when no advance directives exist. Starting with spouses, these acts specify a hierarchy of persons to be consulted. Such persons have acceptable legal standing in making decisions. The theory on which these laws are based is laudable: the person most apt to understand the patient' s style is to make the decision. This, even if by proxy, would foster the patient's ultimate autonomy and would permit each patient to finish his or her "work of art." There is a severe fallacy in such a law: regrettably one's spouse is not under all circumstances the person closest to one (a man who has been estranged from his wife for 5 years and who is now living with someone else is unlikely to appreciate such a choice!). Families do not, in reality, always exist exactly as the law envisions.

Physicians and hospitals have expressed considerable enthusiasm for this surrogate act: it would allow them to receive direction from a legally stipulated person. If the rules were followed, the chance of malpractice suits would, in theory be remote. Furthermore, it is hoped by some physicians that the time used in talking with or arbitrating among many family members could be greatly reduced. In my view, however, it remains the physician's responsibility to ascertain that the legally stipulated surrogate is, indeed, ethically acceptable: that he or she is the person most apt to make the choices that the patient himself or herself would have made. This means far more than following a convenient hierarchical list in lockstep fashion. It implies becoming familiar with a patient's biography as well as with the nexus of relationships in which the patient was and is enmeshed. An attempt to superimpose a given vision of how families "ought to be" on the way a given family in fact is, is to negate personal as well as family autonomy. Discussing possible surrogates with patients, noting the particular personal relations and arrangements, and documenting them in the medical record may greatly serve to promote the patient's good and may, in a much truer sense, foster meaningful autonomy. Choosing the proper surrogate is not materially different from choosing the proper antibiotic: textbooks may indicate that my patient's strep throat should be treated with penicillin but for me to do so without inquiring as to whether that patient is allergic to penicillin would be considered to be malpractice. Likewise, choosing a surrogate (merely because he or she is the "textbook surrogate") is acceptable only when such a generalization is focused on the individual patient and circumstance. Physicians cannot, in attempting to answer ethical or technical questions, turn their judgment over to a neat algorithm and feel that their job is done.

Explanation and dialogue remain critical if a decision made by a surrogate (whether the surrogate is picked by reference to a legally established list or in a somewhat more responsible way) is to be accepted as a proper choice. The process of informing surrogates and engaging in dialog with them, just as that of informing and engaging in dialog with patients who are exerting advanced directives, ultimately remains the physician's responsibility.

Decisions can only be made with proper knowledge and understanding of the medical facts, of prognostic realities, and of possible goals and options. Decisions are not likely to be properly made on the spur of the moment or under the stress of acute illness, fear, and/or pain. Having patients execute an instrument or surrogates make decisions under such conditions (or having them execute such a document without careful deliberation or adequate discussion with those closest to them) may be legally acceptable but is, at the very least, ethically problematic. Having patients execute such documents as part of the hospital admitting process (together with signing a laundry list, providing insurance information, or the telephone number of their aunt) or having them execute such documents a bit later on the ward, but still while hurried, fearful, ill, and, in that sense, coerced makes a sham of the document's value or intent. Executing documents in such a perfunctory or hasty fashion allows the health care team, the hospital administration, and perhaps even society at large to "cop out," to abandon a patient to his or her autonomy, and then to wash their hands of the whole problem, as bureaucrats of health might be encouraged to do."

Last, but not least, advanced directives are executed and choices are made in a community. The interests of family and community are not irrelevant to the decision being made. We are not, as some would have it, "moral strangers"[13] who share no ethical framework and have no common interests or values except the interest to be let alone to pursue our own autonomous choices. Such a minimalist vision of community or of medical practice raptures the tradition of medicine that, albeit paternalistic, claimed to have, and in fact did have, acknowledged beneficent obligations. The vision of community as being composed of such moral strangers is as impoverished as it is false. We are all (whether Americans, Europeans, or Fiji Indians) united by certain inescapable common conditions and interests and, therefore, certain basic values and basic moral framework. We share (thanks to what Kant[14] calls our "common structure of the mind") a common sense of basic logic. Beyond this, however, we are, at the very least, united by a desire to avoid suffering (even when what causes suffering many be different), to pursue our own interests and goals, and, as social animals, to realize ourselves in the embrace of others.[15,16] That may not get us very far toward being moral intimates, but it is a far cry from being moral strangers. While perhaps not moral intimates or even friends, persons are, at the very least, moral acquaintances.[17] As moral acquaintances, we make such decisions knowing quite a few basic things about each other; we respect the basic features that unite us, as well as respecting the uniqueness of each of us that goes beyond such commonalities.

People are social beings, and because they are, they have obligations toward each other. Autonomy does not exist in a vacuum but is developed, enunciated, and ultimately exercised in the embrace of others. To deny the social nexus of autonomy is threatening both to the social nexus and to autonomy. Persons cannot truly exist outside their social nexus or, ultimately, outside their community; in turn, the social nexus and the community cannot develop, thrive, grow, or function without the unique contributions of the individuals within it.[17] When it comes to making decisions for oneself (whether for the here and now or for the distant or not so distant future), one must be mindful of this interdependence. To require families (or communities) to make such decisions totally setting aside any self-interest, or to allow such decisions to be made entirely unmindful of the needs and interests of the community in which such decisions are to be made, is to rip such decisions from the soil that spawned them.

As with all else, the way that advance directives and laws appointing a hierarchy of surrogates are used will determine the merit of the procedure. Medicine has been guilty of crass paternalism, to which such legal instruments are seen as a remedy. Such paternalism (even when in the name of beneficence) was a form of totalitarian control akin to the misuse of alleged beneficence by the Soviet state. Jumping from the frying pan of such a system into the fire of an entrepreneurial system in which consumers freely contract with "bureaucrats" and in which bureaucrats feel no responsibility for caring about patients, but feel responsible merely for adhering to their clients' previously expressed wishes will not improve the matter. Our worship of autonomy and our neglect of beneficence has led to devastating social conditions in this country, a situation to which the 20% of the population who have little, if any, access to timely medical care bear witness. Beneficence implies respect for autonomy: one cannot be truly beneficent without respecting the goals and wishes of another.[18] But having respect for autonomy means more than leaving persons to their own freely chosen fate. Socially, true autonomy outside the context of socks justice is cynical mockery (freedom of speech is of little use to a homeless or hungry person): it implies social justice so that all may enjoy their autonomy. Medically, respect for physician involvement: it implies that physicians genuinely seek to remain in dialogue with their patients and take great care in selecting proper (ethical) surrogates. It is a form of focused physician beneficence: beneficence that is focused on promoting the patient's individual choice and integrating it into the patient's family and community. Beyond this, having respect for autonomy implies a respect for the community without which autonomy is moot. Patients, just as physicians, have responsibilities: responsibilities that transcend cooperating with their physicians only to further their own personal ends. Patients and physicians are not "moral strangers," but are travelers on it perilous journey in a community. In making decisions for patients, the goals, values, and interests of all are legitimate considerations. Advance directives can, if used properly, be vehicles through which dialogue is started and continued or if used improperly, they can foil dialogue and make a mockery of what they were intended to do: to allow an expression of autonomy in the context of others and of the community.

Notes

1. McCloskey EL. Hopes for the PSDA, *Journal of Clinical Ethics* 1991;2:172-173.
2. Cassell EJ. Life as a work of art, *Hasting Center Report* 1984;14:35-37.
3. Loewy EH. Advance directives: A question of patient autonomy, *Cambridge Quaterly* In press.
4. Amundsen DW. The physician's obligation to prolong life: A medical duty without classical roots, *Journal of the History of Medicine* 1977;32:403-421.
5. Edelstein L. The professional ethics of the Greek physician, *Bulletin on the History of Medicine* 1956;30:391-419.
6. Pellegrino ED. Toward a reconstruction of medical morality: The primacy of the act of profession and the fact of illness, *Journal of Medicine and Philosophy* 1979;4:32-55
7. Deichgraber K. Professio medici: Zum vorwort des scribonius largus, *Abh Akad Mainz* 1950;9:856-862.
8. Hamilton JS. Scribonius Largus on the medical profession, *Bulletin on the History of Medicine* 1986;60:209-216.
9. Engelhardt HT. *The Foundations of Bioethics*. New York, NY: Oxford University Press Inc, 1986.
10. Engelhardt HT. Morality for the medical industrial complex: A code of ethics for mass marketing of health care, *New England Journal of Medicine* 1988;319:1086-1089.
11. Relman AS. The new medical-industrial complex, *New England Journal of Medicine* 1980;303:963-970.
12. Cassell EJ. The function of medicine, *Hastings Center Report* 1977;7:16-19.
13. Englhardt HT. *Bioethics and Secular Humanism*. Philadelphia, PA: Trinity Press International, 1991.
14. Kant I. *Kritik der reinen vernunft*. Frankfort am Main, Germany: Suhrkamp, 1984.
15. Loewy EH. The role of suffering and community in clinical ethics, *Journal of Clinical Ethics* 1991;2:83-89.
16. Loewy EH. *Suffering and the Beneficent Community: Beyond Libertarianism*. Albany, NY: SUNY Press, 1991.
17. Loewy EH. *Freedo and Community: The Ethics of Interrelationships*. Albany, NY: SUNY Press, In press.
18. Pellegrino ED, Thomasma DC. *For the Patient's Good: The Restoration of Beneficence in Health Care*. New York, NY: Oxford University Press Inc, 1988.

Chapter 20

Is Truth Telling to the Patient a Cultural Artifact?

Edmund D. Pellegrino

In a 1992 issue of *JAMA*, Antonella Surbone, M.D., describes her dilemma in trying to transfer the ideals of medical ethics she learned in the United States to her native Italy.[1] In the United States, she found truth-telling and respect for autonomy have become virtual moral absolutes. On the other hand, in Italy, families and physicians often shield patients from painful truths and difficult decisions. Dr. Surbone points out, what is beneficent in one country may seem maleficent in the other.

This contrast in moral perspectives, of course, is not unique to the differences between Italy and North America. It has become a world-wide problem as newer models of medical ethics nurtured in the individualistic soil of North America are introduced to other countries with different moral traditions.[2] But similar contrasts may exist within a country, for example, between northern and southern Italy, or between the multiple ethnic groups in the United States.[3] Everywhere, as cultural groups attain freedom of expression, physicians, and patients must relate with each other across ethical barriers especially with respect to the importance of autonomy.

These contrasts raise some provocative questions: Is medical ethics a cultural artifact such that a universal medical ethic is not viable? How should physicians dedicated to the best interests of their patients conduct therapeutic relationships with patients whose cultural values differ materially from their own?

These questions invite a critical re-examination of the foundation and meaning of autonomy and its relationships with truth telling. Such reflection suggests that autonomy is not, and cannot be unequivocally interpreted. Some of the dilemma is more superficial than real and derives from a narrow interpretation of the concept of autonomy.

Autonomy entered medical ethics as part of a system of *prima facie* principles devised to deal with moral pluralism. *Prima facie* principles such as autonomy, non-maleficence, beneficence, and justice are those that ought to be respected unless powerful reasons for overriding them can be adduced.[4,5] In this system, each principle is given equal weight. Priorities among principles can be established only when the detailed circumstances of a particular decision are known. No principle, including autonomy, is granted *a priori* moral hegemony over the others.

The principle of autonomy is grounded in respect for persons and the acknowledgement that as rational beings one of our unique capabilities is for reasoned choices. Through these choices we plan and live lives for which we are morally accountable. Inhibiting an individual's capability to make these personal choices is a violation of his or her integrity as a person and thus a maleficent act.

Source: Reprinted from *Journal of the American Medicine Association*, Vol. 263, No. 13, pp. 1734-1735, with permission from American Medical Association © Oct. 1992.

Autonomy, therefore, is not in fundamental opposition with beneficence as is too often supposed, but in congruence with it. Problems arise when the content of what is beneficent is defined by others such as family members or physicians. This may be warranted when we are mentally incompetent, when our choices harm others, or when we make choices that contravene good medical practice or harm us seriously. In the absence of these limitations competent humans are owed the freedom to define beneficence in terms of their own values. This does not mean that all values are morally equivalent or defensible, but only that as humans we are owed respect for the choices we voluntarily make.

In North America, in the United States in particular, autonomy has tended to become a moral absolute. The reasons for this are multiple. They include improved education of the public, a strong tradition of privacy rights and personal liberty, distrust of authority and the possibilities of medical technology, and the loosening of family and community identification. In this context, truth telling is a necessary corollary, since human capability for autonomous choices cannot function if truth is withheld, falsified, or otherwise manipulated. Truth telling is essential to informed consent, the instrument whereby personal autonomy is expressed in concrete decisions.

Respect for autonomy and truth telling are intrinsic to beneficent medical care for many people in the North American context. It does not follow, however, that this concept of autonomy is always beneficent or that it must be accepted by, or imposed on, everyone living in the United States or elsewhere.

For one thing, autonomous patients are free to use their autonomy as they see fit -- even to delegate it when this fits their own concept of beneficence. Some patients need a more authoritative approach than others. This approach is legitimate when, for example, despite efforts to inform and empower patients to make their own decisions, patients find themselves unable or unwilling to cope with choices. Such patients may feel sincerely that a close friend or family member would be able to make decisions that better protect their values than they could make themselves. Such a delegation of decision-making authority may be explicit or implicit depending on the dominant ethos.

In some parts of Italy, among many ethnic groups in the United States, and in large parts of the world, this delegation of authority is culturally implicit. In such contexts, the uniformity of the practice suggests that delegation of decision-making is an expectation of the sick person that need not be explicit. To thrust the truth or the decision on a patient who expects to be buffered against news of impending death is a gratuitous and harmful misinterpretation of the moral foundations for respect for autonomy. In many cultures clinicians encounter patients who are fully aware of the gravity of their condition but choose to play out the drama in their own way. This may include not discussing the full or obvious truth. This is a form of autonomy, if it is implicitly and mutually agreed upon between doctor and patient. Hoever, autonomy should not be violated by a misconceived attempt to be morally rigorous. Withholding the truth from the patient demands, of course, the utmost care in responding to any occasion when the patient wishes to exert more control.

Among most North American physicians, the withholding of truth, in whole or in part, is a therapeutic privilege accepted as morally licit when we have substantial evidence that offering the patient the truth has a significant probability of causing harm, e.g., emotional damage or suicide. This "privilege" must be used rarely and with utmost care since it is so easily abused.

Treating patients within the conception of beneficence defined by their own cultural ideas is a form of therapeutic privilege. However, a palpable risk of harm in knowing the truth that must exist that must not be outweighed by the risk of withholding the truth. The amount, manner, and timing of truth telling or true withholding are crucial factors for which there is no ready formula.

This autonomy cannot be an absolute principle with *a priori* precedence over other *prima facie* principles. Rather, the judicious exercise of respect for autonomy means that health professionals must act in a manner enables and empowers patients to make decisions and act in a way that is most in accord with their values.

That the patient may draw these values from the circumambient culture does not make autonomy or medical ethics a cultural artifact. Autonomy is still a valid and universal principle because it is based in what it is to be human. The patient must decide how much autonomy he or she wishes to exercise; this can vary from culture to culture.

It seems probable that the democratic ideals that lie behind the contemporary North American concept of autonomy will spread and that something close to it will be the choice of many individuals in other countries. What then does the physician do when a society is in transition as Dr. Surbone suggests is the case in Italy today, or when many different cultures make up one society as is the case in the United States? To preserve both autonomy and beneficence, physicians must get to know their patients well enough to discern when, and if, those patients wish to contravene the mores of prevailing medical culture. This requires a degree of familiarity and sensitivity increasingly difficult to come by, but morally inescapable for every physician who practices in today's morally and culturally diverse world society.

Notes

1. Surbone A. Truth telling to the patient, *Journal of the American Medical Association* 1992;268:1661-1662.
2. Pellegrino ED, Mazzarella P, Corsi P, eds. *Transcultural Dimensions in Medical Ethics*. Frederick, MD: University Publishing Group, In press.
3. Flack HE, Pellegrino ED, eds. *African-American Perspectives on Biomedical Ethics*. Washington, DC: Georgetown University Press, 1992.
4. Beauchamp TL, Childress JF. *Principles of Bioethics*. 3rd Edition. New York, NY: Oxford University Press, 1989.
5. Ross WD. *The Right and the Good*. Indianapolis, IN: Hackett Publishing Company, 1988:33-34.

Chapter 21

Voluntary Risks to Health: The Ethical Issues

Robert M. Veatch

The discovery that health status is affected by personal life-styles and apparently voluntary health risks poses new problems. It has potential impact on clinical practice, health insurance, and theories of health and disease. Five major problems need attention. First, are these health-risk behaviors really voluntary? Five responses are explored: several other models (the medical, psychological, social structural, and multicausal models) all challenge the assumption of voluntary behavior. Second, are some sufficiently in the public interest that they ought to be subsidized? Third, does justice require that persons bear the costs of truly voluntary health risks? Fourth, what policies should apply to cost-saving, health-risk behavior? Finally, does the voluntary health-risks theme make life too rational and calculating? These issues must be dealt with in future health planning and clinical decision making(*JAMA* 243:50-55, 1980).

In an earlier era, one's health was thought to be determined by the gods or by fate. The individual had little responsibility for personal health. In terms of the personal responsibility for health and disease, the modern medical model has required little change in this view. One of the primary elements of the medical model was the belief that people were exempt from responsibility for their condition.[1] If one had good health in old age, from the vantage point of the belief system of the medical model, one would say he had been blessed with good health. Disease was the result of mysterious, uncontrollable microorganisms or the random process of genetic fate.

A few years ago we developed a case study[2] involving a purely hypothetical proposal that smokers should be required to pay for the costs of their extra health care required over and above that of nonsmokers. The scheme involved taxing tobacco at a rate calculated to add to the nation's budget an amount equal to the marginal health cost of smoking.

Recently a number of proposals have been put forth that imply that individuals are in some sense personally responsible for the state of their health. The town of Alexandria, Va, refuses to hire smokers as fire fighters, in part because smokers increase the cost of health and disability insurance (*The New York Times*, Dec 18, 1977, p 28). Oral Roberts University insists that students meet weight requirements to attend school. Claiming that the school was concerned about the whole person, the school dean said that the school was just as concerned about the students' physical growth as their intellectual and spiritual growth (*The New York Times*, Oct 9, 1977, p 77). Behaviors as highly diverse as smoking, skiing, playing professional football, compulsive eating, omitting exercise, exposing oneself excessively to the sun, skipping needed immunizations, automobile racing, and mountain climbing all can be viewed as having a substantial voluntary component. Health care needed as a result of any voluntary behavior

---

Source: Reprinte from *The Journal of the American Medical Association*, Vol. 243, No. 1, pp. 50-55, with permission from The American Medical Association © Jan, 1980.

might generate very different claims on a health care system from care conceptualized as growing out of some other causal nexus. Keith Reemtsma, MD, chairman of the Department of Surgery at Columbia University's College of Physicians and Surgeons, has called for "a more rational approach to improving national health," involving "a reward/punishment system based on individual choices." Persons who smoked cigarettes, drank whiskey, drove cars, and owned guns would be taxed for the medical consequences of their choices (*The New York Times*, Oct 14, 1976, p 37). That individuals should be personally responsible for their health is a new theme, implying a new model for health care and perhaps for funding of health care.[3,4,5,6]

Some data correlating life-style to health status are being generated. They seem to support the conceptual shift toward a model that sees the individual as more personally responsible for his health status. The data of Belloc and Breslow[7,8,9] make those of us who lead the slovenly life-style very uncomfortable. As Morison[3] has pointed out, John Wesley and his puritan brothers of the covenant may not have been far from wrong after all. Belloc and Breslow identify seven empirical correlates of good health: eating moderately, eating regularly, eating breakfast, no cigarette smoking, moderate or no use of alcohol, at least moderate exercise, and seven to eight hours of sleep nightly. They all seem to be well within human control, far less mysterious than the viruses and genes that exceed the comprehension of the average citizen. The authors found that the average physical health of persons aged 70 years who reported all of the preceding good health practices was about the same as persons aged 35 to 44 year who reported fewer than three.

We have just begun to realize that policy implications and the ethical impact of the conceptual shift that begins viewing health status as, in part, a result of voluntary risk taking in personal behavior and life-style choices. If individuals are responsible to some degree for their health and their need for health resources, why should they not also be responsible for the costs involved? If national health insurance is on the horizon, it will be even more questionable that individuals should have such health care paid for out of the same money pool generated by society to pay for other kinds of health care. Even with insurance plans, is it equitable that all persons contributing to the insurance money pool pay the extra costs of those who voluntarily run the risk of increasing their need for medical services?

The most obvious policy proposals -- banning from the health care system risky behaviors and persons who have medical needs resulting from such risks -- turns out to be the least plausible.[10,11] For one thing, it is going to be extremely difficult to establish precisely the cause of the lung tumor at the time the patient is standing at the hospital door. Those who have carcinoma of the lung possibly from smoking or from unknown causes should not be excluded.

Even if the voluntary component of the cause could be determined, it is unlikely that our society could or would choose, to implement a policy of barring the doors. While we have demonstrated a capacity to risk statistical lives or to risk the lives of citizens with certain socioeconomic characteristics, it is unlikely that we would be prepared to follow an overall policy of refusing medical service to those who voluntarily brought on their own conditions. We fought a similar battle over social security and concluded that -- in part for reasons of the stress placed on family members and on society as a whole -- individuals would not be permitted to take the risk of staying outside the social security system.

A number of policy options are more plausible. Additional health fees on health-risk behavior calculated to reimburse the health care system would redistribute the burden of the cost of such care to those who have chosen to engage in it. Separating health insurance pools for persons who engage in health-risk behavior and requiring them to pay out of pocket the marginal cost of their health care is another alternative. In some cases the economic cost is not the critical factor; it may be scarce personnel or equipment. Some behaviors might have to be banned to free the best neurosurgeon or orthopedic specialists for those who need their services for reasons other than for injuries suffered from the motorcycle accident or skiing tumble.

Of course, all of these policy options require not only judgments about whether these behaviors are truly voluntary, but also ethical judgments about the rights and responsibilities of the individual and the other, more social components of the society.

There are several ethical principles that could lead us to be concerned about these apparently voluntary behaviors and even lead us to justify decisions to change our social policy about paying for or providing health care needed as a result of such behavior. The most obvious, the most traditional, medical ethical basis for concern is that the welfare of the individual is at stake. The Hippocratic tradition is committed to having the physician do what he thinks will benefit the patient. If one were developing an insurance policy or a mode of approaching the individual patient; not private practice, paternalistic concern about the medical welfare of the patient might lead to a conclusion that, for the good of the patient, this behavior ought to be prevented or deferred. The paternalistic Hippocratic ethic, however, is suspect in circles outside the medical profession and is even coming under attack from within the physician community itself.[12] The Hippocratic ethic leaves no room for the principle of self-determination -- a principle at the core of liberal Western thought. The freedom of choice to smoke, ski, and even race automobiles may well justify avoiding more coercive policies regarding these behaviors -- assuming that it is the individual's own welfare that is at stake. The hyperindividualistic ethics of Hippocratism also leaves no room for concern for the welfare of others or the distribution of burdens with the society. A totally different rationale for concern is being put forward, however. Some, such as Tom Beauchamp,[13] have argued that we have a right to be concerned about such behaviors because of their social costs. He leaves unanswered the question of why it would be considered fair or just to regulate these voluntary behaviors when and only when their total social costs exceed the total social benefits of the behavior. This is a question we must explore.

Clearly, the argument is a complex one requiring many empirical, conceptual, and ethical judgments. Those judgments will have to be made regardless of whether we decide to continue the present policy or adopt one of the proposed alternatives. At this point, we need a thorough statement of the kinds of questions that must be addressed and the types of judgments that must be made.

Are Health Risks Voluntary? The first question, addressed to those advocating policy shifts based on the notion that persons are in some sense responsible for their own health, melds the conceptual and empirical issues. Are health risks voluntary? Several models are competing for the conceptual attention of those working in the field.

The Voluntary Model

The model that considers the individual as personally responsible for his health has a great deal going for it. The empirical correlations of life-style choices with health status are impressive. The view of humans as personally responsible for their destiny is attractive to those of us within modern Western society. Its appeal extends beyond the view of the human as subject to the forces of fate and even the medical model, which as late as the 1950s saw disease as an attack on the individual coming from outside the person and outside his control.

The Medical Model

Of course, that it is attractive cannot justify opting for the voluntarist model if it flies in the face of the empirical reality. The theory of external and uncontrollable causation is central to the medical model.[14] It is still probably the case that organic causal chains almost totally outside human control account now and then for a disease. But the medical model has been under such an onslaught of reality testing in the last decade that it can hardly provide a credible alternative to the voluntarist model. Even for those conditions that undeniably have an organic causal component, the luxury of human innocence is no longer a plausible defense against human accountability. The more we learn about disease and health and their causal chains, the more we have the possibility of intervening to change those chains of causation. Since the days of the movement for public health, sanitation, and control of contagion, there has been a rational basis for human responsibility. Even for those conditions that do not yet lend themselves to such direct voluntary control, the chronic diseases and even genetic diseases, there exists the possibility of purposeful, rational decisions that have an indirect impact on the risk. Choices can be made to minimize our exposure to potential carcinogens and risk factors for cardiovascular disease. Parents now have a variety of potential choices to minimize genetic disease risk and even eliminate it in certain cases. We may not be far from the day when we can say that all health problems can be viewed as someone's fault-if not our own fault for poor sanitary practices and lifestyle choices, then the fault of our parents for avoiding carrier status diagnosis, amniocentesis, and selective abortion; the fault of industries that pollute our environment; or the fault of the National Institutes of Health for failing to make the scientific breakthroughs to understand the causal chain so that we could intervene. Although there remains a streak of plausibility in the medical model as an account of disease and health, it is fading rapidly and may soon remain only as a fossil-like trace in our model of health.

The Psychological Model

While the medical model seems to offer at best a limited counter to the policy options rooted in the voluntarist model, other theories of determinism may be more plausible. Any policy to control health care services that are viewed as necessitated by voluntary choices to risk one's health is based on the judgment that the behavior is indeed voluntary. The primary argument countering policies to tax or control smoking to be fair in distributing the burdens for treating smokers health problems is that the smoker is not really responsible for his medical problems. The argument is not normally based on organic or genetic theories of determinism, but on more psychological theories. The smoker's personality and even the initial pattern of smoking are developed at such an early point in life that they could be viewed as beyond voluntary control. If the smoker's behavior is the result of toilet training rather than rational decision-making, then to blame the smoker for the toilet training seems odd.

Many of the other presumably voluntary risks to health might also be seen as psychologically determined and therefore not truly voluntary. Compulsive eating, the sedentary lifestyle, and the choice of a high-stress life pattern may all be psychologically determined.

Football playing is a medically risky behavior. For the professional, the choice seems to be made consciously and voluntarily. But the choice to participate in high school and even grade school competitive leagues may not really be the voluntary choice of the student. Then, if reward systems are generated from these early choices, certainly college level football could be the result. The continuum from partially nonvoluntary choices of the youngster to the career choice of professional athlete may have a heavy psychological overlay after all.

If so-called voluntary health risks are really psychologically determined, then the ethical and policy implications collapse. But it must seriously be questioned whether the model of psychological determinism is a much more plausible monocausal explanation of these behaviors than the medical model. Choosing to be a professional football player, or even to continue smoking, simply cannot be viewed as determined and beyond personal choice because of demonstrated irresistible psychological forces. The fact that so many people have stopped smoking or drinking or even playing professional sports reveals that such choices are fundamentally different from monocausally determined behaviors. Although state of mind may be a component in all disease, it seems that an attempt to will away pneumonia or a carcinoma of the pancreas is much less likely to be decisively influential than using the will to control the behaviors that are now being grouped as voluntary.

The Social Structural Model

Perhaps the most plausible competition to the voluntarist model comes not from a theory of organic or even psychological determinism, but from a social structural model. The correlations of disease, mortality, and even so-called voluntary health-risk behavior with socioeconomic class are impressive. Recent data from Great Britain and from the Medicaid system in the United States[15] reveal that these correlations persist even with elaborate schemes that attempt to make health care more equitably available to all social classes. In Great Britain, for instance, it has recently been revealed that differences in death rates by social class continue, with inequalities essentially undiminished, since the advent of the National Health Service. Continuing to press the voluntarist model of personal responsibility for health risk in the face of a social structural model of the patterns of health and disease could be nothing more than blaming the victim,[16,17,18,19] avoiding the reality of the true causes of disease, and escaping proper social responsibility for changing the underlying social inequalities of the society and its modes of production.

This is a powerful counter to the voluntarist thesis. Even if it is shown that health and disease are governed by behaviors and risk factors subject to human control, it does not follow that the individual should bear the sole or even primary responsibility for bringing about the changes necessary to produce better health. If it is the case that for virtually every disease, those who are the poorest, those who are in the lowest socioeconomic classes, are at the greatest risk,[20,21,22] then there is a piously evasive quality to proposals that insist on individuals changing their lifestyles to improve, their positions, and their health potential. The smoker may not be forced into his behavior so much by toilet training as by the social forces of the workplace or the society. The professional football player may be forced into that role by the work alternatives available to him, especially if he is a victim of racial, economic, and educational inequities.

If one had to make a forced choice between the voluntarist model and the social structural model, the choice would be difficult. The knowledge that some socially deprived persons have pulled themselves up by their bootstraps is cited as evidence for the voluntarist model, but the overwhelming power of the social system to hold most individuals in their social place cannot be ignored.

A Multicausal Model and Its implications

The only reasonable alternative is to adopt a multicausal model, one that has a place for organic, psychological, and social theories of causation, as well as voluntarist elements, in an account of the cause of a disease or health pattern. One of the great conceptual issues confronting persons working in this area will be whether it is logically or psychologically possible to maintain simultaneously voluntarist and deterministic theories. In other areas of competing causal theories, such as theories of crime, drug addiction, and occupational achievement, we have not been very successful in maintaining the two types of explanation simultaneously. I am not convinced that it is impossible. A theory of criminal behavior that simultaneously lets the individual view criminal behavior as voluntary while society views as socially or psychologically determined has provocative and attractive implications. In the end it may be no more illogical or implausible than a reductionistic, monocausal theory.

The problem parallels one of the classic problems of philosophy and theory: How is it that there can be freedom of the will while at the same time the world is orderly and predictable? In more theological language, how can humans be free to choose good and evil while at the same time affirming that they are dependent on divine grace and that there is a transcendent order to the world? The tension is apparent in the Biblical authors, the Paleagene controversy of the fourth century, Arminius's struggle with the Calvinists, and contemporary secular arguments over free will. The conclusion that freedom of choice is a pseudo-problem, that it is compatible with predictability in the social order, may be the most plausible of the alternative, seemingly paradoxical answers.

The same conclusions may be reached regarding voluntary health risks. It would be a serious problem if a voluntarist theory led to abandoning any sense of social structural responsibility for health patterns. On the other hand, it seems clear that there are disease and health differentials even within socioeconomic classes and that some element of voluntary choice of life-style remains that leads to illness, even for the elite of the capitalist society and even for the members of the classless society. The voluntarist model seems at least to apply to differentials in behavior within socioeconomic classes or within groups similarly situated. Admitting the possibility of a theory of causation that includes a voluntary element may so distract the society from attention to the social and economic components in the causal nexus that the move would become counterproductive. On the other hand, important values are affirmed in the view that the human is in some sense responsible for his own medical destiny, that he is not merely the receptacle for external forces. These values are important in countering the trend toward the professionalization of medical decisions and the reduction of the individual to a passive object to be manipulated. They are so important that some risk may well be necessary. This is one of the core problems in any discussion of the ethics of the voluntary health-risk perspective. One of the most difficult research questions posed by the voluntary health-risk theme is teasing out the implications of the theme for a theory of the causation of health patterns.

Responsibility and Culpability

Even in cases where we conclude that the voluntarist model may be relevant -- where voluntary choices are at least a minor component of the pattern of health -- it is still unclear what to make of the voluntarist conclusion. If we say that a person is responsible for his health, it still does not follow that the person is culpable for the harm that comes from voluntary choices. It may be that society still would want to bear the burden of providing health care needed to patch tip a person who has voluntarily taken a health risk.

To take an extreme example, a member of a community may choose to become a professional fire fighter. Certainly this is a health-risking choice. Presumably it could be a relatively voluntary one. Still it does not follow that the person is culpable for the harms done to his health. Responsible, yes, but culpable, no.

To decide in favor of any policy incorporating the so-called presumption that health risks are voluntary, it will be necessary to decide not only that the risk is voluntary, but also that it is not worthy of public subsidy. Fire fighting, an occupation undertaken in the public interest, probably would be worthy of subsidy. It seems that very few such activities, however, are so evaluated. Professional automobile racing, for instance, hardly seems socially ennobling, even if it does provide entertainment and diversion. A more plausible course would be requiring auto racers to purchase a license for a fee equal to their predicted extra health costs.

But what about the health risks of casual automobile driving for business or personal reasons? There are currently marginal health costs that are not built into the insurance system, e.g., risks from automobile exhaust pollution, from stress, and from the discouraging of exercise. It seems as though, in principle, there would be nothing wrong with recovering the economic part of those costs, if it could be done. A health tax on gasoline, for instance, might be sensible as a progressive way of funding a national health service. The evidence for the direct causal links and the exact costs will be hard, probably impossible, to discover. That difficulty, however, may not be decisive, provided there is general agreement that there are some costs, that the behavior is not socially ennobling, and that the funds are obtained more or less equitably in any case. It would certainly be no worse than some other luxury tax.

The Arguments From Justice

The core of the argument over policies deriving from the voluntary health-risks thesis is the argument over what is fair or just. Regardless of whether individuals have a general right to health care, or whether justice in general requires the social provision of health services, it seems as though what justice requires for a risk voluntarily assumed is quite different from what it might require in the more usual medical need.

Two responses have been offered to the problem of justice in providing health care for medical needs resulting from voluntarily assumed risks. One by Dan Beauchamp[19,23] and others resolves the problem by attacking the category of voluntary risk. He implies that so-called voluntary behaviors are, in reality, the result of social and cultural forces. Since voluntary behavior is a null set, the special implications of meritorious or blameworthy behavior for a theory of justice are of no importance. Beauchamp begins forcefully with a somewhat egalitarian theory of social justice, which leads to a moral right to health for all citizens. There is no need to amend that theory to account for fairness of the claims of citizens who bring on their need for health care through their voluntary choices, because there are no voluntary choices.

It seems reasonable to concede to Dan Beauchamp that the medical model has been overly individualistic, that socioeconomic and cultural forces play a much greater role in the causal nexus of health problems than is normally assumed. Indeed, they probably play the dominant role. But the total elimination of voluntarism from our understanding of human behavior is quite implausible. Injuries to the socioeconomic elite while mountain climbing or waterskiing are not reasonably seen as primarily the result of social structural determinism. If there remains a residuum of the voluntary theory, then one of justice for health care will have to take that into account.

A second approach is that of Tom Beauchamp,[13] who goes further than Dan Beauchamp. He attacks the principle of justice itself. Dan Beauchamp seems to hold that justice or fairness requires us to distribute resources according to need. Since needs are not the result of voluntary choices, a subsidiary consideration of whether the need results from foolish, voluntary behavior is unnecessary. Tom Beauchamp, on the other hand, rejects the idea that needs per se have a claim on us as a society. He seems to accept the idea that at least occasionally behaviors may be voluntary. He questions whether need alone provides a plausible basis for deciding what is fair in cases where the individual has voluntarily risked his health and is subsequently in need of medical services. He offers a utilitarian alternative, claiming that the crucial dimension is the total social costs of the behaviors. He argues: Hazardous personal behaviors should be restricted if, and only if: (1) the behavior creates risks of harm to persons other than those who engage in such activities, and (2) a cost-benefit analysis reveals that the social investment in controlling such behaviors would produce a net increase in social unity, rather than a net decrease.

The implication is that any social advantage to the society that can come from controlling these behaviors would justify intervention, regardless of how the benefits and burdens of the policy are distributed.

A totally independent, nonpaternalistic argument is based much more in the principle of justice. This approach examines not only the impact of disease, but also questions of fairness. It is asked: Is it fair that society as a whole should bear the burden of providing medical care needed only because of voluntarily taken risks to one's health? From this point of view, even if the net benefit of letting the behavior continue exceeded the benefits of prohibiting it, the behavior justifiably might be prohibited, or at least controlled, on nonpaternalistic grounds. Consider the case, for instance, where the benefits accrue overwhelmingly to persons who do engage in the behavior and the costs to those who do not. If the need for medical care is the result of the voluntary choice to engage in the behavior, then those arguing from the standpoint of equity or fairness might conclude that the behavior should still be controlled even though it produces a net benefit in aggregate.

Both Beauchamps downplay a secondary dimension of the argument over the principle of justice. Even those who accept the egalitarian formula ought to concede that all an individual is entitled to is an equal opportunity for a chance to be as healthy, insofar as possible, as other people.[24] Since those who are voluntarily risking their health (assuming for the moment that the behavior really is voluntary) do have an opportunity to be healthy, it is not the egalitarian dimensions of the principle of justice that are relevant to the voluntary health-risks question. It is the question of what is just treatment of those who have had opportunity and have not taken advantage of it. The question is one of what to do with persons who have not made use of their chance. Even the most egalitarian theories of justice -- of which I consider myself to be a proponent -- must at times deal with the secondary question of what to do in cases where individuals voluntarily have chosen to use their opportunities unequally. Unless there is no such thing as voluntary health-risk behavior, as Dan Beauchamp implies, this must remain a problem for the more egalitarian theories of justice.

In principle I see nothing wrong with the conclusion, which even an egalitarian would hold, that those who have not used fairly their opportunities receive inequalities of outcome. I emphasize that this is an argument in principle. It would not apply to persons who are truly not equal in their opportunity because of their social or psychological conditions. It would not apply to those who are forced into their health-risky behavior because of social oppression or stress in the mode of production.

From this application of a subsidiary component of the principle of justice, I reach the conclusion that it is fair, that it is just, if persons in need of health services resulting front true, voluntary risks are treated differently from those in need of the same services for other reasons. In fact, it would be unfair if the two groups were treated equally.

For most cases this would justify only the funding of the needed health care separately in cases where the need results from voluntary behavior. In extreme circumstances, however, where the resources needed are scarce and cannot be supplemented with more funds (e.g., when it is the skill that is scarce), then actual prohibition of the behavior may be the only plausible option. if one is arguing from this kind of principle of justice.

This essentially egalitarian principle, which says that like cases should be treated alike, leaves us with one final problem under the rubric of justice. If all voluntary risks ought to be treated alike, what do we make of the fact that only certain of the behaviors are monitorable? Is it unfair to place a health tax on smoking, automobile racing, skiing at organized resorts with ski lifts, and other organized activities that one can monitor, while letting slip by failing to exercise, climbing, mountain skiing on the hill on one's farm, and other behaviors that cannot be monitored? In a sense it may be. The problem is perhaps like the unfairness of being able to treat the respiratory problems of pneumonia, but not those of trisomy E syndrome or other incurable diseases. There may be some essential unfairness in life. This may appear in the inequities of policy proposals to control or tax monitorable behavior, but not behavior that cannot be monitored. Actually some ingenuity may generate ways to tax what seems untaxable -- taxing gasoline for the health risks of automobiles, taxing mountain climbing equipment (assuming it is not an ennobling actively), or creating special insurance pools for persons who eat a bad diet. The devices probably would be crude and not necessarily in exact proportion to the risks involved. Some people engaged in equally risky behaviors probably would not be treated equally. That may be a necessary implication of the crudeness of any public policy mechanism. Whether the inequities of not being able to treat equally people taking comparable risks constitute such a serious problem that it would be better to abandon entirely the principle of equality of opportunity for health is the policy question that will have to be resolved.

Cost-Saving Health-Risk Behaviors

Another argument is mounted against the application of the principle of equity to voluntarily health-risking behaviors. What ought to be done with behaviors that are health risky, but that end up either not costing society or actually saving society's scarce resources? This question will separate clearly those who argue for intervention on paternalistic grounds from those who argue on utilitarian grounds or on the basis of the principle of justice. What ought to be done about a behavior that would risk a person's health, but risk it in such a way that he would die rapidly and cheaply at about retirement age? If the concern is from the unfair burden that these behaviors generate on the rest of society, and, if the society is required to bear the costs and to use scarce resources, then a health-risk behavior that did not involve such social costs would surely be exempt from any social policy oriented to controlling such unfair behavior. In fact, if social utility were the only concern, then this particular type of risky behavior ought to be encouraged. Since our social policy is one that ought to incorporate many ethical concerns, it seems unlikely that we would want to encourage these behaviors even if such encouragement were cost-effective. This, indeed, shows the weakness of approaches that focus only on aggregate costs and benefits.

Revulsion Against the Rational, Calculating Life

There is one final, last-ditch argument against adoption of a health policy that incorporates an equitable handling of voluntary health risks. Some would argue that, although the behavior might be voluntary and supplying health care to meet the resulting needs unfair to the rest of the society, the alternative would be even worse. Such a policy might require the conversion of many decisions in life from spontaneous expressions based on long tradition and life-style patterns to cold, rational, calculating decisions based on health and economic elements.

It is not clear to me that would be the result. Placing a health fee on a package of cigarettes or on a ski-lift ticket may not make those decisions any more rational calculations than they are now. The current warning on tobacco has not had much of an impact. Even if rational decision-making were the outcome, however, I am not sure that it would be wrong to elevate such health-risking decisions to a level of consciousness in which one had to think about what one was doing. At least it seems that as a side effect of a policy that would permit health resources to be paid for and used more equitably, this would not be an overwhelming or decisive counter-armament.

Conclusion

The health policy decisions that must be made in an era in which a multicausal theory is the only plausible one are going to be much harder than the ones made in the simpler era of the medical model -- but then, those were harder than some of the ones that had to be made in the era where health was in the hands of the gods. Several serious questions remain to be answered. These are both empirical and normative. They may constitute a research agenda for pursuing the question of ethics and health policy for an era when some risks to health may be seen, at least by some people, as voluntary.

Notes

1. Parsons T. *The Social System*. New York, NY: The Free Press, 1951:437.
2. Stoinfels P, Veatch RM. Who should pay for smokers' medical care? *Hastings Center Report* 1974;4:8-10.
3. Morison RS. Rights and responsibilities: Redressing the uneasy balance, *Hastings Center Report* 1974;1:1-4.
4. Vnyda E. Keeping people well: A new approach to medicine, *Humane Nature* 1978;1:64-71.
5. Somers AR, Hayden MC. Rights and responsibilities in prevention, *Health Education* 1978;9:3739.
6. Kass L. Regarding the end of medicine and the pursuit of health, *Public Interest* 1975;40:11-42.
7. Belloc NB, Breslow L. Relationship of physical status health and health practices, *Preventive Medicine* 1972;1:409-421.
8. Bellow NB. Relationship of health practices and mortality, *Preventive Medicine* 1973;2:67-81.
9. Breslow L. Prospects for improving health through reducing risk factors, *Preventive Medicine* 1978;7:449-458.
10. Wikler D. Coercive measures in health promotion: Can they be justified? *Health Educ Monogr* 1978;6:223-241.
11. Wikler D. Persuasion and coercion for health: Ethical issues in government efforts to change life-styles, *Milbank Memorial Fund Quaterly* 1978;56:303-338.
12. Veatch RM. The Hippocratic ethic: Consequentialism individualism and paternalism, In: Smith DH, Bernstein LM, eds. *No Rush, to Judgement: Essays on Medical Ethics*. Bloomington, IN: The Poynter Center, Indiana University, 1978:238-264.
13. Beauchamp T. The regulation of hazards and hazardous behaviors, *Heath Education Monograph* 1978;6:242-257.
14. Veatch RM. The medical model: Its nature and problems, *Hastings Center Report* 1973;1:59-67.
15. Morris JN. Social inequalities undiminished, *Lancet* 1979;1:87-90.
16. Ryan W. *Blaming the Victim*. New York, NY: Vintage Books, 1971.
17. Crawford R. Sickness as sin, *Health Policy Advisory Center Bulletin* 1978;80:10-16.
18. Crawford R. You are dangerous to your health, *Social Policy* 1978;8:11-20.
19. Beauchamp DE. Public health as social justice, *Inquiry* 1976;13:3-14.
20. Syme L, Berkman I. Social class, susceptibility and sickness, *Am. J Epidemiol* 104:1-8, 1976.
21. Conover PW. Social class and chronic illness, *Internation Jounal of Health Services* 1973;3:357-368.
22. *Health of the Disadvantaged: Chart Book*, publication (HRA) 77-628. Hyattsville, MD: US Dept of Health, Education, and Welfare, Public Health Service, Health Resources Administration, 1977.
23. Beauchamp DE. Alcoholism as blaming tho alcoholic, *Int J Addict* 1976;11:41-52.
24. Veatch RM. What is a 'just' health care delivery? In: Branson R, Veatch RM, eds, *Ethics and Health Policy*. Cambridge, MA: Ballinger Publishing Co, 1976:127-153.

Chapter 22

The Family in Medical Decision-Making

Jeffrey Blustein

Should the authority to make treatment decisions be extended to the competent patient's family? Neither arguments from fairness nor communitarian concerns justify such an infringement on patient autonomy.

Families have traditionally exercised, and continue to exercise, considerable control over medical treatment of minor children. In both law and morality, families (or more specifically, parents) are regarded not just as interested parties whose views should be solicited and taken into consideration, but rather as rightful surrogate decision-makers to whose judgment the physician normally ought to defer. When the patient is an incompetent adult, physicians often consult with family members (that is, children or siblings of the patient, parents, spouse, etc.) about specific medical interventions and even about continuation of treatment, and many physicians are guided by the family's decision if it is not obviously unreasonable and if it does not contradict any previously expressed wishes of the patient. Family involvement is also sought when the patient is a competent adult, not, of course, because the family is given the authority to decide for the patient, but because it is thought that patients may need the emotional support of family members during times of crisis.

The role of the family in treatment decisions for young children has been extensively discussed in the bioethics literature; I will not rehearse the familiar arguments for this general parental authority, nor the reasons for preferring families as proxies for noncompetent adults. I want instead to turn to the case of competent adult patients and critically examine the current system of medical decision-making and its legitimating ethos in the light of the fact that patients are often cared for in the context of the family. I want to ask whether, in view of certain features of the relationship between patients and their families, the principle of patient self-determination at the core of contemporary medical ethics is in need of some serious rethinking. Might it be that family members, by virtue of their closeness to the patient, should not only have some special authority to speak on behalf of patients who are incompetent, but should also share decisional authority with patients who are competent?

A recent proposal that speaks to the family's role in medical decision-making has been advanced by John Hardwig. In his provocative essay, "What about the Family?"[1] he contemplates far-reaching changes in medical practice based on a critique of our prevailing patient-centered ethos. My discussion of his proposal is chiefly designed to pave the way for what I call a communitarian account of the role of the family in acute care decision-making. This account which, I hasten to add, I do not endorse -- has not to my knowledge been taken seriously as a theoretical possibility in the bioethics literature. Since the label "communitarian" is liable to be misunderstood, I should note at the outset that I am not

Source: Reprinted from Hastings Center Report, May-June 1993, pp. 6-13, with permission from The Hasting Center © 1993.

interested in communitarianism as a political theory. Rather, I want to focus on the family as communitarian political writers sometimes think of it, namely, as a model for their conception of the larger society, and on the basis of this understanding of the family, to mount a challenge to the dominant patient-centered ethos that parallels the communitarian critique of liberal political philosophy. This communitarian position resembles Hardwig's proposal in that it does not regard the competent patient as the ultimate decision-maker, but takes it as morally significant for the attribution of decisional authority that his or her life is intimately intertwined with the lives of close others. However, as we will see, the communitarian account is philosophically more radical than Hardwig's challenge to the dominant patient-centered medical ethos.

My own position is that the locus of decisional authority should remain the individual patient, but I also argue that family members, by virtue of their closeness to and intimate knowledge of the patient are often uniquely well qualified to shore up the patient's vulnerable autonomy and assist him or her in the exercise of autonomous decision-making. Families, in other words, can be an important resource for patients in helping them to make better decisions about their care. Recognition of this fact leads to a broader understanding of the duty to respect patient autonomy than currently prevails in acute care medicine.

Family Decision-making and Competent Patients

According to Hardwig, even when the patient is a competent adult, it may be quite appropriate to empower the family to "make the treatment decision, with all competent family members whose lives will be affected participating" (p. 9). This is so because family members have legitimate interests of their own that are likely to be affected in dramatic and profound ways by whatever treatment plan is chosen by or for the patient. Their interests may be affected in these ways because "family," by definition, consists of "those who are close to the patient" and "there is no way to detach the lives of patients from the lives of those who are close to them" (p.6). Since family members must often revise their own priorities and significantly alter their life plans to accommodate the needs of sick or dying relatives, and since the nature and extent of the adjustment depends on the treatment plan that is followed for the patient, it would be wrong categorically to deny family members a role in determining what the treatment will be, how it will be administered, where, and so forth. For one thing, there is a presumption that "the interests of patients and family members are morally to be weighed equally" (p.7), and family decision-making may be necessary to ensure that treatment decisions are fair to all concerned. Even when this is not necessary, the autonomy of other family members would be seriously undermined if the authority to make decisions that cut so deeply into their own lives belonged to the patient alone.

The interests of family members might be self-regarding or other regarding. Particular choices about treatment can seriously affect the lives of family members in many ways, interfering not only with their own personal projects and individual lifestyles, but with their commitments to other family members as well. In any case, they are "separate" in the sense that they diverge from and possibly conflict with patient interests: they are not to be understood as interests in the interests of patients. Of course, those who love the patient also have a direct interest in the protection and promotion of the patient's interests, assuming that the patient has interests that can be protected and promoted. Indeed, this is part of the very meaning of love. But for Hardwig, there can be closeness without love, and even when there is love, there will usually be other interests of family members as well. When all of these interests are taken into account, it may turn out that what is best for the family as a whole is not what is best for the individual patient.

These other interests may be, and frequently are, quite legitimate, and treatment decisions should not be judged morally better or worse solely from the patient's perspective.

Indeed, departures from optimal patient care may be justified "to harmonize best the interests of all concerned or to require significantly smaller sacrifices by other family members" (p.7). Moreover, and very importantly, Hardwig expresses misgivings about the effectiveness of exhorting the patient to consider the impact of his or her decision on the lives of the rest of the family. Patients who seem to be ignoring their family's stake in the outcome of their decision-making process may sometimes respond appropriately to appeals from the physician or other family members, but many patients will be too self-involved to give the interests of others proper consideration or will use their illness as a kind of trump card to dominate the rest of the family. Because of this, Hardwig maintains, we must consider a more radical measure to ensure adequate protection of legitimate family interests, namely, rejection of the prevalent medical ethos according to which the competent patient is always the decisive moral agent. Under this ethos, it is certainly permissible for family members to offer information, counsel, and suasion to patients who must make treatment decisions. But the authority to make the decisions still resides with the competent patient alone, and this Hardwig finds untenable.[2]

The "ethic of patient autonomy" (p.5) allows the competent patient, and the patient alone, to set the terms and conditions of care. Patients may be frightened and distracted by illness and hence in no position to give careful thought to the interests of others, but if their decision-making capacity is judged sufficient for the decision at hand, their wishes prevail. This troubles Hardwig because it mounts to giving patients permission to neglect or slight their moral responsibilities to other family members. Seriously ill patients tend to be self-absorbed and to make exclusively serf-regarding choices about care, and in those cases where "the lives of family members would be dramatically affected by treatment decisions" Hardwig suggests that family conferences be "required" (pp.9-10). These conferences would not merely have an advisory or supportive function: They would be decision-making forums. Patients and other family members would seek to reach a consensus that harmonizes the autonomy and interests of all concerned parties. Failing this, families would be forced "to invoke the harsh perspective of justice, divisive, and antagonistic though that perspective might be" (p.10).

Hardwig's proposal for greater family involvement in medical decision-making, however, runs up against the problem of patient vulnerability: joint family decision-making provides too many opportunities for the exploitation of patient vulnerability. Serious constraints on patient autonomy, such as anxiety, depression, fear, and denial are inherent in the state of being ill.[3] Illness is also frequently disorienting in that patients find themselves thrust into unfamiliar surroundings, unable to pursue customary routines, or to enjoy any significant degree of privacy. For these reasons, the ability of patients to assess their medical needs accurately and protect their own interests effectively is limited and precarious. But if those who are ill and those who are healthy already confront each other on an unequal psychological footing, then family conferences, as Hardwig conceives of them, seem especially ill advised. Weakened and confused by their illness, patients are easy prey to manipulation or coerced by other family members and may capitulate to family wishes out of guilt or fear. (Given that Hardwig would allow even hateful or resentful family members to be included in family conferences, this is not an idle worry.) Family members will understandably not want to be seen by the physician as opposing the wishes of the patient, and so they might exert pressure on the patient to concur with their opinions about treatment. Of course, even as matters now stand, with decision-making not generally thought to belong to the family as a whole, what seems like a patient's autonomous choice often only implements the choice of the others for him or her. But joint family decision-making is likely only to exacerbate this problem and to make truly independent choice even more dubious.

Hardwig, it should be noted, does acknowledge that a seriously weakened patient may well need an "advocate" (p.10), or surrogate participant from outside the family, to take part in the joint family decision. However, this hardly resolves all the difficulties his proposal presents. The presence of an outsider in what is supposed to be a deeply personal and private conference might only create (further) hostility and suspicion among family members. And if consensus in the conference cannot be achieved, the rest of the family could simply overrule the patient's proxy participant, just as it could overrule the patient himself.

From a theoretical point of view, we should, I think, agree with Hardwig about the inadequacy of any view that denies or overlooks the essential interplay between rights and responsibilities. But the practical moral problem as I see it is how to design procedures and structures of decision-making that achieve an acceptable balance between rights and responsibilities, between the important values of a patient-centered ethos and the legitimate claims of other family members. If alternative approaches to medical decision are judged in this light, as Hardwig wants them to be, and not solely in terms of overall happiness or preference satisfaction or the like, then family decision-making for competent patients confronts serious moral objections. For indications are that it will often result not in a mutual accommodation of the autonomy and interests of all affected parties, but rather in a serious erosion of patient autonomy and a subordination of patient interests to the competing interests of other family members.

The Communitarian Defense of Family Decision-making

I have focused on the problems that nonideal, less than fully harmonious families pose for Hardwig's proposal. Critics of the patient-as-primary-agent model might instead restrict their attention to those (admittedly infrequent) cases in which patients belong to close-knit and harmonious families, and with this as their conception of the family, offer a defense of family decision-making that challenges the patient-centered model in a more radical way than Hardwig does. In ideal families, suspicions, resentments, disagreements, and the like, if they exist, are muted and do not set the tone of family life. But more importantly, it may be claimed, the conception of the person that underlies the theory of patient autonomy is patently inappropriate here. The patient is not, as this theory presupposes, an atomic entity, a free and rational choose of ends unencumbered by communal and other allegiances. On the contrary, his or her identity is constituted by family relationships, and he or she is united with other family members through common ends and mutual understanding. In these circumstances, the patient is too enmeshed in a network of relations to others to be properly singled out as the one to make treatment decisions.

I call this the communitarian argument for family decision-making to distinguish it from the argument from fairness and autonomy discussed in the previous section. When I refer below to what "communitarians" say about medical decision-making, I am not thinking of any particular authors who have advanced this position.[4] Rather, I am suggesting that elements of the communitarian view can be taken out of their political context and that a challenge to the prevailing patient-centered ethos can be constructed on the basis of a communitarian conception of the ideal family. Let us look at this challenge more closely.

In acute care settings, the relationship between patients and physicians is, if not exactly adversarial, at least one in which parents should not normally suppose that they and their physicians are participants in a common enterprise with common values and goals. The values involved in medical decision-making are by no means exclusively medical values, but also largely nonnative ones about which patients and physicians frequently disagree. In these circumstances, physicians may attempt to coerce compliance with their wishes, which they are in an advantageous position to do, or to control patient decisions by selective disclosure or nondisclosure of information. In recognition of normative diversity and in the face of various threats to patient autonomy in the caregiving relationship, we invoke the notion of patients' rights. Rights accord patients a protected space in which to make their own choices and pursue their ends free of inappropriate interference from others. Having rights, patients can confront caregivers with the demand that their (possibly conflicting) ends be respected.

Communitarian critics of the traditional ethos of patient autonomy need not deny that patients' rights and patient self-determination play an important role in the caregiving relationship. But, they note, the patient is not always to be thought of simply as the one who is sick or in need of medical attention. If the patient belongs to a close-knit and harmonious family, for example, it is the family as a whole whose values and goals may diverge from those of professional caregivers because such a family is a genuine community, not a mere collection of separate individuals with their own private and possibly conflicting interests. Members of a community have common ends, and these are conceived of and valued as common ends by the members. United by common ends and a common identity, the threats that work against the autonomy of some work against the autonomy of all. Moreover, in these cases the patient would not need to be protected from family pressures for inappropriate treatment. Rather, the family would act as advocate for the patient vis-à-vis the physician, and family decision-making would put patients on a much more equal footing with care.

For communitarians the ethics of acute care, focusing as it does on the individual who is the subject of treatment, rests on a conception of the self that is at odds with how persons define and understand themselves in a community. This is a conception for a world of strangers, where the content of each person's good is, to quote Michael Sandel, "largely opaque" to others, where persons have divergent and possibly conflicting plans and interests, and where their capacity for benevolence is extremely limited.[5] But in the community, of a close and harmonious family these conditions do not obtain. Rather, the defining features of such a family are mutual sympathy, common ends, a shared identity, love, and spontaneous affection. Of course, it is sheer wishful thinking, and cavalier as well, to assume that all families are like this. Family life may instead be fraught with dissension and interests may diverge and conflict. In these situations, questions of justice come to the fore and the importance of individual rights (and individual patient rights) is enhanced. But within the context of a more or less ideal family, the circumstances that make personal autonomy both an appropriate and a pressing concern prevail to a relatively small degree.

For communitarian philosophers, individual rights have no place in intimate harmonious communities. Charles Taylor, for example, suggests that "the whole effort to find a background for the arguments which start from rights is misguided,"[6] and according to Michael Sandel, in "a more or less ideal family situation...individual rights and fair decision procedures are seldom invoked, not because injustice is rampant but because their appeal is pre-empted by a spirit of generosity in which I am rarely inclined to claim my fair share."[7] Rights, as communitarians understand them, are conflict notions, and if they play any role in intimate communities, it is remedial only.[8]

Unlike Hardwig's argent for family decision-making, the communitarian view I have constructed does not claim that families should make treatment decisions because this solves the problem of fairness or because this protects the autonomy of all those individual family members who have a stake in the outcome of treatment decisions. Rather, the argument proceeds from a picture of the family as a community of love where, it is alleged, questions of fairness and individual autonomy normally do not arise and are of minor importance. In the ideal family, there isn't enough of a distinction to begin with between self and others for these concerns to loom large. And this absence of a sharp line separating self and others is not a cause for alarm or a basis for moral criticism of family decision-making, but intrinsic to the nature of community, the experience of which, plainly, is an important good for humans.

The close-knit, harmonious family is a paradigm of community. Here the well-being of one family member does not just have an impact on the well-being of others, for this can happen in families that are no more than associations of individuals (like the ones Hardwig describes). Rather, in families that are genuine communities, individuals identify with one another, such that the well-being of one is part of the well-being of the other. This being so, the communitarian maintains, decisions that importantly affect the well-being of one family member are the province of the entire family. To be sure, in the medical cases there is only one family member, the patient, who literally bears the decision in his or her flesh and bones. But this fact alone, it is believed, does not confer upon the patient a unilateral decision-making right. The right to make the decision is still a right of the family in ideal circumstances -- a group right rather than a right of individuals.

However, since the communitarian argent for family decision-making applies only to families that are communities and not to those that are just collections of individuals whose lives affect each other in major ways, its implications for the practice of medicine will not be as significant as those of Hardwig's proposal. Many families, to acknowledge the obvious again, are not ideal. In addition, physicians frequently have only passing acquaintance with the patient's family and no reliable basis for judging the quality of the patient's relationship with other family members. Even if communitarians reveal genuine inadequacies in the prevalent ethos of patient autonomy and patient rights, physicians will often not be in a position to tell whether, in the particular case at hand, the family is harmonious enough to be entrusted with the authority to make decisions for one of its own. On the other hand, physicians will often have enough information to know that the lives of family members will be seriously affected by treatment decisions, and it is on this fact, not on the existence of a harmonious family, that Hardwig premises the case for joint family decision-making.

Still, the communitarian critique of the dominant medical ethos of patient autonomy and individual patients' rights raises interesting and important philosophical issues. Practical implications aside, the theoretical challenge it poses deserves a response. In what follows, I will try to indicate why I think this challenge fails.

How the Communitarian Challenge Fails

Even in families that are true communities of love, the harmony that exists among their members may not be so thorough going that invocation of individual decision-making rights loses its point. It is not necessary for community that there be complete identity of all ends and unanimity on all matters of value or the good. On the contrary, there is room for significant disagreement about how to rank different components of a common conception of the good, about the proper means and strategies for achieving it, and about whether certain risks are worth taking to achieve common goals. Even the members of a family are in broad agreement about what is of most importance in life, for example, this does not ensure that they will assess the costs and benefits of particular medical treatments similarly. Indeed, given the diversity of human nature and experience, such disagreements are not just possible but to be expected. Absolute harmony in decision-making and thorough going convergence of values are only found in quite extraordinary communities. And this being the case, individual rights can be seen to have an importance the communitarian fails to acknowledge. They are not just claims we fall back on in the unhappy situation where community is lacking or faltering. Additionally, they serve to secure recognition of the diverse values and ends that persist even in intact and well-functioning communities. This lack of homogeneity is glossed over by talk of family rights.

Individual rights have an important place in community because the existence of community does not eradicate serious disagreement about ends, about the relationship between particular choices and shared ends, and so forth. Individual rights are needed because a significant degree of diversity may exist even in a group united by a common conception of the good. But what if, hard to imagine though it might be, there were a community, without such diversity? Would individual rights have much importance in a perfectly homogeneous community like this? Would there be any point in ascribing rights to individual patients, rather than to families, if patients and their family members were in complete agreement about all matters pertaining to the good for themselves? Here if nowhere else, the communitarian would surely argue, individual rights are useless and irrelevant.

This is the conclusion we come to where we adopt a particular conception of rights. We find a clear and succinct statement of this conception in an earlier paper by Hardwig entitled, "Should Women Think in Terms of Rights?" The thrust of this essay, unlike that of "What about the Family?" is communitarian: Thinking in terms of rights rests on a picture, first sketched by Hobbes and then made more palatable by Locke, of the person as atomistic, primarily egoistic, and asocial -- only accidentally and externally related to others. If we are lucky our independent interests may coincide or happily divide in a symbiotic relationship... but we should not expect this to be the normal state of affairs.[9]

The normal state of affairs in a genuine community is quite different, however. Here persons are not just "accidentally and externally related" to each other, but understand themselves as participants in a common enterprise and regard the wellbeing of others as part of their own. No wonder then that rights should seem alien or antithetical to community and, more specifically, ideal familial love.

But communitarians who think of rights only in these familiar legalistic terms underestimate the complexities and possibilities inherent in individual rights. To be sure, rights sometimes function to protect the individual in the pursuit of his or her independent self-interest. But this hardly exhausts their significance. Consider these remarks by Neera Badhwar:

> An ideal family or friendship may wipe out all differences of ends, both final and intermediate, but it cannot wipe out "the separateness of life and experience." Au contraire, it would seem that it is precisely ideal familial love and friendship that will appreciate the "distinction of persons," recognizing the interest of each individual in pursuing a shared good, and her right to do so within the constraints of justice.[10]

On this view, fights are important even in the most closely knit and harmonious community. Even if the lives of persons are inextricably intertwined and their conceptions of the good agree in every respect, they remain numerically distinct persons with their own distinct perspectives on the world and an interest in expressing them. This interest in exercising one's agency in the pursuit of one's ends is not the same as an interest in seeing one's ends realized, for one's ends might be reliable quite independently of the operation of one's own agency. Nor is this interest contingent on one's ends being different from or in conflict with the ends of others.

By linking rights to this fundamental interest in one's own agency, we can explain what is wrong with the communitarian's antipathy to rights. Thinking in terms of rights, on the present account, does not rest either directly or by implication on a picture of the person as atomtic, egoistic, and asocial. It rests rather on a picture of the person as a separate being, with a distinctive personal point of view and an interest in being able securely to pursue his or her own conception of the good. This, by itself, entails neither that one's relationships to others are intrinsic to one's identity, nor that one is only accidentally and externally related to others. In ascribing rights to individuals, we are responding to these basic and universal features of persons.

It may help here to distinguish between having a right and insisting upon or demanding it. The language of demands does seem ill suited to harmonious families. If family members need to insist against one another that they have a right to make their own decisions, then we are probably dealing with a divided and quite antagonistic family. But these observations do not suffice to banish individual rights from harmonious families because the underlying supposition -- that rights must always be linked to demands -- is false. Rights can be expressed in different ways, and what is divisive and antagonistic to community is not the concept of rights, but only a certain way of expressing them. In harmonious families, rights are typically expressed "as reminders -- gentle or forceful, matter-of-fact or emotional -- of legitimate expectations and entitlements,"[11] and as such they play a vital role in the moral lives of families.

The implications of these remarks for a communitarian defense of family medical decision-making are clear. Even in extremely close families, patients may have different priorities from their loved ones and assess life choices in disparate ways, and these differences may surface in disagreements about how, and even whether, patients should be treated. Patients need their own rights regarding choice of treatment not just because family members cannot always be trusted to have the patient's best interests at heart, but because, even in families where trust is not an issue and there is a remarkable measure of agreement on ends and deep mutual affection, other family members may not always concur with the wisdom of the patient's choices. Rights protect patient autonomy and patient interests in these circumstances.

Further, rights for patients would be appropriate and useful even in those quite unusual families where the minimal sort of disagreement just mentioned is absent. For decisions about treatment often have dramatic and far-reaching consequences for the shape, quality, and duration of a patient's life, and individuals have an interest in determining for themselves the course their lives take. The interest in directing how one's life will go in accordance with one's values and preferences exists whether these values and preferences are uniquely one's own or shared with other family members, and it calls for recognition even when there is no disagreement between patient and family over the correct treatment decision. This is why patients have rights as individuals even under the unlikely conditions of absolute intrafamilial harmony: They protect the interests that patients have in exercising their agency.

Important questions remain about how belonging to a harmonious intimate community creates a new identity for the parties involved and about the interplay, for those who belong to such communities, between their interests as single individuals and their interests as members of community. But I believe enough has been said to establish the following, and this is all that is required for my purposes: community does not undermine the normative significance of the individual self nor does it render individual rights otiose.

Family Involvement in the Process of Decision-making

These responses to the communitarian position do not show that patient choices about treatment always trump the choices of family members, and they do not cut against Hardwig's argument for joint medical decision-making by all affected family members. What they show is only that the dominant patient-centered medical ethos cannot be refuted by the sort of all-out attack on the notion of individual rights the communitarian launches. To be sure, an adversarial and legalistic conception of individual rights is ill suited to those cases where family relationships are nonadversarial and there are no deep conflicts of interests, preferences, or values among family members. But if this is the basis for the communitarian claim that community renders individual rights (including patient rights) useless or of minor importance, the communitarian betrays a distorted and incomplete understanding of rights.

Should the choices of competent patients trump the choices of family members, except in the rarest of circumstances? "It is an oversimplification to say of a patient who is part of a family," Hardwig notes, that "it's his life" or "after all, it's his medical treatment" (p.6). Plainly, this by itself hardly shows that patient choices take priority over the choices of others, for when lives are so intertwined that one life cannot be shaped without also shaping the lives of others, it's the lives too. Another approach is to argue for a unilateral decision-making right for patients on the ground that patients have more to lose than their family members. That is, when we measure the sacrifices that family members must make for a patient's health care and the costs to the patient of not receiving the treatment that, other family members aside, he or she would select, the patient's sacrifices almost always outweigh the family's. Of course, the reverberations of patients' self-regarding choices can be so shattering to the lives of other family members that a calculation of relative costs favors the family instead. But familial hardship from this source is usually less of a burden than serious illness, and this difference would be sufficient to establish at least a presumption in favor of patient decision-making.

But if the ethos of patient autonomy survives the challenges I have considered in this paper, it is nevertheless the case that current medical practice and medical ethics can be faulted for not giving the family a more prominent place in medical decision-making for competent patients, and that both family members and patients suffer as a result. For one thing, as we learned from our discussion of Hardwig, because treatment decisions often do have a dramatic impact on family members, procedures need to be devised, short of giving family members a share of decisional authority that acknowledge the moral weight of their legitimate interests. For another, though patients might well benefit from family involvement in the process of formulating views about medical treatment, under the regime of patient autonomy patients tend to be treated for the most part as if they were solitary decision-makers, isolated from intimate others.

The ethos of patient autonomy rightly understood takes seriously the impairments of autonomy that affect us when we are ill. Patients are not ideally autonomous agents but anxious, fearful, depressed, often confused, and subject to ill considered and mistaken ideas. If we are genuinely concerned about ensuring patient self-determination, we will take these factors into account. Here it is necessary to distinguish, as Jay Katz does, between "choices" and "thinking about choices."[12] According to the dominant medical ethos, choices properly belong to the patient alone. At the same time, patients' capacities for reflective thought and effective action are limited and precarious, obliging them to converse and consult with supportive and caring others if they are to make their best choices. Patients' psychological capacities for autonomy can be enhanced by searching conversations with their physicians -- the main point of Katz's book -- and (I would add) by conversations with other family members.

To explain why this is so, we may turn to a characterization of the family found in Nancy Rhoden's influential law review article, "Litigating Life and Death."[13] Her argument, which focuses on decision-making for incompetent patients, finds within family life features that warrant a legal presumption in favor of family choice. Family members are typically the best decision-makers partly because of their special epistemic qualifications: They ordinarily have deep and detailed knowledge of one another's lives, characters, values, and desires. This knowledge might be based on specific statements made by one family member to another, for the intimacy of family life encourages and is partly constituted by the unguarded disclosure of one's most private thoughts and deepest feelings. But there may be nothing specific that was said or done to which family members can point as evidence of another member's preferences. Indeed, their knowledge, acquired through long association and the sharing of intense life experiences, is characteristically of the sort that "transcends purely logical evidence." In addition, family members are the best candidates to act as surrogates for an incompetent patient because of their special emotional bonds to the patient. This is important because possessing deep and detailed knowledge of another can put one in an especially good position to frustrate no less than fulfill this person's desires. Family members, however, can be presumed to have a deep emotional commitment to one another, and this makes it likely that they will put their knowledge to the right use -- that is, that they will decide as the patient would have wanted.

Those features of families that, in Rhoden's view, justify a legal presumption in favor of family decision-making for incompetent patients -- intimate knowledge, caring, shared history -- also provide good reasons for family involvement in the competent patients' thinking about choices. Family members would have no veto power over a patient's decision and would have to honor the choice ultimately made, no matter how foolish or idiosyncratic. But in family conferences, where the process of making a decision is shared, they could encourage the patient to evaluate different treatment options in terms of their impact on the interests of other family members, and could attempt to persuade the patient that the best choice is one that is fair to all affected parties. In some cases, understanding what a particular treatment decision would cost other family members might give the patient a compelling reason to alter an initial choice.

For the physician, the duty to respect patient autonomy has as its corollary a duty to engage in conversation with patients and to encourage and facilitate conversation between patients and other persons to whom they are close (including family members), unless the physician has reason to think that such conversation will not in fact assist the patient in making autonomous decisions. Current medical practice does not in general reflect a commitment to foster this sort of conversation as an integral part of the physician's professional responsibility. But if, as Katz suggests, genuine respect for patient autonomy is shown not merely in accepting patients' yes or no response to a proposed intervention, but rather in facilitating patients' opportunities for serious reflection on their choices, then promoting discussion and dialogue between patient and family is an important part of the physician's duty to satisfy the patient's right of self-determination.

A useful parallel can be drawn here with a central tenet of family medicine. Family physicians stress the importance of adopting a systems approach to health and disease in which the patient is seen as part of a family system. It is the individual patient, not the family unit, that is the primary focus of care, most family physicians will say, but since poor family dynamics can predispose to or cause disease and illness, effective treatment of the patient requires sensitivity to the multiple roles of faulty family relationships in the etiology of disease. In other words, to use language familiar to family physicians, if the physician is to treat "the patient in the family" appropriately, the physician must be cognizant of "the family in the patient."[14] My remarks about promoting and facilitating family involvement in the process of decision-making make a similar point about the importance of physicians' generally extending their attention beyond the individual patient. Only now the rationale for doing so is not that family relationships may contribute to the illness the physician is trying to treat, but that family communication may assist patients in making autonomous decisions about how or whether to treat their illness. The family is the center of most people's lives, for better or for worse, and this means both that the health of individuals is most profoundly influenced by family relationships and that such relationships can play a vital role in restoring the autonomous functioning that illness undermines.

Notes

1. Hardwig J. What about the family? *Hastings Center Report* 1990;20(2):5-10.
2. Hardwig's proposal to "reconstruct medical ethics in light of family interests" (p. 10) is novel in that it rejects the model of patient-as-primary-agent for acute care. Others have argued, along lines similar to Hardwig's, that this is not the appropriate model for home care, where family members share heavily in the burdens of care on an ongoing basis. In the view of Bart Collopy, Nancy Dubler, and Connie Zuckerman, for example, "the ethical problem for home care becomes one of gauging the interplay of agents, the relative weight to be granted to the autonomy and interests of the family vis-à-vis those of the elderly recipient of care." While not disputing the value of the patient-centered model in acute care, these writers argue that decisionmaking in home care should be "an interactive process, involving negotiation, compromise, and the recognition of reciprocal ties." See The ethics of home care: Autonomy and accommodation, Special Supplement, *Hastings Center Report* 1990;20(2):1-16, at 9, 10.
3. See Ackerman TF. Why doctors should intervene, *Hastings Center Report* 1982;12(4):14-17.
4. One author who has advanced something like a communitarian position is Lindemann JN. See his Taking families seriously, *Hastings Center Report* 1992;22(4):6-12.
5. Sandel M. *Liberalism and the Limits of Justice.* Cambridge: Cambridge University Press, 1982:170-71.
6. Taylor C. Atomism, In: Kontos A. ed. *Powers, Possession and Freedom.* Toronto, Ontario: University of Toronto Press, 1979:42.
7. Sandel. *Liberalism,* p. 33.
8. In a similar vein Alasdair McIntyre, taking as his "moral starting point" the "fact that the self has to find its moral identity in and through its membership in communities," attacks the language of rights for its individualism and the a historical and a social conception of the self it expresses. See *After Virtue.* Notre Dame, IN: University of Notre Dame Press, 1981:1-5, 64-67, 204-5.
9. Hardwig J. Should women think in terms of rights? *Ethic 84* 1984;3:441-55, at 446.
10. Badhwar N. The circumstances of justice: Liberalism, community, and friendship, forthcoming in *The Journal of Political Philosophy* 1993;1.
11. Badhwar. *Circumstances of Justice*.
12. Katz J. *The Silent World of Doctor and Patient.* New York, NY: Free Press, 1984:111.
13. Rhoden N. Litigating life and death, *Harvard Law Review* 1988;102(2):375-446.
14. For a critical discussion of the destructive orientation of family medicine, see Christie RJ, Hoffmaster CB. *Ethical Issues in Family Medicine.* New York, NY: Oxford University Press, 1986:68-84.

SECTION 4

PSYCHIATRIC ISSUES

Chapter 23

Cases 4.0

Case 4.1: INFORMED CONSENT FOR DISFIGURING SURGERY

Mike is 52-years-old; he lives with his wife. Their four children are now grown and live nearby.

Mike's medical history includes non-insulin dependent diabetes mellitus, hypertension, angina, and coronary artery disease.

Four years ago, Mike was diagnosed and treated for squamous cell carcinoma of the ethmoid sinus. Treatment included re-section of the tumor and a subsequent course of radiotherapy.

Mike remained symptom free until his admission to the hospital one year ago. At this time, he experienced swelling of his right upper nasal lacrimal region. A day after his admission Mike underwent surgery for recurrent squamous cell carcinoma. ENT and plastic surgery teams performed a bifrontal craniotomy with craniofacial resection, right maxillectomy with orbital exertation, ethmoidectomy, rectus free flap, tensor facial lata graft, spinal drain, tracheotomy, and placement of a central line.

The surgery resulted in marked facial disfigurement. Hair growth occurred on the site of skin grafts inside his mouth and over one eye. In addition, his tongue would involuntarily dart to the side of his mouth. Mike's appearance changed so drastically that he could not recognize the person he had become.

Recently, Mike was readmitted for psychiatric evaluation. During his intake interview, he complained of increased lethargy, poor concentration, and tremors. He reported feelings of low self esteem and attributed them to his radical change in appearance. He also reported a poor appetite due to difficulty he experiences in eating. Mike was extremely distraught over the hair that was growing on the inside of his mouth and over his eye. He said that he feels as if he has the face of a monstrous beast. Mike is concerned that he is not getting better and that he is both an emotional and financial drain on his family. Mike is able to work but has held a series of jobs since his surgery last year. Mike is depressed and now believes that his own death would be best for all concerned.

In your analysis of the case, consider the following questions:

1. Why are human beings so uneasy about physical disfigurement in others and in themselves?

2. Does the concept of "informed consent" require that health care providers (e.g. surgeons) detail all possible adverse affects of medical and surgical procedures?

3. What is the resulting quality of life for patients on whom life-saving measures (e.g. trauma care; reconstructive surgery; burn treatments) have been performed?

4. What have we learned from this experience regarding our relation to our own bodies?

Case 4.2: THE CASE OF LESLIE: SEXUAL HARASSMENT IN CLINICAL ENCOUNTERS

Leslie is a 33-year-old woman diagnosed with bipolar illness and multiple personalities. On a regular basis, Leslie exhibits three distinctive personalities, one of whom includes a five year old girl. Leslie is currently being treated by Dr. Winston, a psychiatrist at the local hospital. Her treatment consists of ongoing psychotherapy sessions and medication.

Dr. Winston is concerned that Leslie is not making progress in their psychotherapy sessions. He raises his concern with Leslie. In response, Leslie reveals for the first time her anguish concerning a scenario which is unfolding with Susan, her long-time and closest friend. Susan has been undergoing therapy with a psychologist in private practice in the area. Susan indicated to Leslie some time ago that she was developing "feelings" for him that were sexual in nature. Susan shared her "feelings" with her therapist who, in turn, acknowledged developing similar "feelings" for Susan. Neither acted on their attraction for a time; recently, however, they did. After one sexual encounter in the office, both thought it best to terminate their therapeutic relationship and cultivate, instead, their friendship, including a sexual relationship. Susan is currently seeking a new therapist with whom to continue her psychotherapy.

Leslie reveals to Dr. Winston that her concern stems from the value she places upon her friendship with Susan. Leslie truly cares for Susan and does not want her to "get hurt." Leslie's anguish stems, moreover, from unresolved issues in her own past. Leslie reveals to Dr. Winston that her former therapist "fondled her" during their sessions. Leslie was 25 at the time. Although she knew that what he was doing to her was "wrong," she never confronted her therapist or reported his activity to anyone. She did not want to risk losing someone who she felt was genuinely concerned about, and responsive to her problems. Leslie's history includes a period of sexual abuse, by a close friend of the family, beginning when she was eight years old and lasting several years.

Leslie's anguish over her friend's sexual involvement with the psychologist prompts Dr. Winston to consider taking action. Following a therapeutic session with Leslie, Dr. Winston contemplates what he should do.

In your analysis consider the following questions: Place yourself in the position of Dr. Winston.

1. What obligations, if any, does this case hold for you?

2. Why is client-therapist sexual contact problematic, ethically?

3. Do you have reason to doubt the validity of Leslie's revelations about her friend's relationship with her respective therapist and/or Leslie's own sexual abuse a child and, more recently, as an adult?

Case 4.3: CONSERVATORSHIP AND SURROGACY

R.C. is an 87-year-old African-American female transferred to the in-patient psychiatric service with a diagnosis of depression. Medical problems include poor nutrition secondary to not eating. She had had several medical admissions for this in recent months. She also has difficulty with ambulation because of a hip fracture 1 1/2 years prior to admission. Prior to her hip fracture she had been independent. She was employed as a cook for many years and was self supporting. Depression had not been a problem until her hip fracture. Three months prior to admission she had been persuaded by her son to move from Oakland to Sacramento to live with him. He felt she was unsafe in Oakland.

At the time of this admission, she was judged to be gravely disabled and thus was under an LPS conservatorship. She was unhappy in the hospital, and cooperated poorly with procedures, pulling out intravenous lines NG tubes etc. Because she was unhappy, her son wished her to be discharged. The son was the attorney-in-fact designated by the patient on a durable power of attorney for health care document executed two years prior to admission.

The team believed that although the patient lacked some capacity for consent for treatment, she maintained some ability to communicate her wishes and was adamant in her verbal refusal of all treatments. Although it was recognized that legally the LPS conservator had full authority to consent or refuse treatment and was in favor of pursuing the course outlined by the physicians, the son opposed such treatment. ECT was the primary consideration for therapy for her.

The caretakers identified the following problems.

1. The extent of the patient's capacity was in question.

2. There was a question of who has legal capacity to consent or refuse treatment when she has both an attorney-in-fact and an LPS conservator.

3. There was serious reflection of the benefit-burden ratio for this patient.

4. In the text of the document of the durable power of attorney for health care form, this patient had explicitly refused NG feedings without qualification. A further difficulty for the primary team was that the LPS conservatorship could be lifted at any time in accordance with the judgment of the primary caretakers.

Used with permission of Christine Rozance, M.D., University of California, Davis, Medical Center.

Case 4.4: THE CASE OF JAMES AND MARY POST

James J. Post is a 46-year-old man. He has been married for 21 years to Mary. They have three children, Tim who is 19, Susan who is 17, and Jane who is 15. Tim is in his second year of college in another city. He no longer lives at home. The girls still live at home. Susan is working, just having completed high school, and Jane is a sophomore in high school. Jim met Mary in the Peace Corps while both were working in Kenya after college. They built what was to all appearances a close and loving family life together, pursuing their careers. They were regular church-goers.

Mary got a degree in health care administration two years ago, and works for a hospital as a vice president. At great personal and family sacrifice, Jim just recently completed his Ph.D. in sociology, and is now employed as a part-time faculty member at a local college. Prior to this, he has worked as a researcher for a health policy foundation.

Both partners sought help from a female psychiatrist for marriage counseling and overload. Mary, especially, initiated this desire for help, since she began having unexplained panic attacks some five years ago. These have been relatively mild, and addressed through psychotherapy. Mary's concerns focused on the lack of intimacy in her relationship with her husband. She has been working on conflict resolution. Jim is an introverted person who strikes the psychiatrist as thoughtful but compulsive, a true perfectionist. This has led to increasing conflicts with Mary, and also with the children. Mary first sought help, in fact, in coping with her son's anger. This was first displayed in high school behavior problems, and later was aimed at her.

Recently the problems Jim has had over the years with alcohol, cocaine, valium, and even smoking, have finally surfaced. He was a heavy user of all these drugs. He has announced to his family that he will seek a divorce, and has found a friend "who understands him better." This is a woman in the department at the college who is a recovering alcoholic. Mrs. "X" is 34-years-old. She is pregnant with her third child, but is thinking of leaving her husband. He is contemplating a move to Oregon for a career change job that has opened up, and she does not want to accompany him.

In one session alone with the psychiatrist, Jim described Mrs. "X" as "teetering on the edge" all the time. Jim sees himself as providing a loving and understanding heart for her problems. He hopes that she will leave her husband and follow her instincts, so they might someday marry. When asked if he thinks his own marriage stands a chance, he responds in the negative, though he agrees that Mary would like to repair it. He doubts whether there really is love after all these years of recrimination and dispute, smoldering anger and resentment, and just plain neglect of one another that came with busy schedules, children, graduate studies, and two career paths.

Just prior to Jim's announcement about his plans for a divorce, his family and co-workers arranged an intervention, to confront Jim with his drinking and drug abuse behavior. Following that, he agreed to voluntarily commit himself at Hazelden in Minnesota, an institution devoted to helping addicts recover. After one week, he left the program, arguing that he felt "confined" there, and that his weekly AA meeting was going to be enough to sustain him. Institutional staff informed Mary that Jim's recovery is in jeopardy by this move. She thinks it is a sign that he still is in denial. Worse still, Mary has evidence that Jim is still drinking from time to time at least, and considers recreational use of cocaine as "no problema!", to use his own words.

Mary is concerned that Jim is not thinking clearly, especially about his new-found "friend." She has started to attend Al-Anon meetings, a group that is aimed at helping co-dependents look at their own behavior and how it contributes to the problems they have had in their lives. Mary is convinced that Jim is to blame for many of the family's problems, and her own lack of self-esteem. She feels that she failed to love him properly, or he would have recognized his own self-destructive path earlier. Although she is counseled to think of alcoholism and drug addiction as a disease, it is hard for her not to assign some free choice to Jim. He was mostly a late-night drinker. His drug use occurred most often when out with buddies. Rarely did he come to bed. He would drink until he fell asleep in front of the TV set. Having a part-time job now meant that he did not have to get up early in the morning. That is when the problem got even worse.

The children's behavior has gotten worse and worse too. Mary thinks that the whole family "has gone down the toilet." Her son, Tim, rarely speaks to her now, and seems to be taking his father's "side" in the pending divorce. He often yelled at her when he was in school, and seems to blame her for the family's unhappiness. She admits that he overheard her often berating her husband during the past several years.

Though both Jim and Mary are of above-average intelligence, the girls have not done well in school. Mary is still close to her youngest, Jane, whom she describes as "very confused." Susan was rarely at home during her high school years. She herself has a drug problem, and has, in her own words, "slept around" a lot. Susan has had two abortions, but now, at least, seems to be holding down a job as a waitress in a local hamburger restaurant.

It is difficult to get Jim to come for a joint counseling session, although the psychiatrist is able to meet with him alone from time to time. Mary sees the psychiatrist twice a week right now. She is deeply into grief and self-pity at present. Although from time to time the children once came for "family sessions," they no longer see the psychiatrist. The family also had to attend meetings called by a certified alcohol counselor, a social worker attached to the police department, after Susan had run away from home with one of her boyfriends, and was later found by the police in the company of an 18-year-old drug dealer. Most of this work was based on establishing rules and limits on Susan's behavior. Neither parent was able to sustain a regular pattern of discipline after the probationary period elapsed.

Jane's sophomore year of high school has been marked by one crisis after the other. She has been disciplined for fighting with a classmate in front of the general assembly room. She is flunking two classes, and has had over 10 unexplained absences from various classes during the first three months of school.

Among the questions on the psychiatrist's mind are:

1. Does Jim's behavior require hospitalization? Should his autonomy be curtailed so that he faces his addiction without denial?

2. Could the psychiatrist treat his wife alone, given the complexity of addiction and its impact on family and society?

3. Can anything of this family's life be salvaged?

4. What should be the goals of therapy for Mary? Jim? The family?

5. What are the pitfalls of confidentiality in dealing with individual family members?

6. Should the psychiatrist also insist on trying to treat the children? If she does, how much can she reveal of the parents' difficulties?

7. If Jim does agree to long-term psychiatric help, what concerns should she have about countertransference in this situation?

8. What rights does society have, considering the social costs of addictive behaviors?

9. Should Jim be forced to be screened for drugs as a condition of employment?

10. What is the difference, if any, between abuse of legal and illegal drugs? Were he solely a cocaine addict, would society treat his addiction differently than it does an alcoholic?

Chapter 24

Sexual Misconduct by Physicians

Gene G. Abel, Drue H. Barrett, and Peter S. Gardos

Introduction

There is long-standing consensus in the medical community that sexual relations with patients are unethical. Yet, this is still an issue of major concern, with numerous physicians being charged each year with sexual misconduct. This paper presents an overview of the literature and introduces a treatment model for professionals with sexual misconduct.

The fields of psychiatry and psychology have taken the lead on trying to understand sexual involvement with patients, hence much of the literature concentrates on psychotherapists. The opportunity and prevalence of sexual misconduct may be greater in these professions; although, most of the information presented will be applicable to any medical professional.

Prevalence

Over half of all psychiatrists will have a patient at some point who was sexually involved with a previous therapist.[1] A number of large surveys have been undertaken in an attempt to assess the extent of sexual involvement between physician and patient.[2,3,4,5] While acknowledging the limitations of survey research, it is striking that in all of these studies a large number of professionals admitted to sexual contact with their patients (as high as 13.7%). Given that these surveys depended upon doctors admitting to having engaged in unethical behaviors, these results are a conservative estimate. In addition, in the one study of its kind, Bajt and Pope[6] found that 24% of psychologists surveyed reported they were aware of instances of sexual contact between therapists and patients who were minors. While this study does not provide information regarding the percentage of therapists engaging in child molestation of their patients, it alerts us to the fact that when discussing sexual exploitation of patients by professionals, children must be included in the analysis.

In a recent review of the literature, Pope[7] attempted to identify predictors of therapist-patient sexual involvement. By far the most robust finding was that in all published studies, male professionals are far more likely than female professionals to have engaged in sexual relations with their patients. No differences were found between specific fields, such as psychiatry or obstetrics, nor were any trends noted related to the educational or professional level of the practitioner. No studies have reported a significant relationship between a therapist's likelihood of engaging in sexual intimacies with a patient and their theoretical orientation. Surprisingly, Gartrell, *et al.*[8] found that those psychiatrists who had been through personal therapy were *more* likely to become sexually involved with a patient. Additionally, therapists who engage in sexual activities with their patients tend to be

---

Source: Reprinted from the *Journal of the Medical Association of Georgia*, Vol. 81, 1992, pp. 237-246, with permission from the Georgia Medical Association © 1992.

significantly older than their patients. Perhaps the single best predictor of a therapist sexually exploiting a patient, is that they had already done so with a previous patient.[9]

A number of recent surveys appear to show an overall decline in the rate of sexual involvement with patients. However, as pointed out by Gabbard and Menninger,[10] "rather than assuming that these data reflect a sudden decline in unethical behavior, it is more convincing to view the trend as reflective of less candid reporting because a number of states are now making therapist-patient sexual relations a felony."

Ethical Guidelines

The ethical guidelines of the American Medical Association as the American Psychiatric Association explicitly state that "sexual activity with a patient is unethical."[11] Similar statements occur in the guidelines of the American Psychological Association[12] and other professional groups. Where the ambiguity occurs regarding professional/patient sexual intimacies is in relation to former patients. There is marked division in professionals' beliefs regarding this behavior. Appelbaum and Jorgenson[13] found considerable variability in ethical, legal, and administrative approaches to involvement with former patients, which they believe stems from confusion regarding the rationale behind such restrictions. The Revisions Task Force of the Ethics Committee of the American Psychological Association has proposed that an absolute prohibition against sex with patients following termination of therapy be made an explicit part of the new ethical guidelines.[14] It is beyond the scope of this paper to describe the numerous arguments for and against post-termination sexual contact with patients; the reader is referred to the above cited sources as well as articles by Gabbard and Pope[15] and Shopland and VandeCreek.[16]

One ethical dilemma faced by many clinicians is that of reporting an errant colleague. Medical professionals have an ethical obligation to expose those colleagues who are in violation of ethical guidelines. Yet, the reporting of sexual exploitation by a fellow professional often conflicts with the obligation to maintain confidentiality. It has been shown that when a psychiatrist is publicly exposed, several colleagues often acknowledge having known about the behavior. Because most of this knowledge comes about in the course of events that fall under the protection of confidentiality, the reporting of such professionals often presents numerous ethical concerns. Frequently, it is easier to do nothing, which seems to have become the excepted norm of the profession.[17] While maintaining a patient's confidentiality is of great importance this should not blind us to other ethical mandates. There are effective ways to mediate both of these very valid concerns. The reader is referred to Stone[17] for a review of this issue.

Etiology

Various authors have attempted to explicate the inner-dynamics involved in professionals who sexually abuse patients. Some have suggested looking at issues such as confusion of therapist's needs with patient's needs, latent hostility, and overzealousness on the part of the therapist.[18] Others have proposed the concept of "lovesickness".[19] Finally, some have offered a breakdown of the therapist's personality into categories such as naive, mildly neurotic, socially isolated, impulsive, and psychotic.[20] However, none of these approaches offers any substantive analysis of data, and at this point, are speculations based upon clinical contact with selected offenders.

One way of conceptualizing etiologic factors in sexual misconduct is presented by Pope and Bouhoutsos[21] and involves an analysis of common scenarios that lead to sexual involvement with patients. These ten situations are: 1) *Role trading* - where the therapist takes on increasingly more characteristics of "patient" with the therapist's wants and needs becoming the focus of treatment; 2) *Sex Therapy* - here the therapist presents to the patient the idea that sexual relations with the therapist is a valid treatment for sexual or other relationship problems; 3) *As if...* - the therapist treats positive transference as if it were the result of something other than transference; 4) *Svengali* - the therapist creates and exploits the patient's excessive dependence; 5) *Drugs* - the use of alcohol or drugs as part of the seduction or as a trade for sex; 6) *True love* - the physician uses rationalizations to discount the professional nature of the relationship and the ensuing dynamics and responsibilities; 7) *It just got out of hand* - this is a failure on the part of the therapist to treat the emotional closeness and attraction that develops with enough attention or care; 8) *Time out* - the main element at work here is the therapist's failure to acknowledge that the therapeutic relationship does not end merely because contact occurs outside of the normally scheduled time and location; and 10) *Hold me* - the therapist takes advantage of the patient's desire for nonsexual contact.

These scenarios represent the tactics used by many professionals enable them to engage in and maintain their unethical behavior. That physicians use these cognitive distortions is further supported by the survey results of Herman, *et al*[22] which showed that offenders believed in certain rationalizations significantly more frequently than non-offenders.

What is most clear is that non-sexual contact frequently proceeds sexual contact.[23] Those therapists who engage in frequent nonsexual touching of their patients are far more likely to subsequently engage in sexual touching with a patient. A good rule of thumb to gauge whether this is indeed a legitimate style of therapy, and not a useful warning sign, is whether this touching is selective, based on the gender and attractiveness of the patient.

Victim Characteristics

It has also been noted that certain types of patients, as well as particular patient-therapist dynamics, are more likely to elicit inappropriate sexual behavior by physicians and therapists. It has been suggested that borderline, and in particular suicidal borderline patients, can be especially effective in manipulating therapists into having sexual relations.[24] These patients have been described as "possessing self-deprecating and hateful internal object relations, primitive defenses such as splitting and projective identification, and ego deficits that cause difficulty in integrating and modulating affect and that can lead to transient psychotic lapses."[24] One needs to be especially aware of counter-transference issues when dealing with borderline patients and to resist the patient's perception of needing the therapist to achieve wholeness. Aside from borderline personality, many victims appear excessively vulnerable, with a great majority being survivors of previous abuse.[25] All of this evidence, however is highly anecdotal and speculative, and the literature on this topic has yet to come up with substantial data regarding a victim profile.

A more fruitful avenue is to examine commonalties and the specific dynamics at play between therapist and patient when sexual boundary violations occur. Several different dynamics have been suggested, the most important being: 1) *power issues* - because of the nature of the physician-patient relationship there is always an imbalance of power and this may not be fully appreciated by the physician or may even be deliberately exploited;[26] 2) *needs of the therapist overcoming needs of the patient* - many times patients endeavor to please their therapists, even at their own expense, and in cases of high need on the part of the therapist, this may translate into sexual misconduct; 3) *transference/countertransference issues* - the reactance of the patient to the physician, as well as the physician to the patient, can be quite powerful; such strong feelings are sometimes misinterpreted as true emotions as opposed to being a result of the therapeutic situation;[27] 4) *repetition compulsion* - patients often re-enact unresolved issues in therapy in an attempt to master them; this is especially the case with incest survivors who may re-create the blurred boundaries of their families; once again the physician needs to be careful not to misinterpret the patient's feelings as if they were unrelated to therapy;[27] and 5) *testing of the therapist by the patient* - as much as the provocative patient may wish to seduce the therapist, often this is in an unconscious attempt to see if the therapist will resist and thus reassure her that her needs and rights will be put first.[28]

Impact on Victim

The impact on the victim of inappropriate sexual behavior by a physician can be quite severe. Feldman-Summers and Jones[29] compared women who had sexual contact with their psychotherapists, women who had sexual contact with some other health care professional, and women who had no sexual contact with either a psychotherapist or any other health care worker. Those women who experienced sexual contact with their psychotherapist reported greater mistrust and anger towards men and therapists, as well as a greater number of psychological and psychosomatic symptoms following the cessation of therapy. Women who had sexual contact with other kinds of health care professionals reported similar reactions.

Feldman-Summers and Jones[29] also noted that the severity of impact of sexual misconduct was significantly related to the magnitude of psychological and psychosomatic symptoms prior to treatment. This is not surprising since those patients who had significant problems prior to sexual contact with their psychotherapist or physician, will then have the additional stressors associated with sexual victimization, and possibly less coping skills to deal with them. In addition, it is likely that due to the inappropriate sexual relationship, the patients did not receive the proper care or attention to their problems. Interestingly, the marital status of the therapist or other health care practitioner also had a significant effect on the impact on the victim. This is likely due to the fact that sexual contact with a married physician brings with it additional feelings of both guilt and anxiety which can be expected to exacerbate previous symptomotology.

Pope[30] has also written extensively about a condition that he refers to as the "Therapist-Patient Sex Syndrome." He states that this disorder is similar to other syndromes such as Battered Spouse or Rape Response Syndrome, and is suffered by many patients who had sexual relations with their therapist. Ten characteristics are said to be associated with the Therapist-Patient Sex Syndrome: 1) *ambivalence*- similar to the reaction of women in other types of abusive relationships, the victim may long to escape the exploitive physician yet fear the separation; 2) *feelings of guilt*- despite being entirely unfounded, most victims feel as if they are in some way to blame for the sexual abuse; 3) *sense of emptiness and isolation*- again similar to survivors of rape or battering, many victims feel emotionally hollow and alone; 4) *sexual confusion*- due to being sexually traumatized, most victims develop a profound confusion about sexuality that can effect their sense of identity; 5) *impaired ability to trust*- having opened themselves up so completely to their therapists only to be followed by betrayed, leaves many women with a lifelong mistrust of professionals and often of other people in general; 6) *identity, boundary and role confusion*- often analogous to incest, roles and boundaries becomes blurred when a physician becomes sexually involved with a patient; this has lasting consequences on the victim's ability to form appropriate boundaries with others and maintain a sense of identity and proper roles in their lives; 7) *emotional liability*- often the experience of having had sex with their physician can be emotionally overwhelming to the patient; 8) *suppressed rage*- victims frequently feel an understandable rage towards the exploitive therapist yet this is often blocked by their feelings of guilt and ambivalence as well as the force and influence of the therapist himself; 9) *increased suicidal risk*- the rage that victims feel may turn to self-destructiveness; feelings of guilt or hopelessness may reach such high levels that suicide may seem to be the only way out; and 10) *cognitive dysfunction*- the trauma caused by inappropriate sexual involvement with a therapist is often so great that cognitive abilities, particularly attention and concentration, are impaired.

Finally, the problems with subsequent psychotherapy have been discussed from the perspective of both the patient and the therapist.[31] Patient issues tend to center around issues of trust, anxiety and guilt. For the therapist, problems revolve around how to best understand and evaluate the patient's past sexual experiences and how to avoid repeating in some way the previous therapist's counter-transference issues.

Treatment Approaches

Pope[32] has stated that "in a search of the literature, I failed to locate any publication presenting principles of therapy to help enable therapists at risk to refrain from engaging in sexual relations with their patients." The situation has not changed much since that time. With the exception of a handful of articles,[20,33] strikingly little has been written regarding treatment possibilities. No treatment outcome studies in this area have been reported. At the Behavioral Medicine Institute of Atlanta we have begun a treatment program which has had success in reintegrating professionals who have engaged in sexual misconduct back into practice. This program is unique in that it integrates multiple treatment components, most importantly a system of surveillance to ensure compliance with treatment objectives (see Table 1). What follows is a description of this program.

A Sexual Misconduct Treatment Program

Once a physician has engaged in sexual misconduct within his practice, is it possible for him to continue in the medical field? Our treatment with such professionals indicates that it is. This treatment has involved an integrated approach with both individual and group therapy elements. The major components of treatment include training in cognitive-behavioral procedures found to be effective in decreasing inappropriate sexual arousal, detailed examination of episodes of sexual misconduct in order to identify antecedents to inappropriate behavior, and increasing the physician's understanding of the impact of his sexual misconduct upon the victim through literature review and attendance at continuing medical education courses. Additionally, the physician is assisted in developing a detailed practice plan specifying how future patients will be protected against sexual abuse. Included in the practice plan are specifics regarding the establishment of a surveillance network which submits data on the appropriateness of the physician's behavior, a system for surveying patient's feedback regarding the physician's professional conduct, and handouts for patients detailing the physician's ethical guidelines for the practice of medicine.

The major objective of therapy is to determine to what extent and under what limitations the physician who has engaged in sexual misconduct may return to practice. Initially therapy is conducted on an individual basis to assess the specifics of the physician's sexual misconduct, and to begin training in cognitive-behavioral procedures aimed at decreasing inappropriate arousal. Additionally, family sessions are used to assess the degree of social support for the physician, to break through the denial and secrecy that typically surrounds sexual misconduct, and to enlist family members in reporting on the physician's progress. As treatment progresses, the physician enters group treatment with other physicians who have been similarly charged with sexual misconduct within their practice. Group therapy focusing on relapse prevention is a long term component of treatment and provides continuity of care and ongoing surveillance to monitor the physician's conduct after returning to practice. Overall, the treatment provided in the sexual misconduct program focuses on developing skills to decrease inappropriate arousal and to allow the physician to return to practice without presenting a risk to patients. Physicians are also referred for individual psychotherapy in order to address the underlying dynamics of their behavior.

TABLE 1 - Components of Sexual Misconduct Treatment Program

1. Cognitive-behavioral treatment
   a. identify antecedents to sexual misconduct
   b. develop alternatives to antecedents
   c. identify grooming behaviors
   d. confront cognitions used to rationalize misconduct
   e. build victim empathy
   f. develop a relapse prevention strategy
2. Review the impact of sexual misconduct on patients
   a. CME course regarding sexual misconduct
   b. literature review and patient's article on sexual misconduct
3. Individual psychotherapy to identify/treat intrapsychic causes of sexual misconduct
4. Installation of a practice plan
   a. possible restriction of patients
   b. modifications of office characteristics or practice setting
   c. surveillance network with feedback from
      1. informed staff and colleagues
      2. patients
      3. professional practice group
5. A summary of all treatment program components advanced to the licensing board of other sponsoring organizations for its review, modification, acceptance or rejection.

I. Cognitive-Behavioral Treatment

Physicians receive cognitive-behavioral treatment using a relapse prevention model to identify antecedents to inappropriate sexual misconduct and to develop alternative responses to these antecedents. Past research has documented the success of cognitive-behavioral techniques in decreasing inappropriate sexual arousal.[34,35] This form of treatment has been used extensively with a variety of forms of sexual behavior (exhibitionism, pedophilia) and includes such procedures as ammonia aversion, covert sensitization, and cognitive restructuring. As utilized within the sexual misconduct treatment program, the main goal of these procedures is to teach the physician how to disrupt inappropriate thoughts, fantasies, or beliefs that have been associated with sexual misconduct with patients. The details of how to conduct these procedures is beyond the scope of this article, however they are well documented elsewhere.[36]

A second approach for identifying antecedents to sexual misconduct is for the physician to write a detailed description of one episode of sexual misconduct. This description is written in the form of a letter to the victim and should explain how the victim was "groomed" by the physician for the purpose of sexual misconduct. This letter is not intended to be mailed to the victim and is not included in the physician's medical record. Physicians find this aspect of therapy to be especially difficult as it directly confronts their images of themselves as a concerned caregivers. For most individuals engaged in inappropriate sexual behavior, denial is a central component. The purpose of writing the letter as if it were to be sent to the victim is to break through this denial and assist the physician in becoming aware of how he actively created an environment in which sexual misconduct could occur. It is especially important to help the physician understand how his behaviors, cognitions, and affect served as manipulations of the patient. The letter is read out loud in the physician group so that others may provide feedback and hear the physician's previous rationalizations. Often, the first attempt at this letter results in apologies to the victim and generalized statements of wrong doing. It is important that the feedback process assist the physician in describing in as much detail as possible the antecedents which allowed him to carry out his sexual misconduct. This element of treatment is based upon the work of Hindman.[37]

II. Development of the Practice Plan

The majority of physician's involved in the sexual misconduct program entered treatment after allegations of sexual misconduct were brought before the medical board and they were forced to terminate practice. They are typically in a position where they have lost their source of income and the support of their medical colleagues. Developing a strategy which would allow return to practice is a major component of treatment and is initiated early so that the elements of the practice plan can be added on as they become more apparent. The purpose of the practice plan is for the physician to demonstrate to potential employers, the medical board and other concerned individuals that he has taken precautions and is able to practice in a safe manner without further incidences of sexual misconduct with patients. Mandatory components of the practice plan include details of how patients will be protected from sexual misconduct, establishment of a surveillance team of coworkers, and development of a patient survey form.

The majority of physicians who have participated in the sexual misconduct program are males who have become sexually involved with adult female patients. A continuum of strategies is available for protecting these patients. One approach is to prohibit the physician from treating female patients. This may be stipulated as a time limited restriction (such as for the first year of return to practice) or as a permanent restriction. The physician is responsible for finding a work setting where access to female patients is highly unlikely, such as the criminal justice system. Another approach is to require that female patients only be seen in the presence of a chaperon who is fully informed about the nature of the physician's prior sexual misconduct. A third approach is to allow the physician to see female patients while structuring the physical environment so that patients are protected. This has included the stipulation that the physician only see patients in an office with a window. The office furniture is arranged so that the physician is always visible to office staff. The office manager is asked to do random observations of the physician, such as noting the amount of time spent with female patients.

An additional method for assuring that the physician is not engaging in sexual misconduct is to inform professionals and paraprofessionals at the physician's work site about the details of the sexual misconduct. Individuals to be informed should be those who are best able to observe the patient physician interaction. At least three of these individuals are asked to act as a supervisory team observing, during the normal course of their day, the physician's interactions with patients and coworkers. It is important that the surveillance team be instructed that they are not to act as detectives, but rather to be informed observers of the physician during their routine interactions with him.

One of the members of the surveillance team should be a individuals on the physician's call group as this person will have direct contact with the physician's patients.

The surveillance team is asked to complete monthly reports of the physician's behavior and to forward this information to the treatment team. The surveillance forms include a description of the physician's typical behaviors which allowed him to engage in sexual misconduct. This is included in order to alert the observers to what behaviors may be indicators of misconduct. This may include spending increased time in sessions, scheduling unusually early or late physical exams, non-billing of patients for unknown reasons, or excessive socializing with patients outside of the professional setting.

These surveillance data are reviewed in a timely fashion and feedback given to the physician regarding the surveillance team's observations. Any report of suspicious or inappropriate behavior is investigated by the treatment team. Additionally, summaries of the surveillance data are forwarded to the state medical board. It is made clear on the surveillance forms that the information provided will not be kept confidential and that the physician is aware and approves of the surveillance system and consents to this information being forwarded to the treatment team and the state medical board. Figure 1 presents an example of the typical surveillance form used with physicians.

Another method of monitoring the physician once he returns to practice is to request that patients provide feedback regarding the physician's professional conduct. This is typically accomplished within the format of collecting information on the patient's satisfaction with the physician's practice. Patients are asked to rate a number of dimensions of the physician's practice, including degree of comfort with the physician, appropriateness of the physician's behavior, satisfaction with the handling of billing issues, and courteousness of office staff. These data are collected every three months on all patients seen within a one week interval. The forms are administered by office staff with the exact week of administration determined by the staff rather than the physician. As with the surveillance data, the treatment team reviews the patient surveys on a regular basis to assess if any complaints of the physician's behavior have been made and the physician is provided with feedback regarding the patient ratings. Figure 2 presents an example of the typical patient survey.

A final component of the practice plan is to ensure that all patients are educated about what constitutes ethical medical care. If patients are knowledgeable of their rights and how to go about reporting unethical behavior they will be better protected within the physician patient relationship. Specifically, patients need to be informed that the medical standards of the American Medical Association specify that sexual contact between a physician and a patient is unethical. To accomplish this, a one page hand out handout summarizing medical ethical standards and patient rights is administered and explained by office staff. Patients may also be asked to sign a form indicating that they have received this information and that its contents have been explained to their satisfaction.

III. Appreciating the Impact of Sexual Misconduct

A variety of tactics are used to assist the physician in appreciating the impact of his behavior upon the patient. Initially, all physicians entering the sexual misconduct treatment program are required to research the psychiatric and psychological literature in order to gain a better understanding of the harmful effects of sexual misconduct on the patient and of the physician patient dynamics which make sexual misconduct more likely. The physician is asked to submit to the treatment team a written summary of this literature.

Additionally, physicians are asked to attend continuing medical education courses specifically dealing with ethical and victim issues. Documentation that the physician has attended this course work is submitted to the treatment team.

Conclusions

There are a number of things that physicians and therapists can do to prevent sexual exploitation of patients. Obviously, one needs to start with oneself. It is important to remember that the vast majority of professionals report feeling sexually attracted at least occasionally to a patient.[22] This in and of itself is normal. What is crucial is to prevent these feelings from escalating into inappropriate behavior. There are a number of suggestions that can help.

Rater's Name:______________________ Date___________

Rater's Signature:____________________

Dr. _______________ has admitted to past inappropriate sexual behavior with adult female patients. In the past this behavior has included sexual misconduct during physical examinations and office sessions. Dr. ___________ reports that in the past this inappropriate behavior might have been recognized because he did not bill such patients; he locked his office door when he was with these patients; he socialized outside the office with these patients, and he saw these patients before 8:00 am, during evening hours, or on weekends.

This form is to be completed by staff who work with Dr.___________ and/or his patients. Your responses will not be kept confidential but will be made available to the licensure board, and Dr. _________'s therapist.

Please evaluate each area of performance by circling the appropriate number.

	Never	Seldom	Usually	Most of the Time	Always
1 Appropriately uses chaperones with female patients................	1	2	3	4	5
2 Keeps office door open while with patients........................	1	2	3	4	5
3 Deals with patients in an ethical manner...............................	1	2	3	4	5
4 Has clear social and physical boundaries established with patients..	1	2	3	4	5
5 Sees patients only during normal business hours.....................	1	2	3	4	5
6 Avoids revealing details about his personal life to patients............	1	2	3	4	5
7 Interacts professionally with female nurses and other office staff.........	1	2	3	4	5
8 Is receptive to feedback from staff about his behavior with patients......	1	2	3	4	5

Please add any specific documents on the back of this page. Dr.________'s signature below indicates his awareness and approval of your surveillance of him and that he agrees to your advancing these reports irrespective of their consequences to him.

____

Physician's Signature

Patient Survey

It is our desire to offer good quality care in a comfortable atmosphere. We value your opinion about how we are doing and would like to have you rate us in a number of areas. Please circle the number which best describes your opinion about your doctor's care and your treatment at our office. Include any comments which you feel would help us improve your treatment.

Your Doctor's Name: ________________

Your Sex: ____ Male ____ Female

Today's Date: ________

Please rate your doctor's performance in the following areas:

	Poor	Good	Fair	Excellent
1. Understanding the nature of my problems .	1	2	3	4
2. Making me feel at ease	1	2	3	4
3. Ability to listen and really hear what I am saying	1	2	3	4
4. Conducting examinations in a professional manner	1	2	3	4
5. Explaining the proposed treatment	1	2	3	4

Please rate the office staff in the following areas:

	Poor	Good	Fair	Excellent
6. General helpfulness of the office staff	1	2	3	4
7. Explaining the "Patient's Bill of Rights" to my satisfaction	1	2	3	4
8. Protecting my confidentiality	1	2	3	4
9. Explaining the billing procedures	1	2	3	4

Please add any comments that you think would help us improve your care or make you feel more comfortable.____

____

____

First, as sexual contact and sexual relationships are often preceded by nonsexual contact and nonsexual dual relationships, it is best to avoid these. Second, monitor your own thoughts, feelings, and impulses toward patients. If in doubt, get supervision. It is common that professionals who end up in sexual relations with patients, hide their encroaching feelings from potential supervisors. Thirdly, establish and publish clear standards for social and physical contact at your work site(s). Review these standards with colleagues and office staff and request feedback to assess compliance with the standards. Fourth, be appreciative of the published literature that reflects the high incidence of professional sexual misconduct with patients. Finally, studies by Borys and Pope,[5] Vasquez[14] and Menninger[38] describe preventive steps such or consumer education, advocacy and self-help groups, resources for impaired professionals, administrative policies, and risk management approaches which might be employed to help prevent professional sexual misconduct.

Notes

1. Gartrell N, Herman J, Olarte S, *et al*. Reporting practices of psychiatrists who knew of sexual misconduct by colleagues, *American Journal of Orthopsy* 1987;57(7):287-295.
2. Stake JE, Oliver J. Sexual contact between therapist and client: A survey of psychologists' attitudes and behavior, *Professional Psychology: Research and Practice* 1991;22(4):297-307.
3. Pope KS. Research and laws regarding therapist-patient sexual involvement: Implications for therapists, *American Journal of Psychotherapy* 1986;40(4):564-571.
4. Pope GG. Abuse of psychotherapy: Psychotherapist-patient intimacy, *Psychotherapy and Psychosomatics* 1990;53:191-198.
5. Borys DS, Pope KS. Dual relationships between therapists and client: A national study of psychologists, psychiatrists, and social workers, *Professional Psychology: Research and Practice* 1989;20(5):283-293.
6. Bajt TR, Pope KS. Therapist-patient sexual intimacy involving children and adolescents, *American Psychology* 1989;44(2):455.
7. Pope KS. Therapist-patient sexual involvement: A review of the research. *Clinical Psychology Review* 1990;10:477-490.
8. Gutheil TG. Patients involved in sexual misconduct with therapists: Is a victim profile possible? *Psychiatric Annals* 1991;21(11):661-667.
9. Brodsky AM. Sex between patient and therapist: Psychology's data and response, In: Gabbard GO, ed. *Sexual Exploitation in Professional Relationships*. Washington, DC: American Psychiatric Press, 1989.
10. Gabbard GO, Menninger WW. An overview of sexual boundary violations in psychiatry, *Psychiatric Annals* 1991;21(11):649-650.
11. American Psychiatric Association. *Opinions of the ethics committee on the principles of medical ethics with annotations especially applicable to psychiatry*. Washington, DC: APA, 1985.
12. American Psychological Association. *Ethical Principles of Psychologists*. Washington, DC: APA, 1981.
13. Appelbaum PS, Jorgenson L. Psychotherapist-patient sexual contact after termination of treatment: An analysis and a proposal, *American Journal of Psychiatry* 1991;148(11):1466-1472.
14. Vasquez MJT. Sexual intimacies with clients after termination: Should a prohibition be explicit? *Ethics and Behavior* 1991;1(1):45-61.
15. Gabbard GO, Pope KS. Sexual intimacies after termination: Clinical, ethical and legal aspects, In: Gabbard GO, ed. *Sexual Exploitation in Professional Relationships*. Washington, DC: American Psychiatric Press, 1989.
16. Shopland SN, VandeCreek L. Sex with ex-clients: Theoretical rationales for prohibition, *Ethics and Behavior* 1991;1(1):35-44.
17. Stone AA. Sexual misconduct by psychiatrists: The ethical and clinical dilemma of confidentiality, *American Journal of Psychiatry* 1983;140:195-197.

18. Gabbard GO. Psychodynamics of sexual boundary violations. *Psychiatric Annals* 1991;21(11):651-655.
19. Twemlow SW, Gabbard GO. The lovesick therapist, In: Gabbard GO, ed. *Sexual Exploitation in Professional Relationships*. Washington, DC: American Psychiatric Press, 1989.
20. Schoener GR, Gonsiorek J. Assessment and development of rehabilitation plans for counselors who have sexually exploited their clients, *Journal of Counsel Dev* 1988;67:227-232.
21. Pope KS, Bouhoutsos JC. *Sexual Intimacy Between Therapists and Patients*. New York, NY: Praeger, 1986.
22. Herman JL, Gartrell N, Olarte, S, *et al.*, Psychiatrist-patient sexual contact: Results of a national survey, II Psychiatrists' attitudes, *American Journal of Psychiatry* 1987;144(2):164-169.
23. Kardener SH, Fuller M, Mensh IN. Characteristics of "erotic" practitioners, *American Journal of Psychiatry* 1976;133(11):1324-1325.
24. Eyman JR, Gabbard GO. Will therapist-patient sex prevent suicide? *Psychiatric Annals* 1991;21(11):669-674.
25. Gutheil TG. Patients involved in sexual misconduct with therapists: Is a victim profile possible? *Psychiatric Annals* 1991;21(11):661-667.
26. Chesler P. *Women and Madness*. New York, NY: Doubleday, 1972.
27. Holtzman BL. Who's the therapist here? Dynamics underlying therapist-client sexual relations, *Smith College Studies in Social Work* 1984;54(3):204-224.
28. Stone M. Boundary violations between therapist and patient, *Psychiatric Annals* 1976;6(12):670-677.
29. Feldman-Summers S, Jones G. Psychological impacts of sexual contact between therapists or other health care practitioners and their clients. *Journal of Consulting Clinical Psychology* 1984;52(6):1054-1061.
30. Pope KS. How clients are harmed by sexual contact with mental health professionals: The syndrome and its prevalence. *Journal of Counsel Development* 1988;67:222-226.
31. Apfel RJ, Simon B. Patient-therapist sexual contact: II. Problems of subsequent psychotherapy. *Psychotherapy and Psychosomatics* 1985;43:63-68.
32. Pope KS. Preventing therapist-patient sexual intimacy: Therapy for a therapist at risk, *Professional Psychology: Res Prac* 1987;18(6):624-628.
33. Pope KS. Rehabilitation of therapists who have been sexually intimate with a patient, In: Gabbard GO, ed. *Sexual Exploitation in Professional Relationships*. Washington, DC: American Psychiatric Press, 1989.
34. Marshall WL, Barbaree HE. Outcome of comprehensive cognitive-behavioral treatment programs, In: Marshall WL, Laws DR, Barbaree HE, eds. *Handbook of Sexual Assault: Issues, Theories and Treatment of the Offender*. New York, NY: Plenum Press, 1990:363-385.
35. Marshall WL. *Effectiveness of Treatment with Sex Offenders,* Presented at the Second International Conference on the Treatment of Sex Offenders, Minneapolis, MN, 1991.
36. Abel GG, Becker JV, Cunningham-Rathner J, Mittelman MS, Rouleau JL, Kaplan M, Reich J. *Treatment of Child Molesters*. Atlanta, GA: Behavioral Medicine Institute of Atlanta, 1984.
37. Hindman J. *Just Before Dawn: From the Shadows of Tradition to New Reflections in Trauma Assessment and Treatment of Sexual Victimization*. Ontario: Alexandria Associates, 1989.
38. Menninger WW. Identifying, evaluating, and responding to boundary violation: A risk management program, *Psychiatric Annals* 1991;21(11):675-680.

Chapter 25

Borderline Personality Disorder: Boundary Violations, and Patient-Therapist Sex: Medicolegal Pitfalls

Thomas G. Gutheil

In an earlier review based on forensic and consultative experience,[1] I addressed certain medicolegal difficulties that emerged in clinical work with patients who have borderline personality disorder. The present review, also based on empirical findings, addresses an important area omitted from detailed consideration in the earlier study: sexual relations between therapist and patient and the related boundary violations commonly seen in conjunction with such relations. I have three points to make here: 1) Patients with borderline personality disorder are particularly likely to evoke boundary violations of various kinds, including sexual acting out in the transference-countertransference; 2) Patients with borderline disorder apparently constitute the majority of those patients who falsely accuse therapists of sexual involvement. (False accusations represent a minuscule fraction of total allegations; the accusation is usually true;) and 3) Therapists can benefit from awareness of certain repeating patterns of errors in therapy and countertransference responses. With this awareness, they can avert the serious outcomes that result from such errors, such as trauma to the patient and/or highly destructive litigation.

One caveat is necessary to prevent misunderstanding. To study the patient-therapist dyad in clinical terms is not the same as indicting the patient (blaming the victim) for some malfeasance, nor is it the same as explaining away, exonerating, or excusing the therapist's behavior. I believe that sex with a patient is never acceptable. This article aims to alert clinicians to a potential pitfall in order to prevent its occurrence.

The Legal Context of Malpractice

In recent years, case law (Roy v. Hartogs[2], for example) has reflected agreement with the ethical codes of all mental health professional societies that sexual relations between clinicians and their patients are at least unethical and, under rare circumstances, criminal. Such relations represent a deviation from the standard of care and a basis for a finding of malpractice if the other requisite elements (damages, for example) are present.[3] Case law dramatically fails, however, to reflect the actual scope of the problem[4,5,6,7] because of the large number of episodes never reported at all and the substantial number of filed legal cases-probably but not probably the majority -- that are settled out of court. (An unknowable but probably small fraction of these cases might have been settled for legal strategic reasons even though the clinician was not culpable.)

For symmetry, note that Stone[8] has offered a typology of therapists and situations most commonly associated with patient-therapist sex, and others, such as Gartrell *et al.*,[4] have

Source: Reprinted from *American Journal of Psychiatry*, Vol. 146, No. 5, pp. 597-602, May 1989, with permission from the American Psychiatric Association © 1989.

empirically studied the therapists involved. In contrast, the present review examines the other side of the dyad and the pathological interaction between patient and therapist.

The Clinical Context: Relevant Borderline Psychodynamics

The psychodynamics of borderline personality disorder have been well described elsewhere (by Kernberg[9] and Shapiro[10], for example) and will not be rehearsed here. For completeness, note that nondynamic issues may play a role in accounting for the high numbers of patients with borderline personality disorder who are involved in patient-therapist sex. It may be important (Alan A. Stone, M.D., personal communication) that psychotic patients are not perceived as attractive and that neurotic patients are clear enough to know better than to become sexually involved. Thus, the field may be left to patients with borderline personality disorder through a kind of diagnostic default, as it were.

In any event, dynamic factors are clearly powerfully operative in the cases described in the literature. Empirically, those features of patients with borderline personality disorder which are most relevant here are borderline rage, neediness and/or dependency, boundary confusion, and manipulativeness and entitlement.

Borderline Rage

Borderline rage is an affect that appears to threaten or intimidate even experienced clinicians to the point that they feel or act as though they were literally coerced -- moved through fear -- by the patient's demands; they dare not deny the patient's wishes. Such pressure may deter therapists from setting limits and holding firm to boundaries for fear of the patient's volcanic response to being thwarted or confronted. Of course, such fear ultimately derives from the therapist's conflicts over sadistic countertransference feelings, which patients with borderline personality disorder are particularly prone to evoke.

At other times, therapists who would ordinarily reflect back personal inquiries about themselves may feel actually trapped or pressured by the patient's potential rage into unusual and inappropriate degrees of social interaction with the patient or of self-disclosure, such as discussing their own marital difficulties. Intimidation may be further reinforced by latent and implicit or oven suicide threats.

In a different context the patient with borderline personality disorder may express rage in a vengeful manner by filing a specious suit. As will be explored later in this paper, this particular form of vengeful hostility predominates in the group of false accusations.

Neediness and/or Dependency

Neediness and/or dependency are dynamics that call forth the therapist's nurturant side, at times in ways that foster overinvolvement or overinvestment. The rescue fantasy -- common if not universal in trainees-appears to me to occur particularly frequently in treating those patients with borderline personality disorder who manifest a helpless, waif-like demeanor.[1] The clinician may experience pressure not to disappoint or abandon the patient "as everyone else has done."

In a related manner the patient may wishfully draw from therapy the experience of being promised something -- being offered membership in the therapist's idealized family, for example. Smith[11] has perceptively noted that some patients cherish a related wish, which he termed the golden fantasy: the wishful belief that the therapist will gratify all needs, not just therapeutic ones. Needless to add, a reciprocal narcissistic fantasy may motivate the therapist: the wish to be everything to the patient.

In this regard, Judith Herman, M.D. (personal communication), pointed out that since so many patients with borderline personality disorder have histories of sexual abuse they may have been conditioned to interact with significant others on whom they depend in eroticized or seductive ways. This learned response might provide some of the driving force for boundary violations.

Boundary Confusion
Under stress, patients with borderline personality disorder may lose sight of the me-thee boundary and -- through such recognized mechanisms as fusion and projective identification -- may induce similar confusion in therapists. This confusion may derive from patients' own boundary-blurring interpersonal manner. If the therapist colludes in such boundary confusion, reciprocal perceptions of both the real therapist and the real patient may be powerfully influenced and distorted by the intense affects, longings, and wishes common in patients with borderline personality disorder.

It is just such vulnerability in this group of patients that calls for scrupulous -- even overscrupulous -- attention by the therapist to clarity of boundaries and to preservation of the professional nature of the relationship.

Manipulativeness and Entitlement
Patients with borderline personality disorder who are dysfunctional in many areas of life may still preserve intact powerful interpersonal manipulative skills. They may still be capable of getting even experienced professionals to do what they should know better than to do or -- all too commonly -- what they do know better than to do. Clinicians have rejected early sexual advances from patients with borderline personality disorder, pleading professionalism, only to succumb later, like the alcoholic who, flushed with success at passing a bar, goes back to toast the victory.

On this latter point, I have identified a repeating theme in clinical contexts such as teaching conferences, consultations, and private inquiries. The therapist's near-conscious awareness of deviating from the standards of care, the therapist's countertransference guilt, even the therapist's awareness of overt wrongdoing -- all are commonly conveyed by the therapist remarking at the outset of a conference or consultation, "I ordinarily don't do this... "or "While I don't usually do this with my patients...," or even, "Although I really didn't think I should be doing this...," and similar introductory comments. I view these remarks as pathognomonic of a likely countertransference trouble spot with a probably borderline patient, since the latter appears to generate and invite "not my usual" behavior. This situation appears to draw some of its force from the narcissistic entitlement and consequent sense of specialness of the patient with borderline personality disorder, in which the therapist may wish to share.[1,12,13] This specialness may tempt the therapist to make exceptions for both the patient and himself or herself, to the detriment of both parties. Some of the most destructive dyadic relationships may begin as a mutual admiration society, not recognized as an idealizing transference[14] and its countertransference complement. The doctor, already idealized, is further invited to share in the patient's specialness through a narcissistic seduction.

The narcissistic isolation of the dyad that results from this sort of misalliance appears to account in part for the failure of so many of these therapists to obtain consultation and even to use their own critical judgment. It is as though such measures would break the fragile magic bubble in which all this gratification is occurring.

Some Clinical Material
To illustrate the points in this paper I will use actual but disguised cases that I reviewed in the context of either malpractice litigation (28 cases) or forensic consultations (dozens) to clinicians or patients. All of the cases I will use involved male therapists and female patients with borderline personality disorder (the most common pairing nationally). In the service of confidentiality, all legal cases discussed have either been resolved (won, lost, settled, etc.),

dropped, or dismissed; more than 1 year with no further news or follow-up from the consultee has elapsed for all consultations described.

Some generalizations at the outset may be helpful. All of these cases, true and false accusations alike, were clinically mismanaged in important ways, most commonly through failure to attend to boundaries and to the patients' need for clarity. Thus, as is so often the case, an ostensibly legal issue rests on a clinical one. In some cases the mismanagement appeared to represent the kind of lapse not uncommon even for experienced clinicians in treating these difficult patients; in others, lack of experience, frank ignorance of essential principles of treatment of patients with borderline personality disorder, or countertransference difficulties seemed to predominate.

An interesting element in a number of cases was the patient's history of previous physical and/or sexual abuse. Conceivably, some element of a repetition compulsion was operating there, but the evidence is not decisive on this point.

To bring some validity to the often complex issue of which allegations are true and which are false, I have identified as true those accusations which have been admitted and/or acknowledged by the therapist, and as false those cases in which either the patient retracted the claim and identified it as false or the patient admitted to a disinterested third party that the claim was specious. Although recognizing that this selection method still does not guarantee validity, I believe it will offer sufficient reliability to permit the heuristic implications to be drawn.

False Accusations: Rare Events

To begin for convenience with the far smaller group, false accusations appear to be the product of borderline rage, expressed as vengeful action, coupled with a disregard for truth that is apparently self-justified by the strength of the affect. Snyder[15] discussed this subject under the rubric of pseudologia fantastica or pathological lying, including material related to sexual fantasies. He suggested that this kind of lying may feed self-esteem, serve primitive denial or projective identification, or represent transient loss of reality testing. It is important to consider the context in which such an accusation occurs.

> *Case 1.* A patient with borderline personality disorder became enraged at her physician because she felt he was treating her in a disrespectful manner: in her words, "like a welfare case." She later brought suit against him for sexual molestation. During the discovery phase of the lawsuit, an investigator, who was not known to the patient, visited her under false pretenses and obtained (probably illegally) a tape recording of her admitting that she had been furious with the physician and had fabricated this story in a scheme to "get him good."

> *Case 2.* A psychiatrist had been excessively but not sexually involved with a patient with borderline personality disorder in ways that fed her magical wishes to be a part of his family. He rejected the patient's request to see him on a major holiday, pleading family commitments. Her fantasy rudely shattered, the enraged patient brought litigation for sexual abuse and other specious claims but confided in a fellow patient, who revealed the deceit to the attorney.

Other triggers for false accusations have included borderline rage at bill collection practices, at the therapist's termination of therapy, and at being generally mistreated.

Boundary Violations

Patients with borderline personality disorder are known for their frequent difficulties with boundaries and limits, whether referring to their own ego boundaries, the realistic limitations of reality, another person's capacities, or interpersonal space.[9] What may be less universally acknowledged is that patients with borderline personality disorder possess the ability, as it were, to seduce, provoke, or invite therapists into boundary violations of their own in the countertransference.[16] Thus, the therapists' psychological defects and educational deficiencies aside, these boundary violations seem to derive at least in part from the dynamic forces addressed earlier in this paper. I repeat that these empirical observations neither blame the victim nor exonerate the therapist. They must, however, be understood as temptations to be avoided to prevent mishap.

Case 3. In addition to doing therapy, a psychiatrist gave a patient with borderline personality disorder hundreds of dollars; gave her medications from a supply he had prescribed to himself; and had her stay, at his invitation, in his own house -- in a spare bedroom--during a housing "crisis." The psychiatrist slept on the floor in front of the spare bedroom door so that the patient could not leave without his knowing it. All of these actions were rationalized as being in response to the patient's needs.

Given that patients with borderline personality disorder might well require unusual degrees of clarity about the therapist's role and particular vigilance concerning possible distortions of his or her role functions, this boundary-blurring behavior by the therapist represents an obvious and serious deviation. Similar examples follow.

Case 4. A psychiatrist invited a hospitalized patient to stay rent free at a guest house on his property as a halfway step to discharge to outpatient status.

Case 5. A psychiatrist who was in the habit of having meetings with a patient with borderline personality disorder two to three times a week invited her to see him daily following the week he was away in "compensation." He remarked, "I let her come as frequently as she wanted because I did not want to disappoint her."

These two examples appeared to have as subtext the therapist's conflict over aggression in setting limits and fear of the patient's consequent rage. Similar dynamics appear to foster exchanging of gifts, real and symbolic, between patient and therapist.

Case 6. A psychiatrist participated in long late-night telephone calls to and from a patient with borderline personality disorder while his wife and children slept. He remained blind to the erotic potential of this habit. He also shared many personal, marital, and financial troubles of his own with the patient.

Case 7. A psychiatrist asked an editorially gifted patient to work with him on improving his professional articles for publication.

Patient-Therapist Sex

Clearly, sex between patient and therapist represents, among other things, a severe boundary violation. Its drama, its often traumatic effects on the patient and on future therapy,[17,18,19] and a number of ambiguities in the medicolegal area set this behavior somehow apart.

A surprisingly and regrettably large number of psychiatrists appear to believe, quite incorrectly, that sex with a patient is acceptable as long as therapy has been terminated first.

(Some believe it is acceptable if therapy has been terminated with referral.) This is clearly false. The therapist who stops treatment on June 30 and has sex with the patient on July 1 is clearly violating the fiduciary relationship just as egregiously as if the sex had occurred on June 29.

Audiences at risk management seminars occasionally ask, "How long after therapy is over may one date a patient?" The only unassailable answer, in my opinion, is never. This restraint represents the only infallible approach to liability prevention in this unclear area.

Regrettably, desirable-clarity about sexual behavior may be lost by even experienced clinicians, as in the next example.

Case 8. A patient with very primitive borderline personality disorder was being treated on an inpatient unit. Unit staff had evolved a plan involving giving the patient hugs -- a regressive response -- as a reward, paradoxically, for mature and realistic behavior, despite the fact that this patient had a known history of major psychotic regressions, confusions of fact and fantasy and of intimacy and sexuality, sexual abuse by her family in childhood, and, on one occasion, confessing that she had fabricated sexual accusations for attention. Despite this background, her experienced therapist acknowledged giving her, on various occasions, a large number and variety of hugs, including social hugs, reassurance hugs, goodbye hugs, and congratulatory hugs. On one previous occasion in reaction to a threatened termination of therapy this patient had explicitly accused this therapist of sexual advances. When confronted she retracted the accusation as false and attributed it to a wish to punish yet keep the therapist.

On the particular occasion in question the patient had threatened to commit suicide in the context of a planned termination of therapy and was being seen for a second, extra appointment on the same day as her regular one. During this very session the patient showed impulsivity, loose associations, and serious regression. At the end of the session, the patient requested a goodbye hug and the therapist acquiesced and attempted a social hug. The patient suddenly began to breathe heavily and thrust her pelvis, then drew a vibrator from her purse, which led the therapist to disengage and set a limit. The patient regressed, sobbing and threatening suicide, but refused hospitalization. She then attempted to persuade the therapist to take her home himself rather than have her face the "unsavory characters" found at the bus station. He delayed several times, but then he drove her home from this tumultuous, out-of-control session.

The therapist later stated that he remained unclear about whether all this activity related to termination of therapy or not. His report of the incident reads, "Contrary to [my] usual policy of making a termination session final (especially with a borderline patient) because of the possibility of a misunderstanding, [I] told her [I] would call her to check if she was okay and, if she wanted it...set up one more appointment" (my italics). The patient subsequently accused this doctor of sexual relations both in his office and in the car on the ride home.

Although the patient later retracted as false the specific accusations, I would suggest that the hugging alone, from her viewpoint, represented sexual behavior with this patient. It was a clear boundary violation in this context. The patient's history practically guaranteed confusion as to what was and what was not sex, and the therapist's behavior was ambiguous in the very area where the patient already had problems with clarity. The record, moreover, strongly suggests that the patient was directing the sessions to whatever issues she thought would get the doctor to hug her. As therapy for other goals, the sessions may well have been meaningless. Expecting this patient to distinguish among hugs, no matter how therapeutically rationalized, appears quite unrealistic.

Given the fact that this therapist had already been explicitly accused of sexual misconduct by this very patient, his later boundary violations appear incomprehensible, as well as ill-advised, no matter how nonconstructively gratifying for both parties this activity may have been. I infer from the data that the patient's desperation, suicide threats, sense of urgency, and neediness were sufficient to overcome even heightened caution.

Case 9. A psychiatrist, responding to the alleged sexual naivete of a patient with borderline personality disorder, gave her anatomy lessons on both their naked bodies. He reasoned that as long as they stopped short of intercourse, the behavior was not really sex and thus acceptable. Over time, predictably, the relationship eventually came to include intercourse.

Case 10. Rationalizing the press of scheduling, a psychiatrist saw a patient with borderline personality disorder in the hospital daily for 2- and 4-hour appointments, sometimes running from 2:00 to 6:00 a.m. The relationship eventually became sexual.

Recommendations

"I don't understand why every psychiatrist is not fully forewarned about both sex and rage" (Cornelia B. Wilbur, personal communication).

A number of factors combine to foster the kinds of blind spots and unfortunate consequences outlined in this paper in regard to patients with borderline personality disorder. One such factor, in keeping with Dr. Wilbur's rueful lament, is the relative decline in teaching about psychodynamics, transference-countertransference, and similar issues in many training programs today. For example, the inpatient unit involved in case 8 provided a number of different therapies and therapeutic ideologies, but no dynamic ones.

Clearly, such understanding, although useful and necessary in averting problems, is not sufficient to explain or avert these problems. Psychoanalysts, after all, are not immune to sexual involvement with their patients. Dynamic instructional approaches are, moreover, of no avail with consciously exploitative, predatory therapists, of the sort that Stone[8] described. Fortunately, those individuals are comparatively rare, but weeding them out from the profession would be a laudable goal. Even some faint awareness of transference, with its power to produce flattering attitudes in the patient, and of countertransference, with its potential to trigger the feeling that the therapist and only the therapist can save the patient (drive home, feed, love, provide with the "right kind of sex"), might offer young therapists needed perspective, both at the crisis point and at later junctures in their work.

Some such minimal educational efforts, no matter how antianalytic the training program, appear to be a necessary survival-oriented part of the modern curriculum. In particular, trainees should be told and shown that the impulse to make an exception -- especially with patients with borderline personality disorder -- no matter how plausibly rationalized, is suspect and should set off red flags of caution. Didactic sessions on borderline personality disorder should include as warnings case examples such as those given here. Rescue fantasies should be described in nonjudgmental terms, and their operation and mastery should be explored.

Explicit instruction in practical management of treatment impasses such as those noted here (suicide threats, wishes to be driven someplace, etc.) is equally essential. I have referred to this management dimension as clinical administration.[20] This involves alliance-based interaction and intervention in the patient's physical behavior, such as setting limits and placing some responsibility for the solution of reality problems on the patient.

From a preventive viewpoint, the clinician encountering a transference that becomes eroticized would do well to begin regularly presenting the case to a colleague, supervisor, or appropriate consultant. In addition to providing valuable input and perspective, such consultation opens the case up and avoids the dangerous insularity of the treatment dyad that often promotes boundary violations. Not only does this approach prevent the illusion that the dyad is encased in a magic bubble from forming but -- through this very openness -- may also offer some possible defense against false accusations of sexual misconduct.

Finally, reality issues such as the trauma to the patient[17] and the serious legal consequences should be articulated. Sex with a patient is ultimately bad for the patient, no matter how good it feels, and a malpractice suit for sex is devastating to the doctor's career, affecting registration and licensing. These deterrents should be explicitly described.

The educational approaches outlined here may be helpful for those situations where therapists are on the verge of losing perspective, succumbing to the force of countertransference, or simply getting carried away. Under those circumstances, education, anticipation, and forewarning may serve the clinician and the patient well.

Notes

1. Guthell TG. Medicolegal pitfalls in the treatment of borderline patients, *American Journal of Psychiatry* 1985;142:9-14.
2. *Roy v Hartogs*, 366 NYS 2d 297 (Civ Ct, NY, 1975); affirmed on condition of remittitur, 381 NYS 2d 587 (Sup Ct, NY, 1976).
3. Guthell TG, Appelbaum PS. *Clinical Handbook of Psychiatry and the Law*. New York, NY: McGraw-Hill, 1982.
4. Gartrell N, Herman J, Olarte J, *et al.*, Psychiatrist-patient sexual contact: Results of a national survey, I: Prevalence, *American Journal of Psychiatry* 1986;143:1126-1131.
5. Perry JA. Physicians' erotic and nonerotic physical involvement with patients, *American Journal of Psychiatry* 1976;133:838-840.
6. Kardener SH, Fuller M, Mensh IN. Characteristics of "erotic" practitioner, *American Journal of Psychiatry* 1976;133:1324-1325.
7. Kardener SH. Sex and the physician-patient relationship, *American Journal of Psychiatry* 1974;131:1134-1136.
8. Stone AA. *Law, Psychiatry, and Morality: Essays and Analysis*. Washington, DC: American Psychiatric Press, 1984.
9. Kernberg O. *Borderline Conditions and Pathological Narcissism*. New York, NY: Jason Aronson, 1975.
10. Shapiro ER. The psychodynamics and developmental psychology of the borderline patient: A review of the literature, *American Journal of Psychiatry* 1978;135:1305-1315.
11. Smith S. The golden fantasy: A regressive reaction to separation anxiety, *International Journal of Psychoanalysis* 1977;58:311-324.
12. Pollack I, Battle W. Studies of the special patient, *Archives of General Psychiatry* 1963;9:344-350.
13. Main TF. The ailment, *Br J Med Psychol* 1957;30:129-145.
14. Adler G. Valuing and devaluing in the psychotherapeutic process, *Archives of General Psychiatry* 1970;22:454-461.
15. Snyder S. Pseudologia fantastica in the borderline patient, *American Journal of Psychiatry* 1986;143:1287-1289.
16. Stone MH. Boundary violations between therapist and patient, *Psychiatr Annals* 1976;6:670-677.
17. Collins DT, Mebed AAK, Mortimer RL. Patient-therapist sex: Consequences for subsequent treatment, *McLean Hospital Journal* 1978;3:24-36.
18. Ulanov AB. Follow-up treatment in cases of patient/therapist sex, *Journal of the American Academy of Psychoanalysis* 1979;7:101-110.
19. Apfel RJ, Simon B. Patient-therapist sexual contact: Psychodynamic perspectives on the causes and results, *Psychother Psychosom* 1985;43:57-62.

20. Guthell TG. On the therapy in clinical administration, part II: The administrative contract, alliance, ultimatum and goal, *Psychiatry Quaterly* 1982;54:18-25.

Chapter 26

Rational Suicide and Psychiatric Disorders

Edwin Schneidman

To the Editor: Because Conwell and Caine quote me appositely in their Sounding Board article "Rational Suicide and the Right to Die" (Oct. 10 issue),[1] I am emboldened to comment on their remarks. They write:

> The concept of rational suicide is elusive and controversial. A pioneer in the study of suicidal behavior, Edwin Schneidman, captured this quality when he said, "It is not a thing to do while one is not in one's best mind. Never kill yourself when you are suicidal."[2]

Of course, I believe that. What I am not so sure about is what follows in their article.

The burden of their presentation is that the crux of suicide prevention lies in the diagnosis (and treatment) of affective disorders. I do not believe this is necessarily so. Forty years of practice and research as a suicidologist have led me to believe that the assessment and treatment of suicidal persons is best conceptualized not in terms of psychiatric nosologic categories (such as one finds in the Diagnostic and Statistical Manual), but rather in terms of psychological pain and thresholds for enduring that pain.

Some suicidal persons have psychiatric disorders. Many suicidal persons are depressed. Most depressed patients are not suicidal. (One can live a long, unhappy life with depression.) But it is undeniable that all persons -- 100 percent -- who commit suicide are perturbed and experiencing unbearable psychological pain. The problem of suicide should be addressed directly, phenomenologically, without the intervention of the often obfuscating variable of psychiatric disorder.

In human beings pain is ubiquitous, but suffering is optional, within the constraints of a person's personality. Just as it is important to distinguish between the treatment of physical pain and the treatment of suffering,[3] so there are also important differences between the diagnosis of depression and the assessment of psychological pain. A focus on mental illness is often misleading. Physicians and other health professionals need the courage and wisdom to work on a person's suffering at the phenomenological level and to explore such questions as "How do you hurt?" and "How may I help you?" They should then do whatever is necessary, using a wide variety of legitimate tactics,[4] including medication, to reduce that person's self-destructive impulses. Diagnosis should be adjunctive to a larger understanding of the person's pain-in-life.

Source: Reprinted from *The New England Journal of Medicine*, Vol. 326, No. 13, pp. 889-890, with permission from The New England Journal of Medicine © March, 1992.

Notes

1. Conwell Y, Caine ED. Rational suicide and the right to die -- reality and myth, *New England Journal of Medicine* 1991;325:1100-3.
2. Schneidman ES. Some essentials of suicide and some implications for response, In: Roy A, ed. *Suicide*. Baltimore, MD: Williarns & Wilkins, 1986:1-16.
3. Cassell EJ. *The Nature of Suffering: And the Goals of Medicine*. New York, NY: Oxford University Press, 1991.
4. Shneidman ES. Aphorisms of suicide and some implications for psychotherapy, *American Journal of Psychotherapy* 1984;38:319-28.

Chapter 27

Does Depression Invalidate Competence? Consultant's Ethical, Psychiatric, and Legal Considerations

Ernlé W. D. Young, James C. Corby, and Rodney Johnson

The ethical principle of respect for autonomy has come into its own in American medicine since World War II as equal in importance to the traditional medico-moral principles of non-maleficence and beneficence.[1] Respect for autonomy provides the ethical underpinning for the patient's right to exercise an informed choice -- whether to consent to or refuse recommended medical treatment.[2] However, an informed choice demands a certain level of competence.[3] As the following four cases illustrate, there may be times when depression can render problematic a patient's ability to comprehend the consequences of a choice, giving rise to the question: Does depression invalidate competence?

Four Cases in Which Depression Could Be Thought to Invalidate Competence

1. *Quadriplegic*: The depressed quadriplegic patient with amyotrophic lateral sclerosis (ALS) who wished to be extubated and allowed to die.

   A 33-year-old man, diagnosed seven years ago with ALS, had became progressively paralyzed. After becoming paraplegic, he was still able to work (and find meaning in life) as a cartoonist. Even after becoming quadriplegic, he continued cartooning with a mouthstick. Eventually, however, this became impossible. He was admitted to the ICU when he could no longer breathe without ventilatory assistance. He agreed to a two-week trial on the ventilator. At the end of this period, he asked to be extubated and to be allowed to die, saying that the quality of his life as a ventilator-dependent and completely paralyzed patient was unacceptable to him. When faced with this request, the medical resident called for a psychiatric consultation. The psychiatrist pronounced the patient depressed and, therefore, incapable of taking a decision to die. At this point, an ethics consultation was invited.

Psychiatric Comment: The finding of depression, per se, did not mean that the patient necessarily was incompetent. There are two distinct issues here for a psychiatric consultant to address. The first is whether or not a diagnosis could be made of a mental disorder. And second, if so, did it significantly interfere with the patient's decision to refuse further ventilatory assistance? Like most psychiatric disorders, depression has a wide range of severity. In the most severe forms, the patient is overtly psychotic and out of touch with

Source: Reprinted from *Cambridge Quaterly of Healthcare Ethics*, Vol. 2, 1993, pp. 505-515, with permission of Cambridge University Press © 1993.

reality.

The task of the consultant in this case was to render an informed opinion about whether the severity of this particular patient's depression sufficiently compromised his competence to comprehend the consequences of his decision for his care and for his life. In the absence of a finding of incompetence, the patient had a right to refuse further aggressive medical treatment. Given the clinical situation, extubation certainly seems a "reasonable" choice by the patient. However, if the psychiatric consultant's examination revealed an overt psychosis with psychotic symptoms that directly and significantly influenced the extubation decision, then a substituted judgment ought to have been obtained.

The psychiatric consultant's job is to protect the patient from the disease; hence the need to be alert to any situation where the disease, and not the patient, seems to be making the decision.

2. *Amputee.* The amputee who, post-operatively depressed, attempted to extubate saying he wanted to die.

A 57-year-old man with Burger's disease came into the hospital for amputation of his left leg, at the thigh, because of serious circulatory problems. Post-operatively, he was in the ICU on a ventilator (the expectation being that he would only require ventilatory support for 3-4 days). On the first day, he extubated himself saying that he wanted to die. The nursing staff reintubated him, and called for an ethics consultation. Was he competent to refuse further aggressive treatment?

Psychiatric Comment: The suddenness of the patient's decision, and the fact that it seemed out of character for the patient, alert us to the possibility that some extrinsic factor might have caused his competence to be compromised. We presume that the medical staff had ruled out metabolic problems, adverse medication reactions, or complications from the surgery as causal factors. It might have been useful to have obtained a psychiatric consultation prior to the ethics consultation, in order to assess confounding psychological issues such as the patient's vulnerability to the enforced isolation and dependency occasioned by the ventilator or to the significance he himself attached to the loss of a limb. Because of the gravity of the patient's expressed wish, a high standard of competence should be required. For the same reason, stability of the decision over time is necessary. Many emotionally overwhelming situations that predispose patients to impulsive decision-making resolve merely with the passage of time, as irrational fears are tempered by reason or reassurance. Happily, it was anticipated that the period of intubation would be brief. This made it likely that the situation was likely to resolve spontaneously.

3. *Elderly Patient.* The elderly patient with a history of delusional depression, who stopped taking Haldol, and then had a "vision" in which she was told that she was no longer to eat or drink.

Two weeks later, the board and care facility where she was living had her admitted to the medical center because of severe malnutrition and dehydration. On admission, a nasogastric tube and an intravenous line were placed, to provide her with nutrition and hydration. She consented to these measures, but refused to eat or drink on her own. Since she could no longer stay in the hospital once she was stabilized, the question of how to manage her care in the long-term was addressed. After psychiatric evaluation, two options were discussed: electro-convulsive therapy (ECT), to get her to start eating and drinking voluntarily; or surgical placement of a gastrostomy feeding tube. The board and care facility was reluctant to take her back with a G-tube, so there was strong pressure from psychiatry to go ahead with ECT. At this point an ethics consultation was invited. The patient explained that she was willing for a G-tube to be inserted, but refused ECT. She said it would "make her forget her vision," which was very important to her. Was she competent to refuse ECT?

Psychiatric Comment: I have had personal experience with similar patients who were successfully treated with ECT. We are told that this patient had a history of similar episodes of delusional depression. Major mood disorders tend to wax and wane; in the more severe forms of the illness, patients may become psychotic and experience delusions. Treatments are helpful but often not completely effective.

I remember one patient who begged him to authorize ECT treatments because his "voices" told him that he was totally evil and deserving of the worst punishment imaginable. He begged for ECT as a punishment for his sins. Because of the severity of his illness, he lost his capacity to appreciate that he was ill, and thus was incapable of meaningful consent to (or refusal of) treatment. His illness was making the decision, eroding his autonomy. His self was no longer meaningfully present as the autonomous decision-maker.

Apparently the patient in this case was in a similar predicament: in the grip of a terrible illness which distorted her sense of self to the point of psychosis. Her decisions were unduly influenced and, in fact, were probably determined by the symptomatic "vision" that occurred in the context of her illness, untreated once she stopped taking her medication. The patient was no longer present, only her illness. Categorically it can be stated that she lacked any meaningful ability to consent to or refuse treatment. She could thus neither refuse nor accept ECT.

Legal Counsel: A court proceeding would have been necessary to confirm her incapacity to make the treatment decision, and then ECT could have been pursued with substituted decision-makers. Special informed consent laws apply to ECT in California. If either the patient's attending physician or attorney believes that the patient does not have the capacity to give a written informed consent to the ECT, then a court hearing must be held to determine that issue. If the court finds that the patient does not have the capacity to give consent, then the special informed consent process can proceed with the responsible relative, guardian, or conservator.[4] While waiting for that judgment to be handed down, she could have been treated vigorously with antipsychotic and antidepressant medications and maintained through G-tube feeding on the medical ward. Once medically stabilized, she could then be transferred to a psychiatric unit, hopefully to receive her court-ordered ECT treatments.

4. *Suicide Attempt.* The quadriplegic survivor of a suicide attempt who resisted reintubation after accidentally being extubated.

This 45-year-old man, depressed because he had lost his job and because his wife had left him, taking with her their 2-year-old daughter, attempted suicide by shooting himself in the mouth with a 0.38 caliber revolver. Instead of killing himself, he completely destroyed the second cervical vertebra (C-2), rendering himself immediately quadriplegic. In the ICU, on a respirator, he accidentally became extubated. When the nurses attempted to reintubate him, he resisted as vigorously as he could, indicating afterwards, by means of signing, that he wished to be allowed to die. At this point, an ethics consultation was invited. The question was, was he competent to refuse further aggressive treatment?

Psychiatric Comment: This man was suicidal. His feelings probably reflected his inability to deal with the situational losses he had sustained. He deserved the treatment usually given all suicidal patients: time in a protected environment to be assisted in coming to terms with the reality of his losses. Hopefully, he would accept treatment and it would be helpful.

The question posed is the competence of the patient at the time of the ethics consultation. From a practical perspective, in California (as in most other states) his immanent suicidality would pre-empt the issue of competence. The situation was that of a psychiatric and medical emergency. Emergency measures such as intubation were required to stabilize the situation and save his life. California law[5] would permit involuntary hospitalization for a total of thirty-one days, after which the patient would be permitted to leave. If subsequent observed behavior revealed immanent suicidality, the patient could be hospitalized again for a total of thirty-one days -- and so on.

The man's actual competence may, in fact, be difficult to determine. The psychiatric consultant needs to be on the alert for signs of impaired reality testing, such as psychosis, and should ascertain whether the patient appreciated the reasons for his treatment and understood the risks and consequences of refusing treatment. There should also be a determination of the extent to which the patient's mental disorder -- in this case, an adjustment disorder with depressive features -- influenced the decision to refuse treatment. All these factors would enter into a global assessment of the patient's competence to refuse life-sustaining treatment. Again, given California law, even if he were found competent to refuse treatment a determination of immanent suicidality could still result in an involuntary hospitalization for a maximum of thirty-one days.

I would have tried to err on the side of the patient's welfare, and would likely argue that the suicidality, occasioned by the pain of the recent and obviously overwhelming series of losses, was irrational and was thus significantly impairing his competence. The patient was not choosing against life, but against the pain of his losses. He had not yet learned what life awaited him as a quadriplegic who had had time to adjust to his multiple severe losses. While he might remain suicidal if that life, ultimately, was unacceptable to him, at the time of the evaluation he deserved the chance to find this out. Hopefully, in the future worst case in which he remained suicidal, there would be some acceptable and legal path to assist him to end his life.

Issues Emerging From An Analysis of These Cases

These cases prompted a discussion between an ethicist (EWDY), a psychiatrist (JCC), and legal counsel (RJ) about six issues that appear germane to the subject of depression and competency.

The first is the fairly narrow meaning of competence within the context of medical decision-making

Ethicist: The patient does not necessarily have to be broadly competent, i.e. competent to drive an automobile or an airplane, or competent to make complicated financial deals. All that is required is, (1) that the patient understand the situation and why certain treatments are either being given or proposed; (2) the implications or consequences of either accepting or refusing these treatments.

A "sliding scale" model of competency such as that proposed by Ruth Macklin,[6] attempts to avoid two types of error: that of disqualifying a competent person from participating in treatment decisions, on the one hand and, on the other, that of failing to protect an incompetent person from the harmful effects of a bad decision. The model proposed is as follows:

Standard 1: (the least stringent) applies to medical decisions that are low-risk and are objectively in the patient's interest. The cognitive requirement is that the patient be aware of the general situation, and the decisional component is satisfied by the patient's assent to the intervention.

Standard 2: requires that the patient understand the risks and outcomes of treatment options, and then be able to make a choice based on this understanding. The patient need not be able to articulate conceptual or verbal understanding, but should be able to grasp the physician's explanation with strong feelings and convictions. This standard should be applied when the illness is chronic rather than acute, or if the treatment is more dangerous or offers less certain benefit to the patient.

Standard 3: (the most stringent) applies to treatment situations in which there is little uncertainty about a correct diagnosis, the available treatment is effective, and death is likely to result from refusal of treatment. Here, the patient must be able to appreciate the nature and consequences of the decision being made. The patient must be able to give reasons for the decision. Persons suffering from mental or emotional disorders that compromise their ability to appreciate their situation or to make rational decisions fail to meet this standard.

Psychiatrist: It is important to realize that the courts have defined consent and competence across a broad continuum,[7] at least for decision-making in the case of psychiatric patients. In fact, it has varied from Standard 1 (mere failure to evidence refusal) to Standard 3 (the highest level of competence). It seems reasonable to insist on a progressively more stringent test of competence as the stakes become higher in terms of the patient's welfare. It is important to remember that in the case of psychiatric illnesses, the tendency for low self-esteem or for anger to turn against the self or against the medical decision-makers may further diminish the patient's ability to judge the relative risk *versus* benefit ratio of an offered treatment. In these cases, the physician must be extremely careful and consider whether a substituted judgment should be obtained.

Legal counsel: In California, substituted decision-making usually takes one of three forms when the patient is not competent to make medical (but not necessarily mental) treatment decisions. First, the patient may have appointed an individual to make medical decisions through a durable power of attorney for health care. Second, under certain circumstances the nearest relative can make such decisions. Finally, through a court proceeding, a treatment order, or the appointment of a conservator or guardian with the authority to make medical decisions can be obtained.[8]

The issue of restricted domain of competence is certainly relevant to psychiatric patients. Many psychotic patients who grossly distort many areas of reality remain competent in the limited sense of deciding about medical treatments.[9] The finding of psychosis does not preclude competence, per se, but merely alerts the examiner to a higher potential risk of impairment. The nature of the psychosis is all important, and this can only be ascertained by talking with the patient and considering each patient in a case by case manner.

A second issue is that of what might be regarded as appropriate versus inappropriate situational responses by patients.

Ethicist: In case 1, the patient's response to his situation seems entirely appropriate. He had been sustaining progressive losses for seven years, and had abundant time both to attempt to maximize and to assess his quality of life -- as he himself defined it. His situation was indeed depressing, as it would have been for anyone confronted by it. It would not seem to me, therefore, that his depression invalidates his competence to refuse further ventilatory support.

In case 2, this appears to be an inappropriate situational response. A conversation with the patient revealed that he was afraid his wife would leave him now that he only had one leg. Before acceding to his request to be allowed to die, the situation demanded that his wife be afforded the opportunity to tell him that she would continue to love him and stand by him despite that fact that he only had one leg. (She did this, and his attitude towards continued ventilatory support changed abruptly; he became completely compliant and, in due course, was extubated and later discharged home.)

In case 3, the patient seems competent to consent to the placement of a gastrostomy tube and to refuse electro-convulsive therapy. But her situational state of mind seems also to be strongly determined by her psychosis. I begin to feel out of my depth.

Psychiatrist: In situations where there is an obvious psychiatric disorder, I think it is wise to err on the side of requesting psychiatric consultation for a second opinion about potential impairment of competence. I remember one situation where a detailed mental status examination was required to discover that the patient's paradoxical refusal of critical treatment was totally determined by the fact that the patient's auditory hallucinations--her "voices" -- told her to refuse. The patient herself wished to have the treatment, but was terrified of challenging the "voices."

Ethicist: In the fourth case, the patient's depression seems clearly to be a response to his situation. As irresponsible as it would be to accede immediately to his request to be allowed to die, so it would seem to be inhumane and paternalistic to refuse to respond to it indefinitely. Obviously, he needs first to have attempted rehabilitation therapy, and to have attempted to rediscover some meaning in life as it now is, before it could possibly be said that his was a competent refusal of ventilatory support. The question I struggle with is, For how long? How long do we continue to impose our will on his in the belief that he is incapable of making an informed choice because of his situational depression?

Legal Counsel: You may wish to work in the avenues afforded legally in such cases: "If the treating staff and the patient continue to disagree, the patient may resort to a judicial process." In *Bouvia v. Superior Court*,[10] a 28 year-old patient suffering from cerebral palsy from birth and quadriplegic sought a court order to have her nasogastric tube removed. Even though the treating physicians believed she was trying to commit suicide, the court entered such an order after finding no evidence of suicidal intent. Or a conservator may evidently be appointed, and would ultimately have to make the decision.[11]

Psychiatrist: The question of how long do we wait also bothers me. Because I practice in California, the ethical dilemma is eased by the legal reality of state statutes which prevent psychiatrists from involuntarily confining suicidal patients for longer than thirty-one days. Since this man will be unable voluntarily to leave any treatment setting without assistance, the staff are potentially in a most difficult situation. There may be massive resistance from treatment staff and treatment institutions which might make it difficult in the extreme for this patient to have any real chance of acting on a decision to kill himself -- even if that decision were competent. He will probably need legal assistance to protect his right to refuse life-sustaining treatment. Hopefully, he would agree to counseling and empirical trials of antidepressant medications. These might restore a sense of meaningful existence, even in his compromised situation.

A third issue is whether the patients' circumstances are reversible or irreversible.
Ethicist: From my limited knowledge, reactive depressions usually have a specific event as the precipitating factor, and usually last one to three months. Chronic depressions last much longer, and are more difficult to treat. In all four cases, depression was an appropriate accompaniment to loss. The question is, is the loss "reversible" or "irreversible." In cases 1 and 4, it was probably irreversible. But in case 4, is it not too soon to allow the patient to choose to die? In cases 2 and 3, the circumstances were possibly reversible. Depending on the reversibility or irreversibility of the circumstances, the depressed person's refusal of treatment may have to be over-ridden. Which brings me back to the question, For how long? This is especially difficult in case 4.

Psychiatrist: Clearly, inappropriate situational responses do alert us to the possibility that an incompetent decision has been made. Typically, people act reasonably, and true to character. Most competent decisions seem appropriate when viewed from both the patient's and the physician's perspectives. However, we must be particularly careful when "appropriate" decisions have grave consequences. This is because the term "appropriate" necessarily invites the physician to put herself in the patient's situation. Sometimes severely ill patients handle their situations far better than we could ever imagine handling them ourselves.

In psychiatry, the term "countertransference" is used to describe how one's own character and personal psychological issues can distort perceptions and judgments. Physicians must be aware of their own countertransference issues; these potentially influence their assessment of a patient's treatment decision. In psychiatry, strong countertransference responses are frequently encountered in the responses of medical staff to suicidal patients, and range from hostility to over-identification. I think that there is the potential problem of what I term "countertransference compassion" for medical staff in dealing with these terrible clinical situations.

The countertransference concept must also be considered in any situation of substituted judgment. The task of the substitute decision-maker is to make the decision most in accord with the patient's preferences -- so far as these preferences can be determined. This means acting as the patient would have acted.[12] Only when the patient's preferences cannot be known should the decision-maker use his own preferences -- putting himself in the patient's shoes. The ability to use the patient's preferences rather than one's own is dependent on one's awareness of one's own countertransference responses and their contribution to the decision-making process.

Even when a patient's preferences cannot be known, a substitute decision may be strongly biased if countertransference issues are not examined, as in the situation where the decision-maker's personal history loads the issue of withdrawing care, one way or the other. A psychiatric consultant should ideally be well positioned and by training equipped to assist medical staff and family members with this difficult role.

Legal counsel: Mental rights advocates[13] have asserted as the overriding principle the deprivation of freedom inherent in involuntary confinement. They have successfully imported the procedural due process (right to representation, hearings, etc.) found in other areas (e.g., criminal penalties) where involuntary confinement occurs into treatment decisions for mental disorders.

Psychiatrist: Their countertransference response is to promulgate regulations which are so restrictive that many psychiatrists feel that patients are being allowed to "rot with the rights on." That is to say, the protection of individual autonomy is so absolutistic that the patient-benefiting principle (beneficence) is overridden, restricting treatment and often equating treatment with brief and often inadequate confinement.

With respect to the issue of reversibility, there is simply no way to be sure that a depression is irreversible other than to treat it vigorously. Even chronic "characterological" depressions can surprise experienced clinicians by responding nicely to antidepressant medications.

While losses may be irreversible, the mental state produced by these losses is typically reversible -- to a large extent. Even irreversible circumstances may be accompanied by reversible states of depression. There is no way to tell, ahead of time. We are left to treat as best we can, and allow the passage of time to define which depressions are truly irreversible. Just as I did not feel that we should simply equate depression with incompetence, I do not feel that irreversible circumstances should be equated with irreversible depressions.

On the other hand, the fact of irreversibly compromised circumstances does seem to limit the losses occasioned if a patient's incompetent decision to refuse treatment is mis-identified as competent and is thus respected by the treatment staff. The issue of irreversibility is particularly salient in the area of terminal care. In California, we are witnessing increasing efforts by the lay public to legalize physician-assisted suicide for terminal patients.[14] Reversibility is what distinguishes the non-terminal suicidal patient who would be involuntarily confined from the terminal suicidal patient who may be assisted in his suicide. Case 4 puts the issue rather nicely: What should we do with the suicidal, apparently terminally miserable, but not clearly terminal patient?

Fourthly, these cases remind us that we have constantly to balance the ethical principles of nonmaleficence, beneficence, and respect for autonomy.

Ethicist: Although, as has been mentioned, respect for autonomy has become a highly prized ethical principle in American medicine in the latter half of the twentieth century, it is neither the only ethical principle nor the one that necessarily trumps all others. Physicians must also be attentive to the principles of non-maleficence (requiring the avoidance of harm to the patient and the alleviation of suffering) and beneficence (mandating the attempt to preserve life), as well as to the proportionality of harms to benefits. Too readily respecting a patient's autonomy may result in avoidable harms, as in the second and third cases. To defer respecting a patient's right to choose for too long may equally harm the patient, as in the fourth case. It seems that as the likelihood of harms increases, so the more stringent the standard for competency must be -- as in Ruth Macklin's "sliding scale."

Psychiatrist: I tend to agree. The issue of autonomy as an overriding principle is necessarily delimited by the clinical reality of the patient. Autonomy rests on the substrate of patient mental competence. Disease, particularly mental illness, threatens this substrate. The other two principles, nonmaleficence and beneficence, seem to rest on the substrate of provider professional and ethical competence.

Fifthly, different responses are required of caregivers in emergent and non-emergent situations.

Ethicist: In emergent situations, the general rule has to be that of doing everything necessary to stabilize the patient, and then to evaluate. Therefore, all attempted suicides brought into the emergency department have to be treated aggressively, the presumption and hope being that, with appropriate support, therapy, and counseling, they will see the world differently and choose life over death. Suicidal ideation in the non-emergent situation may be very different. It may be entirely rational, even though the person wishing to die may be chronically depressed (as in case 1). Here, the irreversibility of the situation which produces the depression may also provide grounds for respecting the autonomy of the person who wishes to die.

Legal counsel: The initial decision about competence was stated quite strongly, and bothered me for that reason. The practitioner must keep one eye on the legal framework when approaching such cases. For example, initially the decision was that the patient was not competent to make the decision to withdraw life support. But in documenting such a conclusion in the medical record, room must be left for deciding later that circumstances have changed, and that the patient is now competent. What factors were listed initially? How have these factors changed?

Psychiatrist: As a psychiatrist, I would make the additional point that any patient with a chronic depression or suicidal state of mind should be offered treatment for depression, including antidepressant medications and counseling. If competent, he or she would then have the option of refusing treatment. If not competent, a substitute decision-maker should be chosen to make the treatment decision. If a competent patient, who wants life-sustaining treatments stopped, refused antidepressant treatments I personally would have difficulty assisting their decision. Given the subtleties of clinical depression, I would hope that I was offered antidepressant treatment before I chose such a course of action for myself.

Sixth and finally, family members and friends can serve as important checks and balances on a patient's competency.

Ethicist: Family members and friends can provide a larger context in which to make an assessment of a depressed person's treatment choices. In case 1, the family was extremely supportive: his mother, father, sister, as well as the nurses who had cared for the patient at home all agreed that the patient was making a reasonable choice, entirely consistent with the effort he had made over the past seven years to discover meaning in his life and with his own self-definition of quality of life. This made the eventual decision easier. In case 2, the patient's wife was equally helpful, both in resisting the suicidal impulse and in reassuring the patient that she would continue to love him with one leg. In case 3 thee was no family. In case 4, the wife had contributed to the present problem and was not at all available. In all cases, family members and friends can provide and invaluable check on reality and balance to impulsive or hasty decisions.

Psychiatrist: I concur. Family and friends, if available, can alert the physician to any decision which seems "out of character" for the patient, and thus more suspect of being incompetent. Also, the mobilization of the patient's support system and their supportive presence can shore up a failing sense of self, remind a patient of meaning systems and identities overwhelmed by the impact of the immediate situation, and lessen the forces that compel the patient to choose suicide.

Concluding Remarks

Psychiatrist: My major comments in these cases seem to focus on the need to offer depressed or suicidal patients treatment for their depressions. Clinical, biological, or endogenous depression can never be decisively ruled out as a contributing factor in any request for withdrawal of life-sustaining treatment. So I would treat vigorously, and allow ample time for treatment to be effective (three to four weeks minimum). My duty to my patient as a physician requires me to make sure that the patient, and not the illness, is making this mortal decision to end a life. I repeat what I said earlier: the psychiatric consultant's job is to protect the patient from the disease by ensuring, so far as possible, that the patient, rather than the disease, makes the decision.

Ethicist: Of course, this presupposes the sovereignty of the medical model. Eric Cassell makes the point, somewhat humorously, that illness is what a patient has when he or she goes to a physician; he or she returns home with a disease.[15] The fact that a discrete disease can be named and studied scientifically creates in contemporary medicine a tendency to treat the disease, rather than the patient. All who cherish the notion that the art of medicine is as important as the science must resist this tendency. Part of the art of medicine may consist of recognizing that a time may come in the course of an illness when the disease can no longer be separated from the patient: the illness is so pervasive and profound that it "takes over" the patient's life--dominating his or her worldview, attitudes, actions, and sense of self. Quadriplegia may well have that effect eventually. Whereas the physician may want to continue regarding the disease as an adversary, to be driven back or at least held at bay by all means possible, the patient may have come to the point where death is preferable to a life so dominated by the illness. At such a juncture, the ethicist may have to stand with the patient against the physician. Whereas the physician is concerned not to have the disease speak for the patient, the ethicist may have to ensure that the voice of the patient with the illness is clearly heard. I wonder how patients can be treated vigorously for their depressions when this is not what they want?

Legal counsel: This can be done only by utilizing the legal process for holding the patient involuntarily and treating the mental disorder. In this regard, the amount of time the patient can be held and treated is limited, and may or may not furnish sufficient time for successful treatment.

Psychiatrist: I also briefly discussed countertransference issues which would seem to be endemic in the arena of terminal care. Substitute decision-making requires that family members and the treatment staff try to "put themselves in the patient's shoes." Psychiatric consultants, trained to recognize countertransference issues, could provide assistance with this difficult role of substitute decision-maker.

Notes

1. See Rothman DJ. *Strangers at the Bedside*. New York, NY: Basic Books, 1991; and Young EWD. *Alpha and Omega: Ethics at the Frontiers of Life and Death.* Reading, MA: Addison-Wesley, 1989.
2. See Faden RR, Beauchamp TL. *A History and Theory of Informed Consent.* New York, NY: Oxford University Press, 1986.
3. For the purpose of this paper, "competence" is used in the legal sense of "capacity for consenting or refusing medical treatment," and not in the legal sense of competence to continue to manage one's affairs as in a conservatorship proceeding. In California, capacity for treatment decisions is generally defined as the ability to understand the nature and consequences of treatment to which one is asked to consent, or the refusal of that treatment. California Association of Hospitals and Health Systems, *Consent Manual*. 19th ed. at 15.
4. California Welfare and Institutions Code, Section 5326.7.
5. An individual can be held involuntarily if the individual is a danger to self or others or gravely disabled as a result of a mental disorder, and treated for that mental disorder. The procedure to justify such involuntary treatment increases as the length of stay, i.e., 72 hours, 14 days, 14 more days. California Welfare and Institutions Code, Section 5150 *et seq.*

6. Macklin R. *Mortal Choices: Ethical Dilemmas in Modern Medicine.* Boston, MA: Howard Mifflin Company, 1987:91-93. This approach was suggested earlier in a paper by JF Drane. Competency to give an informed consent, *Journal of the American Medical Association* 1984;252:925-7.
7. Roth LH, Meisel A, Lidz CW. Tests of competency to consent to treatment, *American Journal of Psychiatry* 1977;134:279-284. See also Kentsmith DK, Salladay SA, Kiya PA, eds. *Ethics in Mental Health Practice*. Orlando, FL: Grune & Stratton, Inc., 1986:83-108.
8. California Association of Hospitals and Health systems, *Consent Manual* 199, 19th Edition:Chap. 5.3.
9. For example, in California an individual may retain the right to make medical decisions even when a conservator has been appointed to make financial and other decisions for the individual. California Probate Code, Section 2354.
10. 179 Cal. App. 3d 1986:1127.
11. *Conservator of Drabick*, 200 Cal. App. 3d 185 (1988) -- affirming the authority of the conservator to withdraw life sustaining treatments.
12. California Association of Hospitals and Health Systems, *Consent Manual*, 1992, 19th Edition:Chap. 5.3.
13. Lawyers have often helped mental rights advocates, but mental rights advocates are not necessarily lawyers.
14. An initiative that would have allowed physician assisted death on the November, 1992, ballot in California was defeated. The Hemlock Society has stated that it intends to pursue another such ballot measure in California.
15. Cassell EJ. *The Healer's Art*. Cambridge, MA: MIT Press, 1985.

Chapter 28

The Many Faces of Competency

James F. Drane

The doctrine of informed consent, less than twenty-five years old, creates many dilemmas because it tries to balance very different values -- specifically, on one side beneficence (health or well-being); on the other, autonomy (or self-determination). Most of the ethical commentary on informed consent and a majority of the court cases deciding consent questions have focused on the physician's responsibilities to disclose information and to keep the medical setting free of coercion. But more and more frequently clinical questions arise about the capacity or competence of a specific patient to give an informed consent.

If the patient is not competent, then his or her consent does not constitute an authorization to treat, no matter how thorough the disclosure or how free from coercion the medical setting. Incompetence also calls into question a patient's refusal of treatment. Patient competence in effect is a condition for the validity of consent. Incompetence both reveals a new obligation to identify a surrogate and provides a basis for the physician to set aside the informed consent requirement in favor of what he or she thinks is best for the patient.

Only recently have scholars begun to pay attention to this element in the informed consent doctrine. Loren Roth, Paul Appelbaum, Alan Meisel, and Charles Lidz found that different clinicians use very different tests to judge competence.[1] They reduced these to five categories: (1) making a choice; (2) reasonable outcome of choice or ability to produce a reasonable choice; (3) choice based on rational reasons; (4) ability to understand the decision-making process; and (5) actual understanding of the process. Later, Appelbaum and Roth suggested four possible standards for judging competency: (1) evidencing a choice; (2) factual understanding of issues; (3) rational manipulation of information; and (4) appreciation of the nature of the situation. They found any one of the four to be acceptable, as long as it was justified by a reasonable policy perspective.[2] Other authors have argued for a single standard: For Grace A. Olin and Harry S. Olin, competence means ability to retain information. For Howard Owens reality testing is the standard. Bernard Gert and Charles Colvet in their book, *Philosophy in Medicine*, helped clarify the term by showing different ways competence is used in ordinary and professional language. Alan A. Stone has written extensively on informed consent and severely criticized court decisions that extended competency even of involuntary mental patients to refuse treatment. Mark Siegler made important conceptual points about the meaning of competency, and more than any other writer connected the issue to the medical setting in which it emerges.[3]

Finally, the President's Commission for the Study of Ethical Problems in Medicine and Biomedical and Behavioral Research in a recently published report discussed competency, which the Commission prefers to call decision-making capacity.[4] The Commission spelled out

---

Source: Reprinted from *Hastings Center Report*, Vol. 15, No. 2, pp. 17-21, with permission from The Hastings Center © April, 1985.

the components of competency or decisional capacity: the possession of a set of values and goals, the ability to communicate and understand information, and the ability to reason and deliberate.

Although they did not adopt any one of the standards listed by Roth and Appelbaum, the Commissioners were very critical of the first two tests: "evidencing a preference" and "reasonable outcome" of the patient's decision.

Despite all the work done to date, the competency question remains unsettled. What should the standard for competence be in order to ensure valid consent or refusal of consent to medical procedures? To be acceptable, any standard of competence must meet several important objectives. It must incorporate the general guidelines set out in legal decisions; it must be psychiatrically and philosophically sound; it must guarantee the realization of ethical values on which the consent requirement is based; and it must be applicable in a clinical setting.

In practice some tests seem too lenient and expose patients to serious harm. Others seem too stringent and turn almost all seriously ill patients into incompetents, thereby depriving them of rights and dignity. The solution proposed here is based on no one standard, but works out a sliding scale for competency. Accordingly as the medical decision itself (the task) changes, the standards of competency to perform the task also change.

The Competency Assessment

As long as a patient does or says nothing strange and acquiesces to treatment recommended by the medical professional, questions of competency do not arise. These questions arise usually when the patient refuses treatment or chooses a course of action which, in the opinion of the physician in charge, threatens his or her well-being. Either consenting to treatment or refusing consent may raise a suspicion of unreasonableness. More careful evaluation is then called for before a final determination of competency is made.

Competency assessment usually focuses on the patient's mental capacities: specifically the mental capacities to make a particular medical decision. Does this patient understand what is being disclosed? Can this patient come to a decision about treatment based on that information? How much understanding and rational decision-making capacity is sufficient for this patient to be considered competent? Or how deficient must this patient's decision-making capacity be before he or she is declared incompetent? A properly performed competency assessment should eliminate two types of error: preventing competent persons from deciding their own treatments; and failing to protect incompetent persons from the harmful effects of a bad decision.

The assessment process leads to a decision about a decision. A good clinical determination must balance the different and sometimes competing values of rationality, beneficence, and autonomy. Rationality, or reasonableness, is an underlying assumption in competency determinations. In an emergency we presume that a rational person would want treatment and the informed consent requirement is set aside. But rationality cannot be set aside in nonemergency settings. A particular medical setting establishes certain expectations about what a reasonable person would do, and these expectations play an important role in competency determinations.

The patient's well-being (beneficence) also has to be considered in assessing competence. The same laws that establish right to give or refuse informed consent express concern about protecting patients from the harm that could result from serious defects in decision-making capacity. Finally, a competency assessment must respect the value of autonomy. Patients must be permitted to determine their own and a decision cannot be set aside simply because it differs from what other persons think is indicated.

A Sliding-Scale Model

How should the physician proceed when deciding on a patient's competence? The model purposed here posits three general categories of medical situations; in each category, as the consequences flowing from patient decisions become more serious, competency standards for valid consent or refusal of consent become more stringent. The psychiatric pathologies most likely to undermine the mental capacities required for each type of decision are listed in the tables.

A number of assumptions underlie the use of a sliding scale or variable standard rather than one ideal competency test. First, the objective content of the decision must be taken into consideration so that competency determinations remain linked to the decision at hand. Second, the value of reasonableness operates at every level. When people sit down to play chess, certain expectations are created even though no particular decisions are required. If, however, one player makes peculiar moves, the other will have to wonder whether his partner is competent or knows what he is doing. Something similar is assumed in the patient-physician partnership. Third, the reasonableness assumption justifies some paternalistic behavior. The physician or another surrogate is authorized by this model to decide what is best for the patient who is incompetent. In more cases than a patient-rights advocate would prefer, the patient's decision is set aside in favor of beneficence. The clinical values of health and patient well-being are balanced with the libertarian values of autonomy and self-determination.

Easy, Effective Treatments

Standard No. 1. The first and least stringent standard of competence to give a valid consent applies to medical decisions that are not dangerous and are objectively in the patient's best interest. Even though these patients are seriously ill, and thereby impaired in cognitive and volitional functioning, their consent to an effective, safe treatment is considered informed so long as the patient is aware of what is going on. Awareness, in the sense of being in contact with one's situation, satisfies the cognitive requirement of informed consent. Assent alone to the rational expectations of others satisfies the volitional component. When an adult goes along with what is considered appropriate and rational, then the presumption of competency holds. Higher standards for capacity to give a valid consent to this first type of medical intervention would be superfluous.

Consider the following two examples. Betty Campbell, a twenty-five-year-old secretary who lives alone, has an accident. She arrives at the hospital showing signs of mild shock and suffering from the associated mental deficiencies; but her consent to blood transfusion, bone-setting, or even to some minor surgery need not be questioned. Even though there is no emergency, if she is aware of her situation and assents to receiving an effective, low-risk treatment for a certain diagnosis, there is no reason to question her competence to consent.

Phil Randall's situation is quite different. A twenty-three-year-old veteran who has been addicted to drugs and alcohol, he is on probation and struggling to survive in college. When Phil stops talking and eating for almost a week, his roommate summons a trusted professor. By this time Phil is catatonic, but the professor manages get him on his feet and accompanies him in a police car to the state hospital. The professor gets through to Phil sufficiently to explain the advantages of signing in as a voluntary patient. Phil signs his name to the admission form, authorizing commitment and initial treatment. His consent to this first phase of therapy is valid because Phil is sufficiently aware of his situation to understand what is happening, and he assents to the treatment. Later on, when his condition improves, another consent may be required, especially if a more dangerous treatment or a long-term hospitalization is required. The next decision will require a higher degree of competence because it is a different type of task.

Having a lenient standard of competence for safe and effective treatments eliminates the ambiguity and confusion associated with phrases like "virtually competent," "marginally competent," and "competent for practical purposes." Such phrases are used to excuse the common sense practice of holding certain decisions to be valid even though the patients are considered incompetent by some abstract standard, which ignores the specific rusk or type of medical decision at hand.

The same modest standard of competence should apply to a dying patient who refuses to consent to treatments that are ineffective and useless. This is the paradigm case in the refusal-of-ineffective-treatment category.

Most of the patients who would be considered incompetent to make treatment decisions under this first category are legally incompetent. Those who use psychotic defenses that impede the awareness of their situation and any decision-making ability are the only other patients who fall outside the wide first criterion. Even children who have reached the age of reason can be considered competent. According to law however, those below the ages of twenty-one or sometimes eighteen are presumed incompetent to make binding contracts, including health care decisions.

But exceptions are common. The Pennsylvania Mental Health Procedures Act (1976), for example, decided that fourteen-year-old adolescents were competent to give informed consent to psychiatric hospitalization. Adolescents are also considered competent in many jurisdictions to make decisions about birth control and abortion. I am suggesting that, for this first type of decision, children as young as ten or eleven are competent.

Authors like Alexander M. Capron, Willard Gaylin, and Ruth Macklin support a lowering of the age of competency to make some medical decisions.[5] The President's Commission also endorses a lower age of competence. The physician, however, cannot ignore the law and must obtain the consent of the child's legal guardian. But if a minor is competent or partially competent, there is good reason to involve him or her in the decision-making process.

Less Certain Treatments

Standard No. 2. If the diagnosis is doubtful, or the condition chronic; if the diagnosis is certain but the treatment is more dangerous or not quite so effective; if there are alternative treatments, or no treatment at all is an alternative, then a different type of task is involved in making an informed treatment decision. Consequently, a different standard of competence is required. The patient now must be able to understand the risks and outcomes of the different options and then be able to make a decision based on this understanding. In this sorting, competence means ability to understand the treatment options, balance risks and benefits, and come to a deliberate decision. In other words, a higher standard of competence is required than the one discussed above. Let me give some examples of this type of decision, and the corresponding competency standards.

Antonio Marachal is a retired steel worker who has been hospitalized with a bad heart valve. Both the surgeon and his family doctor recommend an operation to replace the valve. Mr. Marachal understands what they tell him, but is afraid of undergoing the operation. He thinks he'll live just as long by taking good care of himself. His fear of surgery may not be entirely rational, but the option he prefers is real and there is no basis for considering his refusal to be invalid because of incompetence.

Or consider Geraldine Brown, a forty-year-old unmarried woman who is diagnosed as having leukemia. Chemotherapy offers a good chance for remission, but the side effects are repugnant and frightening to her. After hearing and understanding the diagnosis, alternatives, risks, and prognosis, she refuses, deciding instead to follow a program that centers on diet, exercise, meditation, and some natural stimulants to her immune system.

A Sliding - Scale Model for Competency

STANDARD NO. 1

Objective Medical Decisions

A. *Incompetent*			B. *Competent*
unconscious severe retardation small children total disorientation severe senile dementia autism pschotic defenses denial of self and situation delusional projection	Consent effective treatment for acute illness diagnostic certainty high benefit/low risk limited alternatives severe disorder/major distress/immediately life-threatening	Refusal ineffective treatment	children(10 and above) retarded(educable) clouded sensorium mild senile dementia intoximcated conditions listed under #2 and #3 (A & B)

Competency Standards

Minimal Reguirements:

1. *Awareness*: orientation to one's medical situation
2. *Assent*: explicit or implied

STANDARD NO. 2

Objective Medical Decisions

A. *Incompetent*		B. *Competent*
severe mood disorders phobia about treatment mutism short term memory loss thought disorders ignorance incoherence delusion hallucination delirium conditions listed under #1 (A & B)	consent or refusal chronic condition/doubtful diagnosis uncertain outcome of therapy for acute illness balanced risks and benefits: possibly effective, but burdensome high risk, only hope	adolescent (16 and over) mildly retarded personality disorders: narcissistic, borderline and obsessive conditions listed under #3 (A & B)

Competency Standards

Median Requirements:

1. *Understanding*: of medical situation and proposed treatment
2. *Choice*: based on medical outcomes

STANDARD NO. 3

Objective Medical Decisions

A. *Incompetent*			B. *Competent*
indecisive or ambivalent over time false beliefs about reality hysteria substance abuse neurotic defenses: intellectualization repression dissociation acting out mild depression hypomania conditions listed under #1 and #2 (A & B)	consent ineffective treatment	effective treatment for actue illness diagnostic certainty high benefit/low risk limited alternatives sever disorder/major distress/immediately life-threatening	above legal age reflective and self-critical mature coping devices: altrusim anticipation sublimation

Competency Standards

Maximum Requirements:

1. *Appreciation*: critical and reflective understanding of illness and treatment.
2. *Rational decision*: based on relevant implications including articulated beliefs and values

Objectively, the standard medical treatment is preferable to what she decides, but informed consent joins objective medical data with subjective personal factors such as repugnance and burden. In this case, the objective and subjective components balance out. A decision one way or the other is reasonable, and a person who can understand the options and decide in light of them is competent.

Although ability to understand is not the same as being capable of conceptual or verbal understanding, some commentators assume that the two are synonymous in every case. Many would require that patients remember the ideas and repeat what they have been told as a proof of competence. Real understanding, however, may be more a matter of emotions. Following an explanation, the patient may grasp what is best for her with strong feelings and convictions, and yet be hard pressed to articulate or conceptualize her understanding or conviction.

Competence as capacity for an understanding choice can also be reconciled with a decision to let a trusted physician decide what is the best treatment. Such a choice (a waiver) may be made for good reasons and represent a decision in favor of one set of values (safety or anxiety reduction) over another (independence and personal initiative). As such, it can be considered an informed consent and create no suspicion about competence.

Ignorance or inability to understand, however, does incapacitate a person for making this type of decision. This is especially so when the ignorance extends to the options and persists even after patient and careful explanation. Patience and care may sometimes require that more than one person be involved in the disclosure process before a person is judged incompetent to understand. An explanation by someone from the same ethnic, religious, or economic background may also be necessary.

Dangerous Treatments

Standard No. 3. The stringent and demanding criterion for competence is reserved for those treatment decisions that are very dangerous, and run counter to both professional and public rationality. Here the decision involves not a balancing of what are widely recognized as reasonable alternatives or a reasonable response to a doubtful diagnosis, but a choice that seems to violate reasonableness. The patient's decision now appears irrational, indeed life-threatening. And yet, according to this model, such decisions are valid and respectable as long as the person making them satisfies the most demanding standards of competence. The patient's decision is a different type of task than the others we have considered. As such, different and more stringent criteria of capacity are appropriate.

Competence in this context requires an ability on the part of the decision-maker to appreciate what he or she is doing. Appreciation requires the highest degree of understanding, one that grasps more than just the medical details of the illness, options, risks, and treatment. To be competent to make apparently irrational and very dangerous choices, the patient must appreciate the implications of the medical information for his or her life. Competence here requires an understanding that is both technical and personal, intellectual and emotional.

Because such decisions contravene public standards of rationality, they must be subjectively critical and reflective. The competent patient must be able to give reasons for the decision, which show that he has thought through the medical issues and related this information to his personal values. The patient's personal reasons need not be scientific or publicly accepted, but neither can they be purely private or idiosyncratic. Their intelligibility may derive from a minority religious view, but they must be coherent and follow the logic of that belief system. This toughest standard of competence demands a more rational understanding: one that includes verbalization, consistency, and the like. Some examples will illustrate.

Bob Cassidy, an eighteen-year-old high school senior and an outstanding athlete, is involved in an automobile accident which has crushed his left foot. Attempts to save the limb are unsuccessful, and infection threatens the boy's life. Surgeons talk to parents who immediately give permission for amputation of the leg below the knee. Since Bob is legally no longer a minor, however, his consent is required for the surgery, but he refuses. "If I cannot play sports, my life is meaningless," he says. First the doctors try to talk to him, then his parents, finally some of his friends. But he refuses to discuss the matter. When anyone comes to his room he simply closes his eyes and lies motionless. "If they cannot make my foot as good as before, I want to die," he tells them. "What good is it to live with only one leg? Without sports I can't see anything worth living for." Bob is using unhealthy coping behavior to handle his situation. He refuses to consider the implications of what he is doing and shows signs of being seriously depressed. No arguments or justifications are offered to counter the indications of immaturity and mild emotional illness. For these reasons he is incompetent for the task he presumes to undertake.

Charles Kandell is a Jehovah's Witness and refuses a blood transfusion after a bad accident at his job. He is not yet in shock, but will shortly be in danger of death. His wife: and family support his refusal and pledge to help care for his children. The doctor asks Charles if he fears judgment from God if blood were given against his will. He is adamant, explaining to the medical group that he has lived his life by these beliefs, knows the possible consequences, and holds eternal life to be more important than life here on earth. This decision meets the high standards required for such a decision, and should be respected as a competent refusal.

A patient need not have a serious psychiatric pathology in order to be considered incompetent to make such serious decisions. On the other hand, not every mental or emotional disturbance would constitute incompetence. A certain amount of anxiety, for example, accompanies any serious decision. A patient may suffer some pain, which would not necessarily impair such a decision. Even a degree of reactive depression may not incapacitate a patient for this type of decision. But any mental or emotional disorder that compromises appreciation and rational decision making would make a person incompetent. Persons, for example, who are incapable of controlling their destructive behavior cannot be considered competent to decide about treatments that have destructive features. Consequently, a patient who is hospitalized for a self-inflicted injury would not be considered competent to refuse a life-saving treatment. And dangerous decisions that are inconsistent with life-long values are strongly suspect as being products of incompetence.

The paradigm case of consent to ineffective treatment is a decision to engage in a high-risk drug trial unrelated to one's own illness.

Objections to the Sliding Scale

Certain objections to this sliding scale notion are easy to anticipate. Libertarian thinkers will see it as justifying paternalistic behavior on the part of physicians and diminishing the patient's discretion to do whatever he or she prefers no matter what the consequence. True, by these standards some patient decisions would not be respected, but competency was originally required and continues to be needed in order to set aside certain dangerous and harmful decisions. This model provides guidelines for determining which patient decisions fall within the original purpose for a competency requirement. Besides, the sliding scale provides a justification even for decisions that are considered by some to be irrational. Instead of limiting freedom, it safeguards patient autonomy while balancing this value with well-being.

Admittedly, in the least stringent category the outcome, which is beneficial to the patient, plays a role in establishing the rationality of the decision and the competency of the decision-maker. The President's Commission rejected a standard based on outcome for the following reason: If only the physician can determine outcome, and outcome constitutes the only test of a competent choice, then competence is a matter of doing what the doctor thinks best. But outcome is not the standard of competence in this model, rather it is an important factor in only one class of medical decisions. In other decisions patients may competently go against medical assessment of outcome. In fact, a decision that leads to an outcome that professionals and nonprofessionals alike would consider the most unacceptable -- unnecessary death -- can be considered a valid and competent option according to this model.

Objections will also bc raised against the most stringent standard for judging competence. If every patient must understand thoroughly and make a rational decision in order to be considered competent, then too many people will be considered incompetent. Consequently, the medical delivery system will be clogged with surrogate decision-making, and many patients will be robbed of dignity and self-determination. The most stringent standard in this model requires just such capacities for competence, but only in cases where the patient has most to lose from his or her choice. If patients in category three suffer a decline in autonomy (and they do because some decisions will not be respected), this is balanced by a gain in beneficence.

Balancing Values

A balancing of values is the cornerstone of a good competency assessment. Rationality is given its place throughout model. Not only does the sliding scale reflect a rational ordering of things, but reasonableness is an underlying assumption for each standard of competence. Maximum autonomy, however, is also guaranteed because patients can choose to do even what is not at all beneficial (participate in an experiment which has little chance of improving their condition) or refuse to do what is most beneficial. Finally, beneficence is respected because patients are protected against harmful choices, when time are more the product of pathology than of self-determination.

Notes

1. Roth LH, Lidz CW, Meisel A. Toward a model of the legal doctrine of informed consent, *American Journal of Psychiatry* 1977;134:279-84, 285-89; Appelbaum PS, Roth LH. Clinical issues in the assessment of competency, *American Journal of Psychiatry* 1981;138:1462-67; and The dilemma of denial in the assessment of competency to refuse treatment, *American Journal of Psychiatry* 1982;139:910-13.
2. Appelbaum PS, Roth LH. Competency to consent to research, *Archives of General Psychiatry* 1982;39:951-58.
3. GA Olin, HS Olin. Informed consent in voluntary mental hospital admission, *American Journal of Psychiatry* 1975;132:938-41; Owens H. When is a voluntary commitment really voluntary? *American Journal of Orthopsychiatry* 1977;47:104-10; Culver C, Gert B. *Philosophy in Medicine.* New York, NY: Oxford University Press, 1982; Stone A. The right to refuse treatment, *Archives of General Psychiatry* 1981;38:358-62; Stone A. Informed consent: Special problems for psychiatry, *Hospital and Community Psychiatry* 1979;30:231-37; Siegler M. Critical illness: The limits of autonomy, *Hastings Center Report* 1977;7:12-15; and Siegler M, Goldblatt AD. Clinical intuition: A procedure for balancing the rights of patients and the responsibilities of physicians, In: Spicker SE, Healey JM, Engelhardt HT, eds., *The Law-Medicine Relation: A Philosophical Exploration* Dordrecht, Holland: D. Reidel Publishing Co., 1981.
4. The Presidents Commission for the Study of Ethical Problems in Medicine and Biomedical and Behavioral Research. *Making Heath Care Decisions*, Vol. 1, Washington, DC: U.S. Government Printing Office, 1982.
5. Gaylin W, Macklin R, eds. *Who Speaks for the Child?* New York, NY: Pienum Press, 1982.

SECTION 5

ADULT MEDICINE

Chapter 29

Cases 5.0

Case 5.1: SICKLE CELL CRISIS IN PREGNANT JEHOVAH'S WITNESS

You have learned from a staff member that a Jehovah's Witness patient is in your hospital's Ob-Gyn unit. She is currently in a very painful sickle-cell crisis and is 24 weeks along in her pregnancy. Her hemoglobin has dropped so low that the physicians are worried about the fetus dying (it is 5.2 at the last reading). As a Jehovah's Witness, however, she has, in the past, refused and currently refuses a blood transfusion. That is no problem, except that the reason she is in the Ob-Gyn unit is for a Caesarean Section. She required one for her earlier and only other known pregnancy six years ago.

Ms. M. is not married. Her extended family accompanied her and reinforces her decision to refuse a transfusion. One member of the family said they were there because years ago, during a sickle cell crisis, she "broke down and asked for a transfusion." The family wants to insure that this does not happen again.

Ms. M. is 36-years-old and not in good health. In addition to her sickle cell disease, she suffers from high blood pressure (she is on medications to control it), diabetes (adult onset, controlled -- from time to time -- by diet), obesity (she weighs 310 pounds at 5' 4"), and arthritis in her knees.

The reason for the phone call to you is that the anesthesiologist, who was to assist at the C-Section, is deeply concerned. If the C-Section is done without transfusion, enough blood might be lost that the mother would die. At the very least, the anesthesiologist believes that not to give a transfusion would constitute a failure of practicing the standard of care. Yet, to give a transfusion would violate the patient's deepest religious values and her right to determine her care. Transferring Ms. M to another hospital would seem to be a way out, yet her health is such that a transfer would constitute a kind of abandonment, and may leave the hospital open to a lawsuit. Transferring Ms. M. would endanger both the patient and the fetus. Dr. Charleston, the anesthesiologist, is aware of recent court cases that upheld the right of the patient to make religious choices even when they had obligations to children. She is also aware of the possibility of getting a court order to transfuse the mother in order to save the fetus. Yet, her quandary remains: even with such a court order, once the umbilical cord has been cut, the patient's life would no longer be tied to the life of the fetus. Could one still give the patient a blood transfusion when necessary during the final stages of the operation and early recovery?

Consider the following questions:

1. Do you support Ms. M's refusal of the blood transfusion?

2. Should a patient's religious values affect a physician's determination of medical care?

3. How does the fact that Ms. M is pregnant influence your decision in this case?

Case 5.2: SUICIDE ATTEMPT AND EMERGENCY ROOM ETHICS

After the car that he is driving at high speed hits a telephone pole, Mr. D. is brought to the hospital emergency room in serious condition. The physicians who examine him recommend surgery to repair a major internal hemorrhage. But the sixty-eight-year-old man refuses, saying that he wants to be "left alone to die." The physicians also learn that three weeks earlier Mr. D. was diagnosed as having carcinoma of the tongue. He has refused surgery for the lesion and has asked his own physician not to tell his wife that he has a fatal disease.

The hospital physicians believe that Mr. D. will die without surgery for the hemorrhage, and they call a psychiatric resident to evaluate the patient. Dr. M. interviews Mr. D. and finds him coherent, rational, and alert. Mr. D. describes himself as a man who values independence. He feels he has a good professional life as an engineer, and a good personal life with his wife and two children. He expresses some sadness at his situation, but says, "I have had a good full life and now it's over."

Dr. M. suggests, and Mr. D. does not deny, that the automobile accident was a deliberate suicide attempt. What should Dr. M. recommend? That the patient's treatment refusal for immediate surgery be accepted as the act of a rational person? That the refusal not be honored, and a court order sought on the ground that a presumed suicide attempt is per se evidence of mental illness?[1]

Case 5.3: A SURGEON'S QUALITY OF LIFE

A surgeon named Tom was 35 years old, and the single-parent of a 14 year old boy. Tom kept himself in great shape, running each morning for 10 miles, and lifting weights in the evening at his local health club.

One morning while jogging, Tom was hit from behind by a truck. The force of the impact broke his neck at the C5 disc. He was immediately paralyzed from the jaw down.

After being stabilized at the hospital, Tom was brought to the spinal cord injury service of the V.A. hospital. During a bout with pneumonia, he begged his neurologist not to treat him. He said he wanted to be allowed to die. The neurologist refused. This refusal was based in the neurologist's mind on the "ambivalence" expressed by the patient. Tom said he did not want to live this way, but when he had difficulty breathing, he requested help.

The surgeon allowed only Tom's parents to visit him, but not his son. Tom claimed that he had nothing to live for, and that he particularly did not want his son to see him in this condition.

A second major crisis occurred. After an operation to fuse the discs to prevent further damage --an operation agreed to by the patient only after many days of discussion--Tom suffered a respiratory arrest. After resuscitation, Tom saw two of his own classmates who now practice at the V.A. hospital in question, and who were involved in the resuscitation attempt. Tom cried bitterly to them about his status, and begged them not to do it again.

After further stabilization, Tom was taken permanently off a ventilator, and a more complete discussion with the neurologists took place again. Tom's view of his quality of life included the following features:

- The social position of a surgeon in society, one that he could no longer exercise.
- Fatherhood, which he identified with being actively supportive to his son throughout his teens and into adulthood.
- His own sexual prowess, now permanently inoperative. He can no longer have a relationship with a woman, especially with his girlfriend.

The neurologist and other doctors on the case consider these identifications of self-worth to be somewhat superficial. What about the courage he might demonstrate to his son? Wouldn't that be more important? And perhaps the patient could learn, too, that he has value simply by being a human being. With his mental ability and medical experience, maybe he could help others who are in a similar condition.

Furthermore, as the physicians caring for one of their own honestly admit, as they look into Tom's eyes, they see themselves and recognize their own ambiguity about self-image and value. It seems important to them to convince Tom to live, not only for his own growth as a human being, but also for their peace of mind. They also admit that their surgeon-patient knows as well as they do that he will eventually die of pneumonia, since his muscles for breathing are completely dead.

Tom continued to demand no resuscitation or any other measures to prolong his life if he should suffer another respiratory arrest or even an infection. Additionally, he asked his primary physician to assist him in committing suicide. Tom was declared mentally competent following a psychiatric consultation.

You are Tom's primary physician. What will you do?

What factors will you consider in your deliberation?

Case 5.4: THE HIV POSITIVE PHYSICIAN

Dr. Whitney is a general practitioner in a small town in Iowa. He has lived there for ten years. Dr. Whitney first moved to the town to fulfill his obligation with the National Health Service Corps. He liked the area and decided to stay. Dr. Whitney married a local resident and they now have two children, ages 5 and 3. Both Dr. Whitney and his wife are actively involved in community affairs.

Recently, a Red Cross Blood Drive was held in town. Dr. Whitney and his wife participated in the blood drive. The blood was sent to a nearby city for routine testing. Dr. Whitney was later notified that he tested positive for HIV.

Dr. Whitney was devastated. Like many rural areas, this region of Iowa suffers from a severe shortage of practicing physicians. Being the sole physician within a 75 mile radius, Dr. Whitney provides a broad range of much needed services to his patients. For example, Dr. Whitney performs minor surgery; he also delivers babies, and when necessary, he performs caesarean sections.

What should Dr. Whitney do about his practice? He knows that if he informs his patients of his HIV status, they might refuse to be treated by him. His professional career would be seriously threatened. The social consequences for his family are quite serious if knowledge of his HIV status is made public. In addition, the hospital could suffer grave financial loss because patients might go to facilities in other towns to receive care.

Consider the following questions:

1. Who should Dr. Whitney inform that he is HIV positive?

2. What personal and societal values and professional obligations are important to consider in this case?

3. Should Dr. Whitney continue to practice? Should he restrict his practice in any way?

Case 5.5: NO ADVANCE DIRECTIVE

DP is a 68-year-old white male with a history of a Myocardial Infarction 4 years ago who presented to the hospital after previous diagnostic work-up had revealed significant vascular disease in three coronary vessels. This level of recurrence required coronary artery bypass grafting (CABG). Preoperatively, the patient had refused to sign any advance directives, stating that this was a "routine operation" and further, upon discussion of possible negative outcomes, that "nothing dangerous like that is going to happen to me."

The operative course was complicated by damage to the left phrenic nerve resulting in paralysis of the left hemidiaphragm. On the second through the sixth postoperative days, attempts to wean DP from the ventilator were made; however, they were unsuccessful. On the seventh postoperative day, DP's ventilator status worsened, he became confused and at times unresponsive, he began to spike fevers, and had several episodes of shaking chills. Sputum and blood cultures revealed a gram negative pneumonia and septicemia; chest x-rays revealed severe consolidation in the left lower lung lobe correlating with a severe pneumonia.

Empiric intravenous antibiotic regimes were started. However DP's respiratory condition and mental status did not improve: he continued to require increasing assistance from the ventilator and was now completely unresponsive, even to painful stimuli. Clinical neurological exams and CT scan revealed cerebral infarction most likely secondary to the septicemia. Over the course of the next day DP began to show signs of septic shock and the ICU team noted EKG changes consistent with severe cardiac ischemia/infarction.

In light of the start of multiple organ system failure and the impending cardiovascular system collapse, the ICU team decided to approach the family with the possibility of establishing Do-Not-Resuscitate (DNR) orders for the patient. DP's wife supported this option, emotionally stating that "while I cannot bear to just let my husband die, I know he wouldn't want to live this way".

DP's children (age 36 and 39) disagreed with their mother's position, stating "Our father means the world to us -- you have to try to save him, even if it means using a life support machine." Attempts to get the family to think alike about this matter failed. The chaplain and the ethics consult team were called.

What should be done?

Submitted by Kevin Bock

Case 5.6: **THE RELUCTANT FATHER**

HG was a 63-year-old man who underwent an exploratory laparotomy for a colon carcinoma. This was found to be locally invasive and unresectable and he had multiple metastases to his liver. Preoperatively, he gave no evidence of bleeding or obstruction from the tumor. Post-operatively, his course was a difficult one, in part, because of significant cardiac disease, diabetes, and chronic pulmonary disease. Two weeks post-operatively, HG was still requiring intravenous fluids, on total parenteral nutrition, and requiring antibiotics for an urinary tract infection.

He was quiet, pleasant, and undemanding person. His daughter was a lawyer, who lived out-of-town and visited him once a week. After he had been in the hospital for 3 weeks, the daughter requested of the attending surgeon that he give her father a lethal dosage of Morphine in order to "save him from continued misery." The surgeon, of course, refused.

The following week, the daughter requested that no further drug treatments be utilized for her father, even if he were to sustain another treatable infection. The patient was still arousable, and he informed the surgeon that he indeed did want antibiotic therapy for any potentially reversible infection. This confirmed the surgeon's experience with the patient as an individual with insight who knew he would eventually die, but who wished to continue any reasonable therapy that made him comfortable.

He was slightly depressed at this time. The therapeutic plan was to stabilize the patient and return him home for the estimated 2 to 3 months of life. The following week the daughter visited the patient again, this time for several hours. Soon after the daughter left, the patient called in the surgeon to tell him that he wanted no more antibiotics should he have even a reversible infection. Since this was a reversal of his earlier wishes, the surgeon spoke at length to him, a process made more difficult because of his weakened condition and pain medications. The patient remained resolute, underscoring his determination by requesting that, "I wish to be given enough Morphine to end this suffering."

The attending surgeon was puzzled and concerned by this change of heart. He had recently finished reading some short stories by a fellow surgeon, Richard Selzer, one of which closely paralleled this case, except that the surgeon in that case knew his patient better. The surgeon refused the dying patient's request, but wondered afterwards whether it was cowardice or conviction that led him to the refusal. Other concerns of the surgeon were:

1. Was the patient indeed giving an informed consent and exercising autonomy when he asked outright not to receive antibiotics for serious infections?

2. What is the moral difference between honoring this request and the more direct action of an overdose of Morphine, since both would in all likelihood bring about the patient's death? Many ethicists and some judges see no moral or legal distinction between leaving someone to die and actively assisting them, since the end result is the same.

3. The patient had given his daughter the power of attorney for health care, should he become incompetent. Did her initial request that her father be given a lethal dose of Morphine vitiate her capacity to act in his presumed best interest, even though he remains insistent that she be his spokesperson when he is unable to give his own opinions? What kind of problems would the surgeon inevitably face when the patient became comatose?

4. Since the patient, in the surgeon's opinion, was not terminally ill and had some hope for restoration of function and discharge, must the surgeon follow the patient's instructions not to receive antibiotics for reversible infection?

Case 5.7: **RATIONAL SUICIDE?**

The patient is a 58-year-old white female who was diagnosed one year ago with Type III gastric adenocarcinoma. She was not considered an operable candidate at the time of diagnosis due to the presence of metastases to her liver and peritoneum. During the past year, she has been hospitalized on several occasions and the patient's condition has deteriorated greatly. She has received radiation therapy for obstruction and chronic bleeding at the primary cancer site with some alleviation of symptoms. During the past year, she became severely depressed. She lived alone, has never been married, and has no known living relatives.

Due to the fact that her dysphagia, nausea, vomiting, and intractable pain had increased in their frequency and intensity during the past two weeks, the patient decided that she no longer wanted to live. She contacted a lawyer whom she had known for several years and had a Living Will written up. In the Living Will, it was clearly stated that no extraordinary measures were to be instituted to keep her alive in the event that she was hospitalized and unable to communicate her wishes to the physicians.

Unbeknownst to the lawyer, the real reason the patient had the Living Will written up was to secure that her suicide attempt would be allowed to succeed if she were to be discovered before death overcame her. The patient planned on taking her life with the surplus of pain pills she had accumulated over the past year. Before taking the pills, the patient wrote a letter to her lawyer detailing her suicide plan so that the lawyer could have the proper authorities remove her corpse. She planned on the letter taking the average three days to be delivered to her lawyer. However, the letter was received earlier than expected.

Upon receipt of the suicide note, the lawyer called 911 and had the paramedics rush to the patient's house. There they found the patient comfortably lying on her bed, unconscious, but still breathing slightly. The patient was brought to the Emergency Room and was treated for her overdose.

Upon fully awakening, the patient became enraged with the doctors and her lawyer for not allowing her to die.

1. Should she have been left alone?

2. Should her lawyer have ignored the letter and not notified authorities?

3. Even if he did do so notify them, should the doctors in the emergency room have resuscitated her?

Based on a case presented by Scott B. Cienkus,
1993 4th year medical student

Case 5.8: INFORMED CONSENT IN RESEARCH

A drug company has manufactured a drug which it hopes will be helpful in the treatment of patients with migraine headaches. The drug is manufactured by the Micetich and Marshall Drug company (M and M Drug Company). The drug has not yet been named and is known by the acronym "AP." AP is considered an experimental drug in the treatment of migraine headaches. AP is a tablet which is taken once every morning. The M and M Drug Company has approached you to see if you would be willing to conduct a clinical trial testing the efficacy of AP in decreasing the frequency of migraine headaches.

Patients who have migraine headaches at least once a month will be eligible to participate in a double blinded, placebo controlled trial. Prior to participation, the patient must have a normal physical examination and normal blood count and serum tests of liver function. The patient will be observed for three months. During this time the frequency and severity of migraine headaches will be determined. Following this observation period, the patient will be randomized to receive either AP once a day or an identical looking placebo once a day for a period of 6 months. The trial will be double blinded (neither doctor nor patient will know what drug the patient is taking). The patient will be asked to keep a diary of the frequency and severity of migraine headaches during the study period.

At the end of the six months, the patient will stop taking the tablets but will continue to keep a diary of the frequency and severity of migraine headaches for the next 4 months.

The physician will collect the data and send it for analysis to the drug company. The company will determine statistically if AP is superior to the placebo in reducing the frequency and severity of migraine headaches in a susceptible patient population. It is anticipated that to detect a 20% decrease in the frequency of migraine headaches, 50 patients will receive the placebo and 50 patients will receive the drug, AP.

AP is a compound which is well tolerated when taken orally once a day. In over one thousand subjects who have taken the drug, approximately 14% have complained of side effects. These side effects include: mental disturbance (3.4%), headache (2.8%), nausea and vomiting (3.3%), sleep disturbances (1.1%), itching or rash (1.2%), anxiety or depression (1.0%), vertigo (0.6%), dry mouth (0.5%), and hot flashes (0.1%), asymptomatic elevation of the liver enzymes which is reversible (1.0%) and agranulocytosis which may be life threatening (1 case in 20,000 administrations of AP).

The patient will keep the diary and will visit the doctor monthly. Complete blood counts and blood liver function determinations will be performed every week for the first two months the patient receives the drug and then once a month for the remaining four months of drug administration. These tests and the doctor visits will be done at no cost to the patient. If the white blood cell count falls to less than $4x10^9$/liter and/or the transaminases rise to twice the upper limit of normal, the patient participation in the study will be discontinued.

Pregnancy is an absolute contraindication to participation in the study and effective means of birth control must be used since the effect of AP on the fetus is not known.

The Department will be paid $1,000.00 for each patient who completes the study.

1. The physician agrees to participate in the trial. His Institution receives Federal Funds. What regulations govern his actions with respect to the conduct of this study?

2. The attached informed consent document is submitted. Is it appropriate? Explain.

INFORMED CONSENT

Patient's Name:______________________________________Date:__________

Project Title: AP in the Treatment of Migraine Headaches

AIMS OF PROJECT

The purpose of this project is to see if a new drug, AP, taken once a day orally is helpful in reducing the frequency and the severity of migraine attacks.

PROCEDURE

You will undergo a physical examination and testing of your blood. If you and your blood are normal, you will keep a diary of the frequency and severity of migraine headaches for three months. Then you will take a pill once a day and keep the diary. We will see if the frequency and the severity of your headaches are less while you take the pill. You will take the pill for six months and then stop. You will then keep the diary for another four months so that we can see if your headaches become worse when the pill is stopped.

SIDE EFFECTS

The side effects associated with AP are as follows: mental disturbance, headache, nausea and vomiting, sleep disturbances, itching or rash, anxiety or depression, vertigo, dry mouth and hot flashes.

POTENTIAL BENEFITS

There is a good chance that AP will decrease the headache that you are having.

FINANCIAL RISKS

You will not be charged for any of the tests or the medication or the doctor's fees.

CONSENT

I have fully explained to ____/the nature and purpose of the above described procedure and the risks that are involved. I have answered and will answer all questions about the study to the best of my ability.

____

Signature of Doctor

I,____have been fully informed of the above-described procedure with its possible benefits and risks. I give permission for my participation in this study. I know that ___________________________ and his associates will be available to answer any questions I may have. If, at any time, I feel my questions have not been adequately answered, I may request to speak with a member of the Medical Center Institutional Review Board. I understand that I am free to withdraw this consent and discontinue participation in this project at any time without prejudice to my medical care. I have received a copy of this informed consent document.

I understand that biomedical or behavioral research such as that in which I have agreed to participate, by its nature, involves risk of injury. In the event of physical injury resulting from these research procedures, emergency medical treatment will be provided at no cost, in accordance with the policy of__________________________. No additional free medical treatment or compensation will be provided except as required by Illinois law.

In the event I believe that I have suffered physical injury as the result of participation in the research program, I may contact the Chairman of the Institutional Review Board for the Protection of Human Subjects at the Medical Center, at 999-9999.

I agree to allow my name and medical records to be available to other authorized physicians and researchers for the purpose of evaluating the results of this study. I consent to the publication of any data which may result from these investigations for the purpose of advancing medical knowledge, providing the name of any other identifying information (initials, social security number, etc.) is not used in conjunction with such publication. All precautions to maintain confidentiality of the medical records will be taken. I understand, however, that the Food and Drug Administration of the United States Government is authorized to review the records relating to this project.

____

(signature: patient/legal representative)

____

(signature: witness to signature)

Notes

1. Jellinek M. A suicide attempt & emergency room ethics, *Hastings Center Report* August 1979.

Chapter 30

Surrogate Decision-Making for Incompetent Adults: An Ethical Framework

Dan W. Brock

MY ROLE in this discussion is to add a philosophical perspective to the consideration of surrogate decision-making. In the medical ethics literature a substantial, though not universal, consensus has developed that health care decision-making should be shared between the physician and the competent patient. Typically, in medical practice, the physician brings his or her knowledge, training, expertise, and experience to the diagnosis of the patient's condition and provides the prognoses associated with different treatment alternatives, including the alternative of no treatment. The patient brings his or her own aims and values to the decision-making process and ideally evaluates the alternatives, with their particular mixes of benefits and risks.[1]

What values underlie a commitment shared decision-making, and what ends are we seeking to promote with it? The first, and most obvious, is the promotion and protection of the patient's well-being. Shared decision-making rests in part on the presumption that competent patients who have been suitably informed by their physicians about the treatment choice they face are generally, though of course not always, the best judges of what treatment will most promote their overall well-being.[2] The other value is respecting the patient's self-determination. I mean by self-determination the interest of ordinary persons in making significant decisions about their own lives themselves and according to their own values. It is by exercising self-determination that we have significant control over our lives and take responsibility for our lives and the kind of person we become. These then are the values that guide shared decision-making.

For incompetent patients we still want shared decision-making, but then the patient lacks the capacity to participate and a surrogate must take the patient's place. My aim in this paper is, therefore, to sketch an ethical framework for surrogate decision-making about medical treatment for incompetent adults and for thinking about the ethical issues that arise in that decision-making.[3] Surrogate decision-making should seek to extend the ideals of health care decision-making for competent adults, with suitable changes required by and reflecting the patient's incompetence. Before considering who should be a surrogate and how the surrogate should decide, we must consider which patients should have a surrogate to decide for them.

Determining Incompetence

In health care, if the patient is competent, the patient is entitled to decide and to give or refuse informed consent to treatment. If the patient is incompetent, a surrogate must be selected to decide for the patient. The concept, standards, and determination of competence

Source: Reprinted from *The Mount Sinai Journal of Medicine*, Vol. 58, No. 5, pp. 388-392, with permission from The Mount Sinai Medical Center © Oct. 1991.

are complex; and there is space here to emphasize only a few important points about competence and incompetence (see especially 3, ch. 1). Adults are presumed to be competent unless and until found to be incompetent. In questionable or borderline cases, competence should be understood as decision-relative, that is, a patient may be competent to make one decision but not another. First, decisions can vary in the demands they make on patient, for example, in the complexity of the information relevant to the choice. Second, from the effects of medications, disease, and other factors, patients can change over time in the capacities they bring to the decision-making process.

Three distinct capacities are needed for competence in treatment decision-making: The capacity for understanding and communication; the capacity for reasoning and deliberation; the capacity to have and apply a set of values or conception of one's good. Though people possess these capacities in different degrees, it is important to recognize that the determination of competence is not a comparative judgment. Because the competence determination in health care (and in the law) is used to sort the patient into either the class of patients who are competent to decide for themselves or into the class of patients who must have a surrogate to decide for them, it must be recognized as a threshold determination. The crucial question about competence in borderline cases then is how defective or impaired a person's decision-making must be to warrant a determination of incompetence.

Two central values are at stake when a patient is judged competent or incompetent, and so two kinds of dangers should be balanced in that determination. One value is protecting the patient from the harmful consequences of his or her choice when the patient's decision-making is seriously impaired. The other value is respecting the patient's interest in deciding for him or herself. The dangers to be considered are failing adequately to protect the patient from the harmful consequences of a seriously impaired choice, which must be balanced against failing to permit the patient to decide for him or herself when sufficiently able to do so. There is no unique objectively correct balancing of these two values and dangers. Instead, the proper balancing is inherently an ethically controversial choice.

Process as the Standard

The evaluation of a patient's competence should address and evaluate the process of the patient's decision-making; the standard should not be an outcome standard that simply looks to the content of the patient's choice. Given the values at stake in the competence determination, it follows that the standard for competence should vary according to the consequences for the patient's well-being of accepting his or her choice. The standard should vary along a continuum from high (when the choice appears to be seriously in conflict with the patient's well-being) to moderate (when the patient's choice appears to be comparable to other alternatives in its effect on the patient's well-being) to low (when the choice will clearly best serve the patient's well-being).

One controversial consequence of this account of the competence determination is that a patient might be competent to consent to a particular treatment, but not to refuse it, and vice versa. This follows from two facts. First, the process of reasoning to be evaluated will inevitably be different if it leads to a different choice. Second, the effects on one of the values to be balanced (the patient's well-being -- if the patient's choice is accepted) can be radically different depending on whether the patient has consented to or refused the recommended treatment. Treatment refusal may reasonably trigger an evaluation of the patient's competence, though it should also trigger a revaluation by the physician both of the treatment recommendation and of the communication of that recommendation to the patient; some studies have shown that the most common cause of treatment refusals is failure of communication between physician and patient, and most refusals are consequently withdrawn when the recommendation is better explained.[4]

The critical question to answer is: Does the patient's choice sufficiently accord with the patient's own underlying and enduring aims and values for it to be accepted and honored, even if others, including the physician, may think it not the best choice?

Selecting a Surrogate

Assume now that a patient has been found incompetent to make a particular treatment choice, so that a surrogate must act for the patient. Who should serve as surrogate? What standards should guide the surrogate's decision? If we are to respect the incompetent patient's wishes, then the surrogate should be the person the patient would have wanted to act as surrogate. In a number of states, by executing a Durable Power of Attorney for Health Care (DPOA), it is possible for a person, while competent, to legally designate a surrogate who will make health care decisions in the event of later incompetence. This document also allows a person to give instructions to the surrogate about one's wishes concerning treatment. Ethically, an oral designation by a person of a surrogate should have nearly the same weight as a formal DPOA. Competent patients should be encouraged to designate who will decide for them in the case of later incompetence. In fact, physicians have a responsibility to seek this information early in treatment and while patients are still competent, especially if a period of later incompetence is likely.

Often an incompetent patient will not have explicitly designated a surrogate. It is then reasonable and common to act on a presumption that a patient's close family member is the appropriate surrogate. (In most jurisdictions, a close family member lacks explicit legal authority to act as the patient's surrogate until formally appointed by a court as the guardian. States should consider adopting legislation like the recently enacted Health Care Decisions Act in the District of Columbia which formally authorizes a family member to act as surrogate for an incompetent patient without recourse to guardianship proceedings.) Only the most important considerations that support this presumption for a family member acting as surrogate can be discussed here. First, usually a family member will be the person the patient would have wanted to act as surrogate for him or her. Second, the family member will know the patient best and will be most concerned for the patient's welfare. It is important to underline that the claim is only that the practice of using a close family member as surrogate will result overall in better decisions for patients than any feasible alternative practice, such as appointing an attorney to act as the patient's guardian. Third, in our society the family is the central social and moral unit assigned responsibilities to care for its dependent members. Although dependent children are the most obvious example, dependent adults are another important instance of this responsibility. The family is also the main place in which most people pursue and realize the values of intimacy and privacy. Both to fulfill these responsibilities and to realize these values, the family must be accorded significant, though not unlimited, freedom from external oversight, intrusion, and control.

These grounds for presuming a close family member to be an incompetent patient's surrogate do not imply that such a surrogate must always make the optimal choice. On the other hand they also make it clear that family members' authority as surrogate decision-makers is limited. When the grounds do not hold -- for example, when there is no close relation between patient and family member, or when there is a clear conflict of interest between patient and family member -- the presumption for family members as surrogates can be rebutted. In such cases, an incompetent patient's physician can have a positive responsibility not to allow the family member to act as surrogate.

Sometimes no family member is available to serve as surrogate. Most reasons that support a family member serving as surrogate will then also support using a close friend who is available and willing to serve. When no family member or friend is available, institutional flexibility is desirable because of the wide range of different decisions that must be made.

Institutions only need a settled and public policy insuring that decision-making in such cases does not become paralyzed from lack of a natural surrogate. For example, a hospital might have a policy for a specified range of decisions (such as decisions to forgo life-sustaining treatment or resuscitation) requiring that the attending physician's proposed decision be referred to the chief of service who could review the decision and take any further steps deemed appropriate (perhaps referral to an ethics committee or to the courts).

How Surrogates Should Decide

Advance Directives

What standards should a surrogate employ in deciding for an incompetent patient? Three ordered principles can guide decision-making: advance directive, substituted judgment, best interest. These are ordered principles in the sense that the surrogate should employ the first if possible; if not it, then the second if possible; and if neither the first or second can be used, then the third.

The advance directive principle tells the surrogate that if there is a valid advance directive from the patient, there is a strong presumption that it should be followed. Formal advance directives take two principal forms, living wills and durable powers of attorney for health care. Living wills are given legal force in approximately 40 states; DPOAs, at present, have legal force in far fewer jurisdictions.

Several common features limit the usefulness of living wills. I shall mention two. First, they are usually formulated in vague terms for describing both the patient conditions ("terminally ill") and the treatments ("extraordinary measures," "aggressive treatment"). Because they are executed well in advance of the decision to be made, this is to some extent inevitable and means that others must interpret how the should now apply. Second, probably in response to worries about potential abuses, enabling statutes in many states place limitations on the circumstances in which living wills can either be executed (for example, the person must already have been diagnosed as terminally ill with death imminent) or applied (for example, the decision cannot cover nutrition and hydration). When persons follow these restrictions and limitations, in many circumstances their living wills will fail to apply. Since living wills are rarely brought into court for enforcement, but function primarily as a means of informing others about the patient's wishes, restrictive formulations may be inadvisable.

Except for those who have no surrogate, DPOAs are the more desirable form of advance directive for most persons. First, they allow a person to give more detailed instructions to the surrogate about wishes regarding treatment, though it is important to avoid letting greater detail narrow the application of the instructions. Second, they address the issue of later interpreting the patient's instructions by allowing the patient to designate the interpreter.

Although there is a strong presumption that a valid advance directive should be followed, there are reasons why advance directives should not have the same degree of binding force as the contemporaneous decision of a competent patient. The decision of a competent patient can be made attending to the full and detailed context, whereas advance directives must inevitably be formulated before the precise context of future decisions is known. This means that occasionally a treatment decision will arise in circumstances radically different from those imagined by the patient when executing the advance directive; in such cases, following the letter of the directive may be contrary to following its spirit. Moreover, concern over whether the patient would have changed his or her mind about treatment does not arise for a competent patient. Finally, a decision contrary to his or her interests usually will be challenged by the caregivers, thereby testing understanding and resolve to an extent not possible with advance directives. Despite these limitations, there are good reasons to accord a strong presumption to any patient's advance directive.

Substituted Judgment

At present, and probably for the forseeable future, most patients do not have advance directives. Then the substituted judgment principle should be followed. This principle tells the surrogate to attempt to decide as the patient would have decided, if competent, in the circumstances that now obtain. In effect, the principle directs the surrogate to use his or her knowledge of the patient and the patient's aims and values to infer what the patient's choice would have been.

Physicians have an important responsibility in helping surrogates to understand their role in applying substituted judgement. Rather than asking, "What do you now want us to do for your mother?" the physician should say, "You, of course, knew your mother better than I did, so help us decide together what she would have wanted done for her now." Confirmation that asking the right question matters in the choices surrogates make can be found in Tomlinson.[5] This substituted judgment approach is helpful for arriving at decisions which are more in accordance with the patient's wishes. The approach also has the practical advantage of making the psychological and emotional burdens easier for surrogates to carry and facilitating their effective participation in decision-making.

"Do everything" is nearly always an inadequate and unhelpful answer. Surrogates should be assured that appropriate care will always be given, including all care needed to maintain the patient's comfort and dignity. But what care is appropriate will often change with changes in the patient's condition and prognosis, and surrogates must be helped to understand that all possible care is not automatically appropriate care.

Two features of substituted-judgment decision-making should be explicitly noted. First, the substituted-judgment model will let surrogates take account of how the interests of others will be affected by the decision, to the extent there is evidence that the patient would have weighed those interest. Second, it will allow surrogates to assess the patient's quality of life, both at present and as it will be affected by treatment decisions, according to the patient's own values. For consideration of forgoing life-sustaining treatment only a limited judgment of quality of life is relevant: Is the best anticipated quality of life with life-sustaining treatment sufficiently poor that the patient would have judged it to be worse than no further life at all? No judgment about social worth or the social value of the patient are warranted under substituted judgment.

Best Interest

When no information is available about what this particular patient would have wanted in the situation at hand, the "best interests" principle directs the surrogate to select the alternative that furthers the patient's best interests. This, in effect, amounts to asking how most reasonable persons would decide in these circumstances, an approach which is justified by the absence of any information about how this patient differs from others. Treatment choices based on best interests can be especially difficult when reasonable persons can and do disagree about the choice. It is, therefore, important, where possible, to avoid having to appeal to best interest by determining patients' wishes about future treatment options when patients are still competent.

Ordering These Three Principles

Strict ordering of these guidance principles would be an oversimplification. Evidence bearing on the patient's wishes concerning the decision at hand, whether from an advance directive or from the surrogate's knowledge of the patient, is not either fully determinate and decisive on the one hand, or completely absent on the other. Instead, such evidence ranges along a broad continuum in how strongly it supports a particular choice. In all cases, physicians and surrogates should seek confidence that the choice made is reasonably in accord with the patient's wishes or interests. The better the evidence about what this particular patient would have wanted, the more one can rely on it. The less the information and evidence about what this patient would have wanted, the more others must reason in terms of what most persons would want.

What constitutes adequate evidence about the patient's wishes has been an issue in several recent court cases, most notably the O'Connor case in New York and the Cruzan case in Missouri, recently upheld by the U.S. Supreme Court.[6] In the New York case, the court imposed an extremely high standard of evidence for forgoing life-sustaining treatment by surrogate order, requiring clear and convincing proof that the patient had made a settled commitment, while competent, to reject the particular form of treatment under circumstances such as those now obtaining. Where there is any significant doubt, the court reasoned, the decision must be on the side of preserving life. This decision set a very difficult standard in New York for patients and their surrogates to satisfy, and thereby establishes a strong presumption in favor of extending the lives of incompetent patients with life-sustaining treatment. In Cruzan, the U.S. Supreme Court upheld the right of the State of Missouri to impose this same strong presumption, though without endorsing the wisdom of doing so.

Such a presumption undervalues patients' interest in self-determination and fails to recognize adequately the extent to which patients' well-being is determined by their own aims and values. But is it not reasonable, the Court might ask, always to err on the side of preserving life when there is any doubt about the patient's wishes? Several decades ago, when medicine only rarely had the capacity to extend life in circumstances where doing so would have been unwanted and no benefit to patients, such a policy would have been reasonable. Medicine, however, has vastly enlarged its capacities to extend life. Patients' lives can now often be extended when they would not want this done, and, as a result, New York's and Missouri's strong presumption in favor of extending life, when there is any significant doubt about the patient's wishes, can no longer be justified.

Though the U.S. Supreme Court found no constitutional bar to the clear and convincing evidence standard, good reasons remain for other states not to adopt it.

Conclusion

I want to conclude with a plea for "preventive ethics" aimed at reducing the necessity to resort to surrogate decision-making. This can only be accomplished by persons, while still competent, talking with their physicians and families about their treatment wishes should they become seriously ill. Such preventive measures are especially appropriate for persons with chronic, progressive diseases in which both a possible period of incompetence and the nature of later treatment decisions likely to arise are relatively predictable. Physicians have an important role in encouraging their patients to reflect on their wishes and to make those wishes known to those who are likely to be involved in their treatment decisions. The need for surrogate decision-making in health care will never be eliminated, nor can all difficult decisions be avoided. But it should be possible greatly to reduce the number of cases in which physicians and surrogates must decide about an incompetent patient's care in the absence of knowledge of the patient's wishes when that information could have been obtained earlier had it been sought.

Notes

1. Some respects in which this division of labor is oversimplified are explored in Brock DW. Facts and values in the physician/patient relationship, In: Veatch R, Pellegrino E, eds., *Ethics, Trust, and the Professions*. Washington, DC: Georgetown University Press, 1991.

2. For a discussion of different kinds of cases in which competent patients make irrational choices, and the responsibilities of their physicians in such circumstances, see Brock DW, Wartman SA. When competent patients make irrational choices, *New England Journal of Medicine* 1990;322:1595-1599.
3. I draw freely here on prior published work I have done on this topic, some of it collaborative work with Allen Buchanan. See especially Buchanan AE, Brock DW. *Deciding for Others: The Ethics of Surrogate Decisionmaking*. Cambridge, England: Cambridge University Press, 1989.
4. Applebaum PS, Roth LS. Treatment refusal in the medical hospital, In: *President's Commission for the Study of Ethical Problems in Medicine and Biomedical and Behavioral Research. Making Health Care decisions: The Ethical and Legal Implications of Informed Consent in the Patient-Practitioner Relationship*. Vol. 2 Appendices. Washington DC: U.S. Government Printing Office, 1982.
5. Tomlinson T, *et al.* An empirical study of proxy consent for elderly person, *Gerontologist* 1990;30(1):54-60.
6. *In re O'Connor*. No. 312 (NY Court of Appeals, October 14, 1988); *Cruzan v. Director*. 110 Sct 2841 (Missouri Department of Health, 1990).

Chapter 31

Management of the Severely Anemic Patient Who Refuses Transfusion: Lessons Learned during the Care of a Jehovah's Witness

John Votto

> As for any man . . . who eats any sort of blood, I shall certainly set my face against the soul that is eating the blood, and I shall indeed cut him off from among his people.--Leviticus 17:10

The Jehovah's Witnesses is a Christian sect that was founded in the late 1870s by Charles Russel in Pittsburgh, Pennsylvania. What began as a small Bible study group evolved into a religious sect that currently includes over 2.6 million members worldwide. The refusal of Jehovah's Witnesses to receive blood transfusion dates back to a 1945 church decision[1] and has often resulted in controversy and conflict with the health profession. Such cases present the physician with ethical, medicolegal, and clinical challenges. An example of such a case and a review of the literature are presented.

Case Report

A previously healthy 74-year-old Jehovah's Witness man was admitted with a 3-day history of passing blood through the rectum. Upper endoscopy showed no source. He was taken to the operating room on the day of admission because of continued bleeding and because he had signed a statement refusing blood transfusion. He underwent a subtotal colectomy with ileorectostomy to control the bleeding. No malignancy was found. His hematocrit fell from a preoperative value of 0.27 to 0.15, and he was sent to the intensive care unit for further management.

The patient was sedated and on full ventilatory support. A pulmonary artery catheter was placed, allowing continuous monitoring of mixed venous oxygen saturation and determination of cardiac output. An arterial line was inserted, and transcutaneous oxygen saturation was continuously monitored. Oxygen delivery and consumption were determined periodically. Parenteral hyperalimentation was begun, and metabolic measurements were analyzed weekly. Phlebotomies were minimized and tests were combined when possible. On hospital day 3, the hematocrit dropped to 0.11, the patient's lowest value. Neuromuscular blocking agents, intravenous iron, erythropoietin, and vitamin K were administered. Inspired oxygen concentrations of 50% to 60% with positive end expiratory pressure were administered and resulted in PO2 values of 300 to 350 mm Hg. Cardiac outputs consistently ranged from 10 to 12 L/min. Daily nutritional requirements exceeded 2000 calories.

Source: Reprinted from *Annals of Internal Medicine*, Vol. 117, No. 12, pp. 143-149, with permission from University Press of America © Dec. 1992.

One week after admission, the patient developed an upper gastrointestinal bleed despite prophylaxis. The hematocrit remained in the range of 0.13 to 0.15. Neuromuscular blocking agents were briefly withdrawn on hospital day 10, with a subsequent fall in mixed venous saturation and cardiac output. Electrocardiographic and echocardiographic studies confirmed anterior wall ischemia and hypokinesis. The patient stabilized as he was paralyzed again, and his hematocrit at this time was 0.17. On hospital day 21, paralytic agents were safely withdrawn. He had a very slow recovery of neuromuscular function and also developed Pseudomonas aeruginosa pneumonia, which required 3 additional weeks of ventilatory support and antibiotic therapy before extubation could occur. He was discharged to an extended care facility for continued rehabilitation 17 days later, on hospital day 58, with a hematocrit of 0.28. At 6-month follow-up, he was doing well at home with no gastrointestinal complaints and his hematocrit was 0.37.

History and Philosophy

Jehovah's Witnesses arc deeply committed to the nets of their faith, which include the refusal of blood transfusion. Their position is based on several biblical passages forbidding the eating of blood, which they interpret to preclude transfusion of blood. They all hope of eternal life will be forfeited if transfusion is accepted. They readily accept other forms of medical therapy, however, and clearly are not suicidal or believers in "faith healing."[2]

Two recent cases emphasize the importance of understanding and continuously clarifying the wishes of a Jehovah's Witness patient.[3,4] Each report describes Jehovah's Witnesses who, on the advice of their physicians, preoperatively donated blood for later use. However, after conferring with church members, they refused autotransfusion, and their surgery had to be rescheduled.

Such scenarios might be avoided with some understanding of the philosophy of Jehovah's Witnesses regarding transfusion (Table 1). Whole blood and its components are clearly prohibited, whereas the acceptance of albumin, immune globulin, hemophilia preparations, vaccines, sera, and organ transplants is an individual decision. Autotransfusion of banked blood or blood products is prohibited because they believe that blood that has left the body is best discarded. Blood remaining in circulation within the body, such as during cardiopulmonary bypass, plasmapheresis, or dialysis is acceptable to many Witnesses. Nonblood plasma expanders, erythropoietin, and the new fluorinated blood substitutes are also generally accepted. Because so much of their philosophy is left to personal discretion, the importance of open and continuous communication between physician and patient cannot be overstated.

Medicolegal and Ethical Issues

Major medicolegal and ethical issues surround Witnesses' refusal of blood transfusion, often to the great frustration of their caretakers. The 1914 trial of Schloendorff v. Society of New York Hospital was a landmark case regarding the necessity for patient consent before the performance of procedures.[5] Although the patient lost the case, Judge Cardozo's concluding statement, "Every human being of adult years and sound mind has a right to determine what shall be done with his own body," formed the basis for subsequent rulings regarding an individual's right to refuse specific therapies. The courts have since invariably upheld the right of competent adult Witnesses to refuse transfusion. This right is often denied, however, in cases of "compelling state interest," such as those involving pregnant women or a parent whose children would become wards of the state should he or she die. In the 1944 case of Prince v. Massachusetts,[6] the approach with respect to children of Jehovah's Witnesses was defined: "Parents may be free to be martyrs themselves. But it does not follow that they are free in identical circumstances to make martyrs of their children."

Physicians must weigh two conflicting ethical principles when treating an anemic Jehovah's Witness: 1) beneficence (the duty of the physician is to do what is good for the patient) and 2) respect for autonomy (the right of a patient to make choices that affect his or her body). Two basic viewpoints based on these principles are outlined by Jonsen,[7] who defines the paternalistic view as "the practice of disregarding a person's own choices for his or her own benefit" and the nonpaternalistic view as "the physician's duty to respect the competent patient's wishes." Along with most ethicists today, Jonsen favors the latter view in the matter of the Jehovah's Witness because the patient has defined refusal of blood as a higher good than life itself.

A more complex ethical question arises when a Witness refuses blood transfusion but demands alternative therapies of questionable benefit, many of which may be quite expensive. Chervenak and McCullough dealt with this issue in a recent report,[8] advocating the physician's right to autonomy in practicing reasonable medical care: "Physicians may justifiably limit patients' refusals of medical interventions when the refusal is based on a negative right to noninterference coupled with a request for an unreasonable alternative."

Table 1. Philosophy of Jehovah's Witnesses Regarding Transfusion Therapies

General accepted
Crystalloids
Ringer's lactate
Normal saline
Hypertonic saline
Colloids
Dextran
Gelatin
Hetastarch
Perfluorochemicals
Erythropoietin
Generally not accepted
Whole blood and its components
Packed red cells
Leukocytes
Platelets
Plasma
Autotransfusion of blood or blood components
Individual decision
Cardiopulmonary bypass
Dialysis
Plasmapheresis
Immune globulin
Vaccines
Sera
Hemophilia preparations
Transplants

Most clinicians would agree that such moral and ethical issues are the most challenging and frustrating aspect of caring for Jehovah's Witnesses. This is emphasized in a recent poll of European intensivists:[9] Sixty-three percent would administer transfusion to an exsanguinating Jehovah's Witness despite the patient's refusal. Understandably, these physicians felt morally obligated to administer transfusion, but, disturbingly, 26% admitted they would never inform the patient that a transfusion had been given.

To our knowledge, although several U.S. court cases have upheld the Witnesses' right to refuse transfusion,[10,11] few have resulted in a cash award. A recent Canadian case[12] found that a physician clearly disregarded a patient's well-documented advance directive and awarded the patient a settlement. However, the physician was not found medically negligent. Practitioners should be aware of the potential liability inherent in such cases, and appropriate documentation of every decision should be made.

Clinical Management

The clinical management of the anemic Jehovah's Witness and, indeed, any anemic patient refusing transfusion depends much on the patient's underlying physiologic status and the acuity of his or her condition. Adaptive mechanisms leading to improved cardiac output and oxygen extraction will occur in otherwise healthy patients and may be sufficient to sustain life at remarkably low hemoglobin values.[13]

Table 2. Management of the Anemic Jehovah's Witness

Considered Therapy	Effect of Therapy
Minimize blood loss	Higher hemoglobin levels and improved
Reduce iatrogenic loss	and improved oxygen delivery
Microchemistry analyzers	
Pediatric-sized blood samples	
Analyze necessity of tests	
Sterile reservoirs	
Reduce hemorrhagic loss	
Hemodilution	
Red cell scavenging devices	
Hypotensive anesthesia	
Desmopressin	
Progesterone	
Maximize blood production	Higher hemoglobin levels and
Erythropoietin	improved oxygen delivery
Intravenous iron dextran	
Nutritional support	
Maximize cardiac output	Enhanced cardiac output and
Volume expansion	improved oxygen delivery
Hemodilution	
Increase oxygen content	Increased dissolved oxygen content
Oxygen	and improved oxygen delivery
Fluorinated blood substitutes*	
Decrease metabolic rate	Reduce oxygen consumption
Hypothermia	
Paralysis, sedation	

Patients with chronic anemia should be evaluated to rule out treatable causes such as iron, folate, or vitamin B12 deficiency, as well as erythropoietin-responsive conditions such as chronic renal failure and zidovudine-induced anemia.[14] However, for patients with acute anemia who do not stabilize with volume replacement or for patients with a compromised cardiovascular status, more aggressive management may be indicated.

Extensive invasive and noninvasive monitoring of the critically anemic patient refusing blood transfusion is now possible, although at some risk and expense. Effective management of such patients depends simply on maximizing oxygen delivery and minimizing oxygen consumption. Various approaches to achieving these goals are summarized in Table 2.

Minimizing Blood Loss

"Iatrogenic anemia" is a well-documented problem in the intensive care unit. One recent study of intensive care-unit patients with in-dwelling arterial lines found that they were phlebotomized an average of four times a day, resulting in a mean blood loss during their total hospital stay of almost 1 litre.[15] One approach to this problem includes the use of newly available wholeblood microchemistry analyzers. These portable devices can be used at the bedside and require only 1 mL of blood to determine blood gas values, electrolyte levels, and the hematocrit.[16] If this technology is not available, pediatric-sized samples should be drawn using 5-mL evacuated tubes and 3-mL EDTA (ethylenediaminetetraacetic acid) tubes, which will reduce the volume of blood drawn by 40% to 45%.[15] The necessity of doing phlebotomies should be critically reviewed, and tests should be combined whenever possible. If arterial lines are in place, sterile reservoirs are recommended to avoid the need to discard blood before sampling. In our patient, pediatric-sized samples were drawn from such a line for determination of electrolytes, blood urea nitrogen, and creatinine approximately three times a week, with hematocrit values estimated from arterial blood gases drawn approximately every other day. Such conservative blood-saving measures are applicable to all patients, given our limited blood supply and the substantial risks of transfusion.

Efforts to minimize intraoperative blood loss in Jehovah's Witnesses have been numerous. Hemodilution has been advocated in the belief that any blood lost would contain fewer red blood cells per unit volume.[17] Other benefits include reduced blood viscosity, increased cardiac output, and improved microcirculatory flow.[18] Preoperatively, hemodilution has been achieved by expanding intravascular volume with infusion of crystalloid or colloid solutions.[17] This results in hypervolemia, however, and can only be done electively in patients who are cardiovascularly fit. Ingenious techniques have been developed that allow some blood to be diverted intraoperatively while maintaining normal intravascular volume with crystalloid or colloid infusions.[19,20] Such normovolemic hemodilution techniques may be safer and can be used emergently if necessary. The diverted blood is maintained in continuous contact with the patient's circulation and can be reinfused later without violating religious beliefs. Postoperatively, hemodilution has been maintained in anemic Witnesses with good results.[21,22]

Red cell salvaging devices such as the Haemonetics 30 blood cell processor (Braintree, Massachusetts) have been useful in reducing blood loss in Jehovah's Witnesses undergoing open-heart surgery[23,24] and are acceptable because the salvaged blood is maintained in continuous contact with the circulation. Complications associated with the use of these devices include coagulation disturbances and hemolytic reactions.

Hypotensive anesthesia has been safely used to reduce intraoperative blood loss in Jehovah's Witnesses.[25] The development of improved monitoring devices and new hypotensive agents has led to a renewed interest in this technique, once regarded with disfavor because of the associated high complication rate. Mortality rates currently range from only 0.1% to 0.5%, with morbidity rates ranging from 1% to 2%.[26,27,28] Serious complications, such as myocardial infarction, cerebrovascular accidents, and permanent renal insufficiency are rare.

Acute tubular necrosis and deep venous thrombosis have been reported,[25] but are not common. Impressive reductions in operative blood loss (range, 40% to 50%) have been seen in various controlled studies using this technique.[25,29]

Desmopressin has proved to be effective in reducing bleeding after cardiopulmonary bypass.[30] It has been administered both intraoperatively and postoperatively to Jehovah's Witnesses in an attempt to improve hemostasis and to reduce blood loss.[31,32] In fact, at one major institution, Witnesses receive desmopressin as part of routine postoperative care.[33] Desmopressin is given intravenously for 20 to 30 minutes in doses of 0.3 μg/kg body weight. Its major risk is its prothrombotic potential; thus, caution is indicated in patients with underlying vascular disease. For menstruating patients, progesterone is another drug that can be administered to minimize blood loss.[34]

Maximizing Blood Production

Erythropoietin is the primary hormonal regulator of red cell hematopoiesis and is now available due to recombinant DNA technology. Although the formulation contains a small amount of albumin, it is accepted by most Jehovah's Witnesses because the albumin is simply a carrier for the hormone and does not actually "feed" the body. Several reports document the use of erythropoietin in critically ill, anemic patients who refuse transfusion.[4,34,35,36,37,38] The management of such patients often includes driving PaO2 to supranormal levels, thereby blunting the primary stimulus for erythropoietin production. Hormonal replacement therapy in these situations may therefore be especially beneficial.

Little information exists regarding the dosing of erythropoietin in anemic patients without renal disease. Data from patients with renal failure reveal a dose-dependent response; doses of 50 units/kg given intravenously three times a week yield a significantly increased hematocrit within 4 weeks, and larger doses of 150 units/kg produce a substantial rise in hematocrit within 2 weeks.[39] Patients with erythropoietin levels of less than 500 U/L generally respond well, whereas anemic patients whose erythropoietin levels are already elevated may require much higher doses.[40] According to the literature, physicians using erythropoietin in severely anemic Jehovah's Witnesses have generally followed these guidelines; however, slightly higher doses, varying from 100 units/kg to 300 units/kg, have been used.[4,34,35,35] Both intravenous and subcutaneous routes of administration have been reported, with the subcutaneous route offering the obvious benefit of being easier and less costly to administer, as well as possibly providing more sustained plasma erythropoietin levels.[40] Patients are usually treated daily for several days, then three times a week, with careful attention given to nutritional support and iron replacement. In most cases, the hemoglobin rises to acceptable levels within 3 weeks. In our patient, erythropoietin doses of 75 to 100 units/kg were administered three times per week, resulting in a rise in hematocrit from 0.11 to 0.22 after 4 weeks.

Adverse effects with erythropoietin are uncommon, and, indeed, our patient tolerated it well. Careful monitoring of iron stores is recommended. Accelerated hypertension has been noted in patients with renal failure, but it is not known whether this complication occurs in patients without preexisting hypertension. Seizures and thromboses of fistulae have occurred with rapid rises in hematocrit; thus, caution is recommended when administering large doses. Occasional allergic reactions, including the development of urticarial and maculopapular rashes, have been noted. Bone marrow studies show no mutagenic effects in patients treated for 8 weeks.[39] Currently, erythropoietin comes in vials of 2, 3, 4 or 10 million units, at a hospital cost of approximately $10 per 1000 units.

Although the oral route of iron administration is preferred for most patients, intramuscular and intravenous routes have been used in the treatment of severely anemic, critically ill patients who have poorly functioning alimentary tracts. Intramuscular injections of iron are generally avoided because of volume restrictions, muscle mass limitations, and local adverse reactions. Dudrick and coworkers[41] reported relatively good efficacy and safety when intravenous iron was administered to six patients with acute severe anemia who refused blood transfusion. The required total iron replacement dose was derived from the following formula:

$$\text{Fe (mg)} = 0.3 \times \text{body weight (lb)} \times \left(100 - \frac{\text{hemoglobin (g/dL)} \times 100}{14.8}\right)$$

The dose of iron dextran (in mL) was calculated by dividing the amount of required iron (in mg) by 50 (mg/mL) and was infused with total parenteral nutrition solution over a mean treatment period of 23 days. Previous studies reported safe and effective doses of iron dextran to include up to 100 mg of iron per litre of total parenteral nutrition solution; however, in the study by Dudrick and coworkers,[41] a maximum dose of 500 mg/L was safely infused over 8 to 12 hours. The mean hemoglobin level in their study group rose from 5.0 g/dL to 10.6 g/dL over an average of 23 days. Because our severely anemic patient had a nonfunctioning gastrointestinal tract, intravenous iron was administered and the hematocrit rose from 0.11 to 0.22 after 4 weeks. Because erythropoietin was also given, the effect of each agent on hematopoiesis could not be differentiated.

Iron dextran is not labeled for intravenous use but may be administered intravenously at the discretion of the physician. Adverse effects, although uncommon, may be severe. Most worrisome is the possibility of anaphylactoid reactions, which occurred in 2 of 87 patients in one study.[42] Therefore, it is recommended that a test dose of 30 mL of iron dextran solution be given over a 2-minute interval and that the patient be observed for 1 hour. Oxygen and a syringe containing epinephrine should be available for immediate use. In this same series, a delayed reaction of myalgias, arthralgias, and fever occurred in slightly over one third of the patients. Premedication with aspirin, diphenhydramine, or steroids did not prevent these symptoms, but patients responded well to nonsteroidal therapy. No adverse reactions were noted in our patient.

The success of such sophisticated therapies as iron dextran and erythropoietin depends highly on the adequate provision of substrates and energy necessary for erythropoiesis. The importance of adequate protein supply, particularly amino acids, in sustaining red blood cell production has been documented in several studies involving animals.[43,44] In the study by Dudrick and coworkers,[41] anemic patients were treated with intravenous iron, and the previously healthy patients with good nutritional status responded much more rapidly to therapy than did the patients with chronic disorders.[41] Metabolic cart studies may help determine the surprisingly high caloric requirements of such severely anemic patients. For instance, our paralyzed patient required over 2000 calories per day, an amount that we might have underestimated had it not been for the metabolic measurements.

Maximizing Cardiac Output

Maintenance of circulating blood volume and, therefore, cardiac output is an obvious therapeutic objective in any critically anemic patient. Crystalloid solutions alone may be insufficient because of rapid extravascular redistribution; thus, synthetic colloids may be required.

Currently available synthetic plasma volume expanders include hydroxyethyl starch (HES) 450/0.70, HES 264/0.43, dextran 70, dextran 40, urea-bridged gelatin, and modified fluid gelatin. Dextran 40, HES 264/0.43, and the gelatins are potent oncotic agents but have very short half-lives, with only 7% to 12% of the administered dose remaining intravascular after 24 hours.[45] Dextran 70 and HES 450/0.70 are less potent oncotic agents but have a longer lasting effect, with approximately 20% to 30% remaining intravascular 24 hours after infusion.[45]

Side effects of colloid solutions include anaphylactoid reactions, which are most severe with dextrans but overall are rare. Hemostatic defects occur primarily with dextrans but also with the other macromolecules. The case of a Jehovah's Witness patient who developed a severe coagulopathy after receiving two litres of HES 450/0.70 underlines the importance of avoiding massive infusion of any synthetic colloid as the sole fluid to prevent hypovolemia.[46] Modified fluid gelatin may be the safest macromolecule in this respect because volumes of up to four litres have been infused in less than 24 hours with no effect on coagulation.[47] Its short half-life, however, militates against this benefit.

Increasing Oxygen Content

Normally, oxygen content of blood depends mostly on oxygen bound to hemoglobin, with only a small amount (1% to 2%) composed of dissolved oxygen. In severely anemic patients, however, dissolved oxygen may contribute up to 25% of the oxygen content. Therefore, attaining supranormal PO2 values in severely anemic patients may significantly improve oxygen carriage to the tissues. This benefit must be balanced against the risks of oxygen toxicity, and, as mentioned previously, the suppression of erythropoietin release. Conceivably, oxygen transport could be further augmented with the use of a hyperbaric chamber, which has been used to sustain life without hemoglobin.[48] These chambers are not indicated in the management of anemic Jehovah's Witnesses because toxicity precludes their prolonged use.

The development of an effective blood substitute would be a "special boon to Jehovah's Witnesses."[49] Two areas of current research include the hemoglobin solutions that bind and carry oxygen in a manner similar to red blood cells and fluorocarbon emulsions, which carry dissolved oxygen in a manner similar to plasma.

Human hemoglobin solutions have yet to be developed for routine clinical use, although research in this area is being actively pursued. The recently reported production of human hemoglobin using genetically engineered pigs[50] is a particularly exciting achievement because such a therapy would most likely be acceptable to Jehovah's Witnesses, and, more important, would be unlikely to transmit blood-borne viruses. The efficacy of human hemoglobin solutions, however, is limited by their poor release of oxygen to tissues. They also have several potential side effects, including renal toxicity; transmission of infection; allergic reactions; and coronary, renal, and peripheral vasoconstriction.[51] Modifications of human hemoglobin solutions are currently being undertaken in the hope of overcoming these obstacles.[50,52]

Of the fluorocarbon preparations, only Fluosol DA 20% (FDA-20) (Alpha Therapeutic, Los Angeles, California) has been used clinically. Unfortunately, FDA-20 is limited by a relatively low perfluorocarbon content and, therefore, low oxygen carrying capacity. High PO2 values are necessary to maximize its limited ability to carry oxygen. Further, its dose-dependent half-life ranges from only 6 to 24 hours. Anemic patients refusing blood transfusion would require frequent infusions of this product, a process not yet tested, possibly because of fears of volume overload and increased toxicity. Currently, FDA-20 is approved for use only in patients undergoing percutaneous angioplasty, where small doses are administered over a short period of time.

Several investigators have examined the effects of a single dose of FDA-20 (varying from 20 to 40 mL/kg, depending on the study) on anemic patients refusing transfusion.[53,54,55,56,57,58] Significant improvement in oxygen content and oxygen consumption after FDA-20 infusion was shown in a minority of patients and was not impressive. This effect peaked between 6 and 12 hours after FDA-20 administration and was nonexistent at 24 hours. The contribution of

FDA-20 to overall oxygen content was greatest in the most anemic patients, ranging from 5% to 15%. Its contribution to oxygen consumption was more significant, ranging from 17% to 28%, which may reflect improved microcirculatory oxygen delivery to poorly perfused tissues, a benefit attributed to the small size and low viscosity of FDA-20 particles. Side effects from FDA-20 in these studies were rare.

Reactions to the test dose usually manifested as chest pain, and none were life-threatening.[53,54,55,56,57,58] Reactions to full-dose therapy were transient; the most serious complication, an abnormal hematologic profile, occurred in a patient who received the maximum allowed dose of 40 mL/kg.[55] This patient's extremely slow recovery from anemia prompted the investigators to caution against use of massive doses of this drug. A transient fall in leukocyte count and mild elevation of liver function tests have been occasionally noted.[54,56] A rapid infusion rate (25 mL/min) was associated with hypotension in one patient, who later tolerated infusion at 10 mL/min.[56]

Fluosol DA 20% is made by the Green Cross Corporation in Osaka, Japan, and can be obtained for compassionate use from the Alpha Therapeutic Corporation, Los Angeles, California, at a cost of $1800 for 1500 mL of emulsion (approximately one dose). However, because of its short duration of action and limited oxygen carrying capacity, its use in the management of severely anemic Jehovah's Witness patients is not advised. It is hoped that future generations of perfluorocarbons having longer half lives and greater oxygen carrying capacity will be developed for such cases.

Decreasing Metabolic Rate

Deliberate mild hypothermia has been successfully used in the intraoperative and postoperative management of anemic Jehovah's Witnesses.[20,21] A target core temperature of 30 to 32 °C is usually chosen because oxygen consumption is reportedly reduced to 48% below control values at this temperature,[59] and cardiac side effects are uncommon.[60]

Oxygen delivery is affected in several ways during hypothermia. The oxy-hemoglobin dissociation curve shifts leftward, favoring the affinity of hemoglobin for oxygen, but no evidence of impaired tissue oxygen extraction has been found. In fact, one study showed that during hypothermia, tissue affinity for oxygen may increase to the same degree as that of hemoglobin.[61] The solubility of oxygen increases as body temperature is lowered, enhancing dissolved oxygen content. A potential detrimental effect is that blood viscosity increases as temperature fails. Deliberate hypothermia is therefore usually accompanied by hemodilution to counteract this phenomenon.

Neuromuscular blocking agents with sedation and ventilatory support have been used in severely anemic Jehovah's Witnesses in an attempt to minimize oxygen consumption.[21,22] Our case shows how important this therapy can be, because the patient experienced almost immediate cardiac ischemia when the paralytic agent was prematurely withdrawn. Paralysis is especially beneficial in hypothermic patients because shivering can significantly increase oxygen consumption. The paralytic agent of choice in patients with altered renal or hepatic function is atracurium. Pancuronium and vecuronium are commonly used in patients with normal hepatorenal function. As in our patient, prolonged paralysis occasionally results in a delayed recovery of muscle function.[62,63,64,65,66,67] Regarding this complication, the particular paralytic used is not as important as the duration and degree of paralysis. Therefore, daily periodic twitch monitoring is advised to determine the minimum amount of necessary drug. Other medications that affect the neuromuscular system, such as steroids and aminoglycosides, should be avoided. Range-of-motion exercises may help prevent muscle atrophy caused by disease[65] and physical and occupational therapy are recommended when paralytic agents are withdrawn.[62] In most cases, the paresis is temporary, with full recovery of muscular function.

Summary

Proper management of the severely anemic patient refusing blood therapy requires an astute clinician who understands the patient's philosophy and appreciates the often conflicting medicolcgal and ethical aspects of their care, as well as the therapeutic options that are currently available. In caring for such patients, the clinician should heed the wise advice of William Osler, who once said it was more important to know "what sort of person has the disease than what sort of disease the person has."

Notes

1. Immovable for the right to worship, *Watchtower* 1945;66:195-6.
2. *Jehovah's Witnesses and the Question of Blood.* New York, NY: Watchtower and Bible Tract Society of New York, Inc., 1977.
3. Oneson R, Douglas DK, Mintz PD. Jehovah's Witnesses and autologous transfusion [Letter], *Transfusion* 1985;25:179.
4. Green D, Handley E. Erythropoietin for anemia in Jehovah's Witnesses, *Annals of Internal Medi*cine 1990;113:720-1.
5. *Schloendorff v. Society of New York Hospital*, 105 N.E. 92 (1914).
6. *Prince v. Commonwealth of Massachusetts*, 321 U.S. 158 (1944).
7. Jonsen AR. Blood transfusion and Jehovah's Witnesses, *Critical Care Clinicain* 1986;2:91-100.
8. Chervenak FA, McCullough LB. Justified limits on refusing intervention, *Hastings Center Rep*ort.
9. Vincent JL. Transfusion in the exsanguinating Jehovah's Witness patient -- the attitudes of intensive care doctors, *Eur J Anaesthesiol*ogy 1991;8:297-300.
10. *Wons v. Public Health TR. of Dade County*, 541 So.2d 96 (Florida 1989).
11. *Nicoleau v. Fosmire*, 551 NE2d 77 (New York 1990).
12. *Shulman v. Malette and others*, 47DLR18 (1988).
13. Welch HG, Meehan KR, Goodhough LT. Prudent strategies for elective red blood cell transfusion, *Annals of Internal Medicine* 1992;116:393-402.
14. American College of Physicians. Practice strategies for elective red blood cell transfusion, *Annals of Internal Medi*cine 1992;116:403-6.
15. Smoiler BR, Kruskall MS. Phlebotomy for diagnostic laboratory tests in adults, *New England Journal of Medicine* 1986;314:1233-5.
16. Chernow B, Salem M, Stacey J. Blood conservation--a critical care imperative [Editorial], *Critical Care Medi*cine 1991;19:313-4.
17. Trouwborst A, Hagenouw RR, Jeekel J, Ong GL. Hypervolaemic haemodilution in an anaemic Jehovah's Witness, *Br J Anaesthiology* 1990;64:646-8.
18. Messmer K. Hemodilution, *Surg Clin North American* 1975;55:659-78.
19. Khine HH, Naidu R, Cowell H, MacEwen GD. A method of blood conservation in Jehovah's Witnesses: In circulation diversion and refusion, *Anesth Analg.* 1978;57:279-80.
20. Lichtiger B, Dupuis JF, Seski J. Hemotherapy during surgery for Jehovah's Witnesses: A new method, *Anesth Analg.* 1982;61:618-9.
21. Lichtenstein A, Eckhart WF, Swanson K, Vacanti CA, Zapol WM. Unplanned intraoperative and postoperative hemodilution: Oxygen transport and consumption during severe anemia, *Anesthesiology* 1988;69:119-22.
22. Nearman HS, Eckhauser ML. Post-operative management of a severely anemic Jehovah's Witness, *Critical Care Medi*cine 1983;11:142-3.
23. Olsen JB, Alstrup P, Madsen T. Open-heart surgery in Jehovah's Witnesses, *Stand J Thor Cardiovasc Surg* 1990;24:165-9.
24. Lewis CT, Murphy MC, Cooley DA. Risk factors for cardiac operations in adult Jehovah's Witnesses, *Ann Thorac Sur*gery 1991;51:44850.
25. Nelson CL, Bowen WS. Total hip arthroplasty in Jehovah's Witnesses without blood transfusion, *J Bone Joint Surg [Am]* 1986;68:350-3.
26. Enderby GE. A report on mortality and morbidity following 9,107 hypotensive anaesthetic, *Br J Anaesthiology* 1961;33:109-13.

27. Hampton HJ, Little DM. Complications associated with the use of "controlled hypotension" anesthesia, *Arch Surgery* 1953;67:549-56.
28. Larson AG. Deliberate hypotension, *Anesthesiology* 1964;25:682-706.
29. Davis NJ, Jennings JJ, Harris WH. Induced hypotensive anesthesia for total hip replacement, *Clin Orthopedics* 1974;101:93-8.
30. Salzman EW, Weinstein MJ, Weintraub RM, Ware JA, Thurer RL, Robertson L, *et al.* Treatment with desmopressin acetate to reduce blood loss after cardiac surgery, *New England Journal of Medicine* 1986;314:1402-6.
31. Martens PR. Desmopressin and Jehovah's Witness, *Lancet* 1989;1:1322.
32. Stone DJ, DiFazio CA. DDAVP to reduce blood loss in Jehovah's Witnesses [Letter], *Anesthesiology* 1988;69:1028.
33. Cooper JR Jr. Perioperative considerations in Jehovah's Witnesses, *Int Anesthesiol Clin* 1990;28:210-5.
34. Koestner JA, Nelson LD, Morris JA Jr, Safcsak K. Use of recombinant human erythropoietin (r-HuEPO) in a Jehovah's Witness refusing transfusion of blood products, *J Trauma* 1990;30:1406-8.
35. Law EJ, Still JM, Gattis CS. The use of erythropoietin in two burned patients who are Jehovah's Witnesses, *Burns* 1991;17:75-7.
36. Boshkov LK, Tredget EE, Janowska-Wieczorek A. Recombinant human erythropoietin for a Jehovah's Witness with anemia of thermal injury, *Am J Hematology* 1991;37:53-4.
37. Johnson PW, King R, Slevin ML, White H. The use of erythropoietin in a Jehovah's Witness undergoing major surgery and chemotherapy [Letter], *Br J Cancer* 1991;63:476.
38. Jim RT. Use of erythropoietin in Jehovah's Witness patients, *Hawaii Med* Journal 1990;49:209.
39. Stone WJ, Graber SE, Krantz SB, Dessypris EN, O'Neil VL, Olsen NJ, *et al.* Treatment of the anemia of predialysis patients with recombinant human erythropoietin: A randomized, placebo-controlled trial, *American Journal of Medical Science* 1988;296:171-9.
40. Erslev AJ. Erythropoietin, *New England Journal of Medicine* 1991;324:1339-44.
41. Dudrick SJ, O'Donnell JJ, Raleigh DP, Matheny RG, Unkel SP. Rapid restoration of red blood cell mass in severely anemic surgical patients who refuse transfusion, *Archives of Surgery* 1985;120:721-7.
42. Auerbach M, Witt D, Toler W, Fierstein M, Lerner RG, Ba!lard H. Clinical use of the total dose intravenous infusion of iron dextran, *Journal of Laboratory Clinical Medicine* 1988;111:566-70.
43. Whipple GH, Robscheit-Robbins FS. Amino acids and hemoglobin production in anemia, *J Exp Medicine* 1940;71:569-83.
44. Anagnostou A, Schade S, Ashkinaz M, Barone J, Fried W. Effect of protein deprivation on erythropoiesis, *Blood* 1977;50:1093-7.
45. Mishler JM 4th. Synthetic plasma volume expanders--their pharmacology, safety and clinical efficacy, *Clinical Haematology* 1984;13:7592.
46. Lockwood DN, Bullen C, Machin SJ. A severe coagulopathy following volume replacement with hydroxyethyl starch in a Jehovah's Witness, *Anaesthesiaolgoy* 1988;43:391-3.
47. Edwards JD, Nightingale P, Wilkins RG, Faragher EB. Hemodynamic and oxygen transport response to modified fluid gelatin in critically ill patients, *Critical Care Medicine* 1989;17:996-8.
48. Boerema I, Meyne NG, Brummelkamp WK, Bouma S, Mensch MH, Kamermans F, *et al.* Life without blood: A study of the influence of high atmospheric pressure and hypothermia on dilution of blood, *Journal of Cardiovascular Surgery* 1960;1:133-46.
49. Gonzalez ER. Fluosol--a special boon to Jehovah's Witnesses [News], *Journal of the American Medical Assocation* 1980;243:720,724.
50. Moffat AS. Three li'l pigs and the hunt for blood substitutes [News], *Science* 1991;253:32-4.
51. Alsop KS, Condie RM. Current status of hemoglobin-based resuscitative fluid: A review, *Laboratory Medicine* 1987;18:444-8.
52. Pool R. Slow going for blood substitutes [News], *Science* 1990;250:1655-6.
53. Spence RK, McCoy S, Costabile J, Norcross ED, Pello MJ, Alexander JB, *et al.* Fluosol DA-20 in the treatment of severe anemia: A randomized, controlled study of 46 patients, *Critical Care Medicine* 1990;18:1227-30.

54. Tremper KK, Friedman AE, Levine EM, Lapin R, Camarillo D. The preoperative treatment of severely anemic patients with a perfluorochemical oxygen-transport fluid, Fluosol-DA, *New England Journal of Medicine* 1982;307:277-83.
55. Ohyanagi H, Nakaya S, Okumura S, Saitoh Y. Surgical use of fluosol-DA in Jehovah's Witness patients, *Artificial Organs* 1984;8:10-8.
56. Waxman K, Tremper KK, Cullen BF, Mason GR. Perfluorocarbon infusion in bleeding patients refusing blood transfusions, *Archives of Surgery* 1984;119:721-4.
57. Tremper KK, Lapin R, Levine E, Friedman A, Shoemaker WC. Hemodynamic and oxygen transport effects of a perfiuorochemical blood substitute, fluosol-DA (20%), *Critical Care Medicine* 1980;8:738-41.
58. Gould SA, Rosen AL, Sehgal LR, Sehgal HL, Langdale LA, Krause LM, *et al.* Fluosol-DA as a red-cell substitute in acute anemia, *New England Journal of Medicine* 1986;314:1653-6.
59. Michenfelder JD, Uihlein A, Daw EF, Theye RA. Moderate hypothermia in man: Haemodynamic and metabolic effects, *Br J Anaesthesiology* 1965;37:738-45.
60. Thompson R, Rich J, Chemlik F, Nelson W. Evolutionary changes in the electrocardiogram of severe progressive hypothermia, *Journal of Electrocardiology* 1977;10:67-70.
61. Longmuir IS. The effect of hypothermia on the affinity of tissues for oxygen, *Life Sciences* 1962;1:297-300.
62. Gooch JL, Suchyta MR, Balbierz JM, Petajan JH, Clemmer TP. Prolonged paralysis after treatment with neuromuscular junction blocking agents, *Critical Care Medicine* 1991;19:1125-31.
63. Op de Coul AA, Lambregis PC, Koeman J, van Puyenbroek M J, Ter Laak HJ, Gabreels-Festen AA. Neuromuscular complications in patients given Pavulon (pancuronium bromide) during artificial ventilation, *Clin Neurol Neurosurg* 1985;87:17-22.
64. Margolis BD, Khachikian D, Friedman Y, Garrard C. Prolonged reversible quadriparesis in mechanically ventilated patients who received long-term infusions of vecuronium, *Chest.* 1991;199:877-8.
65. Kupfer Y, Okrent DG, Twersky RA, Tessler S. Disuse atrophy in a ventilated patient with status asthmaticus receiving neuromuscular blockade, *Critical Care Medicine* 1987;15:795-6.
66. Segredo V, Matthay MA, Sharma ML, Gruenke LD, Caldwell JE, Miller RD. Prolonged neuromuscular blockade after long-term administration of vecuronium in two critically ill patients, *Anesthesiology* 1990;72:566-70.
67. Partridge BL, Abrams JH, Bazemore C, Rubin R. Prolonged neuromuscular blockade after long-term infusion of vecuronium bromide in the intensive care unit, *Critical Care Medicine* 1990;18:1177-9.

Chapter 32

Suffering as a Consideration in Ethical Decision-Making

Erich H. Loewy

Ethics committees and ethics consultants are becoming more involved in helping individuals make decisions and in advising institutions and legislatures about drafting policy. The role of these committees and consultants has been acknowledged in law, and their function is generally considered salutory and helpful. Ethics consultants and committees, furthermore, play a critical role in educating students and members of the hospital community and the public at large. Moreover, many ethicists engage in scholarly activities to expand the boundaries of our understanding and, in turn, facilitate our capacity for helping. The role of the ethicist and of the ethics committee is thus manifold.[1,2] Ethics committees and ethics consultants somehow "in competition" is a mistaken notion: When ethics committees, ethics consultants, and the community work smoothly together, much good can be accomplished.[3]

As a teacher to medical students, a lecturer in various contexts, a member of ethics committees, a consultant in specific cases, and a theorist, I have been struck by the need for some framework of decision-making. I have watched as myself and others have grappled with difficult cases, all of us agonizing over what almost invariably is far from an ideal answer. I have been impressed that few if any of us ever invoke let alone explicitly appeal to the traditional formal principles of ethics, such as autonomy or beneficence, or to the other explicit principles of what has come to be called the "Georgetown Mantra." Such principles have great importance when we teach: they allow students to become familiar with some of the basic problems and questions and serve as a helpful and proper heuristic device. Although such principles are important and often helpful as a tacit background, they often fall short and are therefore rarely explicitly used when it comes to making specific decisions in particular cases.

In this paper, I: 1) briefly examine some of the traditional frameworks for decision-making; 2) suggest and very briefly sketch a different type of framework that in my experience is far more frequently used even though it may not be explicitly acknowledged; and 3) develop the applicability of such a theoretical framework to actual decision-making.

Frameworks of Decision-Making

When ethicists see formal consultations in hospital settings or when ethics committees deliberate about cases, a framework of reasoning about such cases is essential. This framework is also necessary when policy decisions must be made or advice about making policy decisions must be given, without some sort of framework.

Source: Reprinted from *Cambridge Quarterly of Healthcare Ethics*, Vol. 1, No. 2, pp. 135-142, with permission from Cambridge University Press © Spring, 1992.

Some have argued that "no framework is needed," and that problems dealing with ethical issues in patient care are solved best solely by paying strict attention to the particulars of each individual case. Even here, however, the lack of a framework constitutes a framework; a schema by which decisions can and ought to be made. If I say that I will judge each situation confronting me capriciously or according to what my emotions tell me (going by what I feel is "right" and eschewing what I feel to be wrong: using my "gut feelings" in other words), I am in fact utilizing a framework. Although such a framework is actually a totally subjective and in that sense intuitive approach, it is a framework nevertheless. A largely subjective and intuitive framework denies the need for disciplined reasoning, therefore such a framework is basically anti-intellectual.

Problems of medical diagnosis and treatment cannot properly be left to caprice or be made emotionally or idiosyncratically. Diagnostic and therapeutic decisions must be defensible by appeal to certain accepted "facts" (changeable as these may be over time) and to accepted standards of reasoning. Ethical decisions associated with medical treatment are often, if not almost invariably, decisions that profoundly influence further technical medical decisions. These ethical decisions must also be defensible by an appeal to certain standards. By their nature, capricious, purely emotional, or idiosyncratic decisions cannot easily be defended.

Arguments for casuistry or virtue ethics have recognized the need for some sort of framework.[4,5] Those favoring a casuistic approach have concluded that although overt principles are not needed, cases can be worked out by using "rules of thumb," which themselves emerge from working out a host of similar cases, cases that if solved well provide rules for then solving similar cases. To casuists, the framework itself evolves from the particular disposition of a category of cases.[6] In many respects, this approach is similar to that of virtue ethics, in which good solutions are made by virtuous people and good solutions are defined as those solutions virtuous people make. Judgments evolve out of the cases themselves, and making such judgments makes one more skilled in dealing with cases of a similar kind. As appealing as such arguments are, they contain a serious if not fatal flaw: what constitutes a good solution has to be a prior assumption. A "good solution" that merely serves the patient's "biomedical good," regardless of other considerations, is quite different from a "good solution" that serves the patient's self-selected goals.[7] A framework for what is good (and conversely for what is bad) is still needed. Without it, persons could well become increasingly skilled ("virtuous") in solving particular cases in particular ways and could evolve rules of thumb from this process. But without a framework or reference as to what goals "good solutions" are to serve, ethically unacceptable solutions could easily be made and made more and more "skillfully." What many would consider unacceptable ethical solutions could give rise to what most would consider ethically unacceptable rules of thumb. Such solutions and such rules of thumb could then be unwittingly institutionalized.

A tendency to appeal to strict principles and to reduce each particular case to such principles has never been a very workable solution. Persons of goodwill, even when they believe in different principles, commonly arrive at the same decision when considering particular cases or problems. When they begin to argue their case by appealing to diverse principles, however, disagreements occur.[8] Blindly following rules or strictly adhering to prescribed preordained principles "works" only because it provides a "solution," which is then often judged "good" or "bad" in accordance with the very principle from which it is derived.

When we grapple with ethical problems in the clinical setting and strive towards finding a "right" solution, we will generally be sorely disappointed. Most cases seen by consultants or referred to committees are not cases in which "good" answers are easily at hand; rather, choices between various undesirable alternatives must be made. Consultants and committees do not properly make specific decisions. Rather, consultants and committees serve as advisors and facilitators who help guide, rather than make, decisions. They are, in a sense, geographers of decision-making, who help the decision-makers to do three things: 1) determine where they are (the technical "facts" and the technical options of a case); 2) determine what goals are possible (prognostic facts) and what important values are to be served; and 3) select a course of action (point out the terrain along possible roads and help make a selection) connecting these two points.[9] Unless where we are and where we are going are agreed upon, a proper road cannot be chosen.

Solving problems, as John Dewey pointed out long ago, is a tentative activity. Solutions are solutions not in the sense of final answers or in the sense of establishing immutable truths but rather are tentative hypotheses. Inquiry serves to make indeterminate situations more determinate.[10,11] Such situations are more determinate because they work better in the context in which they are used in dealing with the situation at hand not because they are unalterably true or "right." "Working better" denotes that such a solution provides a resolution of a problem and can then be used to further inquiry, learning, and growth. Frameworks of decision-making (some might call them principles) are critically important as tools or guide posts facilitating the decisions made but are not meant to be applied as straight jackets limiting options and inquiry.

Suffering as a Possible Framework

Traditional frameworks have left us with few guidelines. Methodologically, all of them have merit and all can be severely criticized. In real situations, few if any ethicists or ethics committees directly appeal to specific principles. Such appeals, in my experience, are most often made by those with the least experience and are rarely made by people who have dealt with such problems extensively. More experienced people may have internalized such principles and may be applying them tacitly to the problem at hand. When questioned about this, however, the majority of ethicists will deny any appeal to such principles.

A utilitarian framework for making individual decisions, as useful and indeed indispensable as it may be for decisions of macro-allocation, serves poorly when individual decisions must be made. A Kantian reliance on respect for persons, although frequently serving as a tacit background for making such decisions, has certain glaring difficulties. Reducing cases to such principles often yields humanly unsatisfying results.

Over the years, I have taught medical ethics at my school of medicine and have watched and participated in the deliberations of several ethics committees. I have performed formal ethics consultations in three hospitals. In addition, I have given a series of[12] lectures dealing with ethical theory and foundational issues in bioethics to a developing ethics committee in one of our smaller institutions and have then helped them begin to reason through cases. Although a thorough understanding of ethical theory and traditional principles is not only extremely helpful but essential in promoting an understanding of particular cases, it is an incomplete framework for dealing with most actual cases. After watching and analyzing the process over the years, I am convinced that a deeper framework is more helpful and is, indeed, what is often consciously and unconsciously appealed to.

An example may be helpful. One of the cases brought to me was a gentleman who was evidently dying of cancer. Because he wanted to live as long as possible, he had been given extensive chemotherapy and radiation. To facilitate adjuvant therapy, the patient was given hyperalimentation. Although he knew by the time of this story that chemotherapy and radiation had failed to control the disease, he pinned his hopes on the belief that hyperalimentation could prolong his life for some time. His physician (who knew the patient well and had engaged in an almost ideal ongoing dialogue with him) was troubled; the patient had repeatedly asked to be reassured that hyperalimentation would continue his life and, although his physician was certain that hyperalimentation served no useful purpose, he dreaded its being stopped. The physician was troubled because he had not "really told him the truth" but had allowed the patient to continue (and had perhaps even had supported him) in his evident error. The patient seemed to cling to the notion of hyperalimentation with the desperation of a drowning man clinging to a life preserver. His physician, fully aware that respect demands truth telling, could not get himself to tell him the truth.

An appeal to the principle of truth telling or to autonomy in such a case is unsatisfying. One could, of course, appeal to beneficence. However, such an appeal would clash with the principle of autonomy and fail to yield a useful answer. What, specifically, would the content of such beneficence be, how would it "play itself" out? The physician in our case was troubled but quite convinced that in this particular case he was bound to allow the patient to remain in his wrong belief. Why?

One of the most fundamental questions in ethics is what gives an entity moral standing. Why is it that we look at kicking a football as exercise or as part of a game but look at the kicking of a dog or child as a morally unacceptable act? Using Kantian respect, which would give such respect (or moral standing) to entities having the capacity to self-legislate, would not solve our problem. It might explain why kicking the child is immoral but would (at least according to Kant, albeit that I strongly disagree) not explain why kicking a dog would have similar standing. Self-legislation is a higher capacity, one which Kant (albeit not I) would not grant to any but to humans. Further, many humans lack that capacity: 6-month fetuses, infants, the permanently vegetative or comatose, the severely demented or mentally retarded, and many of those who appeal their actions only to authority (religious fundamentalists, in that sense, generally cannot be considered self-legislating persons). Although the moral standing of such beings may be different, few would deny them all moral standing. Furthermore, most persons would give at least some moral standing to animals: torturing dogs, birds or monkeys would be considered morally reprehensible by almost all people.

An entity's capacity to suffer gives it moral standing. In a recent work, I described the biological foundations enabling suffering and analyzed the concept. Although suffering cannot be reduced to its biological substrate, the presence of the substrate is a necessary but insufficient condition for suffering to occur.[12,13]

Things that can suffer have moral standing. They are, as I have termed it, of "primary moral worth." Such moral worth cannot, of course, be absolute; if it were, no distinction among any of the many entities that have such capacity (parakeets, dogs, monkeys, and college students) could be made. It is a *prima facie* condition; having the capacity to suffer and having primary worth means, ethically speaking, that acceptable reasons for causing suffering must be given. Having the capacity to suffer, so to speak, gives such entities "their day in court." Beyond that, it counsels that even when causing or allowing suffering is ethically unavoidable and necessary, it must be kept to a minimum. The capacity to suffer makes objects that are acted upon subjects that are acted with. The capacity to suffer is basic to "having a life." Without such a primitive capacity, the higher capacity of having hopes, aspirations and life plans cannot occur. Having the capacity to suffer is what begins to distinguish "being alive" from "having a life."[14,15]

Objects that lack a capacity to suffer are not necessarily without value. In such cases, the valuation by those who have primary worth, almost by reflection, gives these objects value. Such objects, of "secondary worth," can have two types of value: material (what Kant calls "market value" or "Marktpreis") or symbolic or aesthetic (what Kant calls "affective value" or "Affektivpreis").[16] The value of such objects (be they material or symbolic) can be either positive or negative. Obviously, hierarchies of value must be established as guidelines in making practical decisions. Such hierarchies are made by communities in an ongoing dialogue and are not immutable or absolute. Certain guidelines for making such judgments have been suggested.[17,18]

The capacity to suffer is one that many ethics consultants and ethics committees use in grappling with specific cases. Time and again the conversation around committee tables or with patients and families revolves, overtly or tacitly, around suffering. For most people, prevention of the suffering of themselves or their loved one is the value ultimately pursued. After the medical determination of "where one is" (what are the "facts" and the options of the case) has been made and while attempting to determine where to go and what means to employ to get there, prevention of suffering, rather than the traditional principles of ethics, is almost always the prime consideration. The "common man" (as Kant would call such a person) knows this implicitly.[19]

The way we look at a framework of suffering is critically dependant upon our sense of community. If our community is only an association of people who safeguard one another's freedom, a quite different sense of obligation develops than if we envision our community as being far more involved. A community as a loose association of persons who, because of fear of one another, have formed a compact promising merely to leave each other alone so as to better get on with their lives, is a community in which liberty is of paramount importance emerges.[20,21] Obligations in such minimalist communities are purely those of safeguarding one another's freedom: We are obligated not to interfere with our neighbors' freedom and they are similarly obligated to us; communities are constituted merely to safeguard the liberties of all their members. Individuals who wish to extend their obligation and to help their neighbors are free to do so, but doing so is a supererogatory act rather than one founded on an ethical obligation.

In the medical setting, physicians are obligated to their patients and patients to their physicians purely by explicit contract; physicians are "bureaucrats of health" who give whatever services patients want as long as patients (through insurance or otherwise) pay for such services.[22] Physicians do the best (technical) job they can, not primarily to discharge beneficent obligations (though they are personally free to adopt such an ethic) but to fulfill their contractual obligations and, of course, to attract more business. They are not only bureaucrats but, and properly so, entrepreneurs of healthcare.[23]

In minimalist communities, freedom is a "side-constraint," that is, it constrains or limits all other ethical decisions.[24] An ethic based on suffering would make little sense in a community in which the only ethical obligation is safeguarding each others' liberty: the suffering of another might, but need not, bother me, and even if it did it could confer no obligation on me. Persons are and must be left entirely free to suffer.

An ethic based on suffering makes sense only when it is embedded in a more generous conception of community. Infants are born into larger or smaller communities and are critically dependent upon nurture and beneficence if they are to survive. At birth and for a few months thereafter, infants have no sense of self; they and the world are one and the same thing. Their sense of selfhood, their notion of others, and consequently their sense of autonomy necessarily emerges in the embrace of nurture and beneficence. When such a sense begins to develop, older infants and children still are critically dependent upon the sustenance and help of their communities. As a sense of others develops, moreover, a "primitive sense of pity" emerges. This sense of pity or compassion is a "natural repugnance" (la répugnance naturelie) to see the suffering of others, which Rousseau also speaks of as "l'impulsion intérieur de la compassion."[25,26] Such a sense is the driving force ("Triebfeder") of ethics, the impulse that motivates us to initiate the moral question of how my action will affect others.[27,28]

A primitive sense of pity may be the thing that not only urges persons to worry about ethical questions but causes communities to institutionalize such concerns in ethics committees and to embody them in ethics consultants. Beyond this, however, a sense of compassion can be reenforced or attenuated by experience and education. Properly conceived, education can go far in fostering this sense and channeling it into useful activities.[29] Education, in that sense, is a life-long activity. By working with particular cases and by using an ethic of suffering, ethics committees naturally sharpen and enhance the compassion of their members and, indirectly by their daily activity, engender sensitivity and compassion in others.

Concrete Decisions

Using suffering as a framework will help ethics committees or ethics consultants make decisions. Such decisions, however, require more than just a framework. The way in which such decisions are made--the formal conditions, as it were, must rely on "just process," the procedure wherein all those legitimately concerned (patients, health professionals, families in their wider sense and even communities) have their proper role to play. Facts and pertinent moral values must be fully presented, precedents must be considered, subtle coercion must be guarded against, and all must be given adequate time to present their points of view.[30] In conducting this process and facilitating decisions, one must carefully look at the particulars of specific cases, and suffering can be a useful principle. Notions of primary and secondary worth can also help in sorting out practical situations.

An example may help. A man is admitted to the ICU of a hospital following a head-on collision. Although unconscious and on a ventilator, his physicians at first judge his prognosis as fair. As the case develops, it becomes evident that the patient is permanently comatose and because of severe cerebral injury will probably be permanently ventilator dependent.

A patient whose prognosis is fair or even unknown is rightly considered to have primary worth, as would a patient temporarily under anesthesia. Barring a patient's known prior wishes to the contrary, such a patient deserves and must ethically receive full therapy regardless of ability to pay, the family's wishes, or the fact that a critically ill patient might benefit from the salvage of organs. When, however, patients become brain dead or permanently comatose or enter the permanently vegetative state, they lose primary and assume secondary worth. As an organ donor, material worth is positive; others who are of primary worth may benefit greatly. As one who consumes resources, material worth is negative. Additionally, such a patient has symbolic worth: to loved ones as well as to the community as a symbol of others who are of primary worth.

Using such considerations in dealing with the practical cases we are called upon to help with on the ward can be most useful. Decisions of this sort, however, require a sense of community and must be subject to fair process. Organ donation or the consumption of resources is of critical concern to the community, and consideration of such aspects in decision-making is an expression of such an ethic at work. In a larger sense, we cannot as a community condone the wasting of organs or of resources that others in the community could use. Where we draw the line (how we go about harvesting organs or how we decide to establish a "cutoff" point beyond which futile medical care is no longer given) is a communal activity; an activity that is properly made prior to the specific decisions that ethics committees or ethics consultants help to fashion. Fair process must involve all concerned with the decision: the physician, the healthcare team, and the family. Physicians cannot paternalistically ignore the concerns of others, and the patient and the family cannot, within this ethical concept, treat members of the healthcare team as merely bureaucrats of health. The proper role of physicians and other healthcare workers is to honestly make the others aware of the medical "facts": the diagnosis, prognosis, and technical options of the case. Determining the goal and the means of getting to the goal is a joint activity between the "experts" in the case and the others involved in the decision. Medical "experts" are here to explain the realm of the possible: what can and what cannot be done. All must engage in a mutual exploration of values so that a decision acceptable to all concerned can be made.

In such a process, communities (when functioning well, advised but not controlled by "experts") play their tacit role in all decisions. Communities have, prior to specific decisions, set the framework of what is and what is not acceptable. Communities may, for example, determine that persons who are brain dead are considered legally dead and will, therefore, no longer be supported. They could and should decide whether keeping permanently vegetative and permanently comatose persons alive is a justifiable community expense or whether the monies (billions per year in the United States alone) might better be spent elsewhere. Such communal decisions are the framework within which specific decisions are then made. Using fair process and utilizing a framework of suffering may help make such communal decisions just as it helps in making individual decisions. Of course, communal decisions are just as changeable and as subject to learning and growth as are specific decisions.

Notes

1. Churchill LR, Cross AW. Moralist, technician, sophist, teacher/learner: Reflections on the ethicist in the clinical setting, *Theoretical Medicine* 1986;7(1):3-12.
2. Glover JJ, Ozar DT, Thomasma DC. Teaching ethics on rounds: The ethicist as teacher, consultant and decision maker, *Theoretical Medicine* 1986;7(1):13-32.
3. Loewy EH. Ethics consultation and ethics committees: A functioning model for reaching consensus, *HEC Forum* 1990;6:351-9.
4. Jonsen AR, Toulmin S. *The Abuse of Casuistry*. Berkeley, CA: University of California Press, 1988.
5. Maclntyre A. *After Virtue*. Notre Dame, IN: Notre Dame Press, 1981.
6. Maclntyre A. *After Virtue*. Notre Dame, IN: Notre Dame Press, 1981.
7. Pellegrino ED, Thomasma DC. *For the Patient's Good: The Restoration of Beneficence in Health Care*. New York, NY: Oxford University Press, 1988.
8. Toulmin S. The tyranny of principles, *Hastings Center Report* 1981;11(6):31-9.
9. Loewy EH. Ethics consultation and ethics committees: A functioning model for reaching consensus, *HEC Forum* 1990;6:351-9.
10. Dewey J. *The Quest for Certainty*. New York, NY: GP Putnam's Sons, 1980.
11. Dewey J. *Logic, the Theory of Inquiry*. New York, NY: Henry Holt, 1938.
12. Loewy EH. The role of suffering and community in clinical ethics, *The Journal of Clinical Ethics* 1991;2(2):in press.
13. Loewy EH. *Suffering and the Beneficent Community: Beyond Libertarianism*. Albany, NY: SUNY Press, 1991.
14. Rachels J. *The End of Life*. New York, NY: Oxford University Press, 1986.
15. Kushner T. Having a life versus being alive, *Journal of Medical Ethics* 1984;1:5-8.
16. Kant I. Grundlegung zur metaphysik der sitten, In: Wilhelm Weischedel, ed. *Immanuel Kant Kritik der Praktischen Vernunft, Grundlegung zur Metaphysik der Sitten. Band VII*. Frankfurt a/M, Germany: Suhrkamp Verlag, 1989.
17. Loewy, EH. *Suffering and the Beneficent Community: Beyond Libertarianism*. Albany, NY: SUNY Press, 1991.
18. Loewy, EH. *Community, Communities and Suffering*. Albany, NY: SUNY Press (in preparation).
19. Kant I. Grundlegung zur metaphysik der sitten. In: Wilhelm Weischedel, ed. *Immanuel Kant Kritik der Praktischen Vernunft, Grundlegung zur Metaphysik der Sitten. Band VII*. Frankfurt a/M, Germany: Suhrkamp Verlag, 1989.
20. Hobbes T. *Leviathan*. New York, NY: Collier Books, 1962.
21. Nozick R. *Anarchy, State and Utopia*. New York, NY: Basic Books, 1974.
22. Engelhardt HT. *The Foundations of Bioethics*. New York, NY: Oxford University Press, 1986.
23. Engelhardt HT. Morality for the medical-industrial complex: A code of ethics for the mass marketing of health care, *New England Journal of Medicine* 1988;319(16):1086-9.
24. Nozick R. *Anarchy, State and Utopia*. New York, NY: Basic Books, 1974.

25. Rousseau JJ. Du contra social, In: Grimsley, R, ed. Oxford, England: Oxford University Press, 1972.
26. Rousseau JJ. *Discours sur l'Origine et les Fondements de l'Inegalite parmi les Hommes*. Paris, France: Gallimard, 1965.
27. Loewy, EH. *Community, Communities and Suffering*. Albany, NY: SUNY Press (in preparation).
28. Schopenhauer A. Samtliche W, eds. *Preisschrtift über die grundlage der moral*. Frankfurt a/M, Germany: Band III, 1986.
29. Rousseau JJ. *Emile: ou, De l'education*. Paris, France: Garnier Freres, 1957.
30. Hampshire S. *Innocence and Experience*. Cambridge, MA: Harvard University Press, 1989.

Chapter 33

The Relief of Suffering

Eric J. Cassell

The relief of suffering is considered one of the primary aims of medicine. However, what suffering actually is and what physicians must do specifically to prevent or relieve it is poorly understood. Because of this, the most well-intentioned and best-trained physicians may cause suffering inadvertently in the course of treating disease and may fail to relieve suffering when that might otherwise be possible.

Suffering must be distinguished from pain or other symptoms with which it may be associated. Although physicians, patients, and the medical literature generally link pain and suffering, they are distinct phenomena. For example, patients may tolerate severe pain without considering themselves to be suffering, if they know the source of the pain, that it can be controlled, and that it will come to an end. However, even apparently minor pain or other symptoms may cause suffering if they are believed to have a dire cause (eg, a malignant neoplasm), if they are viewed as never-ending, or if patients consider the symptom (and themselves) to be beyond help, or if their condition is considered hopeless. Suffering may occur in the absence of any symptoms whatsoever, e.g., when one is forced to witness helplessly the pain of a loved one. Indeed, helplessness itself may be a source of suffering.

Suffering may occur in relation to any aspect of a person.[1] The word "person," as used herein, refers to all the possible dimensions of an individual. As such, it is larger than and includes the self or personality. A simple topography of person would include personality and character; the lived past; the family's past; associations and relationships with family and others, culture, and society; the person's work and social roles; body image; the unconscious mind; political affiliations; the secret life (which everyone has, whether in reality or in dreams); the perceived future; and the transcendent or spiritual dimension, lending to each person the sense of being greater and more lasting than an individual life.

Sickness, with its pain, dyspnea, weakness, nausea, and the whole panoply of symptoms and disabilities, is important because of what it does to the person, not merely because of its effect on the person's body. Suffering occurs (clinical observation suggests) when the illness or its symptoms threaten not only interference with some aspect of person -- virtually any illness does that -- but when it destroys or is perceived to destroy the integrity of the person through its effects. Most generally, suffering can be defined as the state of severe distress associated with events that threaten the intactness or wholeness of the person. Suffering continues until the threat is gone or the integrity of the person can be restored in some other fashion. Thus, although pain or other symptoms may, as examples, disrupt a person's relationships with others, interfere with someone's ability to work, or make the patient's usual presentation to the world impossible, the sickness usually does not cause suffering until the

---

Source: Reprinted from *Archives of Internal Medicine*, Vol. 143, pp. 522-523, with permission from Archives of Internal Medicine © March, 1983.

patient believes that the changes will continue into the future. Silently or otherwise, patients will continue to suffer until they no longer believe the disruptions to be enduring, come to see the possibility of being whole again, or believe themselves to be total, intact persons, despite the loss of some aspect of themselves or their function. As all physicians know, the capacity of persons and of the human spirit to overcome sickness and loss is wonderful beyond words.

It has always been important for physicians to relieve suffering, but understanding what suffering is and what to do about it has a special urgency in this era. A new category of patients exists for whom the potential for suffering is enormous -- the chronically severely sick patient whose life medical technology can now prolong. The most obvious cases involve patients with metastatic disease whose malignant neoplasm and complications are partially controlled. For example, a woman with surgical stage II endometrial cancer with notable myometrial invasion, who had radiation after her hysterectomy, was given cisplatin and doxorubicin hydrochloride therapy, when intestinal obstruction and an abdominal mass heralded recurrence. Size had a good response to chemotherapy.

After one year, "second look" laparotomy disclosed a return of the tumor. Postoperatively a small bowel fistula and sepsis developed. Because of total parenteral nutrition and antimicrobial agents, she was discharged from the hospital five weeks after undergoing an operation and she looked well and vigorous. Soon the original fistula reopened, followed by several others, and she died at home six weeks later. With such a patient, the number and severity of symptoms, the quantity and cost of medical care, the toll on the patient, family, and friends, are well known to physicians. These cases are common and are the results of current therapeutic gains. A similar situation pertains to some patients who have end-stage congestive heart disease, chronic obstructive pulmonary disease, neurologic diseases, or multiple coexisting diseases. The essential point is not merely the chronicity, which is not new, but the long duration of severe and demanding sickness previously associated only with acute, short-lived illness.

It is also true that the survivors of such illness, either the families or the patients (if they live) do not have good memories of the medical care given. This is especially unfortunate because the care of seriously ill patients frequently demands enormous dedication as well as skill. However, the survivors recall inadequate pain relief, long waits for simple services, an endless parade of seemingly (to the patient) unnecessary procedures, impersonal attention, changing house staff and tangled lines of command, and inadequate information and explanation ranging from what Willard Galen, MD, calls "truth-dumping" to halftruths and lies.

It is a sad fact that such serious illnesses are often characterized by sorrow and pain. However, it is an even greater misfortune when medical care fails to relieve such misery, and it is still worse when it adds to it. I believe that three interlocking principles of treatment will permit physicians to take better care of these sick patients while greatly reducing the suffering of the patients and their families. The first principle is that diagnostic and therapeutic goals should be set in terms of the patient not the disease. The second principle is to maximize the patient's function not the length of life. The third is to actively minimize the patient's and the family's suffering. These three principles cannot really be separated from one another because they derive from the more basic understanding that physicians take care of sick persons not diseases. Since patients generally know best what their goals are, which functions matter most to them, and when they are suffering, following these principles inevitably means working with patients and their families.

While space does not permit great detail, I shall attempt to illustrate what these principles might mean practically.

1. Diagnostic and therapeutic goals should be set in terms of patients not diseases. For example, when the patient is seen with tissue-proved, widespread metastatic cancer, the search for the primary tumor site does not contribute to therapeutic planning, but it does increase the patient's discomfort, fears, length of hospital stay, and costs. However, even in cases of advanced malignant neoplasma, radiation to the spine may avert paraplegia and permit death from a more tolerable complication, e.g., hypercalcemia. When gangrene of a foot occurs as part of the terminal illness of a patient with diabetes, benign mummification is often preferable to amputation. Thus, choosing a more comfortable mode, time, or place of death should be considered an appropriate goal. When the aims of treatment are primarily patient oriented, then the support mechanisms of the family, group, or community are enhanced rather than interfered with by medicine and its technology. Such planning is not lesser medicine; it is medical care that is appropriate to the particular patient with a particular disease in a particular life situation. As such, it requires considerable knowledge of the patient, the disease, and the situation.

2. Maximize function not the length of life. Patients with illnesses of the kind that I am discussing do not often return to normal work or recreation. However, with skillful treatment, help, and encouragement, they may return to their homes and a useful place in the family structure. For this to be possible, the usual intrusiveness of medical care must be greatly reduced. This means reducing hospital stays to a minimum, reducing the frequency of office visits by using the telephone and house calls as a substitute, employing home care units, and teaching the family to provide care. This strategy involves risk to the patient. Infection may not be detected as early, bowel obstruction may occur, the patient may fall, the wrong medication might be taken, congestive heart failure may go undetected, diabetic control may be inadequate, and so on. However, if one works with the patient, and family as partners, these worrisome possibilities usually do not occur with greater frequency than in the hospitalized patient, and the patients are vastly more comfortable and content. One is, after all, avoiding the alternative risks of greater suffering.[2] The patient is in this way given the opportunity to live as well as is possible, despite a terminal illness. While risks can be discussed with the patient or a family member, the physician should not unduly alarm the patient with fears of complications. Such fear can be as crippling to the patient as the event itself. For example, a patient with metastatic disease to the bone had a pathologic fracture of the femur pinned. But the patient was kept bed bound and chair bound because of her physician's fears of another fracture. If such a patient is to return to any degree of function, that kind of risk must be taken. When making these decisions, one must consider the actual probabilities, not merely unusual possibilities. In general, care of this sort develops one's prognostic sense to a high degree. Sometimes, as with high-dose steroids in late-stage cancer, therapeutic maneuvers should be planned that have only the patient's sense of well-being in mind. However, it is important not to start therapies employed in these situations for symptomatic relief that one cannot easily discontinue, eg, use of a respirator or total parenteral nutrition.

3. Actively minimize suffering. Suffering is an individual matter that must be seen as distinct from physical symptoms, even though they may be its source. One can only know the source of suffering by asking the patient; what the physician or even the family believes is causing suffering may not be a reliable guide. However, adequate

pain relief is a hallmark of good care in the sick patient. The proper dose of analgesic is that which relieves pain, something to which only the patient can testify. By proper manipulation of analgesics, e.g., phenothiazines, hydroxyzine hydrochloride, methylphenidate hydrochloride, or dextroamphetamine sulfate, pain can usually be relieved without too much sedation or other side effects. Constipation must be attended to. Giving oral analgesics is almost always satisfactory in adequate dosage (eg, 300 mg of meperidine hydrochloride by mouth is the equivalent of 75 mg by injection), but the family or the patient can be instructed in the use of subcutaneous morphine sulfate. As pain can usually be controlled, so too can many other symptoms; however, minimizing suffering does not stop here. The goal is to maintain the intactness and integrity of the person in the face of severe or increasing sickness and a deteriorating body. Any aspect of personhood -- emotional, social, physical, familial, or private -- may provide the locus of intervention. As in all medical care, the relationship with the patient provides the vehicle for minimizing suffering. That our skills are not equal to the task and our knowledge is inadequate is unfortunate, but this is no different a situation than that pertaining in other areas of medical care throughout the history of medicine. The crucial first step is an understanding that the relief of suffering is a proper goal of medicine.

Notes

1. Cassell EJ. The nature of suffering and the goals of medicine, *New England Journal of Medicine* 1982;306:639-645.
2. Saunders C. *The Management of Terminal Disease*. London, England: Edward Arnold Publishers, 1978.

Chapter 34

The Blood Transfusion Taboo of Jehovah's Witnesses: Origin, Development and Function of a Controversial Doctrine

Richard Singelenberg

Introduction

Part of the underlying tension between religious healing and secular medicine can be found, in particular, within non-mainline Christianity. Certain biblical doctrines as interpreted by followers of particular religious groups, were, and still are, at odds with established medical practice, creating "a degree of tension between the medicine of the soul and the medicine of the body."[1] Accordingly members of Christian Science hold that their faith is "a panacea (...) and the only real remedy for sin, disease and death."[2] Rather than consult secular physicians, orthodox believers would prefer to seek healing from the movement's practitioners. Faith healing or the conviction that the supreme being punishes the sinner by sending illness, thus causing them to reject "worldly" health care, can be found among conservative Pentecostalists within the Holiness Church.[3,4] Similarly, based on the Mathian verse "persons in health do not need a physician", fundamentalistic groups within the Dutch Reformed Church in the Netherlands refused to have their children vaccinated against poliomyelitis in the 60s and 70s, as well as during an eruption of the measles in February 1988.[5]

Perhaps the best known example of this general phenomenon is the blood transfusion refusal of Jehovah's Witnesses. Promulgating the rule in 1945, the Watchtower Bible and Tract Society (hereafter "the Society"), generated one the most controversial issues on the interface of religion and health care. Based on Genesis 9 verse 4, Leviticus 17 verses 11 and 12, and the Pauline New Testamentary reiteration in Acts 15, the Society declared that, irrespective of the mode of consumption, the eating of blood was an unscriptural practice.[6,7] Besides the array of scriptural references, the Witnesses have at their disposal legitimizing the regulation, they feel heavily supported by extra-doctrinal arguments. The second part of the 80s provided them, from their point of view, with a powerful secular ally: AIDS emerged as a macabre confirmation of the doctrine.

The first part of the present paper explores origin, development, and the arguments used to justify the prohibition. The second part offers a functionalist analysis of the doctrine. It appears legitimate to wonder why, of the wide range of possible interpretations of divine precepts, the Society has formulated this extended exegesis of the rule to abstain from blood. However, the anthropologist searches for the taboo's implicit meaning, trying to explain an idiosyncrasy within the context of a specific religious system. So, going beyond doctrine, the questions that must be raised are: why was the rule promulgated in 1945 and not earlier

---

Source: Reprinted from *Social Science Medicine*, Vol. 31, No. 4, pp. 515-523, with permission from Elsevier Science Limited © 1990.

(since blood transfusion was already in use at the beginning of this century) and what is its function within the community of believers? In order to grasp meaning and function of the doctrine, it appears useful to apply the concepts of purity and pollution as formulated by the anthropologist Mary Douglas.[8]

As far as I can tell, the blood transfusion doctrine is unique. I found no evidence in ethnography or medical anthropology of an identical taboo.[9]

Origins, Development, and Justification

Prior to its prohibition of blood transfusion the Society had objections to another medical treatment, namely, vaccination and inoculation. To be sure, this disapproval was never framed in an official doctrine based on biblical articles of faith and promulgated like the ruling on blood but the practice was vehemently discouraged. This position emerges most clearly during the 30s in *The Golden Age*, one of the predecessors of *Awake!* A quote may illustrate this: Thinking people would rather have smallpox than vaccination, because the latter sows the seed of syphilis, cancers, eczema, erysipelas, scrofula, consumption, even leprosy, and many other loathsome afflictions. Hence the practice of vaccination is a crime, an outrage, and a delusion.

The treatment was further described as "defiling", "devilish," and "influencing the criminal tendencies of the present generation,"[10] expressions similar to those uttered by resisters of compulsory vaccination in 19th century Britain and Holland.[5,11] In some instances, letters from readers pointed to the biblical foundation of the evil of inoculation, referring to the appropriate text in Leviticus in which the intermingling of animal matter with human blood is prohibited.[12] Besides the perceived dangers of vaccination and inoculation, the markedly cynical writings also breathe of an antagonistic attitude towards the medical profession, the pharmaceutical industry, and, above all, the state as an active agent which compels its citizens to have themselves vaccinated. It is doubtful whether this doctrine enjoyed large support. In one of the first studies of the Witnesses, undertaken in the early 40s, it is noted that the majority of the adherents would accept medical services.[13] Also indicative may be the case of the approximately 4,300 American Witnesses who were in prison as conscientious objectors during World War II.[14] According to Macmillan, member of the Society's leadership, only a small minority concentrated in one prison refused to submit to the vaccinations compulsory for all inmates. It was only after his intervention convincing them there were no scriptural objections that they complied. Of interest, however, is Macmillan's argument for the prisoners' refusal. In his autobiography (one of the few eulogies on the Jehovah's Witnesses which has not been published by the Society), he notes "(...) our boys (...) considered [vaccinations] the same as blood transfusions (...)"[15,16] As the doctrine on blood had yet to be promulgated his assertion may exemplify the psychological repression of obsolete doctrines or unpopular policy and subsequent reinterpretation into acceptable and plausible ideological statements; a mechanism not uncommon among Jehovah's Witnesses and adherents of similar religious groups. In the Society's own official historiography this particular event has been omitted.[17] Furthermore, as noted by Penton, it is not entirely clear whether the aversion against vaccination represented the Society's viewpoint in general or rather a personal grudge of Woodworth, the editor of *Awake!*[18] Macmillan's explanation may therefore reflect the possible disagreement among the Society's leadership among this specific issue. After 1945 the animosity against vaccinations disappeared from the reading matter, but until the 60s it was still considered an act of pollution of blood and body.[19]

The origins of the ruling on the use of blood are somewhat obscure. To be sure, the Society promulgated the doctrine in 1945, but that was not the first time the matter was brought up. As early as 1939, Rutherford, the then president, wrote that 'life is in the blood and that the blood must not be eaten', in answer to a letter of a Witness who wondered if the eating of pork was scripturally allowed.[20] Blood transfusion was not mentioned: a year later he even seemed to be in favour of it.[21] According to Penton the matter did not rise until 1937, the year in which the first large-scale blood bank was established in Chicago, but the author does not elaborate on the Society's reaction (18, p.153). Then, in the December 22, 1943 edition of *Consolation, Awake!*'s immediate predecessor, a short article mentioned the development of a serum against meningitis, which includes horse blood. The writer concluded that "the divine prohibition as to the eating or partaking of blood does not appear to trouble the 'scientists.'" About that time, at the other side of the Atlantic, a Jehovah's Witness, inmate of the women's concentration camp Ravensbrück in Nazi-Germany, one day approached her warden, announcing that the eating of blood-sausage was a violation of the scriptures. According to Deuteronomy 12:24, she declared that "the blood should not be eaten, but should be poured upon the ground as water." So, from now on, she and her fellow believers would abstain from this food, in spite of the alarmingly low rations. This time, even for the cohesive group of Witnesses, things were being pushed too far; according to the warden's eyewitness account, only 25 out of the 275 detained Witnesses followed their inspired "sister."[22]

Nevertheless, *The Watchtower* of July 1, 1945 introduced the prohibition. Ironically, two months later, the Dutch edition of *Consolation* states:

> God never issued provisions prohibiting the use of medicines, injections or blood transfusion. It is an invention of people who, like the Pharisees, leave Jehovah's mercy and love aside.[23]

This notorious quote, often used by the movement's (Dutch) adversaries as proof of doctrinal inconsistency, did not emanate from the Society's headquarters in New York, but was written by its regional editor, who, apparently, was unaware of the new doctrine; a situation unthinkable today and probably a result of post-war communication breakdowns. During the late forties, the Society hardly paid any attention to the new ruling. From 1949 onwards, some back-up material was published, such as the statement by a homeopathic physician, who warned that "complications and chronic conditions follow as a rule those who live long enough to pay the penalty of such repugnant measures."[24] Also, readers started to ask questions about the prohibition. One of them, apparently worried about one of its implications, was reassured by the editorial staff that "human copulation for the reproduction of mankind cannot be viewed as a blood transfusion from the male to the female." According to another reader, the element of "greed," indissolubly bound up with the biblical injunction of blood eating, is absent in transfusions. "How can you say this," was the Society's reply, "For when a doctor tells a patient that he must have a blood transfusion or else he cannot get well and live, what does the doctor create in the patient but a greed for the blood of another human creature?"[25] Hence the theme of patient as vampire emerged, as noted also by Tannahill, and the preamble for the regularly used parallel of blood transfusion with cannibalism.[26]

Until the mid-fifties the issue received only marginal attention in the Society's publications, measured by the number of articles covering the taboo. According to the Society's subject index, during 1946 and 47 nothing appeared in its literature. In 1948 and 49 only four editions paid attention to the issue. In contrast, in 1971 the subject was covered in 16 editions. Gradually, the medical world was confronted with the doctrine, resulting in an increasing tension between two value systems. An extreme example is that of the father and two brothers of a victim of an automobile accident in Texas in 1952, who kept guard in her hospital room to prevent doctors from giving a transfusion, in spite of the fact that the patient herself was not a Witness ([16], p.187). From the medico-legal angle an important ethical problem arose: was the Hippocratic oath more important than individual religious freedom?

In particular, attention was paid to the element of "forced" transfusions as imposed by court orders. In fact, questions were raised of a persons's constitutional rights, resulting in extensive legislative debates.[27,28] Besides, the medical profession was challenged to adapt its skills and technology to a clientele who refused to accept a treatment that had hitherto hardly been questioned. The doctrine unlocked considerable upheaval within, as well outside, the Witnesses's community. Particularly in the case of minor's whose parents refused to consent to the administering of possibly life-saving blood, emotions ran high; more often than not parental authority was temporarily divested by state agencies, to be followed by the forbidden treatment. Reports such as the transfusions forced upon twelve infants in Canada, who were returned dead to their families resulted in bitter legal debates, as the parents were convinced that the transfusions had caused their children's death.[29] Conversely, many press reports voiced the feelings of society at large, appealing to the fundamental values of parental love and care. Not surprisingly, the Witnesses felt they were under siege. The more outside resistance increased, the more vehemently the Society's defense. Opposing doctors were labelled "bloodthirsty physicians," the divesting of parental authority was compared with the "recruitment of the Hitler Youth," while one of the Society's legal counsels qualified the forced transfusions in Canada as a form of "rape."[30]

Until 1960, violation of the injunction had supernatural consequences only. "We will not take any spiritual action against anyone," replied the Society to those who disagreed.[34] The offender eventually had to stand trial before God. Even an "anointed sister," member of the elite of the 144,000 chosen, who had accepted a blood transfusion, did not face expulsion from the Society.[31] All that was to change. In the "Questions from Readers" part in the January 15, 1961 edition of *The Watchtower*, it was stated that the taking of a transfusion would be followed by excommunication (in the Society's jargon "disfellowshipping"). If the offender would refuse to acknowledge his transgression or would persist in accepting or donating blood, he would be considered "a rebellious opposer and unfaithful example to fellow members" and, therefore, should be cut off from them. It is likely that this rigid measure was taken in view of the increasing application of blood transfusions. During the 1960s medical science had progressed rapidly, in particular in the field of cardiac technology. Open heart surgery was brought into American homes via live TV-broadcasts and within a few years heart transplantations would become a fact of life. What these new methods, to overcome hitherto fatal disorders, needed was, first and foremost, blood. From that time on, the Society paid more attention to the matter. Long articles, in which the doctrinal foundations were highlighted and reiterated, possible dangers of the therapy, stories in which Witnesses miraculously survived drastic surgery without transfusions and descriptions of perceived maltreatment, filled the pages of the magazines.

It is beyond the aim of the present paper to describe in detail how the ruling vacillated through the late 1950s and 1960s, in particular if applied to specific cases. Questions like "can one take medicines containing blood products, should a Witness surgeon give a blood transfusion (in the Netherlands a Witness hospital physician solved this dilemma by opting for laboratory research in order to avoid any possible participation in blood therapy)? can a chicken be fed by products containing blood substances," etc, appeared in the "Questions from Readers" pages of *The Watchtower*. One example, taken from a former Society's top-official experiences, may illustrate the rather fluid character of the rule. Hemophiliacs, inquiring on the permissibility if they could accept medication of blood fractions were told that "(...) to accept such blood fractions *one time* could be viewed as not objectionable (...) but to do so *more than once* would constitute a "feeding" on such blood fractions and therefore be considered a violation (...)"[38] Autologous blood transfusion is also forbidden unless the patient's blood continues to circulate through an external surgical device. Prior storage of one's own blood is not allowed by way of "On the earth you should pour the blood out as water" (Deuteronomy 12:16). Nowadays, the ruling's derivatives are more or less left to the individual. The Society has withdrawn from the exegetic casuistry concerning the use of blood products and its wide variety of applications, appealing instead to the Witness's conscience; cases that are not clear cut are in unprecedented "grey area," an indistinct doctrinal territory within an otherwise absolutistic ideological system. Besides, the research involved in checking the purity of products is "not the responsibility of the Christian, for, doing that, it would give him less time to preach."[32,33]

Although the Society's primary justification for the doctrine is based on biblical exegesis, an array of secular arguments usually accompany the scriptural ones. Prior to the outbreak of AIDS, the amount of medical objections was rather limited. Errors can be made in administering an incompatible blood type and the receiver can be infected by hepatitis, malaria and syphilis. A considerable factor in the Society's abhorrence has been (and still is) the practice of some commercial blood banks. For example, in his description of the life style of an American skid row population, the urban ethnographer Spradley reports that "making the blood bank" provides a significant way to obtain alcoholic beverages. According to one of his informants "it is usual to drink some wine before donating blood in order to avoid too much shaking and to calm the nerves." In case the individual has no means to purchase the liquor in advance, the blood bank provides an advance, to be subtracted from the revenues of the donation.[34] The Society's magazines regularly mentioned similar occurrences, yet, statistically, such reports were hardly significant. certainly not within the context of the Western European situation in which blood donation is usually a free gift: Altruism and life-saving are easy competitors for insignificant casualty rates. This draws attention to the Society's decision making which is primarily an American affair.

Besides the perceived hazards for physical health, as emanating from the exploitation of the penurious urbanites, the Society was convinced that blood transfusion would incur mental contamination. So until the 1970s the Society frequently defended its policy by arguing from the perspective of the humoural physiology. The following quote provides an example:

> Some say blood transfusions are harmless. Do you believe that? For 40 years K. was known as an honest man. Then he was given a blood transfusion after a fall. "I learned the donor was a thief" K. told police. "When I recovered I found I had a terrible desire to steal". And steal he did. He confessed to stealing £10,000 in six robberies in three months. K. threatened to sue the doctor who arranged the transfusion, if he receives a severe sentence for his thievery.

To stress the imaginary danger of contagion with less enviable psychological donor traits, in conformity with the biblical adage "the soul of the flesh is in the blood," the Society regularly quoted from a type of literature which in medical circles would probably be considered controversial. So, according to the book "Who Is Your Doctor and Why?":

> blood contains all the peculiarities of the individual from whence it comes. This includes hereditary taints, disease susceptibilities, poisons due to personal living, eating and drinking habits...The poisons that produce the impulse to commit suicide, murder, or steal are in the blood.

In the same edition, a Brazilian medical journal was quoted, according to which: "Moral insanity, sexual perversions, repression, inferiority complexes, petty crimes - these often follow in the wake of blood transfusion." It is important to note how the Society stresses the perceived quality of blood through this negative characterization of the donor. If he is not a criminal, then at least there exists a social distance from the receiver. It is mentioned, for example, that Witnesses will try to protect their children from taking *strange* blood. And in spite of the fact that the donor may be a respectable member of the family, leading an immaculate life, the danger still looms. To make things worse, however, the donor usually is an *unknown* person, perhaps even a convict of a penitentiary or an alcoholic, as the Society reports.[35] With even more horror the Society refers to the use of cadaver blood for transfusion purposes, a method in vogue in the Soviet Union during the 1930s.[36]

The Society has no need to revert to these arguments any more. Obviously, the more widespread blood transfusion were applied, the more adversely medical side-effects became known. The old humoural physiology, presented in the 1961 brochure *Blood, Medicine and the Law of God* has been omitted in the updated version published in 1977 and been replaced by more sophisticated, although still highly selective references. During the late 1970s and 1980s the provocative rhetorics have gradually been replaced by a tone of accommodative restraint, which, for example, emerged in the publication of the viewpoint by the Society's medical staff in *The Journal of the American Medical Association*.[37]

The last part of this decade provides the Witnesses with an even more powerful argument: AIDS has become the ideal case to convince the outside world that the doctrine is legitimate. The macabre relationship "Blood transfusion = AIDS," as back-up argument to the primordial scriptural semantics, facilitates the Society's justification for the rule. Also, recent medical discoveries have demonstrated that controversies now surround the once hardly questioned efficacy of blood transfusion.[38] Special editions of *Awake!* quote medical experts who agree with the Witnesses in their refusal of blood transfusions, as well as scientific articles in which the hazards of the treatment are highlighted.[39] Whether the disease and other recently discovered possibly adverse medical effects diminishes the controversy among the general public, is less clear. For example, in the Netherlands, during spring 1989, a TV-station reported the case of a Witness who died as a result of blood refusal during obstetrical surgery. The program definitely exuded an atmosphere of antagonism towards the prohibition. Not in the least this was probably due to the reaction of an official of the Society's Dutch branch office who asserted that ultimately the decision to refuse blood has to be made by the individual, thereby disclaiming any responsibility on the part of the Society. Similarly, the day after a broadcast of a recent TV-discussion, in which Witnesses defended their point of view, those engaged in house-to-house calls received several scornful remarks. Apparently the majority of medical personnel usually respects the patient's conviction.[40] A leading Dutch anesthesiologist, though, confronted with a fatal surgery as a result of blood refusal, formulated the dilemma pithily: "It's their conviction, but they do it under my nose."

For the individual believer, the doctrine appears to be of minor importance. Although systematic data collection is still in progress, my fieldwork impressions among the Witnesses do not show a particular concern with the rule. Surely the doctrine is not experienced as profoundly as the Kosher dietary laws among orthodox Jews, considering them "conditions for holiness over against profanity and pollution."[41] After all, the major part of the adherents will never directly be confronted with the prohibition. New members know they have to accept the doctrine before they are allowed to gain access in their new religious environment. In order to establish the ideological suitability for entrance, the candidate has to prove agreement with the Society's theology. In addition to an evaluation of the prospective member's general conduct and attitude based on a recruitment and resocialization phase which may vary from a few months to several years, congregation elders examine the neophyte by way of an oral test. These so-called 124 "baptismal questions" cover the entire doctrinal corpus and include several items on the blood issue.[42] If the elders are convinced that the candidate will accept the new belief system, the subsequent *rite de passage* through baptism initiates the inductee into the status of "full-fledged minister." Proselytizing activities then become the most important visible "cognitive commitment" indicator.[43] The blood transfusion matter manifests itself in the background only: the Witness has to fill out a codicil in which it is declared that the bearer of this document will not accept a blood transfusion. Alternatives like dextran or hetastarch are allowed. Further, medical personnel will be discharged of any responsibility for the consequences resulting from this refusal. Except during July and August 1988 when the Society's brochure *Jehovah's Witnesses and the Question of Blood* was discussed world-wide among the more than 3 million Witnesses, the annual renewal of the codicil will be the only ritual confrontation with the doctrine, thus constituting another proof of cognitive commitment.

On the weekly Sunday gatherings, during which topics from the Watchtower are lectured, the matter is sparsely discussed. After all, from the secular point of view, the hazards of refusal have diminished. Medical technology has found alternatives for those refusing blood, not in the least as a result of the guinea-pig position of the Witnesses: how to do major surgery without blood transfusion has been (and still is) a topic for a considerable amount of papers in medical literature.[28,44] In spite of future divine judgement and medical alternatives, whether the Witnesses will persist in a refusal at the crucial moment, in particular if their children are endangered and in need of a transfusion, is a matter of which some are not entirely confident. "Only that moment will show if I am really committed to Jehovah", is a standard reaction of the doubters. Some have bitter memories of the moment when their authority was temporarily divested in order that their child received a transfusion. Yet, others confided to me they felt relieved to be deprived of the ultimate responsibility for life and death. According to dissident sources Witnesses accept blood transfusions. This was confirmed to me by medical authorities although the magnitude seems limited.

It is only when one of the fellow believers is in a physical condition that requires the therapy that some tension in the congregation is noticeable, though the matter will not be on the agenda of the service. Particularly if there is pressure from hospital staff upon a Witness to accept a transfusion, congregation elders and other senior members will assist the patient and immediate relatives in order to reduce all possible doubts. Simultaneously, to the physicians in attendance, they elucidate the Society's viewpoint on this matter, thus providing a protective shield between doctrinal imperatives and secular temptation. It is during such dramatic events and, even more, when the outside world takes offence, that ranks close.

Discussion

Unlike the objections raised against medical treatment uttered by certain members of the religious groups exemplified in the introduction, the Society's present objection against blood transfusion and previous aversion against vaccination are not founded on divine providence or the availability of alternatively spiritual methods. *Pollution*, in particular in the context of *compulsion*, appears to be the key word through which the antagonisms can be understood. As far as vaccination was concerned, the objections appear to have been founded on the perceived polluting characteristics of the substances: the introduction of evil humours into one's system, a conception similar to the argument for vaccination refusal in 19th century Britain(11, p.162).

But above all, it was the *compulsory* character of vaccination that rubbed the Society the wrong way. Stressed particularly in the pre-60s, in the Society's theology, the state and industrial corporations embody Satan, whereas no good could come from academic professionals. These ideological adversaries, in the shape of public health authorities, the pharmaceutical industry and the medical profession, compelled its citizens to take an evil drug. As Smith notes, "Compulsory vaccination represented a new, and for many people, the first, intrusion into the family of state authority (...) raising fundamental issues about authority and morals" (11, p.159,161). To be sure, in the U.S. state vaccination had caused a considerable number of casualties during the first decades of this century and some medical authorities held extreme views on the eradication of germs. The Old Testament scriptural back-up, brought out at a later stage, only emphasized the polluting aspects of vaccination, thus reiterating the importance to distance oneself from secular dirt; to reject vaccination was part of rejecting the world. The opposition against vaccination never received the aura of divine sanctioning. After all, in certain cases, *public* health was involved. Besides, as noted previously, it is questionable if the opposition was unequivocally supported by the Society's leadership.

If vaccine and inoculant are perceived to pollute the receiver, the same can be said about blood. Ubiquitously, blood has a disquiet cultural connotation, specifically within the religious domain. "Blood is perceived as being simultaneously pure and impure, attractive and repulsive, sacred and profane; it is at once a life-giving substance and a symbol of death."[45] Its metaphorical importance has been widely documented in the ethnographic literature. Blood points to group identity, it is the idiom of kinship, which in its turn constitutes the elementary fabric of social organization. Alliances between groups or individuals or between their deities are often established by a covenant in which blood plays a crucial role. In present-day western societies, its importance is obvious from proverbial expressions like "blood will tell," "blood is thicker than water," etc, let alone the sinister applications in racial ideologies. The closed character of the Indian caste system, for example, is based on the idea that parental blood is transferred to the offspring; the purity of a caste is defined by the purity of the blood of each individual member. Pollution of an individual's blood means a stain on the whole caste.[46] Related to our subject-matter, a blood transfusion in India is a family affair; a patient accepts blood only from his next of kin. This cultural concept of blood pollution may have been the reason behind the murder of two English medical students who transfused their own blood to a patient in an Indian operating theatre.[47]

In the Society's blood transfusion doctrine, this consanguinity aspect plays a partial role. As shown above, the Society often stressed the questionable characteristics of the donor category, transferring its evil qualities into the believer's bodily system. Reception meant individual, and accordingly, group pollution. The analogy with the Indian caste is obvious. However, a significant flaw emerges: why is transfusion *among* Witnesses not allowed? It should be noted that defection among the Society's adherents is considerable.[15,26,38,57] In the view of the Society, apostate members belong to the realm of Satan. Though the transfusion might have been life-saving, the thought of a believer who once received blood from someone who is now in the devil's category, is almost an obscenity within the Society's ideological schemes. Insiders, thus, can also defile, so a absolute prohibition is the most secure defense for spiritual pollution.

Even more important for our discussion is the entwined relationship between blood and war. It points to the socio-historical setting in which the doctrine emerged. Blood transfusion had a definite martial component. World War I had been the first large-scale test-case for blood transfusion, followed by the Spanish Civil War. Surely the Society regards the labeling of Jehovah's Witnesses as "pacifists" a defilement,[48] but the army is considered an odious institution at the disposal of a reprehensible state authority. When, during World War II, the American population was regularly incited to donate blood for its injured soldiers, it is imaginable that this patriotic climate, ideologically anathematized by the Society, provided the breeding ground on which the prohibition crystallized. To put it bluntly: blood donation was considered an act of sacrifice to a false deity.

In this way blood, transfusion was part of nationalistic manifestations like flags, national anthems, and armies. To make things worse, other adversaries like politicians, the established churches and the world of entertainment participated in the blood donation campaigns, rendering the act even more loathsome,[49] to be compared with one of the explanations of the Jewish pork taboo: Pork is impure because the hostile Canaanite neighbours eat it.

The above may explain the choice for this specific taboo, but not *the reason* to implement it. To explore this question, I will turn to the thought-provoking theoretical framework of Mary Douglas. A central theme in Douglas's work is the relationship between symbolic and social order in different cultural systems. In her seminal study, *Purity and Danger,* she presents a thought-provoking analysis of the symbolic meaning of pollution. Departing from Durkheim's view that religion expresses social experience, Douglas hypothesizes that rituals of pollution mirror concerns of the social order, creating "unity in experience," and providing "positive contributions to atonement" (8, p.2). For Douglas, the human body mirrors the surrounding society and, as such, symbolizes social structure. The body's orifices and emissions are society's margins, representing points of entry or exit to social units. Social dangers, threatening the structure, are reflected in the polluting bodily orifices and substances. Basing her assertions mainly on ethnographic material from India she connects the elaborate purification rituals of specific castes with their perceived minority position within the system of Hindoo castes. Also the Israelites seem to conform to the hypothesis in view of the relationship between their status as a "hard pressed minority" and "their care for the integrity, unity and purity of the physical body," thus considering "blood, pus, excreta, semen, etc" as polluting substances (8, p.124.)[50] As such, rules of pollution and purity are instrumental in creating structural boundaries around group members and "(...) expected to be found in situations were the social order is threatened."[51]

It is exactly this situation in which the Jehovah's Witnesses found themselves when the doctrine was promulgated. For the Witnesses, World War II marked the climax of their persecution when in Nazi occupied Europe they were put in concentration camps. This had already been preceded by opposition in other parts of the world during the 30s. Because of the Society's ideological rejection of state authority, the Witnesses were harassed for their alleged anarchistic, communist or whatever perceived extremist political stance. Since, the refusal to salute the flag, not to sing the national anthem, to oppose the established churches and to be a conscientious objector are, in a patriotic atmosphere, obvious indicators of deviant social behavior. Add to that the fierce opposition they encountered as a result of their contentious missionary zeal and the picture emerges of a religious minority to be regarded as the most persecuted group of Christians in the twentieth century (18, p.130).

Though specific local hostility may have contributed to the sect's cohesion on a regional or national level, and the recognition that fellow believers were in more or less comparable trouble elsewhere, it is not clear whether the Society, as a world wide movement, was a cohesive unity. It is conceivable that external threat, more than internal theology, supported the mutual solidarity among members. Surely the act of proselytizing was an ideological necessity welding people together, but it lacked the sacral symbolism that divides the pure from the impure. In the terminology of Douglas, the element of "holiness" was lacking (8, p.49). "Holiness," or its Hebrew original meaning "to set apart" was needed in order to re-establish the movement's universal collective identity; a clear doctrine of purification, connoting a rule of mental and physical hygienics was called for. Blood was decided upon. That is to say, the complete avoidance of it. In that way it is functionally analogous with the Jewish dietary laws: its observance means an encounter with the supreme being.

As such, rules of pollution and purity are instrumental in creating structural boundaries around group members. And, the more distinctive when formulated into divine precepts, the clearer the dividing lines between the faithful and those excluded.[52] For the faithful, the relinquishing of this possibly life-saving medical therapy can be considered a sacrifice as part of the price of membership, thus increasing motivation to remain participant (43, p. 505). The annual renewal of the codicil can partially be considered a test of their cognitive commitment. For the inductee the prohibition can also be considered a barrier prior affiliation. Not until the recruit's motivation is at its maximum full membership is possible.[53] In that way the rule functions as one of the Society's selection criteria: Its endorsement by the individual far surpasses non-committal membership. It is unlikely, however, that the majority of the recruits deal with this specific issue at great length. After all, cognizance of the doctrine is only one part in a usually protracted introductory period. For it is more than doctrinal attraction that ties an individual to a religious movement: the emotional dimension may play an even more important role than the cognitive. In Kanter's scheme this component underlies the community's "cohesion commitment": "(...) the attachment of an individual's fund of affectivity and emotion to a group" (43, p.507). Numerous studies have pointed to the individual's affiliated networks as the primary sources of recruitment to sectarian groups.[54] The new member enters an inner circle in which emotional bonds will be established and reinforced. It is when the outside world takes offence at the blood doctrine that the solidarity of the group becomes visible. As such the blood transfusion has an important secondary function: the opposition reinforces the Witnesses's internal cohesion by distinguishing even more clearly between purity and pollution. The Society's abhorrence of blood also emerges in the annual celebration of the Lord's Supper: the drinking of the wine, symbol of Jesus's blood, is only reserved for the remainder of the elect 144,000. For 1989 that meant 0.2% of the Witnesses. In that way the old church maxim "Ecclesia abhorret a sanguine" applies, in the most literal sense, to the Society.

Conclusion

In the 50s Werner Cohn characterized the Jehovah's witnesses as a proletarian movement: a social category not participating in societal institutions. In order to show this social estrangement, such movements had "separation rites" at their disposal, "demonstrative practices by which the proletarians set themselves apart from everyone else."[55] Though this is not the place to argue about Cohn's use of the adjective "proletarian," his observation of the creation of social boundaries is relevant. World rejection, a major ideological characteristic of the Watch Tower Society, appears to be at the root of the prohibition of blood transfusion among the Jehovah's Witnesses. For the Jehovah's Witnesses purity means to be separate from the outside, "the world." "The world" is the major part of mankind with exception of the Witnesses (7, p.427). An array of biblical references indicate that "true Christians," though living *in* "the world" performing their daily human activities are not part *of* "the world," the classic sectarian position as noted by Beckford.[56] For analytical purposes, secular anti-institutionalism and inter-group purity are the rule's two components. The former is rooted in the Second World War, being part of the patriotic complex which already included the state, flag, army and church. The latter seems to have its origins in the Society's pre-war opposition to vaccination: Blood transfusion emerged as a similar act of pollution. The important difference, however, was the rule's radius: it only afflicted individual group members. Public health was not at stake. Furthermore, as in the case of compulsory vaccinations, here also the arch-enemy state intruded into the private domain of the family or the individual by forcing the polluting treatment on the victim.

Since its promulgation in 1945, the scriptural base of the taboo has not changed, in contrast to its implementations and additional, secular arguments. The amount of attention the Society paid to the subject seems directly related to its rate of application in medical practice, where it initially encountered little tolerance. Eventually, doctrinal imperatives were more or less forced to find a compromise with societal acceptation, in particular concerning the ruling's derivatives concerning blood in food and medical products. This more or less conforms to Beckford's remark that the justification on certain doctrinal views was a response "(...) to requests for assistance from individual Jehovah's witnesses." As such, the decision making process may partly have been inspired by "(...) the defending and promoting [of the Society's] interests," characterized by "*ad hoc* responses to immediate problems without an underlying rationale." Tactics and strategy may have prevailed over principle (56, p. 59). These dialectics between legalistic dogmatism and adherents's commitments may have been the reason that the pre-war vaccination objection never received the aura of divine sanction. The same process created the rather unique "grey area": a doctrinal territory on which the Witness had to decide personally. The same applied to the so-called "1975" prophecy: the Society left it to the individual believers to accept or reject the possibility of an apocalyptic event in that year.[57] In spite of these less stable features, the central issue stands its ground through its complementary function. The rule demarcates the believers from the non-believers thus being one the most salient identity markers. Its controversial character contributes to the internal solidarity, since the enemy is an indispensable ingredient of the survival of any millennial movement.

Although, since the 50s the Society's attitude towards the outside world has evolved from a rigid "anti-worldliness" to a moderate "world-indifference" (56, p.47,48), "the world," though still anathema, is a millenarian prerequisite: it must exist to show how evil it is. Simultaneously, as a consequence of some adverse effects of blood transfusion the Society is eager to quote assenting opinions from the hostile external world. And, ironically, even apostate members, actively engaged in opposing the sect, still abhor blood transfusion. As one stated:

> Most Witnesses can forgive adultery, smoking, bad business practices, and above all drunkenness, but they find it virtually impossible to forgive the ban on blood and apostasy. (...) the idea of taking blood is still dreadfully abhorrent to me. I know how an orthodox Jew must feel when asked to eat pork or shellfish.[58]

It is highly improbable that the Society will quote this phrase, in particular the source, in its magazines. After all, the ultimate enemy is needed for contrast, not consent.

Notes

1. Amundsen DW, Ferngren GB. Medicine and religion: Early christianity through the middle ages. In: Marty ME, Vaux KL, eds. *Health/Medicine and The Faith Traditions*. Philadelphia, PA: Fortress Press, 1982:100. See also Amundsen DW. Medicine and religion in western traditions, In: Eliade M. *The Encyclopedia of Religion*, Vol. 9. New York, NY: MacMillan, 1987:319-324.
2. Wilson BR. *Sects and Society.* London: Heinemann, 1961:128-9.
3. Numbers RL, Sawyer RC. Medicine and Christianity in the modern world, In: Marty ME, Vaux, KL, eds. *Health/Medicine and The Faith Traditions*. Philedelphia, PA: Fortress Press, 1982:153.
4. Redlener IE, Scott CS. Incompatibles of professional and religious ideology: Problems of medical management and outcome in a case of pediatric meningitis, *Social Science & Medicine* 1979;13B:89-93.
5. Douma J, Velema WH. *Polio: Afwachten of Afweren*. Amsterdam: Bolland, 1979.
6. *The Watchtower* 1945.
7. Watchtower Bible and Tract Society(WBTS). *Reasoning from the Scriptures* (Dutch edition). New York, NY:1985:81.
8. Douglas M. *Purity and Danger. An Analysis of the Concepts of Pollution and Taboo.* London: Ark Paperbacks, 1984.
9. So far, the rather limited amount of research among the Jehovah's Witnesses by anthropologists concentrates on recruitment, eschatological expectations, ethnographic description of congregational life and the Society's activities in Africa. An initial impetus to analyze the organization's corpus of millenarian symbolism from an anthropological angle is Botting H, Botting G. *The Orwellian World of Jehovah's Witnesses*. Toronto, Ontario: University of Toronto Press, 1984.
10. *The Golden Age*, Jan. 5, 1929; Feb. 4, 1931

11. Smith FB. *The People's Health, 1830-1910.* London: Croom Helm, 1979:158-168.
12. *The Golden Age*, Apr. 24, 1935; Jan 15, 1936
13. Stroup HH. *The Jehovah's Witnesses.* New York, NY: Russell & Russell, 1967:107.
14. Cushman RE. *Civil Liberties in the U.S.* Ithaca, NY: Cornell University Press, 1956:96-97. See also Zygmunt JF. Jehovah's witnesses in the USA 1942-1976, *Social Compass* 1977;24:47.
15. Macmillan AH. *Faith on the March.* Englewood Cliffs, NJ: Prentice Hall, 1957:1988.
16. Whalen WJ. *Armageddon Around the Corner. A Report on Jehovah's Witnesses.* New York, NY: John Day, 1962:186
17. *Jehovah's Witnesses in the Divine Purpose*. New York, NY: WBTS, 1959. *1975 - Yearbook, Dutch edition.* New York, NY: WBTS, 1975:107.
18. Penton MJ. *Apocalypse Delayed. The Story of Jehovah's Witnesses.* Toronto, Ontario: University of Toronto Press, 1985:66.
19. *The Watchtower*, Sep. 15, 1958:575.
20. *The Watchtower*, Feb. 15, 1939:62
21. White T. *A People for His Name. A History of Jehovah's Witnesses and an evaluation*. New York, NY: Vantage Press, 1967:391,ln. 7. White refers to an edition of *The Watchtower*, in which Rutherford reportedly has stated this opinion. However, upon verification this assertion was untraceable. Either a misprint or an incorrect reference has occurred. For the sake of completeness, White's remark has been included.
22. Buber M. *Under Two Dictators.* London: Gollancz, 1949:236.
23. *Vertroosting*(author's translation) Sep. '45:29.
24. *Awake!*, Jan. 8, 1949:12
25. *The Watchtower*, Dec. 1, 1949:368. See also *Make Sure of All Things*. NewYork, NY: WBTS, 1953:48. *The Watchtower(Dutch ed).*, Jul. 15, 1950:229.
26. Tannahill R. *Flesh and Blood. A History of the Cannibal Complex.* London: Hamish Hamilton, 1975:125. *The Watchtower(Dutch ed).*, Oct. 1, 1966:590,591. Also *Life Everlasting - In Freedom of the Sons of God(Dutch ed).* New York, NY: WBTS, 1966:388.
27. McNally JA. *The Right to Die: Non-Consenting Adult Jehovah's Witnesses and Blood Transfusions.* (MA-thesis, Cornell University), Ann Arbor, MI: University Microfilms International, 1970.
28. Bergman J. *Jehovah's Witnesses and Kindred Groups: An Historical Compendium and Bibliography.* New York, NY: Garland, 1984, covers more than 180 references to articles in both medical and law journals.
29. *1979 Yearbook(Dutch ed).* New York, NY: WBTS:199.
30. *Blood, Medicine and the Law of God.* New York, NY: WBTS, 1961:54.
31. *The Watchtower(Dutch ed.)*, Mar. 1, 1959:159.
32. Franz R. *Crisis of Conscience.* Atlanta, GA: Commentary Press, 1983:106-7.
33. *The Watchtower(Dutch eds),* Sep. 15, 1978; Mar. 1, 1965.
34. Spradley J. Down and out on skid road, In: Feldman SD, Thielbar GW, eds. *Life Styles: Diversity in American Culture.* Boston, MA: Little, Brown & Comp., 1975:466.
35. *Awake!*, July 8, 1969:30. *The Watchtower*, Sept. 15, 1961:564. *The Watchtower*, Apr. 1, 1968:210; *Life Everlasting(Dutch eds. my italics)*:337.
36. Wolstenholme GEW. An old-established procedure: The development of blood transfusion. In: Wolstenholme GEW, O'Connor M, eds. *Ethics in Medical Progres.* London: Churchill, 1966:31.
37. *Journal of the American Medical Association* 1981;246:2471-2472.
38. For example, it is assumed that a relationship exists between the administering of donor blood during cancer surgery and the tumor's metastasis, *Ned. T. Geneesk.* 1987;131:1255-1257.
39. *Awake!(Dutch ed).*, Apr. 22, 1986; Oct. 8, 1988.
40. Weinberger M. *et al.* The development of physician norms in the United States. The treatment of Jehovah's witness patients, *Social Science & Medicine* 1982;16:1719-1723.
41. Levin JS, Vanderpool HY. Is frequent religious *really* conducive to better health? Toward an epidemiology of religion, *Social Science & Medicine* 1987;24:596.
42. *Organized to Accomplish Our Ministry(Dutch ed.).* New York, NY: WBTS, 1983:190-1.
43. Kanter RM. Commitment and social organization: A study of commitment mechanisms in Utopian communities, *Am. Sociol. Rev.*, 1968;33:500.

44. Jarvis GK, Northcott HC. Religion and differences in morbidity and mortality, *Soc. Sci. Med.* 1987;25:819.
45. Roux J. Blood, In: *The Encyclopedia of Religion,* 2:254.
46. Östör A. *Concepts of Person: Kinship, Caste and Marriage in India.* Cambridge, MA: Harvard University Press, 1982:13-15.
47. Saunders JB. A conceptual history of transplantation, In: Najarian JS, Simmons RL, eds. *Transplantation.* Munich, Germany: Urban & Schwarzenberg, 1972:19.
48. *The Watchtower(Dutch ed).*, Apr 1, 1951:99.
49. *Awake!*, Aug. 8, 1950.
50. One wonders if there is any relationship between these remarks and the opposition of the residents of Jeruzalem's orthodox quarter Mea Shearim against a governmental anti-poliomyelitis vaccination campaign, as shown by a picture in a Dutch newspaper in October 1988. According to several scholars on Chassidism, there is no foundation in the Mosaic Law whatsoever justifying this protest.
51. Douglas M. *Implicit Meanings. Essays in Anthropology*. London, England: Routledge & Kegan Paul, 1975:55.
52. Caplan L. Introduction. In: Caplan, L. ed. *Studies in Religious Fundamentalism.* London, England, MacMillan, 1987:15.
53. Borhek JT, Curtis RF. *A Sociology of Belief.* New York, NY: Wiley, 1975:99.
54. To mention one example: Stark R, Bainbridge WS. *The Future of Religion.* Berkeley, CA: University of California Press, 1985:Chap. 14.
55. Cohn W. Jehovah's witnesses as a proletarian movement, *The American Scholar* 1955;24:283.
56. Beckford JA. *The Trumpet of Prophecy. A Sociological Study of Jehovah's Witnesses.* Oxford, Longdon: Basil Blackwell, 1975:56.
57. Singelenberg R. It separated the wheat from the chaff: The "1975" prophecy and its impact among Dutch Jehovah's witnesses, *Sociological Analysis* 1989;50:23-40.
58. Penton, personal communication.

Chapter 35

The Physician's Responsibility Toward Hopelessly Ill Patients

Sidney H. Wanzer, et al.

SOME of the practices that were controversial five years ago[1] in the care of the dying patient have become accepted and routine. Do-Not-Resuscitate (DNR) orders, nonexistent only a few years ago, are now commonplace. Many physicians and ethicists now agree that there is little difference between nasogastric or intravenous hydration and other life sustaining measures. They have concluded, therefore, that it is ethical to withdraw nutrition and hydration from certain dying, hopelessly ill, or permanently unconscious patients. The public and the courts have tended to accept this principle. Most important, there has been an increase in sensitivity to the desires of dying patients on the part of doctors, other health professionals, and the public. The entire subject is now discussed openly. Various studies and reports from governmental bodies, private foundations, the American Medical Association, and state medical societies reflect these advances in thinking.[2,3,4,5,6,7,8,9]

The increased awareness of the rights of dying patients has also been translated into new laws. Thirty-eight states now have legislation covering advance directives ("Living Wills"), and 15 states specifically provide that a patient's health care spokesperson, or proxy, can authorize the withholding or withdrawal of life support.[10,11]

The courts have continued to support patients' rights and have expanded the legal concept of the right to refuse medical treatment, upholding this right in more than 80 court decisions.[12] As a general rule, the cases in the early 1980s involved terminally ill patients whose death was expected whether or not treatment was continued, and the treatment at issue -- for instance, prolonged endotracheal intubation, mechanical ventilation, dialysis, or chemotherapy -- was often intrusive or burdensome. The courts recognized the patient's common-law right to autonomy (to be left alone to make one's own choices) as well as the constitutional right to privacy (to be protected from unwanted invasive medical treatment).

Currently, the courts are moving closer to the view that patients are entitled to be allowed to die, whether or not they are terminally ill or suffering. Many recent cases have permitted treatment to be terminated in patients who are permanently unconscious, indicating that the right to refuse treatment can be used to put an end to unacceptable conditions even if the patients are not perceptibly suffering or close to death. In such court opinions, many of which have dealt with artificial feeding, the cause of the patient's death continues to be attributed to the underlying disease, rather than to the withholding or withdrawal of treatment.[13]

Popular attitudes about the rights of dying patients have also changed, often in advance of the attitudes of health care providers, legislators, and the courts. The results of one

---

Source: Reprinted from *New England Journal of Medicine*, Vol. 320, No. 13, pp. 844-849, with permission from The New England Journal of Medicine © March 1989.

public-opinion poll indicated that 68 percent of the respondents believed that "people dying of an incurable painful disease should be allowed to end their lives before the disease runs its course."[14]

Health professionals have also become much more aware of patients' rights. In states with laws legitimizing living wills, hospitals have become responsive to patients' wishes as expressed in their advance directives, and hospital accreditation by the Joint Commission on Accreditation of Health Care Organizations now requires the establishment of formal DNR policies. The frequency with which DNR orders are used in nursing homes has also increased. In 1987, the California Department of Health Services became the first state agency to develop clear guidelines for the removal of life support, including tube feeding, in the state's 1500 nursing homes and convalescent hospitals.[15]

Gaps Between Accepted Policies and Their Implementation

Many patients are aware of their right to make decisions about their health care, including the refusal of life-sustaining measures, yet few actually execute living wills or appoint surrogates through a health care proxy. Although such documents can be very helpful in clarifying the patient's wishes, they are all too infrequently discussed in standard medical practice. Furthermore, at present, advance directives do not exert enough influence on either the patient's ability to control medical decision-making at the end of life or the physician's behavior with respect to such issues in hospitals, emergency rooms, and nursing homes. There remains a considerable gap between the acceptance of the directive and its implementation. There is also a large gap between what the courts now allow with respect to withdrawal of treatment and what physicians actually do. All too frequently, physicians are reluctant to withdraw aggressive treatment from hopelessly ill patients, despite clear legal precedent.

Physicians have a responsibility to consider timely discussions with patients about life-sustaining treatment and terminal care. Only a minority of physicians now do so consistently.[16] The best time to begin such discussions is during the course of routine, nonemergency care, remembering that not all patients are emotionally prepared, by virtue of their stage in life, their psychological makeup, or the stage of their illness. Nevertheless, as a matter of routine, physicians should become acquainted with their patients' personal values and wishes and should document them just as they document information about medical history, family history, and socio-cultural background. Such discussions and the resultant documentation should be considered a part of the minimal standard of acceptable care. The physician should take the initiative in obtaining the documentation and should enter it in the medical record.

These issues are not sufficiently addressed in medical schools and residency programs. Medical educators need to recognize that practitioners may not sufficiently understand or value the patient's role in medical decision making or may be unwilling to relinquish control of the decision-making process. The interests of patients and physicians alike are best served when decisions are made jointly, and medical students and residents should learn to pursue this goal. These topics ought to be specifically included as curriculums are revised.

In general, health care institutions must recognize their obligation to inform patients of their right to participate in decisions about their medical care, including the right to refuse treatment, and should formulate institutional policies about the use of advance directives and the appointment of surrogate decision-makers. Hospitals, health maintenance organizations, and nursing homes should ask patients on admission to indicate whether they have prepared a living will or designated a surrogate. It seems especially important that nursing homes require a regular review of patient preferences, with each patient's physician taking responsibility for ensuring that such information is obtained and documented. In the case of patients who lack decision-making capacity, surrogate decision-makers should be identified and consulted appropriately. (We prefer the term "decision-making capacity" to "competency" because in the medical context, the patient either has or does not have the capacity to make decisions, whereas competency is a legal determination that can be made only by the courts.)

Although we advocate these approaches, we recognize that the mechanisms of appointing a surrogate and executing a living will do present certain problems. Obviously, it may happen that a surrogate appointed previously is unavailable for consultation when problems arise in the treatment of a patient who lacks decision-making capacity. In addition, there is the problem of determining what constitutes an outdated living will or surrogate appointment and how often they need to be reaffirmed. Laws in most states provide that a living will is valid until it is revoked, but patients need to be encouraged to update and reconfirm such directives from time to time.

Settings For Dying

Home

Dying at home can provide the opportunity for quiet and privacy, dignity, and family closeness that may make death easier for the patient and provide consolation for the bereaved. Assuming that a stable and caring home environment exists, emotional and physical comfort is most often greatest at home, with family and friends nearby.

Patients and their families need reassurance that dying at home will not entail medical deprivation. They should be carefully instructed in the means of coping with possible problems, and appropriate community resources should be mobilized to assist them. The provision of care should be guided by the physician and implemented with the help of well-trained, highly motivated personnel from the hospice units that now serve many communities in this country, since home care often becomes too difficult for the family to handle alone. Hospice, a form of care in which an interdisciplinary team provides palliative and support services to both patient and family, is a concept whose time has come.

Recent cost-containment measures for expensive hospital care have given the home hospice movement considerable impetus, resulting in an emphasis on alternatives such as home care.[17] On the other hand, hospice care at home, which should be adequately financed by insurance as a cost-effective way to care for the patient, is often poorly reimbursed, and many hospice programs struggle to stay solvent. There is too much emphasis on reimbursement for high-technology care in the home, as opposed to hands-on nursing care. More adequate financing is clearly indicated for hospice and other home care providers, since it is clear that, overall, care at home usually costs much less than in other settings.

Nursing Home

When an admission to a nursing home is planned for a terminally ill patient, it is important to specify the treatment plans and goals at the outset. The nursing home should inquire about the patient's wishes with regard to life-sustaining procedures, including DNR orders and artificial nutrition and hydration. The patient should be encouraged to execute an advance directive, appoint a surrogate, or both. The possibility that it may be necessary to transfer the patient to a general hospital should be discussed in advance (transfer may become indicated, but usually it is not). All parties should anticipate that the final phases of the dying process will occur in the nursing home without a transfer to the hospital, unless the patient cannot be kept reasonably comfortable in the nursing home.

Even though care can clearly be given more cost effectively in the nursing home setting than in the general hospital, a major drawback to using the nursing home as a place for dying is that often insurance does not cover the cost of the nursing home care (just as it often does not cover the cost of care at home). Currently, there is almost no private insurance for nursing home care, and Medicare now covers only about 3 percent of nursing home days. The rest must be covered by a combination of Medicaid, to be eligible for which a patient must be pauperized, and private pay. It is essential that federal and private health care plans be modified to make nursing home care more accessible to patients of limited means.

Hospital

As much as one-third of the patients cared for at home and expected to die there actually die in the hospital, even when hospice techniques of home care are used. The symptoms or anxiety generated by an impending death may overwhelm the family, and recourse to the hospital is appropriate whenever any treatment program, including a psychosocial one, cannot palliate the distress felt by the patient, the family, or both.

To accommodate such families and patients, hospitals should consider the development of specialized units, with rooms appointed so as to provide pleasant surroundings that will facilitate comfortable interchange among patient, family, and friends. The presence of life-sustaining equipment would be inappropriate in such an environment.

The intensive care unit should generally be discouraged as a treatment setting for the hospitalized patient who is dying, unless intensive palliative measures are required that cannot be done elsewhere. Too often, life-sustaining measures are instituted in the intensive care unit without sufficient thought to the proper goals of treatment. Although the courts have held that in the treatment of the hopelessly ill there is no legal distinction between stopping treatment and not starting it in the first place, there is a bias in the intensive care unit toward continuing aggressive measures that may be inappropriate. Though difficult, it is possible for a patient to die in the intensive care unit with dignity and comfort, since medical hardware itself has no capacity to dehumanize anyone. The important point is that the physician set a tone of caring and support, no matter what the setting.

Although the physicians and nurses in intensive care units may be less prepared than other professionals to switch from aggressive curative care to palliation and the provision of comfort only, they have all seen many situations in which clear decisions to limit treatment have brought welcome relief. Since these care givers often have considerable emotional energy invested in patients who have previously been receiving aggressive curative treatment, they may need consultation with colleagues from outside the intensive care unit to decide when to change the treatment goals.

Treating the Dying Patient -- The Importance of Flexible Care

The care of the dying is an art that should have its fullest expression in helping patients cope with the technologically complicated medical environment that often surrounds them at the end of life. The concept of a good death does not mean simply the withholding of technological treatments that serve only to prolong the act of dying. It also requires the art of deliberately creating a medical environment that allows a peaceful death. Somewhere between the unacceptable extremes of failure to treat the dying patient and intolerable use of aggressive life-sustaining measures, the physician must seek a level of care that optimizes comfort and dignity.

In evaluating the burdens and benefits of treatment for the dying patient -- whether in the hospital, in a nursing home, or at home, the physician needs to formulate a flexible and adjustable care plan, tailoring treatment to the patient's changing needs as the disease progresses. Such plans contrast sharply with the practice, frequent in medicine, in which the physician makes rounds and prescribes, leaving orders for nurses and technicians, but not giving continual feedback and adjustment. The physician's actions on behalf of the patient should be appropriate, with respect to both the types of treatments and the location in which they are given.

Such actions need to be adjusted continually to the individual patient's needs, with the physician keeping primarily in mind that the benefits of treatment must outweigh the burdens imposed.

When the patient lacks decision-making capacity, discussing the limitation of treatment with the family becomes a major part of the treatment plan. The principle of continually adjusted care should guide all these decisions.

Pain and Suffering

The principle of continually adjusted care is nowhere more important than in the control of pain, fear, and suffering. The hopelessly ill patient must have whatever is necessary to control pain. One of the most pervasive causes of anxiety among patients, their families, and the public is the perception that physicians' efforts toward the relief of pain are sadly deficient. Because of this perceived professional deficiency, people fear that needless suffering will be allowed to occur as patients are dying.[18] To a large extent, we believe such fears are justified.

In the patient whose dying process is irreversible, the balance between minimizing pain and suffering and potentially hastening death should be struck clearly in favor of pain relief. Narcotics or other pain medications should be given in whatever dose and by whatever route is necessary for relief. It is morally correct to increase the dose of narcotics to whatever dose is needed, even though the medication may contribute to the depression of respiration or blood pressure, the dulling of consciousness, or even death, provided the primary goal of the physician is to relieve suffering. The proper dose of pain medication is the dose that is sufficient to relieve pain and suffering, even to the point of unconsciousness.

Dying patients often feel isolated and doubt seriously that their physician will be there to relieve their pain when the terminal phase is near. Early in the course of fatal disease, patients should be offered strong reassurance that pain will be controlled and that their physician will be available when the need is greatest. Both the patient and the family should be told that addiction need not be a source of concern and that the relief of pain will have nothing but a salutary effect from both the physical and the emotional standpoint. When possible, pain medication should be given orally to maximize patient autonomy, but usually a continuous parenteral route is needed for the adequate medication of patients in the near-terminal or terminal state. Under no circumstances should medication be "rationed." For episodic pain, patients should be encouraged to take medication as soon as they are conscious of pain, instead of waiting until it becomes intense and far more difficult to control. For continuous or frequently recurring pain, the patient should be placed on a regular schedule of administration. Some patients will choose to endure a degree of pain rather than experience any loss of alertness or control from taking narcotics -- a choice that is consistent with patient autonomy and the concept of continually adjusted care.

If pain cannot be controlled with the commonly used analgesic regimens of mild or moderate strength, the patient should be switched quickly to more potent narcotics. It is important that doses be adequate; the textbook doses recommended for short-term pain are often grossly inadequate for long-term pain in the patient dying of cancer. The physician should be familiar with two or three narcotics and their side effects and appropriate starting dosages. Doses should be brought promptly to levels that provide a reliable pain-free state. Since adequate narcotic management seems to be an unfamiliar area to many physicians, we urge that educational material be distributed to them from a noncommercial source.[19] To allow a patient to experience unbearable pain or suffering is unethical medical practice.

Legal Concerns

The principles of medical ethics are formulated independently of legal decisions, but physicians may fear that decisions about the care of the hopelessly ill will bring special risks of criminal charges and prosecution. Although no medical decision can be immune from legal scrutiny, courts in the United States have generally supported the approaches advocated here.[20,21,22,23] The physician should follow these principles without exaggerated concern for legal consequences, doing whatever is necessary to relieve pain and bring comfort, and adhering to the patient's wishes as much as possible. To withhold any necessary measure of pain relief in a hopelessly ill person out of fear of depressing respiration or of possible legal repercussions is unjustifiable. Good medical practice is the best protection against legal liability.

Preparing for Death

As sickness progresses toward death, measures to minimize suffering should be intensified. Dying patients may require palliative care of an intensity that rivals even that of curative efforts. Keeping the patient clean, caring for the skin, preventing the formation of bed sores, treating neuropsychiatric symptoms, controlling peripheral and pulmonary edema, aggressively reducing nausea and vomiting, using intravenous medications, fighting the psychosocial forces that can lead to family fragmentation -- all can tax the ingenuity and equanimity of the most skilled health professionals. Even though aggressive curative techniques are no longer indicated, professionals and families are still called on to use intensive measures -- extreme responsibility, extraordinary sensitivity, and heroic compassion.

In training programs for physicians, more attention needs to be paid to these aspects of care. Progress has been made in persuading house staff and attending physicians to discuss DNR orders and to include clear orders and notes in the chart about limits on life-sustaining therapies, but patients are too rarely cared for directly by the physician at or near the time of death. Usually it is nurses who care for patients at this time. In a few innovative training programs, most notably at the University of Oregon, the hands-on aspects of care of the dying are addressed,[24] and such techniques should be presented at all training institutions.

Assisted Suicide

If care is administered properly at the end of life, only the rare patient should bc so distressed that he or she desires to commit suicide. Occasionally, however, all fails. The doctor, the nurse, the family, and the patient may have done everything possible to relieve the distress occasioned by a terminal illness, and yet the patient perceives his or her situation as intolerable and seeks assistance in bringing about death. Is it ever justifiable for the physician to assist suicide in such a case?

Some physicians, believing it to be the last act in a continuum of care provided for the hopelessly ill patient, do assist patients who request it, either by prescribing sleeping pills with knowledge of their intended use or by discussing the required doses and methods of administration with the patient. The frequency with which such actions are undertaken is unknown, but they are certainly not rare. Suicide differs from euthanasia in that the act of bringing on death is performed by the patient, not the physician.

The physician who considers helping a patient who requests assistance with suicide must determine first that the patient is indeed beyond all help and not merely suffering from a treatable depression of the sort common in people with terminal illnesses. Such a depression requires therapeutic intervention. If there is no treatable component to the depression and the patient's pain or suffering is refractory to treatment, then the wish for suicide may be rational. If such a patient acts on the wish for death and actually commits suicide, it is ethical for a physician who knows the patient well to refrain from an attempt at resuscitation.

Even though suicide itself is not illegal, helping a person commit suicide is a crime in many states, either by statute or under common law. Even so, we know of no physician who has ever been prosecuted in the United States for prescribing pills in order to help a patient commit suicide.[25] However, the potential illegality of this act is a deterrent, and apart from that, some physicians simply cannot bring themselves to assist in suicide or to condone such action.

Whether it is bad medical practice or immoral to help a hopelessly ill patient commit a rational suicide is a complex issue, provoking a number of considerations. First, as their disease advances, patients may lose their decision-making capacity because of the effects of the disease or the drug treatment. Assisting such patients with suicide comes close to performing an act of euthanasia. Second, patients who want a doctor's assistance with suicide may be unwilling to endure their terminal illness because they lack information about what is ahead. Even when the physician explains in careful detail the availability of the kind of flexible, continually adjusted care described here, the patient may still opt out of that treatment plan and reject the physician's efforts to ease the dying process. Also, what are the physician's obligations if a patient who retains decision-making capacity insists that family members not be told of a suicide plan? Should the physician insist on obtaining the family's consent? Finally, should physicians acknowledge their role in a suicide in some way -- by obtaining consultation, or in writing? Physicians who act in secret become isolated and cannot consult colleagues or ethics committees for confirmation that the patient has made a rational decision. If contacted, such colleagues may well object and even consider themselves obligated to report the physician to the Board of Medical Licensure or to the prosecutor. The impulse to maintain secrecy gives the lie to the moral intuition that assistance with suicide is ethical.

It is difficult to answer such questions, but all but two of us (J.v.E. and E.H.C.) believe that it is not immoral for a physician to assist in the rational suicide of a terminally ill person. However, we recognize that such an act represents a departure from the principle of continually adjusted care that we have presented. As such, it should be considered a separate alternative and not an extension of the flexible approach to care that we have recommended. Clearly, the subject of assisted suicide deserves wide and open discussion.

Euthanasia

Some patients who cannot carry out suicide plans themselves, with or without assistance, may ask their physicians to take a more active part in ending their lives. In the case of suicide, the final act is performed by the patient, even when the physician provides indirect assistance in the form of information and means. By contrast, euthanasia requires the physician to perform a medical procedure that causes death directly. It is therefore even more controversial than assisted rational suicide, and various arguments have been mustered through the years for and against its use.[26,27]

In the Netherlands, the practice of euthanasia has gained a degree of social acceptance. As a result of a 1984 decision by the Dutch Supreme Court, euthanasia is no longer prosecuted in certain approved circumstances. The Dutch government authorized the State Commission on Euthanasia to study the issue, and the commission's report favored permitting doctors to perform euthanasia with certain safeguards, but the Dutch parliament, the States-General, has not yet acted to change the law.

Many Dutch physicians believe, however, that the medical treatments and actions needed to keep dying patients comfortable may at times be extended to include the act of euthanasia. Some of them hold that a continuum of measures can be brought into play to help the patient, and occasionally the injection of a lethal dose of a drug (usually a short-acting barbiturate, followed by a paralyzing agent) becomes necessary, representing the extreme end of that continuum. This occurs between 5,000 and 10,000 times a year in the Netherlands, according to van der Werf[28] (and Admiraal P: personal communication).

The medical community in the Netherlands has developed criteria that must be met for an act of euthanasia to be considered medically and ethically acceptable.[29] The patient's medical situation must be intolerable, with no prospect of improvement. The patient must be rational and must voluntarily and repeatedly request euthanasia of the physician. The patient must be fully informed. There must be no other means of relieving the suffering, and two physicians must concur with the request.

In recent years, euthanasia has been discussed more openly in the United States, and the public response has been increasingly favorable. When a Roper poll asked in 1988 whether a physician should be lawfully able to end the life of a terminally ill patient at the patient's request, 58 percent said yes, 27 percent said no, and 10 percent were undecided. (This poll, taken for the National Hemlock Society by the Roper Organization of New York City, surveyed 1982 adult Americans in March 1988.)

Presumably, the majority of physicians in the United States do not favor the Dutch position. Many physicians oppose euthanasia on moral or religious grounds, and indeed it raises profound theological questions. All religions address the matter of whether it is proper to decide the time of one's death. Whatever attitudes society may develop toward assisted suicide or euthanasia, individual physicians should not feel morally coerced to participate in such approaches. Many physicians oppose euthanasia because they believe it to be outside the physician's role, and some fear that it may be subject to abuse. (Some physicians and laypersons fear that active voluntary euthanasia, as practiced in the Netherlands, could lead to involuntary euthanasia and to murder, as practiced by the Nazis. Ethically, however, the difference is obvious.) In addition, the social climate in this country is very litigious, and the likelihood of prosecution if a case of euthanasia were discovered is fairly high -- much higher than the likelihood of prosecution after a suicide in which the physician has assisted. Thus, the prospect of criminal prosecution deters even the hardiest advocates of euthanasia among physicians.

Nevertheless, the medical profession and the public will continue to debate the role that euthanasia may have in the treatment of the terminally or hopelessly ill patient.

Notes

1. Wanzer SH, Adelstein SJ, Cranford RE, *et al*. The physician's responsibility toward hopelessly ill patients, *New England Journal of Medicine* 1984;310:955-9.
2. Presidents Commission for the Study of Ethical Problems in Medicine and Biomedical and Behavioral Research. *Deciding to Forego Life-sustaining Treatment: A Report on the Ethical, Medical and Legal Issues in Treatment Decisions*. Washington, DC: Government Printing Office, 1983.
3. Office of Technology Assessment. *Life-sustaining Technologies and the Elderly*. Washington, DC: Government Printing Office, 1987.
4. Senate Special Committee on Aging. *A Matter of Choice: Planning Ahead for Health Care Decisions*. Washington, DC: Government Printing Office, 1987.
5. *Guidelines on the Termination of Life-Sustaining Treatment and the Care of the Dying: A Report by the Hastings Center*. Briarcliff Manor, NY: Hastings Center, 1987.
6. Current Opinions of the Council on Ethical and Judicial Affairs of the American Medical Association-1986. *Withholding or Withdrawing Life-prolonging Treatment*. Chicago, IL: American Medical Association, 1986.
7. Executive Board of the American Academy of Neurology. *Position of the American Academy of Neurology on Certain Aspects of the Care and Management of the Persistent Vegetative State Patient*. Minneapolis, MN: American Academy of Neurology, 1988.
8. Ruark JE, Raffin TA, Stanford University Medical Center Committee on Ethics. Initiating and withdrawing life support, *New England Journal of Medicine* 1988;318:2530.
9. Safar P, Bircher N. *Cardiopulmonary Cerebral Resuscitation: An Introduction to Resuscitation Medicine*, 3rd ed. Philadelphia, PA: W.B. Saunders, 1988.
10. Society for the Right to Die. *Handbook of Living Will Laws*. New York, NY: Society for the Right to Die, 1987.

11. *Appointing a Proxy for Healthcare Decisions*. New York, NY: Society for the Right to Die, 1988.
12. *Adult Fight to Die Case Citations*. New York, NY: Society for the Right to Die, 1988.
13. *Right to Die Court Decisions: Artificial Feeding*. New York, NY: Society for the Right to Die, 1988.
14. Associated Press/Media General. Poll no. 4. Richmond, VA: Media General, February 1985.
15. California Department of Health Services. *Guidelines regarding withdrawal or withholding of life-sustaining procedure(s) in longterm care facilities*. August 7, 1987.
16. Bedell SE, Pelle D, Maher PL, Cleary PD. Do-not-resuscitate orders for critically ill patients in the hospital: How are they used and what is their impact? *Journal of the American Medical Assocation* 1986;256:233-7.
17. Bulkin W, Lukashok H. Rx for dying: The case for hospice. *New England Journal of Medicine* 1988;318:376-8.
18. Angell M. The quality of mercy, *New England Journal of Medicine* 1982;306:98-9.
19. Payne R, Foley KM, eds. Cancer pain, *Med Clin North Am* 1987;71:153-352.
20. *Bartling v. Superior Court* (Glendale Adventist Medical Center), 163 Cal. App. 3d 186, 209 Cal. Rptr. 220 (Ct. App. 1984).
21. *Bouvia v. Superior Court* (Glenchur), 179 Cal. App. 3d 1127, 225 Cal. Rptr. 297 (Ct. App. 1986), review denied (Cal. June 5, 1986).
22. *Brophy v. New England Sinai Hosp., Inc.*, 398 Mass. 417,497, N.E. 2d 626 (1986).
23. *In re* Culham, No. 87-340537-AC (Mich. Cir. Ct., Oakland County, Dec. 15, 1987) (Breck J).
24. Tolle SW, Hickham DH, Larson EB, Benson JA. Patient death and housestaff stress, *Clinical Resource* 1987;35:762A abstract.
25. Glantz LH. Withholding and withdrawing treatment: The role of the criminal law, *Law, Medicine and Health Care* 1987-88;15:231-41.
26. Van Bommel H. *Choices for People who have a Terminal Illness, Their Families and Their Caregivers*. Toronto, ON: NC Press, 1986.
27. Angell M. Euthanasia, *New England Journal of Medicine* 1988;319:1348-50.
28. van der Weft GT. Huisarts en euthanasie, *Medisch Contact* 1986;43:1389.
29. The Central Committee of the Royal Dutch Medical Association. *Vision on Euthanasia*. Utrecht, the Netherlands, 1986.

Chapter 36

The Ethics of Withholding and Withdrawing Critical Care

Lee M. Sanders and Thomas A. Raffin

For the 17 centuries since Hippocrates called for "the most desperate remedies in desperate cases,"[1] physicians have adhered steadfastly to two cooperative goals; to prolong life and to relieve suffering. But during the past 50 years, mechanical interventions at the edge of life have thrown those aims into dramatic conflict. Cardiopulmonary resuscitation, mechanical ventilation, feeding tubes, and the intensive care unit have postponed physiologic death for many patients who are anencephalic, comatose, or in a persistent vegetative state or prefer death to a life of suffering and pain. Demands from patients' families and cries for social justice have compelled physicians, hospital personnel, and the Supreme Court to analyze concepts long reserved for university philosophers. Although decisions are made daily to withhold and withdraw life support, society is gradually agreeing upon an ethical framework that balances hopeful science with dignified death. This article outlines that ethical framework, reviews recent legal precedents, and suggests practical guidelines for their application.

Ethical Framework

Modern medical care is governed by two sets of overriding ethical principles. The first set, beneficence and nonmaleficence, applies almost exclusively to the dayto-day actions of physicians, whereas the second set, autonomy and justice, governs more broadly the roles of patients, family, and society in medical decision making. Beneficence, as already introduced, is the physician's responsibility to preserve life, restore health, and relieve suffering, and nonmaleficence refers to its traditional corollary: *primum non nocere* ("first do no harm"). Autonomy is most often invoked to describe a patient's personhood, deserving of dignity and respect. Justice, in the context of medical ethics, most often engenders attention to the fair distribution of medical services and materials.

Beneficence and nonmaleficence attempt to define the boundaries of appropriate medical care and the quality of the dying process. When a physician fails to provide indicated therapy or when a physician provides nonindicated therapy resulting in morbidity or mortality, these principles are violated. The application of these principles is by no means simple. Often one of the provisions of beneficence, prolonging life, comes into direct conflict with another provision, the alleviation of suffering. Clinicians may be seen to violate the nonmaleficence injunction, for example, when they allow a patient in an ICU to continue to suffer with no reasonable chance of improvement.

Autonomy and justice help to identify decision-making authority. The ideal of patient

---

Source: Reprinted from the *Cambridge Quarterly of Healthcare Ethics*, Vol. 2, 1993, pp. 175-184, with permission from Cambridge University Press © 1993.

autonomy frowns on physician paternalism in favor of doctor-patient cooperation, such that ultimate authority arises from the patient. Within this definition of autonomy, the physician is no more than a source of information and reflection. To ensure the greater good of society, however, the principle of justice has been employed to demand more participation from physicians, families, and government in distributing care. Recent controversies among medical societies and congressional committees, for example, have called into question the ability of Medicare and private insurance to continue to pay for an expanding array of critical care services. In this environment, principles of justice demand a more equitable distribution that could place limits on the care demanded by an autonomous individual.

Legal Precedents

Attempts to balance these four principles to the satisfaction of patients, doctors, families, and hospitals have brought a number of precedent-setting cases to the judicial system. All of the cases involve decisions to withhold or withdraw mechanical life support, such as ventilation, nutrition, and hydration. Although many of the resulting decisions apply only locally (for example, to the state of California), they typify national legal opinion. They have helped to establish the definition of death, the right to refuse medical treatment, the authority of substituted judgment, the distinction between advanced and basic life support, and the suggested standards for medical futility.

Before the 1970s, death was traditionally identified as the cessation of the flow of body fluids (i.e., arrested circulation and ventilation), but the advent of CPR and ICUs fostered the need for a more conclusive definition of death that focused on the brain. The 1972 Virginia case *Tucker v. Lower* first upheld the brain-death definition when it acquitted physicians of wrongful determination of death for removing a heart from a donor who demonstrated "irreversible cessation of all functions of the entire brain, including the brain stem."[2] At least 37 states have since adopted a statutory definition of "whole brain death," as recommended by the President's Commission for the Study of Ethical Problems in Medicine and Biomedical and Behavioral Research,[3] and at least 44 states have passed "required request" legislation that requires physicians to offer organ donation information to families of patients declared brain dead.[4,5] The law clearly mandates, then, that physicians may decide when and how to withdraw life support from any patient determined to be brain dead.

By focusing attention on the integrity of the central nervous system, brain-death statutes called into question the value of life support for patients in comas, persistent vegetative states, or states of extreme pain. "What does life support support?" asked ethicist Al Jonsen,[6] and if life depends upon CNS function, under what circumstances can people demand to be removed from life support?

According to recent legal decisions, the province for refusing medical treatment is very broad. In 1986, Elizabeth Bouvia, a young woman who suffered quadriplegia and constant pain as a result of cerebral palsy, received confirmation from the California Court of Appeals to exercise the right to refuse medical treatment, including basic life support, for a nonterminal illness. The constitutionally derived right to privacy, which the U.S. Supreme Court established in 1891, supports the right of a competent individual over 18 years old to refuse treatment. In Ms. Bouvia's case, the California court invoked this right to privacy, stating that the government does not require that "every life must be preserved against the will of the sufferer."[7]

Refusal of medical care may not always arise from the direct wishes of the patient, however, and a series of rulings have set criteria for allowing family members or other legal proxies to act as decision-making surrogates for an incapacitated patient. The first important case to grapple with surrogate decision making was the 1976 New Jersey Supreme Court case of Karen Ann Quinlan, who had lapsed into a persistent vegetative state allegedly following ingestion of alcohol and tranquilizers. Against the hospital, who refused to act on any orders besides the direct wishes of Ms. Quinlan, the court ruled that Ms. Quinlan's parents could exercise "substituted judgment" to remove their daughter from advanced life support. But the case did more than simply confirm the validity of family judgment as a substitute for patient autonomy. It also suggested, in the context of a right to privacy, a qualitative meaning for medical futility. The New Jersey Supreme Court found reason to invoke her family's authority only insofar as it preserved Ms. Quinlan's right to privacy, which the court felt was abrogated under persistent vegetative conditions that did not promise "at the very least, a remission of symptoms enabling a return toward a normal functioning, integrated existence."[8]

During the 1970s, "substituted judgment" was confirmed in three higher court decisions in Massachusetts and New York. In *Superintendent of Belchertown State School v. Saikewicz* (1977), Massachusetts was allowed to withhold treatment for acute myeloblastic leukemia from a mentally retarded patient because the treatment would be painful, poorly understood, and unlikely to produce a cure.[9] In *In the Matter of Dinnerstein* (1978), Massachusetts families were awarded the right to write do-not-resuscitate orders (DNRs) without prior judicial approval for relatives afflicted by Alzheimer's disease.[10] In *Eichner v. Dillon* (1981), a director of a Catholic order was given the right to withdraw a ventilator from a colleague in a persistent vegetative state because when he was competent the patient indicated such wishes and because his physicians considered his state to be medically futile.[11]

In one of the more dramatic victories for substituted judgment, a California murder case gave physicians greater clout in determining medical futility at the edge of life and negated the distinction between basic and advanced life support. In the case of *Barber v. Superior Court* (1983), a district attorney charged two physicians with murder for removing advanced and basic life support from Clarence Herbert, a 55-year-old man who suffered severe brain damage subsequent to a postoperative myocardial infarction. Acquitting the doctors of the murder charges, the California Appeals Court ruled that once family and physicians agree on a treatment course, decisions to withhold or withdraw care do not require prior judicial approval. Following the judgment of the physicians, the court agreed that because Mr. Herbert could never become socially interactive or aware of himself, he could not appreciate life. Furthermore, the court considered irrelevant the distinction between advanced life support (i.e., mechanical ventilation) and basic life support (i. e., hydration and nutrition). Either type of life support, it concluded, should be "evaluated in the same manner as any other medical procedure."[12] When any medical procedure is determined to be futile, its use is discontinued, and for adhering to that standard of beneficence and nonmaleficence, Clarence Herbert's physicians and his family were exonerated.

Two New Jersey Supreme Court cases upheld the right of families to demand withdrawal of any type of life support from patients judged to be in medically futile states. In *In the Matter of Claire Conroy* (1985), this fight to withdraw was subject to the fulfillment of any of three criteria: the patient expressed a wish to discontinue treatment, her values and lifestyle implied such a wish, or the expected net burden of her posttreatment life outweighed the expected benefits.[13] In *In the Matter of Mary Jobes* (1987), the court ruled that no medical institution could refuse categorically to withhold or withdraw life support, and it exempted from criminal prosecution physicians and healthcare workers who act in good faith.

Not all court decisions, however, have been so lenient in granting doctors or families the authority to judge the futility of a patient's condition. More recent precedents have subjected decisions to withdraw life support to the strict standard of "clear and convincing evidence," requiring proof of a patient's specific wishes in specific medical circumstances. In the 1988 case of Mary O'Connor, the New York Court of Appeals refused the right to withdraw a feeding tube from a woman with dementia because her family could not secure "clear and convincing evidence" of her wishes. In practice, families seeking to withdraw a patient's life support can rarely meet the standard. (After watching two relatives die of cancer, for example, Mary O'Connor told her daughter that she did not wish to die in the same slow, agonizing manner, but the court did not consider such evidence "clear and convincing," since Mrs. O'Connor was suffering from a different disease.)

The latest test of the "clear and convincing evidence" standard was brought in 1990 to the U.S. Supreme Court in the case of Nancy Cruzan, a 26-year-old Missouri woman whose parents requested the removal of basic life support when she lapsed into a persistent vegetative state following a 1983 car accident. Ms. Cruzan had left no written advance directive regarding the withdrawal of life support, but even if she had left a living will, the Missouri statutes would have allowed only the removal of advanced life support, not the basic life support (food and water) upon which Ms. Cruzan was dependent. Nonetheless, the courts considered evidence that Nancy Cruzan wanted to die: She had told a housemate that if sick or injured, she would want to continue living only if she could live at least "halfway normally." The trial court considered the evidence "clear and convincing." The appeals court, however, found the evidence insufficient, envisioning a slippery slope for the state-sanctioned murder of incompetent patients "with all manner of handicaps." In a split 5-to-4 decision, the U.S. Supreme Court upheld the Missouri Court of Appeals decision to prolong Ms. Cruzan's life, affirming Missouri's right to apply the standard of "clear and convincing evidence."

In addition to protecting a state's right to apply any evidentiary standard it sees fit, the narrowly split Cruzan decision confirmed two earlier California precedents. First, confirming the Elizabeth Bouvia decision, the Supreme Court found that the Fourteenth Amendment guarantees the right of a competent patient to refuse life-sustaining medical treatment. Second, as in the case of Clarence Herbert, it recognized no relevant distinction between the withdrawal of advanced life support and the withdrawal of basic life support.

The most recent case to consider the withdrawal of life support has reexamined the physician's role in determining medical futility and is further strengthening the authority of family members to exercise substituted judgment. Unlike the case of Nancy Cruzan, in which a family sought to override the state to terminate a patient's life support, in the Minnesota case of Helga Wanglie, doctors attempted to override a family member's wishes to prolong a patient's life. Oliver Wanglie would not allow doctors to remove the ventilator from his 86-year-old wife Helga, who had been in a persistent vegetative state for more than a year. Although the doctors at Minnesota's Hennepin County Medical Center considered Mrs. Wanglie's continued therapy to be medically futile, the district court ruled that Mrs. Wanglie's husband had unchallengeable authority to make decisions to continue her medical care. The Wanglie decision also silenced the attempt to apply notions of distributive justice to limit autonomous decision-making, so long as Helga Wanglie's health insurance continued to pay for her $800,000-a year care.

Practical Consequences

This evolving history of legal precedents points to practical, comfortable guidelines for decisions to withhold or withdraw treatment.[14,15] Patients and potential patients should leave advance written directives about their care, and they should discuss their feelings about life support with family members and with caregivers. Physicians should communicate effectively, solicit peer judgment, and allow adequate time for decision-making.

Patient's Authority

Although physicians may adhere to authoritative opinions, the real authority for decision-making lies with patients. Written directives concerning life support clarify those decisions when they must be made by a family member or an appointed conservator, but a patient's surrogate still holds authority in the absence of such documents. Much controversy in critical care decision-making occurs, as in the Bouvia and Wanglie cases, when authority is challenged. To avoid the potential for such challenges, doctors should encourage all patients to execute a living will or a durable power of attorney. A living will dictates a course of action to be taken in specific or general states of futile medical treatment, but they may often be too vague to be effective.[16] A durable power of attorney for healthcare, which allows a patient to designate a proxy for decision-making, is more useful.

Forty-one states and the District of Columbia recognize living wills as legally binding documents, and 31 states plus the District of Columbia have durable power of attorney legislation. When not approved by state legislation, as was demonstrated in Florida with In the Matter of Francis Landy (1983), a living will cannot be the sole basis for withholding or withdrawing life support.[17] Although these documents are valid only in the state issued, their information is universally invaluable to physicians, families, and courts who must make decisions in the absence of a patient's competent voice.[18] But the paperwork is inert without participation. The Patient Self-Determination Act requires every healthcare facility receiving federal funds to provide information about living wills and durable powers of attorney to all admitted patients.

Physician Communication

Regardless of comprehensive legislation, most decisions to withdraw and withhold care will remain uninformed by advanced directives, and in practice, doctors must continue to oversee the decision-making process without interfering with patient or family authority. When a decision to withdraw life support becomes imminent, for example, a physician must assess the level of a patient's mental competence, which might require seeking opinion from a psychiatrist. If a patient is declared mentally incompetent, physicians must recognize the legal source of substituted judgment: family member or court-appointed conservator. Once a surrogate decision-maker is designated, physicians must provide the information, judgment, and advice necessary for that surrogate to reach a decision in line with the patient's desires. Without infusing extrinsic religious and cultural values, the physician must allow the patient's legal proxy to judge the proportional weight given to prolonging life and to enhancing life. However fully Helga Wanglie's physicians thought they understood the priorities that governed her care, their understanding ran counter to the religious and personal views of Mrs. Wanglie's husband, and his judgment stands -- legally and ethically.

When responding to the patient's and family's needs for information and recommendation at such critical times, physicians must employ exceedingly high standards for communication and judgment. The most vital physician responsibility in decisions to withhold or withdraw critical care is to use effective communication skills. Everybody -- physician, family, and patient -- feels anxious, awkward, and fearful about discussing quality-of-life and quality-of-death issues, but physicians are obligated to take the lead. Because some physicians are more capable communicators than others, physicians should consult experienced facilitators (e.g., social workers, ethicists, chaplains, or psychiatrists) to assist with communication at critical times in healthcare decision-making.

Regardless of outside assistance, effective physician communication may be enhanced by appealing to privacy, simplicity, and honesty in an atmosphere of encouraged participation. Rushed and noisy environments, such as ICUs or hospital corridors, interfere with fruitful communication. Families, already under emotional duress, should be allowed sufficient privacy to comprehend the facts and adequate time to reach fully informed decisions. Providing too many details on clinical methods and prognoses hinders rational decision-making, but a physician's open, honest expression of feelings as well as facts helps patients and families to overcome their initial intimidation. Determining the correct balance between simplicity and

honesty requires that the physician avoid blunt, esoteric vocabulary on one extreme and false optimism on the other.
The only way to remain within these boundaries is to elicit feedback from patients and family, encouraging reiteration and questioning from each individual.

When presenting their recommendations, physicians should include a language of uncertainty alongside a language of time-limited goals. For example, the children of an elderly man in a persistent vegetative state might be told, "In our best judgment, your father has essentially no chance to regain a reasonable quality of life. If we see no improvement over the next 48 hours, we recommend that life support be withdrawn, in which case we expect that he will probably die." Fairness to the legal doctrine of informed consent requires that judgment be couched in terms of uncertainty and that the prognosis of death be made clearly. Providing time-limited goals not only adds simple, concrete information in a confusing environment; it also allows families enough time to reach clear-headed decisions.

Reassessment of priorities is integral to effective communication, because as illness and therapies change so do the relative values on life and quality of life expressed by patients and their families. At a very minimum, then, physicians should solicit family opinions every time a change occurs in a patient's condition or treatment. Physicians should ask families with candor about the patient's perceived goals, about the family members' personal feelings, and about the quality of the dying process. A patient's goal, such as to spend some time reading, is often a convenient tool toward assessing the futility of continued treatment. Sometimes a family's insistence for or against the withdrawal of care may be more a reflection of a family member's emotional discomfort than an indication of the patient's best wishes. Finally, an open dialogue concerning the physiological, spiritual, and cultural components of the dying process is useful to create an understanding between the physician and the patient's family.

Physician Judgment
Before approaching a family or patient, however, the physician must have exercised reasonable clinical judgment in determining the likelihood of benefit from further treatment, and the physician should make clear, in advance, the likely scenarios and choices that may be part of the patient's future treatment course. Such judgment may be corroborated with the Acute Physiology, Age, and Chronic Health Evaluation (APACHE) II guidelines for critical care and with consensus opinions from colleagues. Developed from a data base recording the outcomes of 2,719 ICU patients, the APACHE II classification uses criteria such as age, extent of organ failure, presence of sepsis, and existence of malignancies to determine relative rates of mortality[19] It can be a very useful communication tool to present prognoses to families and to other healthcare personnel. Staff members who feel that their values conflict with those of the patient, family, or other physicians, however, should be excluded from participation, and if this is not practical, they should be given an opportunity to air their differences.

Action: Withholding and Withdrawing Basic and Advanced Life Support
Despite increasing attention to the ethical and legal issues in life support decision-making, few have written about the practical clinical methods for making the process work well from beginning to end.[20] How should physicians act to withhold or withdraw life support? First, physicians must replace the almost reflexive impulse to institute life support measures with a careful decision-making process that incorporates respect for patients' wishes, identification of substituted authority, exercise of good clinical judgment, and clear anticipation of future decision points. By instituting the decision-making process before treatment is begun, physicians allow patients and families options that may be more manageable than those of withdrawing treatment later. Second, once a decision to withdraw life support has been made,

physicians must act in a way that minimizes the patient's suffering, psychological trauma among family members, and disturbing feelings among health care personnel.

Do-not-resuscitate (DNR) orders are the most common means of withholding life support from patients, and they probably deserve more use than is currently demonstrated. Fewer than 20% of hospital patients who receive CPR, an often brutal and invasive procedure, survive to leave the hospital,[21] and most of them are intubated and admitted to the noisy, mechanical world of the intensive care unit, a world that precludes most communication with the patient. Clearly, physicians more open to the possibility of DNR orders can save many patients (particularly the terminally ill and the elderly, chronically ill) from the brutal CPR process and the uninviting world that follows. But studies indicate that DNR directives are often issued late after the patient's admission and without written justification in light of patient-oriented goals.[22,23,24,25] When doctors choose to discuss DNR orders with patients and families, the dialogue should be begun early, and it may be necessary to enlist the judgments of the healthcare team and the communication expertise of an outside facilitator. Once agreed upon, DNR orders should be identified formally to patients and families, and they should be conveyed prominently on medical charts or records to all healthcare staff responsible for the patient's care. Although hospital policies consider DNR status to require the same aggressive treatment granted patients without DNR codes, in actual practice the writing of a DNR order usually leads to less intensive care.

A DNR order may be the best and most common illustration of advanced life support withheld, but initiating treatment besides CPR may also be unnecessary in the case of hopelessly ill patients. Antibiotics administered to comatose patients to combat infection, for example, may pull them back needlessly from a painless death to live out an extra few days in pain. Driven by the impulse to do "everything possible" to prolong physiological life, physicians may place feeding tubes in a patient in a persistent vegetative state, prolonging a treatment course that the patient may have deemed futile. Unless patients or families agree that a procedure will help fulfill patient-oriented goals, instituting that procedure is unacceptable.

Nonetheless, patients will enter treatment courses that they or their families later judge to be not worth continuing. When a patient or family consents to removal of basic or advanced life support in an ICU setting, the methods for withdrawal must be sensitive, first to the patient's suffering and second to the family's psychological experience. All court precedents demand that the same decision-making standards be applied to advanced life support (ventilation) and basic life support (nutrition and hydration), but the emotional distinction between withdrawing artificial respiration and allowing someone to "starve to death" is real. These feelings must be resolved before families can be comfortable with their decision and with the nature of the patient's dying process. When ventilation is removed, it should be weaned gradually over 15-30 minutes, with drugs administered to relieve pain and agonal breathing. To avoid a perception that the patient has been abruptly abandoned, intravenous lines should remain in place, and the physician should remain with the family during the process.

When a brain-dead patient to be withdrawn from life support has healthy vital organs (kidney, heart, lung, pancreas, or liver), most state legislatures require that the family be informed about the options for organ donation. In the spirit of the Patient Self-Determination Act, physicians should be prepared to give information about organ donation, alongside the information about living wills, to all patients admitted to the hospital. In this way, "advance directives" could be promoted in a fuller context and to a more comprehensive audience. Organ donation "to save another person's life" can be a psychologically positive force for families searching for meaning during the grieving process.[26] However, partly because of poor professional communication, fewer than 20% of potential donor families ever authorize donation, and as a result thousands of patients awaiting transplantation die each year.[27]

Conclusion

By attending to the principles of patient autonomy, beneficence, and nonmaleficence, physicians can avoid ethical dilemmas when decisions to withhold or withdraw life support are imminent. Patients or their legal surrogates exercise ultimate authority in determining the course of treatment, and their opinions must be sought early and often. All patients should be encouraged to execute advance directives for medical care. Physicians must take the lead in opening effective communication, and to optimize communication, physicians may enlist an outside facilitator. Final decisions must reflect the relative importance a patient would assign to the quality of life and to the quantity of life. Once the decision to terminate treatment has been made, physicians must be sensitive to the family's experience as well as the patient's experience during the removal of life support.

Notes

1. *Hippocratic Writings.* Chadwick J, Mann WN, translators. New York, NY: Penguin, 1950:207.
2. Paris JJ, Reardon FE. Dilemmas in intensive care medicine: an ethical and legal analysis. *Journal of Intensive Care Medicine* 1986;1:75-90.
3. Guidelines for the determination of death -- report of the medical consultants on the diagnosis of death to the President's Commission for the Study of Ethical Problems in Medicine and Biomedical and Behavioral Research. *JAMA* 1981;246:2184-6.
4. Singer PA. A review of public policies to procure and distribute kidneys for transplantation. *Arch Int Med* 1990;150:523-7.
5. Blumstein JF. Government's role in organ transplantation policy. *J Health Politics and Policy Law* 1989;14(1):15-39.
6. Jonsen AR. What does life support support? *Pharos* 1987;45:4-7.
7. *Bouvia v. Superior Court*, 179 Cal. App. 3d 1127, 1986.
8. *In re Quinlan*, 70 N.J. 10, 355 A.2d 647, 79 ALR3d 205, 1976.
9. Curran WJ. The Saikewicz decision. *NEJM* 1978;298:499-500.
10. Suber DG, Tabor WJ. Withholding of life-sustaining treatment from the terminally ill, incompetent patient: who decides? Part I. *JAMA* 1982;248:2250-1.
11. Areen J. The legal status of consent obtained from families of adult patients to withold or withdraw treatment. *JAMA* 1987;258:229-35.
12. *Barber v. Superior Court*, 147 Cal. App.3d 1006, 1983.
13. Curran WJ. Defining appropriate medical care: providing nutrients and hydration for the dying. *NEJM* 1985;313:25-9.
14. Ruark JE, Raffin TA, *et al.* Initiating and withdrawing life support: Principles and practice in adult medicine, *New England Journal of Medicine* 1988;318:25-9.
15. Raftin TA. Withholding and withdrawing life support, *Hospital Practice* 1991;March:133-55.
16. Bok S. Personal directions for care at the end of life, *New England Journal of Medicine* 1976;295:367-9.
17. Gilfix M, Raffin TA. Withholding or withdrawing extraordinary life support- optimizing rights and limiting liability, *Western Journal of Medicine* 1984;141:387-94.
18. Raffin TA. Value of the living will, *Chest* 1986;90:444-6.
19. Knaus WA, *et al.* Prognosis in acute organ-system failure, *Annals of Surgery* 1985;202:685.
20. Raffin TA, Shurkin JN, Sinkler WS. *Intensive Care: Facing the Critical Choices.* New York, NY: Freeman, 1989.
21. Bedell SE, Delbanco TL, Cook EF, *et al.* Survival after cardiopulmonary resuscitation in the hospital, *New England Journal of Medicine* 1983;309:569-76.
22. Lo B, Saika G, Strull W, *et al.* "Do not resuscitate" decisions - a prospective study at three teaching hospitals, *Annals of Internal Medicine* 1985;145:1115-7.

23. Bedell SE, Pelle D, Maher PL, Cleary PD. Do-not-resuscitate orders for critically ill patients in the hospital-how are they used and what is their impact? *Journal of the American Medical Association* 1986;256:322-37.
24. Youngner SJ, Lewandowski W, McClish DK, *et al*. "Do not resuscitate" orders-incidence and implications in a medical intensive care unit, *Journal of the American Medical Association* 1985;255:54-7.
25. Lipton HL. Do-not-resuscitate decisions in a community hospital-incidence, implications, and outcomes, *Journal of the American Medical Association* 1986;256:1164-9.
26. Batten HL, Prottas JM. Kind strangers: The families of organ donors, *Health Affairs* 1987(summer):35-47.
27. National Organ Procurement Transplantation Network. Data compiled by the United Network for Organ Sharing, 4 February 1991.

Chapter 37

A Surgeon with Acquired Immunodeficiency Syndrome: A Threat to Patient Safety? The Case of William H. Behringer

Evelyne Shuster

A year ago, the New Jersey case of William H. Behringer, the surgeon with acquired immunodeficiency syndrome (AIDS), caused health experts to focus on health care workers infected with human immunodeficiency virus (HIV) and to call for new policies and guidelines to protect patients against infection. After a year of acrimonious debate over the proper approach to the issues discussed in Behringer, no consensus has emerged. The Centers for Disease Control has quietly abandoned its plan to ease its July 1991 guidelines that call for infected professionals to cease performing invasive procedures or disclose their conditions to their patients. It has now decided to let each state set its own rules and regulations in compliance with its guidelines or risk financial penalties.

The issues discussed in Behringer have remained controversial. This case provides an opportunity to identify reasonable actions that may ensure patient safety without inciting public fears, unduly restricting individual freedom, or violating human rights.

Has the time come to reverse our decade-old policy on acquired immunodeficiency syndrome (AIDS) and begin to routinely screen physicians and their patients? Recent surveys[1] indicate that more than 60% of physicians believe that they should be able to order AIDS tests for patients without their consent, and more than half hold that they, themselves, should be subject to mandatory testing for human immunodeficiency virus (HIV). Almost 90% of people have said they want to know their physician's HIV status.[1] With physicians and patients claiming a "right to know," routine or mandatory HIV screening, once widely condemned, has become more appealing to both sides.

On the other hand, the Centers for Disease Control (CDC), which thus far has effectively set AIDS policy for U.S. health care institutions, has consistently advised against HIV screening and recommended universal barrier precautions as the best means of preventing HIV transmission.[2] It has been thought that mandatory or routine screening would not reduce the risks of infection but could further exacerbate an AIDS-related "underclass" in terms of stigmatization, discrimination, and human rights' violations.[3]

Do we need new laws and regulations to control the AIDS epidemic, and if so, what should they be? Among hundreds of thousands of infected people, only five have been identified as presumably having contracted the disease from a health care practitioner, a dentist, Dr. David Acer.[4]

Yet, on January 17, 1991, the day before the CDC published a description of the Acer

---

Source: Reprinted from *American Journal of Medicine*, Vol. 94, Jan. 93, pp. 93-99, with permission from The American Journal of Medicine © Jan. 1993.

case, the American Medical Association (AMA) issued a statement saying:

> Physicians who are HIV positive have an ethical obligation not to engage in any professional activity which has an identifiable risk of transmission of the infection to the patient. Physicians must abstain from performing invasive procedures which pose an "identifiable risk of transmission," or "disclose their seropositive status prior to performing a procedure and proceed only if there is informed consent."[5] (Emphasis added.)

By the end of 1991, when Kimberly Bergalis, the first patient of Dr. Acer to be diagnosed with AIDS, died at the age of 23, the CDC had already published new guidelines recommending that HIV-infected physicians "should not perform exposure prone procedures unless they have sought counsel from an expert review panel and been advised under what circumstances, if any, they may continue to perform these procedures."[6] The CDC further recommended that exposure-prone procedures should be identified by medical/surgical/dental organizations and institutions at which the procedures are performed and that prospective patients should be notified of the health care worker's seropositivity before undergoing these procedures.[6] By October 1991, Congress had passed legislation requiring each state to adopt the guidelines of the CDC or similar guidelines by the following year, or risk losing federal funding for public health programs. Because professional organizations refused to provide lists of exposure-prone procedures, in November 1991, the CDC issued draft revisions of its July 1991 guidelines, now recommending that local committees review HIV transmission from health care workers to patients on a case-by-case basis.[7]

Courts have also begun to take a position. In April 1991, a New Jersey superior court judge rendered an influential opinion on the case of William H. Behringer, a surgeon with AIDS.[8] This was the first superior court to rule on these issues.

After more than a year of controversy over the proper approach to the issues discussed in Behringer,[8] no consensus has emerged. Regulating the practice of HIV-infected health care workers remains among the most contentious medical and public health policy decisions. The New Jersey case illustrates the enormous difficulties to both hospitals and courts in addressing the problems of HIV infected physicians and those with AIDS.

The Surgeon With AIDS: The Case of William H. Behringer[8]

At age 40, William H. Behringer, an otolaryngologist and plastic surgeon, was diagnosed with AIDS at Princeton Medical Center where he was on staff. Concerned that this information could have a devastating effect on his practice, Dr. Behringer sought a transfer to another facility. After attempts at securing treatment elsewhere failed, Dr. Behringer decided that he would be treated at home. Within hours of his discharge, colleagues, friends, and patients knew of his condition. The president of the medical center, Dennis Doody, unilaterally ordered the suspension of his surgical privileges and required mandatory disclosure under the informed consent doctrine. Ultimately, based in part on the AMA's "identifiable-risk" position, the hospital's trustees adopted a policy that stated:

> A physician or health care provider with know HIV seroposivity may continue to treat patients at the Medical Center at Princeton but shall not perform procedures that pose any risk of HIV transmission to the patient.[8] (Emphasis added.)

Dr. Behringer never performed surgery after his AIDS diagnosis. His office practice, where he remained until his death in July 1989, rapidly declined, resulting in emotional suffering and financial loss. The Behringer estate sued the medical center for breach of confidentiality and for violation of the New Jersey Law Against Discrimination (LAD). After a bench trial, Superior Court Judge Philip S. Carchman ruled in favor of Dr. Behringer on the charge of negligence in maintaining confidentiality. However, the judge upheld the hospital's decision to suspend the surgeon's clinical privileges and affirmed a patient's right to know under the doctrine of informed consent. In essence, the court ruled that Dr. Behringer, as a patient, but not as a physician, was entitled to privacy, for once the information about his HIV status was disclosed, there could be no obligation for maintaining confidentiality.

Obviously, patient safety must be a paramount concern to hospitals and physicians. Hospitals and health care providers must take appropriate measures to reduce risks of infection in the workplace. But are exclusion policies and mandatory disclosure appropriate to this goal?

The Court's Opinion

Dr. Behringer consented to be tested for HIV on the condition that the test results remain confidential. The surgeon claimed that, instead, "the results were available for placement on the chart without restriction, and no special measures were implemented to ensure confidentiality."[8] In his words:

> Nothing is clinically gained by charting the test results without restriction. The knowledge of a patient's HIV status should not reduce the need for (universal barrier) precautions that must be taken at all times, and for all patients. When a patient is a practicing physician, special measures need to be implemented to ensure confidentiality. Access to the chart should be limited to persons within the clinical realm having a "need to know", i.e., those persons who demonstrate to designated record-keeper a bona fide need to know. (The) breach of confidentiality was less the charting of the test results per se than it easy access.[8]

Undoubtedly, an essential aspect of the physician-patient relationship is the opportunity to speak freely and openly with each other.[9] Historically, the law has protected physician-patient communication, understanding that confidentiality is necessary to promote effective therapy. Recently, the disclosure of an individual's HIV-related status has been subject to stringent regulation with few exceptions.[10] Statutes have been promulgated to ensure that information gained as a result of HIV testing remains confidential. The legislature has recognized a person's right to privacy and justified disclosure of information only when there is a "compelling need" to know, i.e., when health care workers are directly involved in the patient's care.[10]

On the other hand, Dr. Behringer knew or should have known that, in modern hospitals, almost everyone has access to a patient's medical record.[11] Even if access on the "need to know basis" is strictly regulated, so many people fit into this category that it is unrealistic to believe that strict confidentiality can be ensured. One may question Dr. Behringer's judgment to be tested for HIV at the very medical center where he was also a practicing surgeon. But poor judgment does not relieve the medical center from its obligation to prevent an outright violation of privacy.

Judge Carchman ruled that the patient's trust was violated, his care undermined, and thus, the medical center was guilty of negligence.

Dr. Behringer further contended that mandatory disclosure and the suspension of his medical privileges violated the New Jersey LAD.[12] The LAD (like the federal Americans With Disabilities Act of 1990[13] has established a comprehensive prohibition on discrimination against persons with disabilities and holds that AIDS is a handicap within the meaning of laws prohibiting handicap discrimination. Anti-discrimination laws specifically prohibit employers from discriminating against handicapped persons on account of their handicap, unless the handicap "reasonably precludes the performance of the particular employment."[13] Dr. Behringer noted that there is no scientific or medical evidence that demonstrates significant risks of professional-to-patient HIV transmission. Had it not been for the exaggerated fear, or prejudices associated with AIDS, he would not have been excluded from practicing. His exclusion was therefore discriminatory, absent a demonstration of a "significant risk," or a "direct threat" to others.

Referring to the hepatitis B virus (HBV) model, Dr. Behringer pointed out that, HBV, which is transmitted like HIV, is common among health care workers. Infected HBV patients incur substantial risks of morbidity and mortality. However, there have been "no restrictions placed on HBV-infected physicians."[8] Thus, an exclusionary policy that applies only to HIV infection is unjustified, prejudicial, and discriminatory. Finally, he argued that the risks of professional-to-patient HIV transmission are not so significant as to create an affirmative duty to warn patients about such risks. Nor are they significant enough to warrant a patient's "need to know." In Dr. Behringer's works:

> While a patient might "want" to know the health status of the physician, the risk is not so "significant" that a patient would "need" to know the information because this is not a risk within a reasonable medical opinion.[9] (Emphasis added.)

The court readily recognized that the New Jersey LAD[12] requires an employer to demonstrate a "reasonable probability of substantial harm to others," and "a materially enhanced risk of serious injury" to warrant exclusion. However, having stated these legal requirements, the court practically ignored them, saying "the risk of transmission is not the sole risk involved." Patients can be exposed to the surgeon's infected blood (e.g., surgical accidents), and the mere possibility of exposure is sufficient to make it a significant risk whether or not HIV transmission actually occurred. Thus, not only does the actual risk of HIV transmission need to be considered, but also the effect of HIV exposure on a patient. The impact of (such exposure) is enormous and could be avoided if patients were informed of the surgeon's condition before the procedure occurs, and obviously, before a surgical accident. Notwithstanding what a physician knows or should know about a patient's informational need, he or she must make a reasonable disclosure of the information and those risks which a reasonably prudent patient would consider material or significant to the decision about a course of treatment.[8] (Emphasis added.)

The judge concluded that if any risk of HIV transmission exists, patients, not physicians, should be the "ultimate arbiters." In the judge's words:

> The way to control "any risk" is to reduce it to "no risk at all" and to include in the decision-making process the most critical participant, the patient... If there is to be an ultimate arbiter of whether the patient is to be treated invasively by an AIDS positive surgeon, the arbiter will be the fully informed patient. The ultimate risk is so absolute, so devastating that it is untenable to argue against informed consent combines with a restriction on procedure which present "any risk" to the patient.[8] (Emphasis added.)

Comments

The decision in Behringer manifests a trend that has developed in American society.[14] Within a week of the ruling, the New Jersey Medical Society called for HIV testing of all hospitalized patients and health providers and asked the state legislature to make mandatory screening a matter of law.[15] A bill was passed in the United States Senate calling "for prison terms for physicians who know they are HIV positive, but do not notify their patients"[16] (the bill was ultimately rejected by a House-Senate committee). States have considered -- or passed -- laws requiring physicians to disclose their HIV-infection or barring them from "doing any medical work."[17] A Pennsylvania state superior court has relied extensively on Behringer[8] and ruled that the "disclosure of information regarding the condition of a physician with AIDS."[18] A federal court has upheld the firing of a licensed practical nurse because he refused to disclose his HIV test results.[19] Recently, the executive editor of the *New England Journal of Medicine* defended "a patient's right to know" and called for screening of pregnant women, hospitalized patients, and health care professionals.[20]

This trend raises several questions: Is all of this necessary? Why would we now want to deviate from an AIDS policy that has been thus far reasonably effective? Are exclusionary policies necessary to enhance patient safety and public health? Is informed consent relevant to this debate? What could possibly justify each state having its own set of rules and regulations? Over a decade of widespread HIV infection across the United States, the one identified and reported case of professional-to-patient HIV transmission has been a "mystery, which may never be solved."[21] Two physicians calculated that "the risk of getting AIDS from a physician whose HIV status is unknown is 1 in 21 mission per hour of surgery, and 1 in 83,000, if the surgeon is known to be HIV positive."[22] They concluded that the "risks are clearly low and might have about the same magnitude as fatal injury to the patient en route to the hospital."[22]

Cases such a Behringer[8] and Acer-Bergalis[4] have prompted the CDC to conduct major studies of patients known to have been treated by HIVinfected health care workers.[23] Of 15, 795 patients in 32 practices, the CDC has found only 84 patients to HIV positive, and not one single confirmed case of HIV transmission from a health care worker to patients.[23] As ironic as it might seem, the CDC had provided some reassurance about the risks of physician-to-patient HIV transmission. Despite this reassurance, the CDC has not rescinded its July 1, 1991, guidelines (even though opposition to the guidelines has left them in abeyance) and is now calling for each state and local health department to decide what kind of care HIV-infected health workers can provide. However, should exclusionary policy be adopted?

Exclusionary Policy

Clearly, the court in Behringer has been unable (or unwilling?) to distinguish between the risk of harm, and harm itself, when harm is death caused by AIDS. Studies to date have not implicated HIVinfected surgeons in the transmission of disease to their patients.[24] The CDC, itself, estimated the average risk of sporadic HIV transmission from an HIV-infected surgeon to a patient during an invasive procedure to be 2.4 to 24 per million procedures.[25] Federal and state laws against discrimination support policies of exclusion only when significant risks to others exist.[26] By emphasizing the "significant risk standard," the framers of the laws intend to protect physicians and patients from inchoate public perception and suspicions. The Behringer court, however, took the position that, in the case of AIDS, only a "no risk at all" standard is acceptable. When the slightest possibility of risk, even fear, of being infected exists, the risk must not be taken. Not only is this "zero tolerance" approach toward HIV infection unique in medicine, since it has never been applied to any other clinical context, it is also unrealistic, prejudicial, misleading and unfair. It is unrealistic because risks are intrinsic to living, and individuals routinely accept much greater risks in life. It is prejudicial because patients may subjectively perceive as objectively material and significant the risks of HIV transmission, regardless of probability. Health care workers perceived at a greater risk for HIV infection because of their riskgroup status could be singled out for HIV testing, while others, not so perceived, could continue their practices. It is misleading because policies of exclusion will not substantially increase patient safety, since they only apply to those health care workers whose HIV seropositivity is known to the medical facility. Health care workers whose behaviors put them at significant risk for HIV infection may not want to be tested or learn about the best infection control practices because of fear of being the object of discrimination and losing their jobs. Those who are already infected may not be encouraged to seek treatment, could find ways of protecting their careers, and quietly change the way they do their jobs.[26] It is unfair because health care workers are at significantly greater risks of contracting HIV from patients than patients are of contracting infection from them.[25] Those who are not infected may refuse to treat HIV-infected patients and risk their livelihoods. Those who are infected may be willing to treat infected patients, and thus, would bear all the burden of care. The cost of these policies could ultimately be enormous to society in terms of expenditures, loss of professional resources, social services, delays, or outright refusals to treat HIV-infected patients, and unjust treatment.

The AMA's "Identifiable Risk" Position[5]

The AMA's position on "identifiable risk" creates different problems when it states that physicians must abstain from performing procedures that pose an "identifiable risk" to patients.[5] This position seems to treat all risks the same regardless of probability. A 1 in a billion risk of becoming infected with HIV during a procedure, a 1 in 100,000 risk, or a 1 in 2 risk are all identifiable risks. For instance, the risk of being infected by a surgeon known to be HIV positive and the risk of death from anesthesia during surgery (which is comparatively 10 times greater) are identifiable risks, and thus, they should be considered.[27] For good reasons, the AMA has never claimed that anesthesia should not be administered. Not only does the AMA position foster a false and misleading view that "identifiable risks" can always be eliminated, it also means, taken literally, the end of medicine.

No surgeon would ever operate, no physician would ever diagnose, treat, or prescribe medications, because these activities all involve identifiable risks. Glantz and colleagues[27] pointed out that the AMA may have applied the "identifiable risk" standard to HIV because the organization believes that AIDS should be treated differently from any other type of risk. As an example, 20 patients per day die in New York state as a result of negligence.[28] These deaths are identifiable risks. However, "there has been no response from the AMA calling for measures to reduce the risks, urging physicians to avoid sending their patients to New York Hospitals or requiring physicians who have been guilty of negligence to so notify their patients."[27]

Informed Consent

The patient's "right to know" requirement is equally misguided. Historically, informed consent has been developed to assist patients in making decisions about the benefits and risks of medical treatment, because of the inherent uncertainties of therapy.[29] Patients have a right to know what is materially relevant to a proposed therapy. The informed consent requirement has never been a screening process. Its purpose is not to identify HIV-infected or otherwise unqualified, impaired, handicapped, or dangerous physicians. These problems should be remedied by professional standards and licensing requirements. Surgeons are either qualified or not qualified to operate on patients. If they are unqualified, the patient's consent does not make them qualified. If they are qualified, giving patients a *de facto* authority to disqualify them under mandatory disclosure only promotes unjustified stigmatization and discrimination. If the hospital where a surgeon practices knows the physician is unqualified, it has the obligation and indeed, the responsibility, to prohibit that physician's practicing, and licensing boards should suspend or revoke the license of unqualified physicians. Whether or not patients consent to be treated by an unqualified or dangerous physician does not change the moral and legal responsibility of hospitals to prevent that physician from practicing. For instance, in criminal law, consent has never been recognized as a defense to such crimes as voluntarily and knowingly transmitting HIV to a consenting adult.[30] Thus, by upholding a patient's right to know, the Behringer court misapplied the informed consent doctrine or ignored what the doctrine represents. Had it seriously wanted to protect patients, the court would have focused on infection control strategy, rather than on the infection status of the surgeon.

The risks patients incur in the ordinary course of receiving care far exceed any risks an HIV-infected physician presents.[31] Yet, patients are not routinely informed about all that could adversely affect therapeutic outcomes. The "right to know" requirement that singles out HIV infection while overlooking or choosing to ignore other such significant risks as HBV transmission, a surgeon's wound infection rates, history of substance abuse, financial or family problems, and fatigue or mental stress is discriminatory and prejudicial. For instance, to this date, the medical profession stands accused and condemned, and properly so, of never having responsibly dealt with HBV-infected surgeons, even now that a vaccine is available (Shrager MW, oral communication). Barnes *et al.*[32] observed that the CDC has thus far allowed HBV-infected health care workers to continue full practice, including highly invasive procedures. The risk of HIV transmission should not be trivialized, but it should be addressed in the context of the true issue of patient safety. The "right to know" approach toward HIV infection is a "clear illustration of the double standards at work in HIV-related injuries, a phenomenon that should be tolerated neither by law nor by public health."[32]

A More Reasonable Approach

Modern medical facilities remain hostile to both patients and physicians despite the high standards set for performance, the use of equipment, infection control, and health hazards. To be sure, the risk of HIV transmission in the workplace is real. However, unusual circumstances should not dictate broad policy questions because these circumstances instinctively prompt emotional and phobic reactions that fail to address the central question: how can we best protect patients (and physicians) from HIV infection? The transmission of HIV from health care workers to patients is likely to increase during procedures in which the operative field cannot be fully visualized.[6] Factors like the duration of an operation and/or the frequent use of sharp instruments in body cavities also increase the risks of HIV infection.[6] Therefore, policy makers should turn their attention to those particular practices and procedures that facilitate HIV transmission and to the need for proper disinfection of instruments that otherwise could result in cross contamination from patient to patient. The use of universal barrier precautions, to date, has resulted in a reduction of the frequency of some type of blood exposure.[24] To further reduce this risk, the development of new technologies and techniques should be encouraged. Scrupulously enforced infection control practices of all surgeons, not just those who are HIV infected, could be a far better and more effective means of reducing exposure to blood-borne pathogens than attempts at removing infected health care workers from the workplace. Obviously, the use of precautions will not reduce the frequency of surgical accidents (e.g., needlesticks or other sharp injuries).[24] Thus, there should also be mandatory ongoing education and training of all health care professionals in both hospitals and private practices in the use of instruments and techniques. For example, the New York State Department of Health has called for mandatory infection control training for purposes of licensing of all health care workers, recognizing that "HIV infection alone is not sufficient justification to limit the professional duties of health care professionals unless specific factors compromise a worker's ability to meet infection-control standards or to provide quality patient care."[33] This is, I believe, is a step in the right direction.

Medical centers and service chiefs should: (1) discuss and monitor a physician's competence to perform medical and surgical procedures that lead to HIV transmission; (2) institute good infection control policies and practices; (3) scrupulously examine all surgeons' and physicians' techniques and procedures; and (4) reinforce compliance with then policy of universal barrier precautions and infection control practices. Noncompliance could be deterred by the threat of professional (or legal) sanctions, or other relevant disciplinary actions. All parties need to be educated about the actual risk or absence of risk of HIV transmission and to explicitly agree on the private and confidential nature of these discussions.

There may come a time when it is determined that a significant risk of transmission does exist, despite appropriate precautions and training. For instance, studies of HBV outbreaks have identified certain procedures such a vaginal hysterotomy as inherently more likely to lead to infection in patients. When this determination is established for HIV through prospective studies like those conducted by Tokars *et al.*[34] it would be appropriate to limit the practice of health care professionals to procedures that do not present such risks. But restriction must be addressed within the context of "true" patient safety.

Conclusion

More than a year after the Behringer decision, experts continue to discuss the proper approach to the issues of policy restrictions and patients' right to know, and there have been almost no changes in laws or policies. This is because society is looking for someone to blame, and discrimination and punitive reactions against patients with AIDS have sadly remained prominent almost everywhere. A (mis)perception exists that HIV-infected individuals ought to be punished for their "unacceptable," "dangerous," or "immoral" behaviors. Ultimately, as it is always the case in the time of an epidemic, perceptions are more important to public policymaking than is reality, and public health officials must address these perceptions accordingly. If these perceptions cannot be persuasively dispelled through explicit and culturally appropriate education, i.e., behavioral changes towards patients with AIDS, then sound scientific, epidemiologic, and medical evidence may have only a modes influence on national health policy. Failure to dispel such perceptions could result in more panic and fear among patients and no improvement in the safety of health care for either patients or physicians.

Notes

1. Survey finds doctors and nurses favor getting AIDS tests. *New York Times* 1991 June 15: A-11; Many doctors infected with AIDS don't follow new US guidelines. *New York Times* 1991 Aug. 18:A-20.
2. Centers for Disease Control. Recommendations for preventing transmission of infection with human T-lymphotropic virus type lll/lymphadenopathy associated virus in the workplace, *MMWR Morb Mortal Wkly Rep* 1985;34:681-95.
3. Gostin LO. The AIDS litigation project, A national review of court and human rights commission decisions. Part 1: The social impact of AIDS: Part 2: Discrimination, *Journal of the American Medical Association* 1990;263:1961-70, 2086-92.
4. Centers for Disease Control. Update: Transmission of HIV infection during an invasive dental procedure-Florida, *MMWR Morb Mortal Wkly Rep* 1991;40:21-7, 33.
5. American Medical Association. *Statement on HIV-infected physicians*. January 17, 1991.
6. Centers for Disease Control. Recommendations for preventing transmission of human immunodeficiency virus and hepatitis B virus to patients during exposure-prone invasive procedures, *MMWR Morb Mortal Wkly Rep* 1991;40:1-9. No. RR-8.

7. Centers for Disease Control. Revised recommendations for preventing transmission of human immunodeficiency virus and hepatitis B to patients during invasive procedures, Draft. November 27, 1991.
8. *William Behringer v. The Medical Center at Princeton*. N.J. Superior Court Law Division, Mercer County. Docket No L 88-2550. Decided: April 25, 1991.
9. Annas GJ, Glantz LH, Manner WK. The right of privacy protects the doctor-patient relationship, *Journal of the American Medical Association* 1990;263:858-61.
10. The Confidentiality of HIV-Related Information Act. 35 P.S.: 7601-12 (Purdon Supp. 1991).
11. Siegler M. Confidentiality in medicine -- a decrepit concept, *New England Journal of Medicine* 1982;307:1519-21. Annas GJ. *The Rights of Patients*. Totowa, NJ: Humana Press, 1992:160-74.
12. New Jersey Stat. Ann;10:5-4.
13. *The Americans With Disability Act of 1990*. H. Rept. 101-558. Washington DC: Government Printing Office, 1990.
14. Hopkins to alert patients of doctor who died of AIDS. *The Sun* (Baltimore)1990 Dec. 2:A-1. 5,000 told their doctor had AIDS. *Philadelphia Inquirer* 1991 June 2:A-14. Doctor infected with AIDS virus urges his patients to get tested. *New York Times* 1991 June 17:A-13. Doctor has AIDS virus, 442 are informed. *New York Times* 1991 June 20:A-15.
15. Test all hospital patients for AIDS. New Jersey doctors urge. *New York Times* 1991 May 1:B-1.
16. Medical groups balk at rules for AIDS risk. *New York Times* 1990 Aug. 30:A-1, 19.
17. Many states tackling issue of AIDS-infected health care workers. *Boston Globe* 1991 May 27:29.
18. Application of Milton S. Hershey Medical Center of Pennsylvania State University and Harrisburg Hospital. Appeal of: John Doe, M.D. Pennsylvania. Superior Court. 1991. Lexis 2178.
19. *Leckett v. Board of Commissioners of Hospital* District 1. 909 F 2d 820. 5th cir. 1990.
20. Angell M. A dual approach to the AIDS epidemic, *New England Journal of Medicine* 1991;324: 1498-500. See also: Bayer R. Public health policy and the AIDS epidemic, *New England Journal of Medicine* 1991;324:1500-4, and Brennan TA. Transmission of the human immunodeficiency virus in the health care setting, time for action, *New England Journal of Medicine* 1991;324:1504-9.
21. Palca J. CDC closes the cases of the Florida dentist, *Science* 1992;256:1130-1. See also: Smith TF, Warweman MS. The continuing case of the Florida dentist, *Science* 1992;256:1155-6, and Ou C, Ciesielski CA, Myers G, *et al*. Molecular epidemiology of HIV transmission in a dental practice, *Science* 1992;256:1165-71.
22. Lowenfelds AB, Wormser G. Letter, *New England Journal of Medicine* 1991;326:12.
23. Centers for Disease Control. Update: Investigations of patients who have been treated by HIV-infected health care workers, *MMWR Morb Mortal Wkly Rep* 1992;42:344-6. See also: Mishu B, Schaffner W, Horan JM, *et al*. A surgeon with AIDS. Lack of evidence of transmission to patients, *Journal of the American Medical Association* 1990;264:467-70.
24. Nichols RL. Percutaneous injuries during operation: Who is at risk for what? *Journal of the American Medical Association* 1992;267:2938-9.
25. Bell DM. Human immunodeficiency virus transmission in health care settings: Risk, and risk reduction, *American Journal of Medicine* 1991;91(Suppl 3B):294S-300S.
26. Rogers DE, Osborn JE. Another approach to the AIDS epidemic, *New England Journal of Medicine* 1991;325(11):806-8.
27. Glantz LH, Mariner WK, Annas GJ. Risky business: Setting public health policy for HIV-infected health care professionals, *Milbank Quarterly* 1992;70(1):43-78.
28. Breenan TA, Leape LL, Laird NM, *et al*. Incidence of adverse events and negligence in hospitalized patients: Results of the Harvard Medical Practice Study l, *New England Journal of Medicine* 1991;324:370-6.
29. President's Commission for the Study of Ethical Problems in Medicine and Biomedical and Behavioral Research. *Making Healthcare Decisions*. Washington, DC: Government Printing Office, 1982.
30. When doctor has AIDS, *The National Law Journal* 1991.
31. Daniels N. HIV-infected professionals, patient rights, and the switching dilemma, *Journal of the American Medical Assocation* 1992;267:1368-71.
32. Barnes M, Rango NA, Burke GR, *et al*. The HIV-infected health care professional: Employment policies and public health, *Law, Medicine, and Health Care* 1990;18:311-30.

33. U.S. drops it plans to ease rules on doctors with AIDS. *Washington Post* 1992 June 14:A-9. Altman LK. U.S. to let states set rules on AIDS related health care workers. *New York Times* 1992 June 15:C-7.

34. Tokars Jl, Bell DM, Culver DH, *et al*. Percutaneous injuries during surgical procedures, *Journal of the American Medical Assocation* 1992;267:2899-904. See also: Mandelbrot DA, Smythe RW, Norman SA, *et al*. A survey of exposures, practices and recommendations of surgeons in the care of patients with human immunodeficiency virus, *Surgery, Gynecolog,& Obstetrics* 1990;171:99-106.

SECTION 6

TRANSPLANT

Chapter 38

Cases 6.0

Case 6.1: NONCOMPLIANCE AND KIDNEY TRANSPLANT

R.O. is a 28-year-old male. At age 17, he was diagnosed with ESRD, and went for dialysis. During the next three years, he chronically signed off dialysis early, and was judged to be extremely noncompliant with diet and other medical directions. During this time the staff struggled with offering the option of nontreatment, but decided instead to continue to persuade the young man to stay on dialysis until a kidney became available. Particularly annoying to the staff was the patient's habit of arriving on a day and time other than his appointment, or arriving for his appointment sometimes 30, sometimes 60, and sometimes even 90 minutes late. They wondered if they should have told him to come back on his own day and time, given his extreme noncompliance. That might have been dangerous for his life. Or if he came late for his actual appointment, were they obligated to keep the unit open in "overtime" in the evening in order to give him his full 4 hour dialysis?

Eight years ago, at age 20, he received a living related kidney transplant from one of his brothers. But he recently lost it secondary to medication noncompliance. He is not yet back on dialysis, but will soon have to be. Meanwhile, 4 other brothers are now willing to donate a kidney.

The patient's history is significant for drug abuse, including intravenous cocaine and crack, but he claims to be clear for the last two years.

Some questions that preoccupy the team are:

1. Is the patient a fit recipient for another live donor transplant?

2. Should they require another course of dialysis before they risk the second live donor transplant?

3. If they do, and the patient remains so noncompliant, can they refuse to do a transplant, even though the brothers are willing?

4. Should they consider, instead, a cadaver transplant, that has a slightly less positive outcome, since it would seem only just that the live donor organ be given to someone who is more compliant?

5. Will sharing this discussion and their concerns with the patient be seen as coercive, particularly since he has had a history of drug abuse in the past? Should that history now be ignored? Factored in?

6. If no discussion of these concerns takes place with the patient now, is there not a danger of waiting until he is in "total system failure" later, when he would not be competent to makes his wishes known?

7. Just how sick does an individual have to be before we intervene and place them on dialysis, or later when the disease has run its course, decide to take them off?

In general, is noncompliance a sufficient ethical reason to deprive individuals of lifesaving medical care? Could it ever be used as a general principle of justice in allocating health care?

Case 6.2: **JAY'S LIVER TRANSPLANT**

Jay B. is mellower now that he is 46-years-old. His life has been a course of one crisis after the other. Now he faces the possibility of a second liver transplant. He is sick and scared.

He was born in the Midwest into a family of alcoholics. His Dad, Mom, and 3 brothers all share the family history of abuse. He has abused alcohol for 20 years himself.

Two years ago his liver failed. He stopped drinking at that time. One year later he got hepatitis. This year he was admitted to the hospital with two other life-threatening conditions, esophageal varices that bled uncontrollably, and later, toxic encephalopathy. He has been ready to "hang up the spikes" a number of times.

He was evaluated as a good candidate for a liver and kidney transplant upon his third hospitalization for the year for liver and kidney failure (he was put on dialysis), and pulmonary edema. Waiting much longer would be fatal to him. Normally, centers establish a five-year alcohol-free period before considering individuals as proper candidates. But the medical center evaluating Jay is anxious to become a major transplant center. The transplant physicians here were trained by the major academic centers in the country doing liver transplants, including Stanford and University of Chicago. They were recruited with this aim in mind by the hospital board.

In September, therefore, Jay received his first liver and kidney transplant. The operation "vamperized" the city blood bank. It took 112 units of packed cells, 152 units of frozen plasma, 120 units of platelets, and 107 units of other blood products.

Post-operatively Jay did alright, but the liver and kidney did not function up to capacity. Eventually, the liver failed again, as did his kidney function. The kidney function would probably be reversible if his liver function were normal. Thus, a second liver transplant is being contemplated. The kidney will be assessed if the liver transplant is successful.

There are many other individuals on the list awaiting an available liver. Jay is now only marginally responsive. The team must decide whether to pursue a second liver transplant.

Consider the following questions:

1. Who is and who is not a proper candidate for transplant? Should alcoholism be considered as a disease, or should a time for disease free behavior be set. Was two years enough? Or should the Center have insisted on five?

2. How much treatment for Jay is adequate? What if this liver fails too? Meagan LaRocco, a baby in Chicago got a total of five before she left the hospital alive.

3. How can bleeding the blood bank dry be justified for one patient? But is it right to ask such access questions at the bedside?

More general questions of access to health care bother the team as well. Does it make sense to expend this much energy and care on one individual, when the costs of health care are so prohibitive for so many people? When almost 30 million people cannot gain access to health care, is it right even to start this liver transplant program for the marginal few individuals who might profit from it? In the Oregon plan for allocating medical services for the poor (Medicaid), the principle is used of supplying care first that will benefit the most people with the least risk. Should this not be the primary principle of access to health care?

Case 6.3: A SECOND CHANCE

Sally is an 18-year-old African American female with a congenital kidney defect which required transplantation three years ago. This was accomplished successfully and over the past three years she has been followed closely by her nephrologist. Sally has no other medical problems. She does, however, have the disadvantage of a poor socioeconomic situation.

Her parents had a difficult divorce complicated by bitter feelings and many arguments over custody of the children. Sally resides with her mother, who is deaf, and her two siblings, all of whom are on welfare. Of the four children in the family, three suffered from the same congenital renal problem: Sally, a brother, who died at the age of fifteen because of renal problems, and another brother, who was also transplanted and is currently doing well. Of all the members of the family, it is commonly thought that Sally is the most mature.

In March of last year, Sally was admitted to a university transplant center because of chronic rejection of her transplanted kidney. It was later determined that this rejection was secondary to noncompliance with the prescribed medical regimen. At first she was managed medically with high dose steroids and immunosuppressives, but once it was realized that her rejection had gone too far for conservative management alone, she was immediately put back on the renal transplant list.

Consider these questions:

1. You are a physician and a member of the team at your medical center that decides which individuals will be placed on the list for renal transplants. Should Sally be placed on the list for a second transplant?

In discussing the answer to this question, consider Sally's age and her socioeconomic status. Should the poor, who have less control over resources, be given special attention in this regard? Or should it be the other way around? What factors will you consider in your deliberations?

----

original case by: Sharon E. O'Brien

Case 6.4: THE MENTALLY RETARDED AS ORGAN DONORS

J.S. has been diagnosed with nephrosclerosis caused by hypertension. Mr. S. is 43-years-old and married with a 16-year-old daughter. He has two brothers. His brother Michael is 39-years-old, severely retarded, and mentally incompetent. He has been institutionalized for the majority of his life. Mr. S.'s parents are guardians for Michael.

In July, 1990, Mr. S.'s wife approached the transplant team about the possibility of her husband being evaluated for renal transplantation. During this initial discussion, when the question of a living donor was raised, Mrs. S. said that the family wanted Michael to be the donor.

The transplant team indicated their severe reservations at that time about Michael being an acceptable donor for his brother. The essence of their concern centered on the problem of using patients that cannot consent for themselves to help others, like the problem of conceiving fetuses to function as organ or bone marrow transplant donors that had been in the news at the time.

Nonetheless, Mr. S.'s health has been deteriorating. He had been encouraged since September to begin dialysis but had not done so. On December 17, 1990, Mr. S. was admitted to the emergency room at a suburban hospital where he underwent dialysis.

Mr. S. may be an appropriate candidate for living or cadaver transplantation. To date, he has not pursued evaluation for renal transplantation. Therefore, he is not currently listed on any organ donation waiting list for renal transplant. There are now, however, over 20,000 people in the United States waiting for kidney transplants on that list, and nowhere near enough organs.

Shortly after the wife's indication to the transplant team that the family would like Michael, the retarded brother, to function as a live donor, an ethics consult meeting was held to discuss issues surrounding the use of a retarded person in this way. Present at the meeting were the transplant surgeon, the medicine service, renal dialysis team members, nurses, a psychologist, a social worker, a risk management specialist, two medical students, residents, and the ethics consult service on-call member that month.

Not all individuals have the capacity for self determination; age, illness, or mental disability, for example, influence one's ability to make autonomous decisions. Because of their diminished autonomy, these individuals may be vulnerable to manipulation or coercion. An appeal to the principle of respect for persons requires protection for those with diminished autonomy. In our society, there is a long tradition that guarantees the protection of vulnerable populations such as the mentally retarded, mentally incompetent, children, or prisoners, in the medical arena (see the Belmont Report, National Commission for the Protection of Human Subjects of Biomedical and Behavioral Research, Washington D.C., DHEW Pub. No. (05) 78-0012, 1978).

Michael's high level of mental incompetence and the severity of his mental retardation indicate that he would not be able to participate in a decision concerning his status as an organ donor. Informed consent is not possible because of his inability to comprehend the situation. In some cases involving mental incompetency (e.g., a case in which a patient is terminally ill and comatose), decisions are made for the patient by family members. Normally, in these situations, it is possible to learn how the patient might make a decision concerning medical treatment either by an advanced directive such as a living will, or by examining lifestyle choices and statements made to others. This would constitute the patient's value history. In Michael's case, because of the severity of his mental disability, the family cannot know what Michael would want, either now or in the future.

Further, although Mr. S.'s life expectancy may be increased if he were to be the recipient of an organ from his brother, he could live for an indefinite period of time on dialysis. Additionally, if he chose, Mr. S. could be evaluated for renal transplantation and be placed on a waiting list for a cadaveric organ.

The majority view, then could be summarized as follows: Michael should not be considered as an organ donor for his brother because: (1) he is unable to make autonomous decisions due to his severe retardation; therefore, he cannot provide informed consent; (2) his diminished autonomy requires that he be protected from undue manipulation and harm; and (3) the potential risks for Michael, should he be a donor, outweigh the anticipated benefits for Mr. S.; at this time, Mr. S. has two alternatives for medical treatment (dialysis or cadaver donation).

Despite these arguments, a minority of the individuals present at the ethics consult service meeting thought differently. Their approach was frankly utilitarian. They argued that the risk to Michael would be minimum compared to the long-term benefits of a live-donor transplant for Mr. S. Mr. S.' health has entered a deteriorating phase. Dialysis, although an alternative as present, is a debilitating experience over the long term, especially were Mr. S.

to try to keep his job and maintain his place in his family.

Furthermore, Mr. S.' parents, the legal guardians for Michael, are presumably competent to act in the best interests of Michael by functioning as surrogate decision-makers in this regard. The fact that he cannot consent and is vulnerable is adequately provided for in the law by so designating his parents as legal surrogates in this regard.

Some of the minority were concerned, rather, with the problem of assessing how "connected" Mr. S. might be with his brother, Michael. Did he visit him regularly? Others of the minority thought that this concern was irrelevant to the case. If the parents were proper legal guardians, why could they not consent to the procedure that would bring about the greatest benefit to all parties with the least harm to a fully-functioning person in society, and minimum harm to Michael. They argued further that, were Michael competent, he may very well consent to aid his brother. This altruism ought to be presumed on the part of the mentally retarded, especially since they are recipients of the care and concern of this family and of the community in providing for them in institutions.

What would be your recommendation to the transplant team?

Case 6.5: THE RETARDED AS ORGAN RECIPIENTS

On March 3, an attending pediatric nephrologist initiated an ethics consult to discuss ethical dilemmas associated with the care of a child named Allison. At the time, Allison was 12 years old; she had just been admitted again to a university medical center, but had been followed by the nephrologist and a colleague for one year.

Allison was born with multiple problems. Her primary diagnosis was fetal alcohol syndrome. Following premature birth, she had a large intraventricular hemorrhage leading to marked microcephaly. She is also blind, and is profoundly mentally retarded. Two years ago she was not considered a candidate for repair of severe scoliosis because of poor pulmonary/lung status. She is fed through a gastrostomy tube and is a permanent resident of a state Children's Hospital; she is a ward of the state.

A year ago when she was admitted to the medical center for a kidney biopsy after developing abnormal lab values. The biopsy revealed membranaproliferative glomerulonephritis with scarring. This is a progressive disease.

During the two weeks prior to the current admission, Allison exhibited complications of kidney failure, i.e., hypertension, significant hyperkalemia, and tremors. She receives Apresoline and Kayexalate. Her blood pressure ranges from 113/72 to 140/74. She requires frequent blood tests. When Allison was admitted on March 2nd, she was in renal failure. Tests results indicate that she might be a candidate for a kidney transplantation.

Ordinarily, a patient in Allison's condition would be dialyzed. However, due to her severe retardation, the nephrologist and other staff members are opposed to instituting dialysis. Dialysis three times a week would need to take place at the medical center. Allison would be subjected to extreme discomfort and suffering that she simply could not comprehend.

Originally (over a year ago) the attending physician requested that the Children's Hospital provide some direction regarding Allison's care. Their hospital ethics committee held a meeting on March 3. They were unanimous in their view that it would be inappropriate to "consider Allison for dialysis and eventual transplantation" because it would subject her to "extensive pain and suffering; very frequent blood drawings; surgical insertion and maintenance of dialysis lines; frequent transportation to dialysis center or hospital; extensive and serious complications from immunosuppressive medications; the very real risk of transplant rejection and need for further dialysis and re-transplantation." Moreover, the committee stated that Allison's weak pulmonary and orthopedic status would make all surgical interventions hazardous. The committee requested that Allison's guardian to consider these issues and advise them of any decision about her continued care.

The Assistant Guardianship Administrator of the Department of Children and Family Services (DCFS) stated that, in view of the circumstances, she would not recommend surgical intervention and/or the transplant. However, on April 30, about a month after the original admission, the Administrator called the staff and said that she had spoken with "a physician, an ethicist, and a judge." She said that DCFS may be compelled to consider the transplantation. She said the judge indicated that this decision would be based on the fact that the kidney failure was not a direct result of the Fetal Alcohol Syndrome and that Allison would probably die without a transplant.

Now, a year later, considerable difficulties remain. The medical center ethics consultant met with the managing physician a day after the admission. After hearing about the case, and reading the recommendations of the ethics committee and the guardianship Administrator, she suggested that it had similarities to the Saikewiez (S.) case In that case, S. had been hospitalized from age one because of severe mental retardation. At the age of 67, he was diagnosed with leukemia. The state hospital did not want to subject S. to the pain of chemotherapy. After many disputes, the court ruled in their favor because of the "quality of life" he was likely to experience under treatment. The court's judgment was based on concerns that Saikewicz would not understand the environment and the treatments, and that this would cause him undue fear and suffering.

Comparing the case directly, however, may be difficult. The reason is that adult onset leukemia rarely can be cured. But Allison may receive significant improvement not only in her life-span, but also in the management of her symptoms. The Chidren's Hospital ethics committee noted that drawing blood more than 3 times a week "would be impossible." But without the transplant, she may live out her remaining days in a high technology medical center environment, rather than in her accustomed "home." Further, the Saikewicz case occurred before the Americans with Disabilities Act that forbids discrimination against anyone solely on the basis of their handicap.

In discussing the issue the ethics consultant emphasized the importance of distinguishing between making a quality of life judgment about Allison's status as a mentally retarded person and making a quality of life decision in regard to the pain and suffering she would undergo in dialysis and possible transplantation. In other words, from an ethical standpoint, the decision to withhold therapy from Allison cannot be based on the fact that she is mentally retarded, but rather, because she would be subjected to enormous pain and suffering that she would be incapable of understanding. Additionally, in this case, her underlying physical conditions alone do not appear to suggest that dialysis or transplantation would be indicated.

On March 8, the attending reported that he spoke with the guardian. He mentioned the Saikewicz case to her. She recognized it and said that she would "check it out" -- meaning that she would pursue discussion of whether or not the state had a compelling interest to medically intervene. She appeared very cautious about the hidden "discrimination" she detected in the distinction between the retarded's quality of life and the medical quality of life, as proposed by the ethics consultant. After all, part of Allison's handicap is a result of the circumstances of her birth, over which she had no control. To draw this distinction requires us to abstract from Allison's real life some sort of Platonic ideal wherein her retardation (and other handicaps) are different from her medical conditions. Doesn't the distinction simply reinforce our instincts, she asked? It permits us to do what we want anyway.

The attending physician continues his opposition to transplantation.

What would you recommend?

Chapter 39

Transplant Recipient Selection: Peacetime vs. Wartime Triage

Rosamond Rhodes, Charles Miller, and Myron Schwartz

Transplantation has become the accepted treatment for certain end stage diseases, allocation of cadaver organs has become a crucial moral problem. Concern over the appropriateness of distribution procedures reflects the recognition that allocation must be both just and fair. Selection of organ recipients should be seen as an instance of distributive justice.

The reality of a scarce supply of donor organs in the face of the inexorable progression of end stage organ failure leaves patients dying on waiting lists before receiving transplants. The current U.S. distribution policy gives allocation priority to those critically ill patients who have been shown to have the least chance of achieving one year survival. Conceptually, this approach can be viewed as an attempt to apply the principles of "peacetime triage" where, in fact, the limited organ resource creates a situation more akin to that seen when dealing with casualties on the battlefield.

This paper argues for acknowledging the fact that it is impossible to offer grafts to every patient, and advocates a policy which rationally accommodates the shortfall situation according to the principles of "wartime triage." Without adopting utilitarianism, the policy we advocate uses the concept of benefit as the criterion for patient selection. This policy proposes forgoing transplantation in a group of patients with the least chance of survival, equal in number to the shortfall of donor organs. This would then allow for the transplantation of the remaining candidates by first treating those with urgent need and the rest on a first-come-first-served basis.

Using criteria such as have been developed by Shaw *et al.*, the patients least likely to survive can be identified. Periodic review of referral patterns and deaths on the waiting list enables the refinement of criteria for candidate acceptability according to the wartime triage principle.

The Problem

It is a common assumption in ethics that everyone is due equal access to basic human goods.[1] In our modern society, at least since the French Revolution, health care is counted along with food, shelter, and security as such a basic good. Anyone suffering from a treatable life-threatening disease can, therefore, be seen as having a *prima facie* claim on medical treatment.[2,3,4,5,6]

Since transplantation has become a clinical reality, the obvious implication is that anyone suffering from the failure of a transplantable vital organ should receive a transplant. We

---

Source: Reprinted from *Cambridge Quarterly of Healthcare Ethics*, Vol. 4, 1992, pp. 327-331, with permission from The Cambridge University Press © 1992.

know, however, that everyone who needs an organ cannot be offered one because there are not enough to go around. Emerging from this scarcity is the problem of how to distribute the short supply of transplantable organs. Who should get them? Who should be left out? How should we decide? Should our allocation policy consider patients' past contributions to society, their future contributions, their contribution to their own illness, how long they have already lived, their life expectancy, the urgency of their need, or none of the above? While the distinction between medical and social criteria may not be as sharp as we would like,[7] current policy focuses on medical criteria, reflecting the ethical position that there are no other differences among people so significant as to disqualify some or give preference to others in their access to health resources. In this paper we present and argue for a workable and intuitively satisfying (albeit at times uncomfortable) model for decision making in the allocation of organs that focuses on medical differences while attempting to maximize outcome in a way that is both fair and just.

Examing the Old Rule: Peacetime Triage

While all are due equal access to health care, it often happens that at the moment need arises there is a shortage of either care providers or health facilities, or both. In the emergency room, the doctor's office, and the hospital admissions office, this common problem of short supply is managed without compromising our commitment to meeting the needs of all patients. To save lives and minimize harm, the most urgent cases are taken first, while the less urgent are seen according to the order in which they arrive. In this way, everyone's health care needs receive attention, although some people must wait longer than others. True, we find ourselves annoyed when we must wait for routine care; yet, when waiting to see the doctor for, say, a skin rash, we understand that the person who came in later but is bleeding should be seen before us. We would want the same consideration in the event that we were urgently ill.

This approach serves us well in the distribution of most health care resources; it fails us, however, if we attempt to allocate organs for transplantation in this way. The scarcity of donor organs in the face of the inexorable progression of end-stage organ failure results in the harsh reality that some patients die before receiving a transplant. Refusing to change our approach is futile. It would require us to continue trying to give organs to all candidates but, in fact, allocating the limited supply primarily to those with the most urgent need. The recipients would thus be those critically ill patients who have been shown time and again to have the least chance of achieving one year survival.[8] Meanwhile, the patients in less urgent need, whose chances of success would be far greater, are left waiting on a list to get sicker, either dying or coming to transplant when they themselves are critically ill, thus perpetuating a vicious cycle of medical and ethical failure. We cannot pretend to have no responsibility for such worst case outcomes because, in fact, it is our responsibility. We therefore need to explore the adoption of a new principle for governing organ allocation -- one that may well entail our refusing to offer this treatment to some patients.

Abandoning the Old Rule

We have learned from Kant that "ought" implies "can." In other words, when something cannot be done, it cannot be our duty to do it; our ethical commitments cannot exceed the limitations of possibility. In the context of transplantation, failure to give some people the organs they need, therefore, is not inherently unethical. Failing to distribute the available organs in accordance with the principles of fairness and justice, however, would be wrong.

Fairness demands that we treat people equally. A policy based on fairness alone would place all candidates (for whom the potential benefits of transplantation outweigh risks) on equal footing. A lottery which distributes equally the chance of getting an organ would satisfy the fairness standard. A first-come-first-served arrangement might also count as providing equal treatment (such an approach, however, presumes equal access to health care). By ignoring the differences among candidates -- life expectancy, urgency of need, and likelihood of survival, for example -- we would, however, be ignoring the demands of justice. Justice requires that we give each person what he or she is due. A policy that is both fair and just examines the differences among patients, and then treats similar differences similarly. With this in mind, let us recast our dilemma, using the analogy of triage on the battlefield.

Adopting a New Rule: Wartime Triage

Triage is the process of sorting the sick and wounded on the basis of urgency so that they can be properly directed for care.

For the civilian population in times of peace, American society has deemed health care to be every individual's right and has provided considerable resources to render this care. We have already outlined the way in which we have chosen to distribute these resources, treating the urgently ill first and then giving routine care on a first-come-first-served basis. This might aptly be labeled "peacetime triage" (PTT). Peacetime triage is the guiding principle behind the organ distribution system currently in use in our country. However, the situation with the shortage of organs leading to deaths on the waiting list more closely resembles the predicament encountered by the medic out on the battlefield. Faced with large numbers of casualties and clearly unable to care for all, the medic must devote his efforts to the salvage of those who are most likely to benefit from his intervention while leaving the most critically injured, who have but little hope of survival, to die. We believe that fairness and justice would be best served by applying the concept of "wartime triage" (WTT) to the formulation of a new organ allocation policy. Let us examine how this might work.

Since benefit to the patient is the primary criterion for receiving an organ, the degree of benefit to be expected is the most meaningful and relevant difference among patients; lack of benefit, or degree of medical risk, is the primary basis for rejecting a candidate. Guided by the WTT principle, we would stratify all potential candidates into three groups. A group of patients with the least chance of survival, that is equal in number to the shortfall of donor organs, would first be trimmed from the list; we would forgo transplanting these patients. The remaining candidates would be divided into two groups: those in relatively urgent need, and those more able to wait in line. The patients in these two groups would be transplanted according to the PTT principle.

The WTT concept is not utilitarian, although at first glance it might appear to be. A policy grounded in utilitarian theory would maximize graft longevity by selecting potential candidates according to the likelihood of survival and life expectancy. Utilitarians would offer grafts first to those with the best chance for the longest survival; the young and the healthy would always be taken first, then the older and the less healthy; the old and sick would always be assigned the lowest priority.[9] The WTT principle is essentially different, attempting to maximize outcome in a way that is perhaps more just. The highest-risk patients are denied treatment only to the extent dictated by the organ shortage; all others, sick and well alike, are transplanted according to the PTT guidelines.

Using the greatest medical risk rejection criterion in a WTT-based policy has the significant value of broad intuitive appeal and minimal discomfort of the conscience. What discomfort we do feel arises from our reluctance to refuse treatment to some of those who are in need -- in fact, the neediest. Denying anyone a basic human good should make an ethical being uncomfortable. However, refusing to withhold transplantation from those least likely to benefit in times of organ shortage would clearly be an ethically worse choice because it would cause harm to many more who would likely have derived greater benefit.[8] For this reason, WTT appears to be a principle that could be accepted by policymakers behind the

Rawlsian veil of ignorance.

Painful Selections

How should the WTT model be implemented? Ideally, this would occur at the national level. The United Network for Organ Sharing (UNOS) currently gathers the data that would be required to structure such a system. We know how many patients are listed for transplantation; recent figures enable us to project how many donors will be available and how many patients will die waiting. The expected donor shortfall could readily be estimated. National implementation, however, would require the adoption of a single national waiting list and the promulgation of uniform candidate selection criteria that would eliminate the requisite number of the highest-risk patients from consideration on an equitable basis among centers. We all understand that this may not be easy to actualize.

A simpler way of approximating a WTT-based system can readily be instituted by individual centers. Each transplant center can adopt a survival goal that attempts to balance justice and fairness with the reality of organ scarcity. The likelihood of survival is primarily a function of medical risk factors, although the experience of the transplant team also plays a role. By varying the mix of high- and low-risk candidates, one year survival rates from 60 to 90% could readily be achieved by most centers. Pinpointing the survival goal that will enable a center to distribute all of its organ supply while leaving no likely transplant survivors without an organ is probably as difficult as collecting exactly the amount of manna from heaven so as to meet but not to exceed one's daily needs. Over time, however, this goal can be approached by creating a servomechanism wherein periodic examination of the center's experience as regards candidate selection, deaths on the waiting list, and survival post-transplant leads to periodic adjustment of the goal through revision of candidate acceptance criteria according to the WTT principle.

An extremely important question remains to be asked. Is there a way of assessing risk or likelihood of benefit that can reliably be used as the basis for candidate rejection in a WTT-based model? In a 1989 report, Shaw *et al.* stratified their liver transplant candidates into high-, medium-, and low-risk groups and noted that the actuarial 1-year survival rate for patients scored as having high risk was 44.5%.[8] This high risk group accounted for 21.7% of their series. The medium and low risk groups had survival rates of 85% and 90.4%, respectively. This report suggests that it is indeed possible to preoperatively identify a subset of transplant candidates with a substantially reduced likelihood of survival following transplantation.

There is a second group of patients to be considered in this regard -- patients with diseases like hepatitis-B and hepatocellular carcinoma that tend to recur following transplantation. Although these patients may not be at high risk for perioperative mortality according to criteria such as those developed by Shaw *et al.*, they, nevertheless, have significantly reduced graft and patient survival rates. A more far-sighted view of survivability should be included, as well, in our formulation of WTT.

Reality

We have conceptualized a rational framework for organ distribution. Can it bear up under the weight of reality? For the time being, consideration of recent UNOS statistics suggests that the answer is yes. In 1990, 377 patients died awaiting liver transplantation while 2627 were transplanted, a ratio of 1:7; from January to June of 1991, there were 258 deaths on the waiting list while 1377 patients received transplants, yielding a ratio of 1:5 (personal communication, D. Ferree, Director of Policy Development, UNOS). Admittedly, these numbers do not tell the whole story. Still, they suggest that the current donor organ shortfall is on an order of magnitude of roughly 15%. Shaw's criteria identified 21% of candidates as having significantly increased risk. It appears, therefore, that present estimates of medical risk have the power and reliability to identify a sufficient number of low-survivability candidates to support a WTT-based system.

The number of patients dying on the list is rising as the number of patients listed for transplantation grows. In January of 1990, there were 938 patients listed and awaiting liver transplantation; in January of 1991, there were 1338. Yet, the number of transplants being performed has not increased over the past year. With the proliferation of liver transplantation and the increased awareness on the part of referring physicians of the promise of transplantation, this gap will continue to widen. Furthermore, with earlier referrals, improvements in treatment, and increased experience, the proportion of patients designated as high-risk will likely decrease.

The usefulness of WTT is limited by the number of patients who can be identified as having substantially increased risk. Once all high-risk candidates have been eliminated, estimates of small degrees of difference in probable benefit seem too uncertain a ground for excluding anyone from a potentially life-saving procedure. Using Shaw's criteria, for example, the difference between the 85% survival of the medium-risk group and the 90.4% survival of the low-risk group does not seem significant enough to justify treating needy individuals differently.

Conclusion

Those of us committed to transplantation must address the organ shortage from all angles. We must work to increase the donor supply through professional and public education, through technical and scientific advances such as splitting livers and the future use of xenografts, and, possibly, through legislation. In the face of the growing shortfall, we may be forced to begin factoring economic and social variables into our equation in ways we have to this point carefully avoided. We believe that the WTT model provides a rational foundation for the modification of current organ allocation policy that is firmly grounded in reality and that offers promise of improved outcome while remaining just and equitable.

Notes

1. Foot P. *Virtues and Vices*. Berkeley, CA: University of California Press, 1978:43.
2. Daniels N. Health care needs and distributive justice, *Philosophy & Public Affairs* 1981;10:146-155.
3. Daniels N. Equality of access to health care, *MMFQ* 1982;61.
4. Brody BA. Health care for the haves and have-nots: Toward a just basis of distribution. In: Schelp E, ed. *Justice and Health Care*. Dordrecht, The Netherlands: D. Reidel Publishing Company, 1981.
5. Veatch RM. What is 'just' health care delivery? In: Veatch RM, Branson R, eds. *Ethics and Health Policy*. Cambridge, MA: Ballinger Publishing Company, 1976:131-142.
6. Fried C. Equality and rights in medical care, *Hastings Center Report* 1976;6:29-34.
7. Veatch R. Allocating organs by utilitarianism is seen as favoring whites over blacks, *Kennedy Institute of Ethics Newsletter* 1989;3:1-3.
8. Shaw BW, Wood RP, Stratta RJ, *et al*. Stratifying the causes of death in liver transplant recipients, *Archives of Surgery* 1989;124:895-900.
9. Weinstein MC, Stason WB. Allocating resources: The case of hypertension, *Hastings Center Report* 1977;7:24-29.

Chapter 40

Reevaluation of Organ Transplantation Criteria -- Allocation of Scarce Resources to Borderline Candidates

Owen S. Surman and Ruth Purtilo

Organ transplantation in the 1960s proceeded according to a "lifeboat" ethics formula with physicians acting as "gatekeepers." Selection of transplant recipients is now based on medical urgency and waiting time. Some candidates continue to be given low priority by virtue of psychological impairment. The three As -- advanced age, acquired immune deficiency syndrome (or positive human immunodeficiency virus status), and alcoholism -- also stand out as characteristics that tend to exclude candidates. Cancer is another relative or absolute contraindication to transplantation. This article focuses retrospectively on the psychosocial and medical aspects of the decision to include six patients at Massachusetts General Hospital who were selected for organ transplantation despite their borderline candidacy. The authors introduce four lines of thinking that decision-makers might use to either include or exclude marginal candidates (e.g., the physician's interpretation of what duty requires, the patient's or surrogate's wishes, cost-benefit considerations, or the need for research to improve our scientific understanding of transplantation issues) and discuss an ethical approach that supports each line of thinking. The authors conclude that not all of the ethical approaches lead practitioners and policymakers to the same conclusions regarding the optimum size of or who should be a part of the recipient pool. The future of who receives transplants and why depends, at least in part, on the underlying ethical considerations that are deemed appropriate as determinants of practice and policy.

Organ transplantation is a growing medical field that offers the promise of meaningful life extension to individuals suffering from end organ disease. Advances in transplantation biology may some day allow for reduced cost and easy access to organs from non-human sources. The available technology is costly and dependent on limited access to cadaveric and living human donor organs.

In the 1960s when kidney transplantation emerged from the laboratory, a "lifeboat" ethics approach to resource allocation gave rise to committees, later referred to as "god squads," which endeavored to select organ recipients on a utilitarian, social-worth basis. The current approach to this distribution is defined by the United Network for Organ Sharing (UNOS). Medical urgency and waiting time determine priorities for cadaveric organ transplantation among those who meet medical criteria.

The limited availability of organs for transplantation, the morbidity associated with the waiting period, and the motivation for transplant centers to maintain good outcome statistics make it desirable to select candidates who are likely to be medically compliant and whose health status offers the best long-term prognosis. Thus, operationally, individuals with

---

Source: Reprinted from *Psychosomatics*, Vol. 33, No. 2, pp. 202-212, with permission from University Press of America © Spring, 1992.

multisystem disease, those from lower socioeconomic groups, older patients, and those with psychiatric impairment are less attractive to transplant centers.

The precise criteria for patient inclusion varies among centers and with the volume and experience of activity at a given center. A team with a well-established record of success can more easily include marginal candidates and assess the potential benefit in similar cases. For example, the University Health Center of Pittsburgh has an extensive history of liver transplantation and includes patients with liver failure secondary to alcoholic cirrhosis and hepatitis. Eighty such patients have received transplants to date, with a success rate similar to that of patients from other diagnostic groups.[1,2] Twenty-five transplant recipients at University Health Center of Pittsburgh have been human immunodeficiency virus (HIV) carriers, three with known infection prior to transplantation. Thirteen of the patients were living at a mean follow-up time of 2.75 years. Survival was greater among younger HIV positive patients.[3] Centers across the country acknowledge that otherwise healthy patients age 60 and older may experience an especially smooth post-transplant course with a minimum of rejection (Paul S. Russell, personal communication).

In this article, we draw selectively from experience in organ transplantation at Massachusetts General Hospital (MGH) to look at six cases in which marginal candidates have received organ transplants. We present these cases with an interest in how the selection process occurred and with a view toward clarifying the way in which each of four ethical models could expand or could restrict inclusion of potential organ transplant candidates, especially those candidates with challenging characteristics.

The ethical models we review are paths to decision-making about patient selection. We do not prescribe how these approaches are best combined, but aim to elucidate the process. Ultimately the reasoning behind a given model may have a tautologic function. We make clinical choices based on logic, but may elaborate the logic to justify the choices we make.

Methods

Each case is from the MGH Transplant Unit where one author (OS) participates actively in patient selection and perioperative care and the other author (RP) was available as an ethics consultant.

A patient who potentially might benefit from renal or hepatic transplantation is screened by a nephrologist or hepatologist who presents the case at weekly multidisciplinary transplant unit rounds. If the team agrees initially that the patient meets inclusion criteria, the transplantation surgeons, psychiatrist (OS), and relevant consultants (from endocrinology, infectious disease, nutrition, oral surgery, orthopedics, social service, etc.) assess the patient further. The patient then may be listed directly or reviewed again at team rounds if there is uncertainty about eligibility for transplantation.

Liver transplantation is performed by a four-hospital consortium, the Boston Center for Liver Transplantation (BCLT), which maintains a common set of criteria and meets monthly to review active cases. Selection policy is monitored by an ethics committee that meets quarterly. Both authors have served on this committee.

Case Reports

Case 1. Mr. A., a 60-year-old man, had been transferred from his local medical center with fulminant hepatitis A and progressive hepatic failure. He was a marginal candidate because of his age and level of morbidity. When placed on the recipient list for liver transplantation, Mr. A. was comatose, intubated for respiratory support, and receiving blood products and pressors for active gastrointestinal bleeding. Believing his death was imminent, the patient's wife and children were in contact with a funeral director.

Brief discussion
Age 60 is a relative contraindication for liver transplantation according to BCLT criteria. Although moribund from hepatic failure at the time of transplantation, Mr. A. had been in good general health prior to the onset of hepatitis A and was therefore believed to be a suitable candidate.

Post-transplant course
Six months after transplantation the patient was actively teaching. Stepping from an elevator during a routine follow-up visit, he energetically greeted author OS and proposed a tennis match. Mr. A. returned to academia until he reached retirement age. He continues in full recovery 5 years after his transplant.

Case 2. Mr. W., a 35-year-old man with hemophilia and liver failure secondary to non-A, non-B hepatitis, had become HIV positive prior to his referral for liver transplantation. Criteria for inclusion or exclusion of HIV-positive individuals had not been formalized by the BCLT at the time of consideration of his case. Aside from liver failure and his bleeding diathesis, the patient was in good general health and had enjoyed an active life style. He had excellent social supports and exceptional motivation.

Brief discussion
The team considered that immunosuppression might hasten the clinical presentation of AIDS, but there were no available data for HIV-positive candidates. It was hypothesized but not known if hemophilia would be cured by successful liver transplantation in this highly motivated and informed candidate.

Post-transplant course
The patient experienced full recovery for a year after transplantation. In addition to returning to work, Mr. W. found that he was able to perform many activities previously inaccessible because of the bleeding diathesis, which his new liver cured. He died 2 years after transplantation from AIDS.

Case 3. Ms. C., was a 20-year-old woman with multiple psychiatric hospitalizations and suicide gestures. Her emotional instability and active substance abuse were exclusionary factors for transplantation. Ms. C. was medically unstable on hemodialysis and in need of a kidney for optimal management of renal failure. The patient was an incest victim with poor social supports, active alcohol abuse, recurrent major depression, and anxiety (panic) disorder. Rejection of a prior kidney transplant was a result of noncompliance with prescribed medication. Prior use of steroids for immunosuppression was associated with complex partial seizures.

Brief discussion
Patients with active drug abuse and medical noncompliance are not considered to be suitable organ transplant candidates. However, the team felt a continued commitment to Ms. C. because of her youth, social victimization, and long history of care through the MGH Transplant Unit. The patient's pediatric nephrologist believed she would die if transplantation were not available and proposed total lymphatic irradiation (TLI). This procedure, which has been effective in the treatment of lymphoma, has been advocated in some transplantation situations in an effort to establish relative immunologic tolerance. After a course of radiation, Ms. C. underwent cadaveric transplantation. The team concluded that this might have the

effect of reducing the patient's subsequent steroid requirement. Psychological effects of prednisone had been, in part, responsible for the difficulties that followed Ms. C.'s first transplant. Further, if TLI were successful, the new renal allograft might theoretically withstand subsequent predictable episodes of noncompliance with anti-rejection medication.

Post-transplant course

Despite the success of retransplantation, psychosocial deterioration was progressive and for a time Ms. C. lived in a public shelter. Her primary psychiatric disorder was complicated by excessive alcohol use and cocaine dependency that proved resistant to psychiatric intervention. Ms. C.'s medical noncompliance resulted in chronic allograft rejection. Two and one-half years after receiving her second transplant, the patient returned to hemodialysis. Between April 1989 and August 1991, she required 16 hospital admissions, 9 of which were in psychiatric and drug rehabilitation settings. Psychosocial difficulties were aggravated by a sexual assault that she suffered in April 1989 and by a repeated episode of father-daughter incest. She was able for the first time to make a serious commitment to psychotherapy, but continued suffering led her to a competent decision to withdraw from hemodialysis.

Case 4. Ms. F, a 32-year-old woman who had had three children, the youngest of whom was aged 9 months, presented with cholangiocarcinoma and no preoperative evidence of extrahepatic involvement. Operative findings revealed no gross evidence of extrahepatic cancer, but at least two lymphatic nodes were positive for microscopic disease. Extrahepatic malignancy is an exclusion criterion, but liver transplantation was performed nonetheless, followed by postoperative irradiation.

Brief discussion

A poor prognosis was evident with the finding of extrahepatic lymph nodes positive for cholangiocarcinoma. The patient presented early in the MGH liver transplantation series, and the team had not yet adopted a "first-look" operative approach to treatment of primary hepatic cancer. Neither the patient, a highly motivated former athlete and businesswoman, nor the team was prepared to turn down the donor liver.

Post-transplant course

A vigorous recovery ensued, with 6 months of remission from biliary cancer. Ms. F. died at 8 months following transplantation from recurrent neoplasm.

Case 5. Ms. B., a 36-year-old woman with hypothyroidism and moderate mental retardation (presumed to have been caused by malnutrition), was living with a 90-year-old foster parent and the parent's middle-aged biological daughter when she was evaluated for treatment of chronic renal failure. Despite her IQ of 50, which made her candidacy for transplantation marginal, and a past episode of psychotic depression, the patient was fully active and had a stable relationship with a psychiatrically impaired male with whom she participated in a community support program.

Brief discussion

Ms. B. had a well-established pattern of medical compliance and a capacity for meaningful recovery despite her limitations. She related well to her physicians and, like Ms. C., she was a victim of childhood abuse and neglect. Demonstration of a social bond with her schizophrenic boyfriend ("He thinks he is a machine," she often said with an affectionate chuckle.) was a positive element in her candidacy. The increased relative cost of dialysis was an additional consideration.

Post-transplant course
Following cadaveric renal transplantation and discharge from the hospital, Ms. B. had a brief psychotic episode that responded to low-dose neuroleptic therapy (thioridazine hydrochloride, 150 mg hs). Full recovery followed. The patient developed breast cancer and died 6 years after transplantation.

Case 6. Ms. W., a 34-year-old woman, developed liver failure following a 17-year history of chronic active hepatitis (CAH). She had a stable family environment but a longstanding history of depression and prescription drug abuse unrelieved by a past psychiatric admission of 1 year. Except for a possible eating disorder, Ms. W. was developmentally normal through high school. Analgesic dependency developed during steroid therapy for CAH and in the setting of multiple endodontic procedures. The patient had worked as a medical receptionist but was on long-term disability. Ms. W. had limited social contacts and had marked dependency on her family.

Brief discussion
The chronic psychological impairment of this patient appeared related to the morbidity of CAH. The team considered that replacement of her liver might also relieve or ameliorate psychiatric features of Ms. W.'s illness.

Post-transplant course
Liver transplantation was followed by multiple hospitalizations for rejection and near fatal infectious complications including hepatitis B and necrotizing herpes simplex pulmonary infection. After several months of hospitalization, the patient was able to live independently and drive her own motor vehicle. At 4 years after transplantation, she remains medically disabled but enjoys an increasing sphere of social activity.

Ethical Considerations
These six cases illustrate that some team-centered circumstances (i.e., prior investment in the care of a patient, prior success with similar cases, or motivation to perform a new procedure) may have an impact on the inclusion of candidates otherwise judged to be marginal or even inappropriate for transplantation. Certain patient characteristics such as youthfulness, motivation, and resourcefulness may be of potential prognostic value or evoke a process of altruistic identification.

Further, perception of the patient as a victim may affect the team's response and subsequently influence the size and characteristics of the recipient pool. Above all, the medical model, based on intent to preserve life and relieve suffering, usually creates a bias toward intervention.

Transplant physicians, ethicists, policymakers, and colleagues continue to grapple with the challenge of finding the most ethically defensible approach to the setting of criteria for determining the size and range of candidates in the recipient pool. The development of policy to date has followed the development of the ethical issues surrounding transplantation in general. Fletcher[4] observes that ethical issues and the ensuing policy to deal with them develop in four stages: threshold, conflict, debate, and adaptation. In adaptation, the stage of development of the policy discussed in this article, Fletcher states that "implementation of public policies with administrative and legislative formulations occur in [a] climate of socioethical debate."[4]

In the development of policy regarding the recipient pool, the notion of benefit has evolved and plays a central role in the setting of criteria. Today, the United States health care system has adopted policy based on the type of benefit described in the Report of the U.S. Task Force on Organ Transplantation.[5] The authors use degree of medical need and success in outcome as the primary considerations in determining eligibility criteria. Kamm[6] summarizes,

> The Report's notion of need, roughly equivalent to urgency, is how soon someone would die, or how badly that person's life would go in the future, without the organ. Successful outcome is a function of the additional length and quality of life that someone will have as a result of the transplant, compared to what he would have had without it. The Report does not consider possible conflicts between additional length and quality of life, but clearly the good to the patient, not the good to society, of additional time alive is at issue.[6]

In short, patient-centered medical need is essential to the accepted notion of "benefit" (ANB) and is a precise notion of extended life expectancy and an imprecise notion of enhanced quality-of-life.

One worthwhile method to further refine policy is to continue to refine the notion of benefit. Another method is to examine several different lines of reasoning about who should be in the recipient pool and why and then assess how big the pool would be, given our ANB. In an ANB-based position, only those who meet that particular criterion of benefit would be included. We chose the latter method. Theoretically, eligibility for the recipient pool could require clear evidence of the ANB to the patient or evidence that benefit will at least be marginal, or it may not require evidence of that type of benefit to the patient at all. What governs eligibility is the line of reasoning and the ethical considerations that support it. Our observations of actual factors that influence decisions suggest that, operationally, there is more to the story than a consideration of the presently accepted parameters of benefit. Further, we believe that whereas reliance on the ANB may be fitting in a period of dire scarcity of organs, this situation may change through the development of artificial organs or other means by which the supply-demand ratio may be altered. We believe that in a period of adaptation of the ethical positions arrived at during the past 30 years of thoughtful debate, it is timely to explore four major lines of reasoning that could be applied to the issue and to remark on the influence such reasoning might have on the size and characteristics of the recipient pool. A summary of our discussion is found in Table 1.

Lines of Reasoning About the Recipient Pool

The Physician's Duty Is to Preserve Life and Relieve Suffering

Medical ethics traditionally has entailed a strong duty-oriented approach to reasoning about morally acceptable practices and policies. The physician's duty is to provide the best interventions possible to his or her patient with the understanding that the goals are to act presumptively to preserve life and relieve suffering. Thus, this approach takes into serious account a process of advocacy of "beneficent paternalism."[7] Policymakers must be responsive to this duty (and process) when designing policy. The recipient's claim is based on the urgency of medical need combined with the promise that the patient will not only survive the transplantation but will have a longer, "better" life. Because the quality of life criteria have been so difficult to describe and measure, and early attempts to base decisions on quality of life dimensions have lent themselves to allegations of elitism, the policymaker is currently likely to place more (though not all) weight on the patient's chance of a longer and more active life than on the promise of a better life.

Table 1. Should patient be included in recipient pool using criteria of "Accepted Notion of Benefit?" Findings of a study of the allocation of organ transplants to various recipients

Line of Reasoning	Benefit Certain	Marginal Likelihood of Benefit	Benefit Unlikely
1. Physician's duty	include	include as exception only	exclude
2. Patient's preference	include	include	include
3. Cost-effectiveness	include	exclude	exclude
4. Scientific progress	include	include	include

The approach requires rigorously defining a range of potential recipients and then including any others on a case-by-case exception basis. The reader will find this approach consistent with the Report of the U.S. Task Force on Organ Transplantation described previously. The ANB guides policy and practice in this line of reasoning. Individuals who are viewed as certain to benefit will be in the pool. Those who are judged to be in a position to only marginally benefit may be included but simply as case-by-case exceptions with no effect on the basic policy. If no benefit is foreseen (using the ANB), the individual will not be included. In each of the six cases discussed previously, patients were included when it was established that transplantation provided the greatest hope of meaningful life prolongation and recovery. Not surprisingly, the traditional medical ethic with its emphasis on the duty to preserve life and relieve suffering prevailed in these cases.

The Patient' s Preference

The idea of the patient as a partner in the physician-patient, decision-making process is a modern conception growing out of the belief that respect for others requires that they be self-determining or autonomous agents.[8] Our conviction that this is true is expressed in the health professions' emphasis on the importance of good communication with patients and is formalized in our doctrine and mechanisms of informed consent.

Engelhardt[9] identifies the tension between traditional beneficence and the more recent interpretations of patient autonomy as the root conflict in bioethics, which springs from "the difference between respecting the freedom and securing the best interests of the person." Engelhardt believes that "they summarize under two headings a range of moral problems and concerns."[9]

Nowhere is the potential for conflict between the two more manifested than in the setting of policy regarding the recipient pool for transplantation. Above, we followed the line of reasoning governed by the beneficent paternalism of the traditional professional ethos. Today, the health professional takes informed consent as an indicator of the patient's wishes and hopes that the patient's judgment will coincide with that of the beneficent professional. However, the range and character of a patient's wishes are neither neatly bordered by the information provided within the health care context nor fully conveyed when a consent form has been signed.

In the present climate of health care, the claim of the patient's authority often bears the moral (and, to a more limited but significant degree, legal) stringency of a right. In this patient's rights approach, in which the patient's wishes should govern, Engelhardt is right. This line of reasoning potentially leads one down a path that is irreconcilable with beneficent paternalism. The beneficent paternalism approach, couched within a framework of the duty-driven medical ethic, gives priority to the ANB, whereas the right to autonomy emphasizes the quality of life benefit strictly as it is defined by the patient.

Our discussion provides some clues as to how this patient preference is likely to affect policy. Because the ANB specifies extension of life but only vaguely defines quality of life, almost any version of the "good life" articulated by the patient could count. Therefore, to the extent that the intervention could be judged as consistent with a competent patient's wishes, he or she would have a claim inclusion in the recipient pool. Patients who would clearly benefit (using the ANB), who would only marginally benefit, or even who would not benefit could be included in such a recipient pool. A negative consequence would be that some who might benefit from scarce resources would be displaced by recipients for whom there might be little or no benefit. More research is needed to elucidate the impact of patient preferences on access to transplantation surgery. A consumer responsive health care market would presumably support policy based on patient requests and expectations.

None of the patients in our six cases was included on the basis of this rights reasoning. However, one can speculate that signals sent to the staff by highly motivated and competent patients may reinforce the staff's willingness to respond. Mr. W. (Case 2) and Ms. F. (Case 4) are examples of such patients.

Cost-Effectiveness Considerations

From a cost-effectiveness point of view, physicians attempt to serve societal interests by engaging in practices that will allow servicing the greatest number of those in need at the least possible cost to society. Although it appears at first that the net of potential recipients initially could be cast wide in the utility-maximizing approach, we judge that in the final analysis the physician and policymaker will decide upon a very small pool. The governing fact is that the patient must be a good investment costwise, so that the maximum number of people receiving health care can benefit. Presently, the idea of a good investment is measured partially by the likelihood of positive medical outcome; positive medical outcome is identified with increased length of life and, to a lesser degree, with an increased quality of life. In other words, the ANB is assumed to reflect the indicators of positive outcome. However, a good investment also entails dollar considerations. A preferred patient A must not only be expected to benefit, but also will be more desirable if the benefit comes at less expense than it would for patient B. Among patients who urgently need and would clearly benefit from the transplant, those judged to do so at the least expense would take priority in the recipient pool over similarly needy persons. Persons who would only marginally benefit would be viewed as poor investments and those deemed unlikely to benefit would not be included in the recipient pool. There is also the possibility that some who are ineligible will be seen as good investments, thereby expanding the pool of candidates. For example, in present practice, age greater than 60 is considered a relative contraindication. As we discuss in the next section of this article, some arguments suggest that present age criteria are not utility maximizing. Mr. A. (Case 1) is an example of an older candidate with an excellent outcome. When listed for transplantation, he was at the margin of age restrictions for the BCLT.

From a distributive justice perspective, it can be argued that even effective outcomes after transplantation are achieved at a cost that could be applied to far less costly preventive care. This argument presumes that the apparent savings from eliminating costly procedures would in fact be distributed for primary prevention. Roger Evans (personal communication) has suggested that we should look instead at areas of currently approved health care expenditure that provide little or no benefit. This might lead, for example, to elimination of some types of aggressive cancer treatment (Case 4 might fall in this category) or to curtailment of futile intervention in the intensive care unit setting.

Scientific Progress

Physicians' acquisition of knowledge may be a basis for expanding or constricting the recipient pool based on outcome. The learning process leads to consideration of another form of utility, scientific progress.

Here, the principal utility-maximizing consideration is the generation of new knowledge. The physician and policymaker must make their judgments on the basis of the merit of scientific progress, providing that the risk to the patient is not excessive. Just as the cost-effectiveness line of reasoning emphasizes overall investments in dollar terms, the research progress approach emphasizes progress in scientific knowledge. Patients will be included in the recipient pool not only because of medical need but also if including them might lead to generation of new knowledge or scientific progress. The goal is to help them, but also to generate new knowledge that will help everyone. Individuals who clearly would benefit (using the ANB), those who would marginally benefit, and even those who would clearly not benefit might be included using this criterion.

Potentially lost is the primary focus on a patient's medical need, the orientation one finds in the duty-driven approach. Ms. C. (Case 3) is an example of how both approaches may be combined as innovative therapy. Inclusion of such poor prognosis patients in the recipient pool must be carefully assessed in terms of patient motivation and deeply held expectations of the health care professional as well as from the standpoint of what knowledge we may derive from the intervention.

Summary of Ethical Approaches

From the previously mentioned cases, it is evident that exceptions to the ANB criteria for inclusion in organ transplantation pools do occur in surgical practice. We have examined some of these exceptions from the perspective of various ethical models. The duty-driven orientation is most familiar to the clinician, but in practice all of these ethical models require consideration. The principal lines of ethical reasoning, including: 1) duty-driven, 2) patients' rights-oriented, and 3) utility-driven (by cost-effectiveness or scientific progress criteria) are significant in their potential impact on health care policy. Policy and practice are in turn interactive so that the system at any time is in a state of flux.

Current expansion of the recipient pool for transplantation is occurring in two areas, alcoholism and older age, which may substantially increase the number of eligible candidates. Current thinking related to these two variables merits further elaboration.

Transplantation and Alcoholism

Factors of scarcity and cost have brought attention to liver transplantation for patients with alcoholic cirrhosis and hepatitis, which account for half of all liver failures in the United States. Foremost is the need to avoid discrimination, which occurs when all within a given subgroup are excluded despite the likelihood that some may benefit.[10] Many who are recovering alcoholics continue to maintain sobriety. Data from the University of Pittsburgh thus far indicate a low rate of recurrent drinking in their series,[1,2] yet there is also evidence that substance abuse histories may be associated with higher rates of noncompliance.[11] Our own retrospective data demonstrate a sixfold incidence of allograft rejection from noncompliance among patients with a past history of substance abuse. All but one of the patients (5 of 400 cases reviewed) who did lose a graft were less than 31-years-old.[12] One might then elect to limit organ loss from noncompliance by choosing only substance abusers who were not young. However, youthfulness is a positive feature among potential transplant recipients. Establishment of careful inclusion and exclusion criteria by trained addictionologists professionals may be the best approach.[13]

Lundberg[14] argues on a social worth basis that an alcoholic with liver failure who has made an extraordinary societal contribution might be preferentially treated. There is the possibility that allograft function might be sustained for an extended period even with persistence of active alcohol dependence. Loewy[15] cautions that the doctor-patient relationship must remain exempt from distinctions of social worth, although these may form a basis for macroallocation decisions. One type of macroallocation decision would be to have patients with alcoholic cirrhosis become recipients of hepatic allografts but at a lower priority.[16] From a practical standpoint, this might result in few such patients surviving to become transplant beneficiaries.[17] Cohen *et al.*[18] argue that "there is not good moral or medical reason for categorically precluding alcoholics as candidates for liver transplantation." There is also a risk that such a precedent for exclusion might empower third-party payers to deny medical care on the basis of past alcohol excess or other forms of dietary indiscretion. We know of one instance in which a woman with retrolental fibroplasia lost insurance coverage when her insurer obtained psychiatric records documenting a history of alcohol abuse.[17]

As we ascertained above, it might be legitimate from a utilitarian viewpoint for society to approve transplantation for alcoholics with liver failure. Alcoholism is a disease of denial in which the physician may be the last informed. The occasion of transplantation may lead to greater sensitivity for early recognition and prevention of alcohol abuse and dependency.[17]

Transplantation and Age

Some have argued recently that the high cost of health care among older individuals may be addressed ethically by restricting high technology interventions for this group.[19] Most likely, organ transplantation would fall in this category. It is clear with reference to Mr. A., that if age 60 were the cutoff point many would be lost to treatment who might benefit significantly. The experience at MGH is that survival following liver transplantation among patients over age 60 compares very favorably with that of other age groups.

One may also argue that allocation by age is discriminatory. A counter argument is that all would bear the same potential chronological limitation if the age of 60 were picked as a cutoff point and that it is unrealistic from a distributive justice perspective for patients over 60 to expect to receive equal access. The latter approach must be considered from a cultural perspective. Kilner[20] found, for example, that in a study of health care allocation among healers in rural Kenya, many subjects would treat age preferentially, even if a young person presented earlier for treatment. Age, from this African perspective, was seen as a source of wisdom.[20]

A longer life expectancy and greater productivity among the young, and the grievous nature of death at an early age are additional factors that might pose age-related limits based on scarcity and cost. However, many otherwise healthy individuals with end organ failure are captains of industry or serve in other substantial leadership roles. The death of vigorous people at any age places a burden of bereavement on survivors and there are the significant costs of terminal care. Also, if we argue that organs are a limited resource and transplantation is costly, shall we extend the same logic of exclusion to competition for food and shelter? The old would then go homeless and undernourished for benefit of the young, or older individuals who have accumulated wealth through savings and investment might be asked to forego what might be considered excess funds (beyond the current concept of taxation). Much of eastern Europe was at one point in this century swept up in a doctrine that advocated this type of approach. From a capitalist perspective, organ allocation might better proceed on the basis of market forces that govern other services.

Some believe that health care policy should consider the boundaries of a natural life span, whereas others, like Medawar,[21] have suggested that human longevity is likely to increase as it has in the past century.

Conclusion

Organs for transplantation are a scarce resource at the present time and the surgical technology is costly to implement.

Moral reasoning about who should be included among potential recipients should allow for change in the supply-demand ratio. Such change could occur, for instance, as a result of policy shifts affecting donor organ availability or with advances in transplantation biology that make xenografts possible.

The current system for allocation depends primarily on medical urgency and waiting time. Eligible individuals must often become sicker before an allograft is available.

Patients with histories of substance abuse, advanced age, HIV-positive status, cancer, and mental illness raise concerns about compliance, longevity, and quality of life after transplantation. In each of these categories, it is essential to look at the factors that have an impact on prognosis. Beresford *et al.*[13] have emphasized this aspect in their discussion of selection among potential liver transplant recipients with alcoholic end stage liver disease. Age is being looked at more as a relative circumstance with attention to other prognostic factors in individual cases. The same focus on factors affecting outcome might be extended to inclusion of patients who are HIV positive. According to Robert Rubin (personal communication), who has reviewed survival data on 120 HIV-positive, transplant patients worldwide, one-third are living and well at 5 years, one-third die in the first 6 months after transplantation, and one-third develop clinical AIDS at 2-4 years after transplantation. The challenge, it seems, would be to learn how to predict which of these outcomes would be more probable in individual cases.

Inclusion and exclusion criteria vary among transplant centers and are affected by macroallocation decisions. For example, if centers are held accountable for surgical outcome relative to a national standard, this may militate against decisions to include marginal patients. In contrast, if funding agencies require that centers perform a certain annual volume, this may lead to inclusion of poorer prognosis recipients.

Four morally relevant considerations include allocations governed by medical duty, patients' rights, the overall utility of a cost/benefit ratio measured in dollars, and the utility to scientific progress.

In our four lines of reasoning about who should be included, we show that the patient's rights and scientific progress approaches allow for the greatest inclusion, although there are risks in deviating from the patient-oriented ANB. The distributive-justice (cost/benefit) approach is most restrictive but must allow for the possibility that money and resources will be saved when the otherwise chronically ill achieve active rehabilitation. For example, improved function among the chronically ill may be associated with benefits in the social network (i.e., to friends, neighbors, family, and employers).

In his autobiography Benjamin Franklin said, "So convenient a thing is it to be a reasonable creature, since it enables one to find or make a reason for everything one has a mind to do"[22] (or not to do). According to biographer Piers Brendon, Winston Churchill instructed his research assistant, "Give me the facts, Ashley, and I will twist them the way I want to suit my argument."[23]

In practice, the ethical models that we employ should be considered together. Objectives must include humane care, moral consideration from all perspectives, and appreciation for what is feasible. Scientific progress and changing societal perspectives require that we continually revisit the issues and maintain open inquiry and open exchange of ideas.

Notes

1. Starzl TE, Van Thiel D, Pzakis AG, *et al*. Orthotopic liver transplantation for alcoholic cirrhosis, *Journal of the American Medical Association* 1988;260:2542-2544.
2. Van Thiel D, Gavaler JS, Tarter RE, *et al*. Liver transplantation for alcoholic liver disease: A consideration of reasons for and against, *Alcoholism: Clinical and Experimental Research* 1989;13:181-184.
3. Tzakis AG, Cooper MH, Dummer JS, *et al*. Transplantation in HIV+ patients, *Transplantation* 1990;49:354-358.
4. Fletcher J. Cardiac transplants and the artificial heart: Ethical considerations, *Circulation* 1983;68:1339-1343.
5. U.S. Task Force on Organ Transplantation. *Organ Transplantation: Issues and Recommendations*. Washington, DC: HEW Committee of Public Welfare, April, 1986.
6. Kamm FH. The report of the U.S. Task Force on Organ Transplantation: Criticisms and alternatives, *Mt Sinai Journal of Medicine* 1989;56:207-220.
7. Priester R. *Rethinking Medical Morality: The Ethical Implications of Changes in Health Care Organization, Delivery and Financing*. Minneapolis, MN: Center of Biomedical Ethics, University of Minnesota, 1989.
8. Young E. *Alpha and Omega: Ethics at the Frontiers of Life and Death*. Reading, MA: Addison-Wesley, 1989:30-31.
9. Engelhardt HT. *The Foundations of Bioethics*. New York, NY: Oxford University Press, 1986:66.
10. Merrican KJ, Overcast TD. Patient selection for heart transplantation: When is discriminating choice discrimination? *Journal of Health, Politics, Policy and Law* 1985;10:7-32.
11. Scharschmidt BF. Human liver transplantation: Analysis of data on 540 patients from four centers, *Hepatology* 1984;4(suppl 1):95s-101s.
12. Gastfriend DR, Surman OS, Gaffey GK, *et al*. Substance abuse and compliance in organ transplantation, *Substance Abuse* 1989;10:149-153.
13. Beresford TP, Turcotte JG, Merion R, *et al*. A rational approach to liver transplantation for the alcoholic patient (editorial), *Psychosomatics* 1990;31:241-254.
14. Lundberg G. License to plunder or paint, *Journal of the American Medical Association* 1983;250:2966-2967.
15. Loewy EH. Drunks, livers and values: Should social value judgments enter into liver transplant decisions? *Journal of Clinical Gastroenterology* 1987;9:436-441.
16. Moss AH, Siegler M. Should alcoholics compete equally for liver transplantation? *Journal of the American Medical Association* 1991;265:1295-1298.
17. Surman OS. The morality of transplantation (letter), *Journal of the American Medical Association* 1991;266:213.
18. Cohen C, Benjamin M, and the Ethics and Social Impact Committee of the Transplant and Health Policy Center. Alcoholics liver transplantation, *Journal of the American Medical Association* 1991;266:1299-1301.
19. Callahan D. *What Kind of Life: The Limits of Medical Progress*. New York, NY: Simon and Schuster, 1990.
20. Kilner J. Who shall be saved? An African answer, *Hastings Center Report* 1984;14:18-22.
21. Medawar P. When we are old, *Atlantic* 1984;253:16-21.
22. Franklin B. *Autobiography of Benjamin Franklin*, ed. Pine FW. New York, NY: Henry Holt and Co, 1916:68.
23. Brendon P. *Winston Churchill: A Brief Life*. London: Secker and Warburg, 1984.

Chapter 41

Should a Patient With End-Stage Alcoholic Liver Disease Have a New Liver?

Steven Schenker, Henry S. Perkins, Michael F. Sorrell

Almost 30 years ago Starzl pioneered liver transplantation in the United States. Since then, the field has expanded enormously, with the procedure being done across the world, some 1,700 transplants were carried out in the United States alone in 1988, with overall 5years survival reaching 70%.[1] With this new hope for patients with life-limiting liver disease, new concerns have emerged. One of these, which is addressed in this issue of *Hepatology* by Kumar *et al.*,[2] is the question of liver transplantation in patients with alcohol-induced end-stage liver disease. Should such patients be transplanted? If so, under what conditions and what would be the impact of such a program on other aspects of liver transplantation and health care in general?

These questions, which have evoked much controversy, are of practical significance because excessive consumption of ethanol (alcohol) is the most frequent cause of severe parenchymal liver disease in the United States and the western world. The second most common cause is viral hepatitis advancing to cirrhosis. Much progress has been made in the field of viral hepatitis prevention (i.e., identification of markers for hepatitis B and C), and there is promise for its treatment with antiviral agents.[3,4] By contrast, although there has been a laudable increase in educational efforts with apparent decrease in alcohol consumption and fewer patients dying of alcoholic cirrhosis in the United States,[5,6] progress in the treatment of established alcoholic liver disease has been frustratingly slow.

In the therapy for alcoholic liver disease, cessation of drinking and provision of adequate nutrition have been time-honored and logical remedies. Abstinence has been shown to prolong life in most such patients,[7,8] except in a few studies of individuals with very severe hepatic dysfunction and bleeding esophageal varices.[9] These patients may have passed the point of no return. How often cessation of alcohol intake in such individuals can be promoted is uncertain, with some estimates of only about 25% to 50%.[10,11,12,13] The figures seem to vary with the population studied, the definition of abstinence and the duration of assessment. Whether major reduction in alcohol intake (but not complete abstinence) would be feasible and therapeutically sufficient as a fall-back position has been hotly debated. This view is supported by fragmentary evidence[13] and requires further study.

It is important to emphasize that severe acute alcoholic injury (alcoholic hepatitis) and chronic end-stage alcoholic cirrhosis are not the same entity, although the former is often superimposed on and leads to the latter. The acute lesion is potentially reversible, and there are no data to our knowledge on the value of hepatic transplantation in this entity. Liver transplantation in alcoholic patients reported here[2] apparently refers not to patients with

---

Source: Reprinted from *Hepatology*, Vol. 11, No. 2, pp. 314-319, with permission from Mosby-Year Book, Inc. © 1990.

alcoholic hepatitis but to patients with end-stage cirrhosis.

Acute severe alcoholic liver damage has been treated with propylthiouracil[14] and in some patient subsets with corticosteroids.[15] The former approach is controversial[14,15,16,17] and has not been generally accepted. The latter, while promising, requires further validation and seems to apply only to a group of patients with acute injury per se or when acute injury is superimposed on cirrhosis. Such therapy thus would not be applicable and may not be helpful in the bulk of patients with end-stage chronic alcoholic liver disease. Androgenic hormones have also been suggested as anciliary therapy,[18] but here, too, the data are conflicting,[19] perhaps because of differences in patient selection. Insulin and glucose administration, as possible promoters of hepatic regeneration, have also been tried with some, but not impressive, success.[20,21] Finally, in one large study colchicine has been reported to prolong life in patients with alcohol-induced chronic liver disease.[22] This elaborate and long-term study, which is unlikely to be reproduced soon, has generated much interest in colchicine but has also been criticized on a number of points.[23,24] These include the very high mortality of the control group, loss to follow-up of a number of patients, uncertainty as to ethanol intake in both groups and lack of extensive follow-up histological data. This promising approach,[22] therefore, requires further investigation and confirmation. One can summarize available data by saying that there is currently no proven effective therapy for severe chronic (established) alcoholic liver disease.

Identification of patients with end-stage chronic alcoholic liver disease is usually not difficult. These individuals, as a rule, have some combination of ascites, which is difficult to diurese, bouts of spontaneous bacterial peritonitis, encephalopathy, bleeding esophageal varices and/or renal dysfunction caused by a failing liver. In addition to these clinical signs of terminal liver disease, they exhibit abnormal liver tests with jaundice, hypoalbuminemia and a prolonged prothrombin time.[25] Under such circumstances one can reasonably assume a survival of less than 6 months for most of these patients.[25] With most other chronic liver disease of this magnitude (i.e., in primary biliary cirrhosis), liver transplantation would have been considered overdue. Yet few such patients with alcoholic liver disease have come to transplantation despite a large available pool. A recent informal survey could locate only 98 such patients, or about 5% of a total of 2,132 individuals with liver transplants, and this has been the experience of other large single centers.[1]

Why are these individuals with chronic severe alcoholic liver disease not now considered for hepatic transplantation? The reasons usually cited to a varying extent are: (a) belief that alcoholics have other serious medical problems that worsen their overall prognosis; (b) concern that their addiction to ethanol will cause them to continue to drink and will make them noncompliant with follow-up care; (c) the view of some that alcoholism and ensuing liver damage is a self-inflicted disease and, hence, does not deserve the same medical care as other hepatic disorders; (d) concern that because of donor organ shortage, livers should be transplanted first into other needy recipients who "did not bring the problem on themselves;" and (e) uncertainty as to who would pay the large cost of liver transplantation for alcoholics, many of whom have a low economic base. Although many of these cited reasons are clearly interrelated, we will consider them sequentially for the sake of clarity.

Other Serious Medical Problems in Alcoholics

Clearly patients with end-stage alcoholic hepatic dysfunction also may suffer from other diseases such as cerebral dysfunction caused by ethanol and/or vitamin deficiencies, chronic pancreatitis and, as shown recently, cardiomyopathy and skeletal muscle abnormalities.[26] The exact percentage of such patients with multiple disorders is uncertain and will depend on the severity of the disorders sought and the sophistication of diagnostic techniques used to detect them. For instance, it has been shown recently that, using special tests, as many as one third of apparently wellnourished alcoholics had evidence of cardiomyopathy and one half had skeletal muscle abnormalities.[26] The point of this latest study is that such a diagnosis could be established with available tools and that the problem was subtle enough to be subclinical. Pancreatic disease, likewise, is fairly readily diagnosable if the disorder is clinically significant. Cerebral dysfunction, on the other hand, if present and not responsive to treatment for hepatic encephalopathy, may be difficult to assign to organic brain syndrome caused by alcohol and/or by refractory hepatic dysfunction.

Whatever the cause, such patients with significant cardiomyopathy, pancreatitis and cerebral dysfunction can usually be identified *a priori* and, at least initially, should be excluded from the pool of transplant candidates. It is likely that despite such restrictions many individuals with severe liver disease and no other major organ involvement caused by alcoholism will remain to test our resolve. Moreover, it is essential to remain flexible with the exclusion criteria. Kidney transplantation in diabetic patients and patients with hepatitis B is frequently carried out despite their other risks[27] and one has only to consider the favorable outcome of liver transplants in patients older than 50 years of age (an exclusionary age limit not too long ago) to realize that changes occur in apparent absolutes with the passage of. time and with accompanying advances in knowledge ([1], Starzl TE, *et al. New England Journal of Medicine* 1987;316:484-485, Correspondence). We would conclude, therefore, that other organ damage should be sought diligently and, if identified and found to be clinically significant, should be a relative contraindication to liver transplantation at this time in these patients. However, there should still remain a large pool of patients primarily with alcohol-induced chronic liver damage for whom liver transplantation could be lifesaving.

Continued Addiction to Alcohol Will Result in Therapeutic Poor Compliance

This is a very reasonable theoretical admonition that could have critical prognostic significance, since these patients require continuing immunosuppression and monitoring. So far, as shown in this issue of *Heptalogy* by Kumar *et al.*[2] and commented on earlier by these authors in a much smaller subset of such patients,[28] theory and practice may not coincide. Seventy-three patients with alcoholic liver disease transplanted in Pittsburgh from 1982 to 1988 had a 2-year survival of 71%, similar to a much larger group of individuals with other types of liver disease.[2] Moreover, their quality of life (assessed by work performance and stay out of the hospital) seemed very respectable. This latter is an area that, in our opinion, deserves more detailed study, both in the alcoholics and in comparison to other adult patients undergoing liver transplants. Moreover, surprisingly, return to alcohol consumption was uncommon in the transplanted alcoholics, with a recidivism of only about 11%.[2] This information was obtained, to be sure, from interviews with the patients, their families and their physicians and not from random alcohol assays, which are known to be much more reliable.[29] Thus the impression of low return rate to alcoholism requires further confirmation. Still, the apparent compliance with immunotherapy after transplantation, normal liver tests in most of these patients and the concordant testimony about their abstention from alcohol must be given credence. It may well be that these patients represent a self-selected (motivated) group that responds well to the intensive medical care related to transplantation and the support of their families during this process. Future studies will be needed to confirm the generality of this phenomenon in larger groups of alcoholic patients. Ideally this should include alcohol analyses in blood or urine. Perhaps eventually criteria can be developed for identifying the group(s) with the most favorable outlook.

Although full reports are not yet available, three other groups have also reported in abstract form favorable results with orthotopic liver transplantation in patients with alcoholic cirrhosis, albeit in a small number of individuals. In France[30] 16 patients with alcoholic cirrhosis had 1-year and 2-year survival of 74% and 55%, comparable to nonalcoholics. The frequency of rejection was also similar in both groups, and death in alcoholics was usually due to sepsis. Only two patients returned to alcohol abuse. In St. Louis, all five patients with alcoholic liver disease have survived a mean follow-up of 6 months.[31] Four have returned to full-time employment and none has resumed drinking alcohol. All received extensive counseling. In Ann Arbor, of 66 patients with alcoholic liver disease referred for liver transplantation, 37 have been accepted and 32 transplanted. The 1-year actuarial survival was 76% and only one patient appears to have had a single episode of return to drinking.[32] These three preliminary reports appear to support the conclusions of Kumar *et al.*[2] derived from a larger patient population. In conclusion, it seems that patients who are transplanted for alcoholic liver disease have survival rates comparable to other recipients and, surprisingly, rarely return to significant alcohol abuse. Obviously a longer follow-up period and better monitoring for alcohol are necessary to determine whether these initial favorable outcomes are maintained.

A key issue is which group(s) of alcoholic patients with liver disease should be selected for transplantation. The initial recommendation of the Consensus Conference on Liver Transplantation in 1983 was for a 6-months abstinence period before consideration for transplantation.[33] This would substantially limit patient availability. In the report by Kumar *et al.*, however, the 11 patients who were abstinent less than 6 months before transplantation seemed to do as well in terms of survival as those 62 who were abstinent for more than 6 months.[2] The group that was initially nonabstinent or abstinent for a short time, however, seemed to return to drinking at a higher rate. There seems to be, therefore, a discordance here in that return to alcohol did not adversely affect compliance with management and early survival. The numbers of patients (especially those abstinent for less than 6 months) are quite small, and this issue will need further evaluation. It would have been helpful also to have more information on how the duration of abstinence was validated. Such data are notoriously difficult to obtain.[29] The preliminary reports cited earlier[30,31,32] do not help in this area. Thus the study from France reported only on patients abstinent for 6 months or more,[30] the abstract from St. Louis referred only to patients abstinent for 6 to 24 months,[29] but the Michigan report states that "duration of preoperative sobriety is no longer a selection criterion and in only 5 rejected patients was lack of compliance or poor alcoholic prognosis a selection criterion."[32] Thus, although some of the results favor abandonment of the 6 months or more sobriety criterion,[2,32] in our opinion the data on this are not yet sufficient to be convincing.

In both the Pittsburgh and Michigan studies, extensive pre-transplantation and post-transplantation psychiatric support was given and may have contributed to the favorable outcome in these patients. There is a need to define which type(s) of psychiatric assessments and follow-up in these individuals are optimal and how to select the most suitable candidates for this procedure. Thus the final word on the selection process, in our view, has not yet been spoken, and the issue of length of confirmed abstinence requires more study. The alcoholic who cannot stop drinking and follow a strict therapeutic regimen puts himself and the success of the liver transplant at increased risk. Before liver transplantation any patient should understand his share of the responsibility for the transplant's success and demonstrate the capacity for adhering to a strict follow-up regimen. The alcoholic patient can justifiably be required to demonstrate his commitment to cooperating with the transplantation regimen and his ability to discipline himself. Proper counseling to help him attain abstinence should be available. Intuitively, proof of abstinence and/or future compliance with medical follow-up will help ensure that the donor organs will go to the patients who will benefit the most from them. It will also help to convince the transplant team that abstinence, which may have major beneficial effects in some of these patients,[8] had failed to reverse hepatic dysfunction.

Another important aspect of optimal patient response to major surgery (i.e., liver transplantation) is the nutritional status of the candidate, especially as it influences sepsis and wound healing.[34,35,36] Alcoholics, especially those with alcoholic hepatitis, often have poor nutritional status.[36,37] As evidence of interrelation of liver disease and nutrient processing, the clearance of amino acids *in vitro* and hepatic protein synthesis *in vitro* correlate well with prognosis of patients with liver disease and their survival after transplantation.[38,39] Hence, a period of abstinence may be beneficial in permitting the patient to get over an acute episode of illness, improve his overall nutritional status and thus to help him survive the rigors of this extensive surgery. In the report of Kumar *et el.*[2] there are little data concerning the nutritional assessment of the alcoholic patients transplanted versus those of the other groups. Does this also enter into the selection process? Future studies in this area, too, are needed.

One wonders, of course, about recurrence of liver disease in the transplanted organ. If the return to drinking is infrequent, as suggested by the recent reports,[2,34] this concern would lessen. Moreover, development of alcoholic liver disease, unlike the rapid recurrence of hepatitis B,[40] usually takes years. Transplanted patients with chronic hepatitis B[46] and those with hepatocellular carcinoma or cholangiocarcinoma[41] have a much worse prognosis than alcoholic patients, yet the procedure has evoked less outcry in those individuals.

Alcoholism as a Self-Inflicted Disease

Alcoholism and its consequences is but one of many self-imposed medical problems brought on by human excesses. Others include: (a) drug abuse and often accompanying hepatitis and AIDS; (b) smoking with increasing risk of cardiopulmonary diseases and cancer; (c) obesity with cardiorespiratory consequences; and (d) violent behavior of various types (i.e., hazardous driving) with resulting trauma to self and others. Although one may justifiably regret that our efforts and resources have to be spent on the consequences of these actions, moral indignation does not heal patients. We do not exclude these other types of patients from medical care, including extensive surgery. For alcoholism there is evidence that a genetic component may play a part in the craving for alcohol in some.[42] In some, social and economic pressures may also contribute to alcoholism. Regardless of the role of these factors in alcoholism or other self-caused problems, medical care, in our view, should be directed both at their prevention and their cure. Indeed, this is the accepted standard of medical care to all in need, rooted in the Judeo-Christian tradition of service.[43] The physician's dedication to all patients in need should be grounded in an appreciation of his own vulnerability to disease and in compassion for the sick.[43] These concepts were elegantly discussed by Atterbury in 1986.[44] For this care to end arbitrarily at one point in therapy for some, when other effective options remain and are given to others, seems illogical and unjustified. Is it ethical for physicians to render such moral judgments concerning patient care?

Donor Organ Shortage

It is a natural extension of some of the concerns raised above to allocate donor organs, when in short supply, to recipients felt likely to benefit more from them. In a sense, the value of the patient to society would be weighted to justify receipt of a donor organ. This would delay or limit access of the procedure to those people whose positions, past accomplishments, and expected future merit are judged less beneficial to society. Application of such principles, however, is problem ridden. Consensus about social values is ephemeral and prone to arbitrary decision-making that may be based on sketchy data and bias. We do not believe that such a system is equitable.

Until now there has been difficulty in finding livers in a timely fashion for needy patients. This has been especially true with children when the organ needed had to be of appropriately smaller size. The short preservation time for donor livers had also been a problem. Many of these concerns have begun to abate and others are amendable to solution. Thus the ability to preserve the liver for longer times with the advent of the "Wisconsin solution"[45,46] and the use of reduced size and split liver grafts should increase the pool of available livers.[47] Moreover, the recent discussion about using older donors[2] and living donors for transplantation ([48], Raia S, *et al.*, Lancet 1989;1:497, Correspondence), with the latter actually having been put to practical test in other countries (Raia S, *et al.*, Lancet 1989;1:497, Correspondence), and very recently in ours, may make liver transplantation possible for more children.

The key to organ availability is not selective rationing, but greater procurement through education of the medical community. Too many patients are still waiting for organs. It has been estimated that more than 20,000 people in the United States will suffer brain death from trauma.[49,50,51] Only about 20% of these patients are likely to be organ donors at present. Some 16,000 potentially usable livers will be buried! Although in many situations the circumstances of death may prevent the use of the organs despite best attempts and intentions, surely a portion of these lost tissues can be retrieved. At a recent discussion of this issue it was suggested that knowledge that organs may be transplanted into alcoholics may decrease the supply of willing donors.[52] Although this may be true initially, it is hoped that emphasis on transplantation of organs to "former" alcoholic patients may strike a more responsive chord and may decrease this perception. Thus the key is better education of medical personnel attending these patients and of the public and decreased bureaucracy. Organ availability and allocation likely will remain a problem with their greater use, but it is an issue that can be addressed constructively through scientific advances and more active procurement, aided by wise legislation favoring more donations.

Economics for Alcoholics

The cost of health care has been rising and has been the subject of extensive debate. Allocation of funds within these scarce resources is not easy.[53] Payment for transplantation of the liver has been in the forefront of this debate. What is cost-effective and who should decide? Are we, as a nation, to be relegated to different standards of patient care for the wealthy and the poor? Or are the poor to be made dependent on media hype to collect funds for transplantation? These economic issues become especially difficult when one deals with transplantation in alcoholic patients and the moral stigma (conscious or subconscious) attached to it for many in the decision-making process. The low socioeconomic status of many alcoholic patients and their dependence on Medicaid or increasingly scarce funds available through the Veterans Administration accentuate the possibility of decisions based on economics rather than sound medical judgment. This editorial cannot hope to do more than bring up these issues for others to debate.

Two points, however, may aid in the discussion. First, liver transplantation is no longer an experimental (research) procedure. The survival of 70% over 5 years is comparable to that hoped for in many diseases. It is, thus, a logical therapeutic intervention for many patients and should be accepted as such, regardless of cost.[54] Second, the cost of alternative (often less effective) therapy for many of these patients is not that much lower than the average cost of transplantation. The exact calculations will vary with the patient, the site of his treatment and the duration of treatment used for comparison. Transplantation, on the average, costs about $125,000 and yearly follow-up about $10,000. Cost of management for someone with complicated endstage liver disease may reach $50,000 to $60,000 for the first admission. Assuming survival, recurrent admissions may each add up substantially. Thus costs of these dual approaches may not be too disparate.

In conclusion, it seems that patients with chronic alcoholic end-stage liver disease should not be *a priori* excluded from liver transplantation provided they are carefully screened for other significant organ damage. The issue of duration of abstinence before consideration for transplant and of selection of appropriate subset(s) of patients requires further study.

Certainly, however, evidence of abstinence before transplantation suggests a more responsible attitude on the part of the patient and a greater possibility of postsurgical compliance. The burden of proof rests with those willing to transplant patients without evidence of prior abstinence. Organ availability should improve with further scientific advances and proper education of patients, their families and, especially, their physicians. The question of liver allocation in a specific setting, however, will probably always remain a difficult one. It should be made on a medical, not moral (judgmental), basis. The issue of payment for the procedure in those unable to do so needs to be considered both in the light of the benefits of transplantation and the costs of alternative, less definitive therapy, as well as the basic right of all citizens to equal access to comparable health care. Allocation of resources to such high-tech medicine is a national issue that should be decided for liver transplantation in general versus other fiscal needs, without regard to any social judgment as to alcoholism. Contrariwise, clinical assessment of success rate in such a patient subset would be a valid basis for decision-making. It is hoped that more data and further debate will make the process easier. However, neither of these is likely to ever make it easy. Decisions of this magnitude never are.

Notes

1. Starzl TE, Demetrus AJ, Van Thiel D. Liver transplantation: Medical progress, *New England Journal of Medicine* 1989;321:1014-1022.
2. Kumar S, Stauber RE, Gavaler J, Basista MH, Dindzans V, Schade RR, Rabinovitz M, *et al.* Orthotopic liver transplantation for alcoholic liver disease, *Hepatology* 1990;11:159164.
3. Pertilo RP, Regenstein FG, Peters MG, DeSchryver-Kecskemeti K, Bodicky CS, Campbell CR, Kuhns MC. Prednisone withdrawal followed by recombinant alpha-interferon in the treatment of chronic type B hepatitis: A randomized controlled trial, *Ann Intern Med* 1988;109:95-100.
4. DiBisceglie AM, Kassianides C, Lisker-Melman M, Martin P, Murray L, Hoofnagle JH. A randomized double-blind placebo-controlled trial of alpha-interferon therapy for non-A, non-B hepatitis [Abstract], *Hepatology* 1988;8:1222.
5. Brooks SD, Williams GD, Stinson FS, Noble J. *NIAAA Surveillance Report No. 13. Apparent Per Capita Alcohol Consumption: National, State and Regional Trends, 1977-1987.* Washington DC: US Department of Health and Human Services, Public Health Service, Alcohol Drug Abuse Mental Health Administration, 1989.
6. Grant BF, Zobeck TS. *NIAAA Surveillance Report No. 11. Liver Cirrhosis Mortality in the United States, 1972-1988.* Washington, DC: US Department of Health and Human Services, Public Health Service, Alcohol Drug Abuse Mental Health Administration, 1989.
7. Alexander JF, Lischner MW, Galambos JT. Natural history of alcoholic hepatitis II: The long term prognosis, *Am J Gastroenterol* 1971;56:515-525.
8. Powell WJ, Klatskin G. Duration of survival in patients with Laennec's cirrhosis, *Am J Med* 1968;98:695-716.
9. Pande NV, Resnick RH, Yee W, Eckardt VF, Shurberg JL. Cirrhotic portal hypertension: Morbidity of continued alcoholism, *Gastroenterology* 1978;74:64-69.
10. Vaillant GE, Clark W, Cyrus C, Milofsky ES, Kopp J, Wulsin VW, Mogielnicki NP. Prospective study of alcoholism treatment: Eight-year follow-up, *Am J Med* 1983;75:455-463.
11. Jackson FC, Penin EB, Smith GH, Dagradi AE, Nadal HM. Clinical investigation of the portacaval shunt II: Survival analysis of the prophylactic operation, *Am J Surg* 1968;115:22-42.
12. Conn HO, Lindenmuth WW. Prophylactic portacaval anastomosis in cirrhotic patients with esophageal varices, *New England Journal of Medicine* 1965;272:1255-1263.
13. Borowsky SA, Strome S, Lott E. Continued heavy drinking and survival in alcoholic cirrhotics, *Gastroenterology* 1981;80:14051409.
14. Orrego H, Kalant H, Israel Y, Blake J, Medline A, Rankin JG, Armstrong A, *et al.* Effect of short-term therapy with propylthiouracil in patients with alcoholic liver disease, *Gastroenterology* 1978;76:105-115.

15. Carithers RL Jr, Herlong F, Diehl AM, Shaw EW, Combes B, Fallon HJ, Maddrey WC. Methylprednisolone therapy in patients with severe alcoholic hepatitis: A randomized trial, *Ann Intern Med* 1989;110:685-690.
16. Orrego H, Blake JE, Blendis LM, Compton KV, Israel Y. Long-term treatment of alcoholic liver disease with propylthiouracil, *New England Journal of Medicine* 1987;317:1421-1427.
17. Halle P, Pare P, Kaptein E, Kanel G, Redeher AG, Reynolds TB. Double blind, controlled trial of propylthiouracil in patients with severe alcoholic hepatitis, *Gastroenterology* 1982;82:925-931.
18. Mendenhall CL, Anderson S, Garcia-Pont P, Goldberg S, Kiernan T, Seeff LB, Sorrell M, *et al.* Short-term and long-term survival in patients with alcoholic hepatitis treated with oxandrolone and prednisolone, *New England Journal of Medicine* 1984;311:1464-1470.
19. The Copenhagen Study Group for Liver Diseases. Testosterone treatment of men with alcoholic cirrhosis: A double-blind study, *Hepatology* 1986;6:807-813.
20. Baker AL, Jaspan JB, Haines NW, Hatfield GE, Krager PS, Schneider JF, The University of Chicago Medical Housestaff. A randomized clinical trial of insulin and glucagon infusion for treatment of alcoholic hepatitis: Progress report in 50 patients, *Gastroenterology* 1981;80:1410-1414.
21. Feher J, Cornides A, Romany A, Karteszi M, Szalay L, Gogl A, Picazo J. A prospective multicenter study of insulin and glucagon infusion therapy in acute alcoholic hepatitis, *Journal of Hepatology* 1987;5:224-231.
22. Kershenobich D, Vargas F, Garcia-Tsao G, Tamayo RP, Gent M, Rojkind M. Colchicine in the treatment of cirrhosis of the liver, *New England Journal of Medicine* 1988;318:1709-1713.
23. Grace NM. Colchicine treatment of cirrhosis: Questions, *Hepatology* 1989;9:655-657.
24. Carithers RL Jr. Treatment of alcoholic liver disease, *Practical Gastroenterol* 1989;13:51-56.
25. Schenker S. Alcoholic liver disease: Evaluation of natural history and prognostic factors, *Hepatology* 1984;4:365-435.
26. Urbano-Marquez A, Estruch R, Navarro-Lopez F, Grau JM, Mont L, Rubin E. The effects of alcoholism on skeletal and cardiac muscle, *New England Journal of Medicine* 1989;320:409-415.
27. Degos F, Degott C. Hepatitis in renal transplant recipients, 1989;9:114-123.
28. Starzl TE, Van Thiel DH, Tzabis A, Shunzaburo I, Todo S, Marsh JW, Koneru B, *et al.* Orthotopic liver transplantation for alcoholic cirrhosis, *Journal of the American Medical Association* 1988;260:2542-2544.
29. Orrego H, Blendis LM, Blake JE, Kapur BM, Israel Y. Reliability of assessment of alcohol intake based on personal interviews in a liver clinic, *Lancet* 1979;1:1354-1356.
30. Doffoel M, Wolf P, Ellero B, Vetter D, Jaegle ML, Jaeck D, Cinqualbre J. Results of orthotopic liver transplantation (OLT) in alcoholic cirrhosis, *Journal of Hepatology* 1989;9(Suppl 1):527.
31. Brems JJ, Joshi S, Kane RE, Berman LA, Kaminski DL. Orthotopic liver transplantation: Primary therapy for alcoholic cirrhosis [Abstract], *Hepatology* 1989;10:658.
32. Lucey MR, Merion RM, Henley KS, Campbell D, Turcotte J, Blow F, Beresford T. Selection of patients with alcoholic liver disease for orthotopic liver transplantation [Abstract], *Hepatology* 1989;10:572.
33. Schenker S. Medical treatment vs. transplantation in liver disorders, *Hepatology* 1984;4:102S-106S.
34. Johnson PJ, O'Grady J, O'Calbeg H, Williams R. Nutritional management and assessment, In: Calne R, ed. *Liver transplantation*. 2nd ed. Florida: Grune & Stratton, 1987:103-117.
35. O'Keefe SJ, E1-Zayadi AR, Carraher TE, David M, Williams R. Malnutrition and immunocompetence in patients with liver disease, *Lancet* 1980;2:615-617.
36. Hill GL. The perioperative patient, In: Kinney JM, Jeejeebhoy KN, Hill GL, Owen OE, eds. *Nutrition and Metabolism in Patient Care*. Philadelphia, PA: WB Saunders Co, 1988:643-655.
37. Mendenhall CL, Tosch J, Weesner RE, Garcia-Pont P, Goldberg SJ, Kierman T, Seeff LB, *et al.* VA cooperative study on alcoholic hepatitis II: Prognostic significance of protein-calorie malnutrition, *American Journal of Clinical Nutrition* 1986;43:213-216.
38. Jenkins RL, Clowes GH Jr, Bosari S, Pearl RH, Kehttry U, Trey C. Survival from hepatic transplantation: Relationship of protein synthesis to histological abnormalities in patient selection and postoperative management, *Annals of Surgery* 1986;204:364-374.
39. Pearl RH, Clowes GH Jr, Bosari S, McDermott HWV, Menzoian JO, Love W, Jenkins RL. Amino acid clearance in cirrhosis: A prediction of postoperative morbidity and mortality, *Archives of Surgery* 1987;122:468-473.

40. Schalm S. Liver transplantation of chronic viral hepatitis B, *Hepatology: Rapid Literature Review* 1989;19:3-5.
41. Donovan JP, Zetterman RK, Burnett DA, Sorrell MF. Preoperative evaluation, preparation and timing of orthotopic liver transplantation in the adult, *Seminal Liver Disease* 1989;9:168-175.
42. Goodwin DW. Genetic influences in alcoholism, *Advisor of Internal Medicine* 1987;32:283-297.
43. Churchill LR. *Rationing Healthcare in America: Perceptions and Principles of Justice*. Notre Dame, IN: University of Notre Dame Press, 1987.
44. Atterbury CE. The alcoholic in the lifeboat. Should drinkers be candidates for liver transplantation? *Journal of Clinical Gastroenterology* 1986;8:1-4.
45. Jamieson NV, Sundberg R, Lindell S, Laravuso R, Kalayoglu M, Southard JH, Belzer FO. Successful 24- to 30-hour preservation of the canine liver: A preliminary report, *Transplantation Procedings* 1988;20(Suppl 1):945-947.
46. Todo S, Nery S, Yanoga K, Podesta L, Gordon RD, Starzl TE. Extended preservation of human liver grafts with VW solution, *Journal of the American Medical Association* 1989;261:711-4.
47. Broelsch CE, Emond JC, Thistlethwaite JR, Rouch DA, Whitington PF, Lichtor JL. Liver transplantation with reduced-size donor organs, *Transplantation* 1988;45:519-524.
48. Singer PA, Siegler M, Whitington PF, Lantos JD, Emond JC, Thistlethwaite JR, Broelsch CE. Ethics of liver transplantation with liver donors, *New England Journal of Medicine* 1989;321:620-622.
49. The Council on Scientific Affairs of the American Medical Association. Organ donor recruitment, *Journal of the American Medical Association* 1981;246:2157-2158.
50. Van Thiel DH, Schade RR, Hakala TR, Starzyl TE, Denny D. Liver procurement for orthotopic transplantation: An analysis of the Pittsburgh experience, *Hepatology* 1984;4(Suppl):66S-71S.
51. Merz B. The organ procurement problem: Many causes, no easy solutions, *Journal of the American Medical Association* 1985;254:3285-3288.
52. Seigler M. *Update on hepatic transplantation: Current controversies in liver transplantation. Transplantation of Alcoholics*. Presented at Annual Meetings of the American Association for the Study of Liver Diseases, Chicago, October 28-31, 1989.
53. Welch HG. Health care tickets for the uninsured: First class, coach, or standby? *New England Journal of Medicine* 1989;321:1261-1264.
54. Shaw BW. Starting a liver transplant program, *Seminal Liver Disease* 1989;9:159-167.

Chapter 42

Ethical Issues and Transplantation Technology

David C. Thomasma

Not that long ago, any thought of transferring body parts, or fluids like blood, among individuals was expressed in terms of a nightmare. Consider the problem of involuntary blood transfusions to Count Dracula! Or recall the infamous brain transplant to the brutish body under Dr. Frankenstein's ministrations. The very thought of bodily transference stimulated writers to create monsters. The stuff of evil seemed to surround any attempt. Hubris was considered the evil that exceeded the normal limits of scientific research and development. Transplantation seemed to make humans into gods who defied death but who, like Icarus and his wax wings, flew too close to the sun.

Some of these same fears still exist as modern medical technology zeros in on replacement of almost every part of the body. It has been an awesome accomplishment. Built up gradually by many specialties, today's and tomorrow's abilities are truly staggering. Although none of our transplant technology would be aimed at a single individual, think of what could be replaced even now if it were: heart, arteries, lungs, kidneys, liver, intestines (not very successfully), parts of brain tissue, genetic material,[1] pancreas, bones, bone marrow, cell transplants to aid muscle disorders, skin, corneas, and limbs. What remains for the future are sexual organs, stomach, spinal column, and the whole brain itself. Perhaps before that happens, and the age of Dr. Frankenstein is upon us, we will be able to regenerate the body's own cells and repair ourselves from within. Some advances in this regard with coronary arteries have already occurred.

We are only at the beginning of what we should call the "regenerative phase" of medical advances, and transplant technology is actually only a temporary, albeit important, step towards development of cellular and immunological manipulation.

Resistance Factors

An ethical analysis of transplant technology can begin by examining the resistance factors to the technology for what these factors reveal about human values and the changes they must undergo. Any new technology introduces possibilities, possibilities create choices, choices force decisions, and decisions are made on the basis of values. Ethical issues in transplant technology cover a broad range of clinical and social policy concerns that can be examined from many different perspectives.

Emotional Factors

Many organs transplanted today are deeply bound up the emotional content because they are so closely identified with individual identity.[2] In some cultures, identity and feelings are

---

Source: Reprinted from *Cambridge Quarterly of Healthcare Ethics*, Vol. 4, 1992, pp. 333-343, with permission from Cambridge University Press © 1992.

centered in the abdomen. Livers, pancreases, and kidneys are all part of that "moral center" of human life. In Western civilization, it is the heart, most of all, that symbolizes our feelings, our care and compassion for others, our moral judgment, and our love.

Just as the American Indians would eat the raw heart of a brave buffalo to participate in the greatness of that being or the ancient warriors did the same with the enemy's heart and blood, so too do many people consider a heart or bone marrow transplant as an identity transfer along the rejuvenation that occurs. Reportedly, after a Ku Klux Klan leader, who was traditionally and explicitly racist, learned that his kidney transplant came from a black donor, he transformed his life. He now speaks on behalf of racial harmony. A mother, upon learning that an older son could donate bone marrow for his younger sibling, remarked that she hoped the older's sense of responsibility would also be transferred to the younger son!

Less obvious but equally dramatic identity transformations occur within the context of a "resurrection" experience. Each transplanted individual is saved from death, and many ask themselves what new purpose in life has been granted them. Although the demands of a "medicalized" life, a life of being monitored for rejection and infection, annoys them, they often set out to do new deeds. One of the first liver transplant recipients, Frank Maier, resigned his job as chief of the Chicago Office of Newsweek Magazine and then talked and wrote about his experience in explicitly religious, even liturgical tones.[3] The powerful emotional feedback from audiences led him to explore issues in transplantation further, including the problem of donor families feeling neglected after the donation. He championed their cause as well, again out of a profound realization of his responsibilities once he had been given another chance at life.[4] He has since died.

Medical Factors

Contrast this personal and emotional view of transplant as experienced by donating families and transplant survivors with the more objective view of organs carried into the debate by many physicians, researchers, and ethicists.[5,6] Buoyed by success on almost every front, it is hard not to consider organs as interchangeable body parts. Only the constant effort of the body to reject them functions as a reminder that the Aristotelian theory of essential parts may still hold true. Such parts can only function in terms of the whole organism. Temporary viability obscures that fact only for a while.

Some transplant specialists have dismissed values encrustation of organs, claiming that they are just interchangeable body parts. As one such surgeon declared, "You get a heart, you get a heart. It's just a pump."[7]

It is easy to see why an objective scientific view of organs is prevalent. Scientists can keep brain cells alive in the lab for 3 years. Organs can be preserved for small lengths of time as they are transferred around the country following organ bank routing[8] and are even the basis of court decisions in some instances, when relatives sue to gain access to a scarce resource.[9]

Ethics and Transplantation

Yet this objective view of organs-as-toasters to be traded in on a new model contrasts sharply not only with the identity features already discussed but also with the terrible struggles patients face after the transplant, especially with the medicalization of their lives. As one heart transplant patient put it, "Getting a transplant is not like bringing your radio in for repairs...It takes a will to live..."[10]

These life and death considerations lead to a number of conclusions that must guide organ donation policy, and will lead to the recommendations I make at the end of this essay.

1. Organs carry intensely personal meaning, and therefore can be regarded as a

profound gift to others out of motives of altruism and human solidarity.

2. Gifts cannot be given out of fear or coercion. They must be given freely. Hence, independent of legal constraints on forcing persons to donate, there is a moral need to respect not only the integrity of persons but also the nature of a gift.

3. Thus, any social policy must reinforce altruism while protecting individual rights, especially the right of those who for one reason or another choose not to donate their organs.[11,12,13]

4. Organ transplantation is a social good, a sharing of the body and of life in the human community. It is so successful in saving lives that to waste healthy organs by burying or incinerating them is a social evil.[14]

Social Factors

The greatest social problem is that societies, wishing to protect human rights, construct systems in which the individual or family members must "opt into" donating organs.[15] Because most patients seen as donor-candidates have died of trauma and are younger than most other patients who face death, they usually have not thought much, if at all, about donating organs. The family is at its peak of initial grief and loss, so that discussing donation moments after death is itself indelicate and rude without some intense social warrant. A law requiring such discussion can "excuse" the transplant team from this concern, even though skills are still needed in balancing concern for the family's loss with the potential good for others to be gained by donating organs.

Would it not make sense to change the assumption about donation, given the data of overwhelming support for this action on the part of citizens? A change in the default mode of "opting in" to one of "opting out" would make the task of obtaining organs easier while still protecting the autonomy of citizens who do not wish to donate. This is done in many countries today.

If organ donation is seen as an intensely personal gift, as I have argued, then buying and selling organs would irretrievably damage this important condition of the process. Because of the dramatic shortage of organs (there are 21,000 people in the United States waiting for vital organs; of these, 30% die each year),[16] it is tempting to consider the view that there is nothing illogical or immoral about buying and selling organs.[17,18] If we use the principle that we may sell those aspects of the body that do not diminish the individual (i.e., that can be replenished or regenerated), then in addition to blood, sperm, and ova, we could add portions of the liver and even excess skin (from a major weight loss) to items on sale.[19]

One kidney from a liver donor could be included because the risk is small to the donor compared to the benefits to be gained.

Yet as social policy, rather than philosophical argument, buying and selling organs should be left as an extreme form of inducement as a last resort.[20] Meanwhile, other efforts to stimulate organ donation ought to be tried on the grounds of altruism and social solidarity already adumbrated. Churches and civic organizations could be enlisted in this effort. Inducements to encourage donations might include the following:

1. Those who, in an advance directive, offer their organs in case of their death could receive a reduction in health insurance premiums, especially for catastrophic diseases. Even in countries supplying free health care for all citizens, the reduction in costs of dialysis, etc., that might come with and adequate supply of organs could be passed on in lower taxes for health care or through some other benefit.

2. Those who donate could be offered earlier access (above those who do not donate) to scarce medical care or experimental therapies newly developed. For example, interleukin-2 therapy for terminal cancer might be offered to individuals who have chosen to donate in an advance directive, although it may be too costly to offer the general public in a national health care plan during its experimental phase.

3. Hospitals may create a class of care for designated donors that provides additional amenities (like first-class airfare) that are not essential to the standard of care everyone should receive.

These are but a few of the methods by which society can encourage altruism among its citizens and alone with it, essentially needed organ donation.

Ethical and Religious Concerns

A number of hurdles have been cleared in the United States with respect to organ transplantation. One of these is the definition of death. Each state adopted one or another version of "brain-death" legislation under the guidance of a uniform Natural Death Act Committee composed of legal and medical authorities. In essence, these acts determine that a person has died (and that, with permission, organs can be obtained) when there has been a "cessation of total brain function," or words to that effect, as determined by the latest medical guidelines.

A tiny minority of thinkers continues to consider it murder to take the organs of persons whose hearts have not stopped. Typically, they argue that the cessation of brain function is no more theoretically irreversible than was the stoppage of the heart, now able to be resuscitated. Hence, current guidelines for the cessation of brain function are going to undergo change as we understand cellular function better. In the view of this minority, we are taking the lives of some to benefit others. An immoral means cannot be used, they argue, to obtain a good end.

This argument fails to take into account a fundamental fact. Medical criteria are just that -- criteria society can use to determine the moment of death. The criteria shift over time as does the determination. The criteria for death have included effects of breath on a feather or a mirror all the way to ruling out hypothermia and encephalopathy today. Similarly, the social determination of death changes with the needs of society or the common good. Because of the fear of infection, persons during the Black Plague were considered "dead" much earlier than they might have been in more normal times. One way Italian city-states avoided the devastation that hit the rest of Europe was to board up the whole family of an infected person and burn down their house. In this action, otherwise health but exposed persons were considered "as good as dead."

Because of severe shortage of organs, society may wish to relax its current standard of brain death (the cessation of total brain function, including the brain stem) in favor of one that centers on higher brain function, the part that gives human life its uniqueness and interaction.[21] Most persons, when queried, would not want to live on in a "vegetative" state, unable to perform any distinctly human task. Those patients in this state might be good candidates for organ donation, provided sufficient consent can be obtained ahead of time.[22,23] Ambivalence and confusion about the ethics of this approach would certainly mean that there would be resistance by caregivers at this time.[24]

A major problem underlying the notion of brain death is how transplant technology for both recipient and donor has caused us and continues to cause us to rethink our definition of a person. This definition includes the problem of social value, not only of persons, but of parts of persons. Consider two cases that occurred recently.

The first case involved the conception of a baby to benefit another sibling.[25] A mother, upon learning that her teen-age daughter needed a bone marrow transplant decided to try and get pregnant again so that the baby could donate its bone marrow to, its sibling at birth. While virtually every ethicist would condemn conceiving a fetus just to abort it, say just before 6 months gestation to harvest its brain tissue for that woman's father suffering from Alzheimer's or Parkinson's, this case is much less easy to condemn. In fact, the mother's motives are laudatory. She might save her daughter's life (it is her daughter's only hope). Her baby will be loved not destroyed. The baby may even be proud of its role in attempting to save another's life (although the attempt might fail). Children have been conceived for far less noble reasons than this.

However, the case does raise the philosophical question of whether we can use one person for the sake of another without that person's consent.[26,27,28] This is also the fundamental problem society faces in trying to obtain organs. The common good can require curtailing individual freedoms, but should that include integrity of the body as well? A special case of this question arises in the debate about fetal tissue transplantation. Once the fetus has been aborted electively, would not the common good require the use of that fetus's tissues, such as brain tissue to benefit Alzheimer's and Parkinson's Disease victims or pancreatic tissue to benefit brittle diabetics, on the grounds that the fetus whose life is no longer to be lived "ought" to donate its body to benefit others?[29] If transplant technology stays sufficiently far away from the decision to abort, as it does from the critical care decisions about accident victims, perhaps it can be brought into the case after the death has been determined so as to benefit others.[30] Scientists argue that the 1.5 million abortions performed each year in the United States would provide sufficient "fetal tissue" to benefit those who need its dramatic properties the most.[31]

Part of an answer to this question was provided by a second case that occurred in my home state of Illinois. Tamas Bosze was unhappy in his marriage and moved in with his mistress, Nancy Cuban, after separating from his wife. They had twins, James and Allison Curran. Later, Tamas returned to his wife and son, Pierre. Jean-Pierre contracted leukemia, and Mr. Bosze sued Ms. Curran to have the twins tested as likely bone marrow transplant donors. Jean-Pierre was in good enough condition at the time to have possibly benefitted from the procedure. It was his only hope. The reason Mr. Bosze sued his former mistress was that she refused to have the twins tested on grounds that the bone marrow procedure would expose them to extreme pain and possible infection. Nancy Curran and Tamas Bosze had been involved for 3 years in court actions because she had sued him for child support. A blood test ordered by the court proved he was the father.[32]

The tragedy of this case was that because of the acrimonious relations between Nancy and Tamas, Jean-Pierre's condition could not be addressed. He deteriorated and died at 13 years of age on 19 November 1990; The Illinois Supreme Court upheld the lower court ruling, however, that the right of individual privacy cannot be violated, even to save the life of another. Children cannot be considered "fair game" for others without parental consent. In place of altruism and human solidarity in this case was anger and legal constraints. The risk to the twins was minimal compared to the possible benefit to Jean-Pierre.

Yet the courts made the correct judgment in this case. As I have argued, organs should not be objects of commerce and market conditions. They are part of the identity of persons and constitute their inherent value as individuals.[33]

This assertion brings us to the most difficult problem in transplant technology, the problem of multiple or successive transplants for one individual in the context of scarcity and social justice. The problem can be compounded by an individual's previous patterns of illness. Further, the problem may be given a distasteful "marketing" flavor when health care institutions decide to get into the "business" of transplant because they wish to remain competitive. Consider the following case. I call it the case of Jay's Liver Transplant.

Jay B. is mellower now that he is 46-years-old. His life has been a course of one crisis after the other. Now he faces the possibility of a second liver transplant. He is sick and scared.

He was born in the Midwest into a family of alcoholics. His father, mother, and three brothers all share the family history of abuse. He has abused alcohol for 20 years himself.

Two years ago, his liver failed. He stopped drinking at that time. One year later he got hepatitis. This year he was admitted to the hospital with two other life-threatening conditions, esophageal varices that bled uncontrollably and, later, toxic encephalopathy. He has been ready to "hang up the spikes" a number of times.

He was evaluated as a good candidate for a liver and kidney transplant upon his third hospitalization in 1 year for liver and kidney failure (for which he was put on dialysis) and for pulmonary edema. Waiting much longer would be fatal to him. Normally, centers establish a 5-year alcohol-free period before considering individuals as proper candidates. However, the medical center evaluating Jay is anxious to become a major transplant center. The transplant physicians here were trained by the major academic centers in the country doing liver transplants, including Stanford and University of Chicago. They were recruited with this aim in mind by the hospital board.

In September, therefore, Jay received his first liver and kidney transplant. The operation "vampirized" the city blood bank. It took 112 units of packed cells, 152 units of frozen plasma, 120 units of platelets, and 107 units of other blood products.

Post-operatively, Jay did well, but the liver and kidney did not function up to capacity. Eventually, the liver failed again, and his kidney function began to decline. The kidney function would probably be reversible if his liver function were normal. Thus, a second liver transplant is being contemplated. The kidney will be assessed if the liver transplant is successful.

There are many other individuals on the list awaiting an available liver. Jay is now only marginally responsive.

The team asks itself the following demanding questions:

1. Who is and who is not a proper candidate for transplant? Should alcoholism be taken as a disease, or should a time for disease-free behavior be set? Was 2 years enough? Or should the Center have insisted on 5 years?

2. How much treatment for Jay is enough? What if this liver fails too? Meagan LaRocco in Chicago, a baby, got a total of five livers before she left the hospital alive.

3. How can bleeding the blood bank dry be justified for one patient? But is it right to ask such access questions at the bedside?[34]

Analyzing all the aspects of this case here would take up more space than permitted, but consider the following features.

Jay received his first liver at a Center that violated the current standards of care to leap into this market. Normally patients do not qualify for a liver until they have been drug or alcohol free for 4 years. Yet it is unfair to stereotype and condemn the Center's actions on this basis alone. The current standards for being drug free may simply be a convenient measure for allocating a scarce resource. Such measures can be overridden on a case-by-case basis due to urgency in saving a person's life.

The Center's ambitions may be driven by an intense desire to respect the lives of the most desperately ill human beings. Just as Jean-Pierre's need was greater than the risk to the twins, so too may Jay's need be greater than others on the list to receive a liver transplant. Jay's requirements to live clearly outweigh some artificially imposed allocation standard that does not seem to take into account individual need and an "emergency ethic" for preserving human life.[35]

The point just raised acquires additional poignancy when coupled with the insight that alcoholism is a disease that is extremely difficult to conquer. Jay has been free for 4 months. Admittedly, this is only a brief time. Some people have experienced recovery for over 20 years and then relapsed. Medicine must be free to care for patients without prejudice, the source and origin of disease must not be used as a way to demean persons by cutting back on their care.

At this point we begin to touch on a theological point. The human condition is such that all of us share not only in illness, but also in choices, conscious and subconscious, that may drive us to a compromised state of health. For Jay, it was his alcoholism; for another it may be lung cancer from smoking; for still another it may be diabetes from years of overeating; and for still another, it may be a bleeding ulcer or hypertension. The interplay of life as lived and its many challenges means precisely that the spirit and the body suffer. Just as health care workers cannot dismiss the person with AIDS as unworthy of their care, neither can society condemn Jay and deny his chance for a resurrection by an upfront judgment that his life of dissolution should eliminate him as a candidate for a liver transplant, all other medical indications being equal.[36,37]

But wait! The line of reasoning thus far has totally neglected the role of justice. Allocating scarce organs, especially when one has failed and another is needed, is not a device to denigrate individual need as has so far been implied in the argument. Rather it represents our best effort to fill that need, to meet as many individual needs as possible without harming large numbers of persons.[38,39]

In this respect, denying Jay an initial liver transplant, while harming him, may have provided a success in someone else with the liver he received (we would not have "wasted" a liver on Jay that another might have used successfully), and a second and third liver (that Jay may now need to stay alive) would also have gone to more suitable candidates.

Allocation on the basis of medical indications, then, is as objective a measure as can be used. It differs from utilitarianism in that it tries to avoid spreading around the benefits to statistical others. Rather, the benefits of transplant technology are distributed to those who might best be able to succeed physically and spiritually.

As Professor Erich Loewy has argued, the capacity to suffer is the moral basis of a beneficent community. It has its roots in the very biological capacity to empathize with another's pain and agony.[40] Although all animals can suffer, only human beings can heal one another. For religious believers, this capacity to heal is a participation in a redemptive process that shares mysteriously in the power of God.[41] For those without religious belief, this capacity drives the most fundamental tenets of humanism and health care.[42]

In a situation of scarce resources, such as the lack of an adequate number of organs to benefit even the most likely candidates, the fundamental instincts of human solidarity as just described are ruptured. On the one hand, we must establish just and equitable standards. These will deny organs, then, even to those who desperately need them to live. Jean-Pierre will die; Jay will die. On the other hand, the duty of the State must be to constantly act to eliminate the scarcity so that our allocation measures can consistently and asymptotically approach medical indications alone.

Transplantation technology is a regenerative human good of such a great measure that burying and incinerating good organs is a monumental evil. Every effort of state and church must be made to conceptualize and reinforce our fundamental instincts to share our bodies and our identities[43] at death with others who could live as a result of this gift. Protecting the notion of gift rather than commercializing the process ought to be the front line of attack that the state should employ.

Recommendations

As technological capacity continues to increase worldwide, the current shortage of organ donors is reaching a desperate stage. The following are steps either already in place or proposed to encourage organ donation.

1. Mandate discussion of the possibility of donation with bereaved families (as does a U.S. Federal Law). This is done by a team separate from the one that cared for the patient, so that confusion of concern can be minimalized. The health care team caring for the potential donor will not be seen as vultures ready to pounce on the victim to "harvest" organs, and conflict of interest is avoided.

2. Broach the subject with patients who come to the hospital for routine care, perhaps through the new Patient Self-Determination Act. The hospital ethics committee might assist the directors of the hospital with suggested policy that would protect patient rights while encouraging organ donation.[44]

3. Alter the default mode, so that people would be assumed to "opt into" organ donation unless they "opted out" in documents such as a Living Will or by checking so on the back of their driver's license. Many European countries do make this assumption in their laws. However, in this country it might require a Constitutional Amendment.

4. Continue to refine public policy about multiple transplants for the same patient, particularly if compliance with recognized guidelines has been lacking.

5. Support medical research on gene therapy and other manipulations at the microscopic and cellular level that will eventually bypass transplant technology in favor of autologous processes.

6. Engage churches and civic clubs in efforts to encourage and reinforce a notion of community that would underline our duties to assist one another, with our own bodies if necessary.[45] Imagine what Beethoven's 10th would have been, or 11th or 12th, had he had a chance for a liver transplant![46]

7. Continue to work for refinements in brain-death legislation. Explore the ethics of donating organs through an advance directive prior to the long-term effects of certain irreversible neurologically damaging states, such as endstage Alzheimer's, permanent vegetative state, massive stroke (like that of Sidney Greenspan),[47] and permanent coma.[48] Of course another definition of death confined to higher brain functions would be required.[49]

Conclusion

The value of identity with organs can be used to promote altruism and responsibility to others. Autonomy can be enlisted to create a public commitment to a new default mode of donation with the choice being opting out, rather than opting in. Organs should not be bought and sold as if they were objects unencumbered with values. The moment of death is not a medical but a social decision that can vary as the times and technology change, and what is distinctly human about us is affect and cognition, not possible when the higher brain function has permanently vanished.

Notes

1. Booth W. Genetic therapy ok'd for cancer use. *Chicago Sun-Times* 1990 Nov. 14:26.
2. Childress JF. The gift of life: Ethical problems and policies in obtaining and distributing organs for transplantation, *Critical Care Clinics* 1986;2(1):133-48.
3. Maier F. A second chance at life, *Newsweek* 1988;Sept. 8:52-5, 57, 59, 61.
4. Maier F. A final gift, *Ladies Home Journal* 1990;March:102-11.
5. Singer PA, Lantos JD, Whitington PF, *et al*. Equipoise and the ethics of segmental liver transplantation, *Clinical Research* 1988:539-45.
6. Corry RJ, Mendez R, Friedlaender GE, *et al*. Organ allocation [set of six papers], *Transplantation Proceedings* 1988;20(Suppl. 1):1011-32.
7. Lauerman C. Life after transplant, *Chicago Tribune Magazine* 1987;May 24:10-11.
8. Starzl TE, *et al*. A multifactorial system for equitable selection of cadaver kidney recipients, *Journal of the American Medical Association* 1987;257:3073-5.
9. Turcote JG, Hakala TR, Tzakis A. Patient selection criteria in organ transplantation: The critical questions [Set of 19 articles, commentaries, etc.], *Transplantation Proceedings* 1989;21:3377445.
10. Lauerman, *loc. cit.*
11. Kamm FM. The report of the U.S. Task Force on Organ Transplantation: Criticisms and alternatives, *Mt. Sinai Journal of Medicine* 1989;56:207-20.
12. Daniels N. Justice and the dissemination of "big ticket" technologies, In: Matthieu D, ed. *Organ Substitution Technology: Ethical, Legal, and Public Policy Issues*. Boulder, CO: Westview Press, 1988:211-20.
13. Jonsen A. Ethical issues in organ transplantation, In: Veatch RM, ed. *Medical Ethics*. Boston, MA: Jones and Bartlett, 1989:229-52.
14. Hansmann H. The economics and ethics of markets for human organs, *Journal of Health Politics, Policy and Law* 1989;14:57-85.
15. Childress, J. Ethical criteria for procuring and distributing organs for transplantation, *Journal of Health Politics, Policy and Law* 1989;14:87-113.
16. Elliot D, Fitz B. *A Case of Need*. [Video program on media coverage and organ transplants.] Boston, MA: Fanlight Productions.
17. Hansmann, *op. cit.*
18. Cowan DH, Kantorowitz JA, Moskowitz J, *et al*., eds. *Human Organ Transplantation: Societal, Medical-Legal, Regulatory, and Reimbursement Issues*. Ann Arbor, MI: Health Administration Press, in cooperation with the American Society of Law & Medicine, 1987.
19. Wolinsky H. 2nd living-donor liver patient dies. *Chicago Sun-Times* 1990 Nov. 20:26.
20. Cotton RD, Sandler AL. The regulation of organ procurement and transplantation in the United States, *Journal of Legal Medicine* 1986;7:55-84.
21. Sorenson JH. The determination of death: The need for a higher-brain death concept, In: Monagle JF, Thomasma DC, eds. *Medical Ethics: A Guide for Health Professionals*. Rockville, MD: Aspen Publishers, 1988:234-48.
22. Ivan LP. The persistant vegetative state, *Transplantation Proceedings* 1990;22:993-4.
23. Downie J. The biology of the persistent vegetative state: Legal, ethical, and philosophical implications for transplantation, *Transplantation Proceedings* 1990;22:995-6.
24. Keatings M. The biology of the persistent vegetative state, legal and ethical implications for transplantation: Viewpoints from nursing, *Transplantation Proceedings* 1990;22:997-9.
25. Hamilton D. Mom, 43, having baby to aid dying daughter. *Chicago Sun-Times* 1990 Feb. 16:1.
26. Annas GJ. Siamese twins: Killing one to save the other, *Hastings Center Report* 1987;17(2):27-9.
27. Rosner F, Risemberg HM, Bennett AJ. The anencephalic fetus and newborn as organ donors, *New York State Journal of Medicine* 1988;88:360-6.

28. Caplan AL. Should fetuses or infants be utilized as organ donors? *Bioethics* 1987;1:119-40.
29. Gillon R. Ethics of fetal brain cell transplants, *British Medical Journal* 1988;296(6631):1212-3.
30. Fine I. The ethics of fetal tissue transplants, *Hastings Center Report* 1988;18:5-10.
31. Bauer AR. Fetal tissue transplantation, *Trial* 1990;Jul:22-7.
32. O'Donnell M. Jean-Pierre death ends transplant court fight. *Chicago Sun-Times* 1990 Nov. 20:5.
33. Thomasma DC. *Human Life in the Balance*. Louisville, KY: Westminster Press, 1990.
34. Thomasma DC, Marshall P. *Clinical Medical Ethics Coursebook*. Chicago, IL: Loyola University, 1990.
35. Thomasma DC. *Human Life in the Balance*. Louisville, KY: Westminster Press, 1990:196-226.
36. Loewy EH. Drunks, livers, and values: Should social value judgments enter into liver transplant decisions? *Journal of Clinical Gastroenterology* 1987;9:436-41.
37. Rettig RA. The politics of organ transplantation: A parable of our time, *Journal of Health Politics, Policy and Law* 1989;14:191-227.
38. Blumstein JF. Government's role in organ transplantation policy, *Journal of Health Politics, Policy and Law* 1989;14:5-39.
39. Childress JF. Some moral connections between organ procurement and organ distribution, *Journal of Contemporary Health Law and Policy* 1987;3:85-110.
40. Loewy E. *Suffering and the Beneficent Community*. Buffalo, NY: State University of New York at Buffalo Press, 1991.
41. Pellegrino ED, Thomasma DC. *The Religious Devotion*. New York, NY: Continuum, 1991.
42. Pellegrino ED. *Humanism and the Physician*. Knoxville, TN: University of Tennessee Press, 1979.
43. Thomasma DC. Corpo e persona: Quando scienza e technologia travolgono la compassione umana, *KOS* 1989;5(32):6-7, 10-11, 14, 15.
44. Anonymous. Organ shortage raises questions about rule of ethics committees, *Medical Ethics Advisor* 1990;6(10):133-5.
45. Thomasma DC. The quest for organ donors: A theological response, *Health Progress* 1988;69(7):2224, 28.
46. Anonymous. Theory offered in Beethoven's death. *Chicago Sun-Times* 1990 Oct. 15:20.
47. Long R. Comatose man's death ends right-to-die ordeal. *Chicago Sun-Times* 1990 Oct. 12:4.
48. Thomasma DC. Making treatment decisions for permanently unconscious patients, In: Monagle J, Thomasma DC, eds. *Medical Ethics: A Guide for Health Professionals*. Frederick, MD: Aspen Publishing Co., 1988:186-204.
49. Sorenson JH, *op. cit.*

Chapter 43

The Effect of Race on Access and Outcome in Transplantation

Bertram L. Kasiske, John F. Neylan III, Robert R. Riggio, Gabriel M. Danovitch, Lawrence Kahana, Steven R. Alexander, and Martin G. White

The American Society of Transplant Physicians directed its Patient Care and Education Committee to examine the issue of racial inequality in transplantation. The committee, made up of physicians involved in clinical transplantation, used both published data and personal experience to develop a consensus on the issues and problems related to race in transplantation. This report summarizes the conclusions reached by the committee and outlines the specific recommendations make to the society.

Prevalence and Incidence of End-Stage Renal Disease Among Minorities

To examine the issue of racial inequality in kidney transplantation, it is important to know the incidence and prevalence of end-stage renal disease among minority populations. In the United States, the relative risk of end-stage renal disease is about fourfold higher four blacks than whites (Table 1). The prevalence of end-stage renal disease among blacks is also higher, since blacks, who make up approximately 12 percent of the U.S. population, accounted for 27 percent of the patients with end-stage renal disease in 1987.[9] The higher relative risk of end-stage renal disease among blacks geographically homogeneous, has been found at all ages over 15 years, and has generally been found among both men and women.[1,2,3,4,5,6,7,8,9,10] Although blacks have an increased prevalence of hypertension and diabetes, the increased incidence of end-stage renal disease among blacks cannot be attributed to any one cause of renal disease.[11,12] The relative risk of end-stage renal disease varies with diagnostic category (Table 1).

Other racial and ethnic groups may also be at greater risk of renal failure. For adult Native Americans living in the United States, the overall risk of end-stage renal disease is approximately threefold higher than for whites.[13] This increased incidence has been ascribed to several factors, including a higher incidence of diabetes mellitus and glomerulonephritis.[13,14,15,16,17,18,19] Little is known about the incidence of end-stage renal disease in Hispanic Americans. One study in California reported that the risk of end-stage renal disease among Hispanics was similar to that among other whites,[4] whereas a study in Texas found that the risk was threefold higher.[5]

Race and the Likelihood of Undergoing Organ Transplantation

As compared with whites, a smaller percentage of nonwhite patients on dialysis have undergone kidney transplantation.[8,20,21] Data from the Health Care Financing Administration

---

Source: Reprinted from *The New England Journal of Medicine*, Vol. 324, 1991, 296-301, with permission from *New England Journal of Medicine,* copyright 1991.

(HCFA) indicated that in 1985 blacks accounted for 28 percent of patients with end-stage renal disease, but only 21 percent of those undergoing renal transplantation.[8] Although 24 percent of the recipients of cadaver kidneys were black, only 12 percent of those receiving a kidney from a living donor were black.[8] Thus, a major proportion of the racial differences in the overall rate of transplantation reflected differences in the rate of transplantation from living related donors. More recent 1987 data from the HCFA confirmed these results for blacks (Table 2). In contrast, the number of Native Americans who had primary transplantation of cadaver kidneys or kidneys from living related donors was proportional to the number of Native Americans with new-onset end-stage renal disease and comparable to the corresponding rates among whites (Table 2). Moreover, the proportion of transplantations performed in Native Americans that involved living relat4ed donors was similar to that for whites (Table 2).

Why proportionally fewer blacks have received kidney transplants is unknown. However, differences in the frequencies of ABO blood groups and the major-histocompatibility-complex (MHC) antigens, inadequate financial coverage, knowledge that the outcome after transplantation is worse in blacks than in whites, cultural barriers, and other socioeconomic factors could all affect the rate of transplantation.[22]

Racial Differences in ABO Blood Groups and MHC Antigens

The distribution of ABO blood groups varies according to race (Table 3). Differences in ABO blood groups, in combination with the fact that only 8 percent of donors are black,[23] may cause fewer kidneys to be given to black recipients. The fact that whites (40 percent of whom have blood group A) make up the majority of organ donors suggests that cadaver kidneys will more often go to whites than to blacks (27 percent of whom have blood group A), Native Americans (16 percent of whom have blood group A), or Asian Americans (28 percent of whom have blood group A). Proportionally, almost twice as many blacks (20 percent of whom have blood group B) as whites (11 percent of whom have blood group B) must wait for the relatively small supply of kidneys from donors with blood group B.

There are also racial differences in the distribution of HMC antigens that may influence the matching of donors and recipients.[24,25] For instance, the frequencies of the common MHC antigens A1, A2, B7, and B8 in whites are approximately 25, 47, 19, and 18 percent, respectively, whereas in U.S. blacks they are 7, 30, 15, and 4 percent, respectively.[26] In Illinois, good matches of MHC-antigens were more often obtained from donors and recipients of the same race.[27] Moreover, the lack of MHC alleles common to blacks and whites correlated with the low frequency with which good matches were made for black recipients.[27]

The racial differences in ABO blood groups and MHC pheno-types make it more likely that a candidate for transplantation will receive a well-matched kidney from a member of the same race. A relative lack of minority organ donors decreases the number of well-matched kidneys available for minority recipients. Because ABO compatibility must be satisfied first, matching of MHC antigens is likely to have a relatively smaller influence on racial disparities in the allocation of organs. However, racial differences in ABO blood groups, combined with a priority system for organ allocation designed to favor MHC-antigen matching, may explain why relatively fewer minority patients undergo kidney transplantation, whereas proportionately more minority patients remain on waiting lists for a cadaver kidney (Table 4).

It has been argued that good results can be obtained regardless of how well kidneys are matched and that abandoning or reducing the priority of MHC-antigen matching would increase the number of minority patients undergoing transplantation.[30] On the other hand, matching has a substantial effect on the long-term survival of allografts. Indeed, some investigations have found that inferior graft survival among black organ recipients may have resulted form the fact that blacks received kidneys that were less well matched than those received by whites (see below). Currently, the Organ Procurement and Transplantation Network uses a point system for organ allocation that takes both waiting time and matching of MHC antigens into account. How this point system has affected the availability of kidneys for minorities, as well as graft survival, remains to be determined.

Race and Organ Donation

The number of minority patients who undergo transplantation could be improved by increasing the number of minority organ donors. Moreover, increasing the number of minority donors could allow closer matching and even enhance long-term survival of grafts (see below). Blacks have been found to be less likely than whites to donate a kidney to a relative,[29] and the rate of refusal to allow an organ to be used for cadaver transplantation was found to be twofold to threefold higher among black families than white.[28,31] The results were similar among Hispanics who were potential organ donors.[28,31] Reasons that may make racial or ethnic minorities less willing than whites to donate organs include a lack of awareness of organ-donation programs, religious beliefs, distrust of the medical community, fears that donors will be declared dead prematurely, and a desire to give organs to members of the same minority.[32,33,34,35]

Other Potential Causes of Unequal Access to Transplantation

Few data are available to evaluate whether health care workers less often consider members of racial minorities to be suitable candidates for transplantation. The results of a study from one dialysis center with a large black population showed that most patients were asked whether they wanted to undergo kidney transplantation.[36] This investigation did not examine the effect of race on the reasons given for refusal to undergo transplantation. There have been no systematic studies to determine how the subject of transplantation has been presented to and perceived by minority patients on dialysis.

Ongoing or recent dependence on alcohol or other addictive substances is generally considered to be a contraindication to transplantation. Drug abuse is associated with reduced survival or renal allografts.[37] The prevalence of heroin abuse may be higher in blacks than in whites,[38] and it is possible that a greater proportion of black patients on dialysis are refused transplantation because of suspected substance abuse. However, no data are available on the prevalence of drug abuse among patients of different races who are on dialysis or on the effects of substance abuse on access to transplantation.

Poor compliance with medical therapy is considered by many to be a relative contraindication to organ transplantation. It is possible that a greater prevalence of disadvantageous socioeconomic conditions leads to a greater likelihood of noncompliance among minority patients than among whites. Indeed, the higher rate of noncompliance among minority patients is more a reflection of socioeconomic status than of race.[39]

For many minority patients, Medicaid is the only source of health insurance. Medicaid coverage varies state to state and in general does not cover the cost of renal transplantation completely.[40] Other forms of transplantation may not be covered at all. Private insurance also varies greatly in regard to transplantation coverage, and in some places transplantation coverage, and in places transplantation insurance is available only at extra cost. It seems likely that minority patients often have inadequate coverage for expenses related to transplantation. Education, language, economics, and subtle cultural barriers may also combine with financial hardship to make it more difficult for minority patients to pursue aggressively and ultimately undergo transplantation. Many health care workers may not be aware of or adequately trained to deal with socioeconomic factors that may make it difficult for minority patients to undergo transplantation.

Race and Allograft Survival

Data from renal-transplant registries have demonstrated that allograft survival is reduced in black recipients[9,41,42,43,44,45] (Table 5). Moreover, in a multivariate analysis of risk factors in the era before cyclosporine (1977 to 1982), race had an effect on allograft survival that was independent of MHC-antigen matching, the presence of preferred alloantibodies, and transplantation center.[46] Race had no independent effect on patient survival.[46]

Although graft survival improved substantially after the introduction of cyclosporine, blacks have continued to have lower rates of graft survival than whites (Table 5). In the Collaborative Transplant Study, the lower success rate among blacks was most pronounced in transplantation centers with "fair" results.[44] In centers with "excellent" results, allograft survival was similar in blacks and whites during the first two years after transplantation but was lower in black thereafter. Blacks had a lower proportion of transplants that were well matched,[47] but the degree of MHC-antigen matching did not explain all the racial differences in graft outcome.[44]

Similar results have been reported by the University of California at Los Angeles Transplant Registry (Table 5). There, the difference in graft survival became even more pronounced with longer follow-up.[45] The racial differences in graft survival could not be attributed to differences in MHC-antigen matching, in the original cause of renal failure, or in results among the participating centers. In contrast, the lower rates of graft survival among blacks as compared with whites in the precyclosporine era were largely explained by a center effect.[48]

Recent data from the HCFA confirmed that long-term survival of renal allografts was lower among black than white Medicare beneficiaries who received kidneys from either living related donors or cadavers between 1977 and 1987.[9] Although the overall rate of graft survival has improved in the past decade, blacks have continued to have uncorrected three-year and five-year survival rates for kidneys from living related donors or cadavers that are at least 10 percent lower than those for whites.[9] The fact that black transplant recipients fared less well than whites was also reflected by the larger number of days after transplantation that blacks were hospitalized.[9] There was no difference in patient survival between blacks and whites.[9,44-46]

Studies of the effects of race on allograft survival in individual centers have produced conflicting results.[29,49,50,51,52,53,54,55,56,57,58,59,60,61,62] Several centers have reported similar rates of allograft survival among blacks and non-blacks.[50-53,56,60,61] Different explanations have been given for the lack of an effect of race on allograft survival in these centers. It has been suggested, for example, that newer immunosuppression regimens incorporating cyclosporine have overcome the effects of inferior MHC-antigen matching in black recipients.[51,52] An emphasis on follow-up care after transplantation and efforts to improve patient compliance may have contributed to comparably good rates of allograft survival among blacks and whites.[60,61] Some of the centers that reported a lower rate of allograft survival among blacks than whites[54,55,57,59,62] found patient noncompliance to be a major factor.[57,59]

Relatively few studies have examined allograft survival in nonblack minorities. Among 935 Hispanics who underwent renal transplantation between 1984 and 1988, the rate of graft survival was comparable to that among 12,373 other whites (UCLA Transplant Registry).[45] The results were also similar for Hispanics and other whites receiving cadaver kidneys at the University of California[29] and the University of Miami.[59] At the University of Texas, survival of primary cadaver renal transplants was higher in Hispanics than in other whites.[63] Asian Americans have had survival rates of cadaver allografts that were similar to those among whites.[29,48,64] Whether matching, underlying renal disease, compliance, or other socioeconomic or biologic factors explain the differences in the rates of graft survival among minorities is unknown.

Race and Pancreas and Liver Transplantation

There are few data concerning racial issues in the transplantation of organs other than the kidney. Data from the International Pancreas Transplant Registry revealed that only 1 of 342 transplant recipients from the three predominant Midwestern centers (all having a low black population) was black, whereas 20 of 318 recipients (6.3 percent) at the other 38 institutions were black.[65] The fact that only 3 percent of all pancreas transplantations performed in the United States were carried out in blacks suggests that blacks have received a lower-than-expected number of pancreas transplants.[65]

At the University of Pittsburgh, among 1,429 liver transplantations performed between 1981 and 1988, only 8.4 percent of the recipients were black and 6.6 percent were Hispanic, Asian, or Native American.[66] Since the rate of death from liver disease has been reported to be higher among blacks than among whites, and over 12 percent of the population in the United States is black, the proportion of liver-transplant recipients who were black was lower than expected. The two-year rate of survival among adults who underwent liver transplantation was less than 50 percent in blacks, as compared with 70 percent in nonblack recipients ($P<0.02$).[66]

Why proportionally fewer blacks than whites have undergone pancreas and liver transplantation is unknown. Many of the socioeconomic factors causing racial discrepancies in renal transplantation may also apply to the transplantation of other organs. In addition, the reluctance of third-party payers to finance pancreas and liver transplantation may have been a further barrier to transplantation in minorities. Whether the recent decision by Medicare to cover part of the costs of liver transplantation in adults will affect the distribution of organs remains to be determined.

Conclusions

The Patient Care and Education Committee of the American Society of Transplant Physicians reached the following conclusions. First, in the United States end-stage renal disease is more common in racial minorities than in whites. Second, fewer blacks than whites in the United States undergo kidney transplantation. It is likely that both biologic and socioeconomic differences between blacks and whites contribute to this inequality. Third, the rate of survival of renal allografts is lower among blacks than whites. The reasons for the lower rate of graft survival among blacks may include greater disparities in both known and unknown MHC antigens, patient noncompliance, and socioeconomic factors. Fourth, there are insufficient data to draw firm conclusions about renal transplantation in nonblack minorities in the United States. The rate of allograft survival among Hispanics and Asians appears to be similar to that among non-Hispanic whites, but the relatively low rates of organ donation and limited access to transplantation may be problems for these minorities. Finally, the problems of racial and ethnic inequality that characterize kidney transplantation are present or even magnified for the transplantation of other organs.

Recommendations

The following recommendations ere made by the Patient Care and Education Committee. First data from the Organ Procurement and Transplantation Network and other sources should be used to examine carefully how differences in ABO blood groups and MHC tissue antigens may influence the rate organ transplantation among minority patients. Second, the process of selecting patients on dialysis for renal transplantation should be examined critically. Well-designed studies that include direct interviews of patients and health care providers are needed to determine why suitable candidates for transplantation remain on dialysis. Third, the effect of variations and inconsistencies in public and private health insurance programs that may limit minority access to transplantation needs to be assessed. Fourth, the process that leads to the placement of patient eligible for transplantation on a waiting list should be examined, since factors that influence this process may create a more favorable position for one patient than another. Fifth, the reasons why blacks who undergo renal transplantation have lower rates of graft survival than whites and other minorities need further study. In particular, the effect on graft survival of patient education after transplantation, of follow-up, and of compliance issues should be addressed. Sixth, the information needed to assess the effect of race on the transplantation of nonrenal organs should be collected by the Organ Procurement and Transplantation Network. Access to transplantation, the source of organ donors, and outcome all need to be examined for minority candidates for nonrenal transplantation.

Although it is important to collect the information needed to answer critical questions regarding race and transplantation, the present lack of data should not delay potentially beneficial action. Efforts to increase the number of organ donations (those make by living related donors or obtained after death) from members of racial minorities is a strategy that should yield immediate dividends. This approach should increase the number of suitable organs available for minority candidates without sacrificing the benefits of matching. Finally, health care providers should increase their advocacy role to assist patients ill equipped to understand, accept, or comply with the complicated issues of transplantation and its follow-up. Any and all barriers imposed by ignorance or misunderstanding on the part of health caregivers and patients alike must be identified and eliminated by an intensive educational process.

Table 1. The relative risk of end-stage renal disease by diagnosis for minorities compared to whites.*

Location (Reference)	Date	Group	Total No. with ERSD (All Groups)	Relative Risk[t] Hypertension	Diabetes	Glomerulonephritis	All Causes	Age	Sex
Southeastern MI(Easterling[1])	1973-1975	Blacks	711	16.9	3.3	2.7	3.8	NO	NO
Michigan (Weller *et al.*[2])	1974-1981	Blacks	7000	10.9	3.8	1.7	4.3	YES	YES
Alabama (Rostand *et al.*[3])	1974-1978	Blacks	296	17.7	3.4	3.3	4.2	NO	NO
California (Ferguson *et al.*[4])	1980-1985	Blacks	NA	4.4	2.6	3.3	2.9	NO	NO
Texas (Pugh *et al.*[5])	1978-1984	Blacks	7027	10.9	4.3	2.6	4.4	YES	NO
Pennsylvania (Mausner *et al.*[6])	1974	Blacks	355	NA	NA	NA	5.6	YES	YES
Eastern U.S.(Sugimoto & Rosansky[7])	1973-1979	Blacks	88968	6.5	2.5	1.5	2.1	NO	YES
United States (Eggers[8])	1980	Blacks	9310	6.6	2.9	1.9	2.8	NO	NO
United States (HCFA[9])	1984	Blacks	26336	7.7	3.7	2.6	3.8	YES	YES
United States (HCFA[9])	1987	Blakcs	33578	6.6	3.8	2.3	3.8	YES	YES
Caifornia (Ferguson *et al.*[4])	1980-1985	Hispanics[a]	NA	NA	NA	NA	.09	NO	NO
Texas (Pugh *et al.*[5])	1978-1984	Hispanics[b]	6986	2.6	6.1	2.3	3.0	YES	NO

* Abbreviations: ESRD denote end-stage renal disease, NA = not available, HCFA= Health care Financing Administration.

t As compared with that for whites.

a. Hispanics were defined as individuals identified as of Spanish or Latin American descent.

b. Hispanics were defined as individuals who designated themselves as being of Mexican origin in the 1980 U.S. census.

Table 2. Race and the likelihood of receiving a cadaver or living-related renal transplant in 1987*

	White	Black	Native American	Asian	Other/ Unknown	Total
New ESRD pts	21966	9119	330	529	2493	34437
First cadaver transplants	3958	1223	59	148	224	5612
First cadaver transplants per new ESRD pts (%)	18.0	13.4	17.9	28.0	9.0	16.3
First living-related transplants	1312	160	18	22	100	1612
First living-related transplants per new ESRD pts (%)	6.0	1.8	5.5	4.2	4.0	4.7
Percent of transplants from living-related donors (%)	24.9	11.6	23.4	12.9	30.9	22.3

*Data from the Health Care Financing System, 1987.[9]
Abbreviations: ESRD, end-stage renal disease; pts, patients.

Table 3. Distribution of ABO blood groups in the United States by race*

ABO Group	Frequency in US Population (%)	White	Black	American	Oriental	Native
O	45	49	79	40		
A	40	27	16	28		
B	11	20	4	27		
AB	4		4	<1	5	

*Adapted from the Technical Manual of the American Association of Blood Banks (22).

Table 4. Comparison of patients who received or waited to receive a cadaver renal transplant by race.

	New York (28)	Los Angeles (28)	Miami (28)	Illinois (27)	San Francisco (29)
Black					
Transplanted	28	13	22	--	14
Waiting	35	19	34	40	19
White					
Transplanted	47	51	42	--	52
Waiting	46	47	34	52	49
Hispanics					
Transplanted	17	24	33	--	15
Waiting	15	26	31	7	17
Orientals					
Transplanted	--	--	--	--	11
Waiting	--	--	--	1	13
Other					
Transplanted	7	10	2	--	8
Waiting	4	6	2	--	2

Values are the percent of all patients who received a cadaver transplant (first row) and the percent of all patients on the cadaver waiting list according to race.

Table 5. Influence of race on cadaver renal allograft survival.

			Number		1yr Graft Survival (%)		3yr Graft Survival (%)		Treated with
Investigation	Centers	Years	White	Black	White	Black	White	Black	Cyclosporine
UCLA (41)	100+	1970-75	3581	978	47	37	35	25	-
KTHS (42)	42	1974-76	1173	292	51	44	40	34	-
SEOP (42)	39	1977-80	942	607	59	50	50	41	-
HCFA (43)	--	1977-80	5578	1624	58	50	47	40	-
CTS (44)	259	1983-88	24072	1807	--	--	70	50	+
UCLA (45)	100+	1984-88	12373	2963	77	70	65	49	+
HCFA (9)	--	1985	5366	1473	77	71	64	53	+/-

Abbreviations: CTS, Collaborative Transplant Study; KTHS, Kidney Transplant Histocompatibility Study; SEOP, South Eastern Procurement Foundation; HCFA, Health Care Financing Administration; UCLA, University of California at Los Angeles Registry

Notes

1. Easterling RE. Racial factors in the incidence and causation of end-stage renal disease (ESRD). *Trans Am Soc Artif Intern Organs* 1977;23:28-33.
2. Weller JM, Wu SC, Ferguson CW, Hawthorne VM. End-stage renal disease in Michigan: Incidence, underlying causes, prevalence, and modalities of treatment, *Am J Nephrol* 1985;5:84-95.
3. Rostand SG, Kirk KA, Rutsky EA, Pate BA. Racial differences in the incidence of treatment for end-stage renal disease, *N Engl J Med* 1982;306:1276-1279.
4. Ferguson R, Grim CE, Opgenorth TJ. The epidemiology of end-stage renal disease: The six-year South-central Los Angeles experience, 1980-85, *Am J Public Health* 1987;77:864-865.
5. Pugh JA, Stern MP, Haffner SM, Eifler CW, Zapata M. Excess incidence of treatment of end-stage renal disease in Mexican Americans, *Am J Epidemiol* 1988;127:135-144.
6. Mausner JS, Clark JK, Coles BI, Menduke H. An areawide survey of treated end-stage renal disease, *Am J Public Health* 1978;68:166-169.
7. Sugimoto T, Rosansky SJ. The incidence of treated end stage renal disease in the eastern United States, *Am J Public Health* 1984;74:14-17.
8. Eggers PW. Effect of transplantation on the medicare end-stage renal disease program, *N Engl J Med* 1988;318:223-229.
9. United States Renal Data System. *USRDS 1989 Annual Data Report*. Bethesda, MD: The National Institutes of Health, National Institute of Diabetes and Digestive and Kidney Diseases, 1989.
10. Eggers PW, Connerton R, McMullan M. The Medicare experience with end-stage renal disease: Trends in incidence, prevalence, and survival, *Health Care Financ Rev* 1984;5(3):69-88.
11. McCellan W, Tuttle E, Issa A. Racial differences in the incidence of hypertensive end-stage renal disease (ESRD) are not entirely ezplained by differences in the prevalence of hypertension, *Am J Kidney Dis* 1988;12:285-290.
12. Cowie CC, Port FK, Wolfe RA, Savage PJ, Moll PP, Hawthorne VM. Disparities in incidence of diabetic end-stage renal disease according to race and type of diabetes, *N Engl J Med* 1989;321:1074-1079.
13. Newman JM, Marfin AA, Eggers PW, Helgerson SD. End stage renal disease among Native Americans, 1983-86, *Am J Public Health* 1990;80:318-319.
14. Megill DM, Hoy WE. Risk factors for renal disease in a Native American community, *Transplant Proc* 1989;21:3902-3905.
15. Hoy WE, Megill DM, Hughson MD. Epidemic renal disease of unknown etiology in the Zuni Indians, *Am J Kidney Dis* 1987;9:485-496.
16. Teutsch S, Newman J, Eggers P. The problem of diabetic renal failure in the United States: An overview, *Am J Kidney Dis* 1989;13:11-13.
17. Nelson RG, Bennett PH. Diabetic renal disease in Pima Indians, *Transplant Proc* 1989;21:3913-3915.
18. Smith SM, Tung KS. Incidence of IgA-related nephritides in American Indians in New Mexico, *Hum Pathol* 1985;16:181-184.
19. Hoy WE, Smith SM, Hughson MD, Megill DM. Mesangial proliferative glomerulonephritis in Southwestern American Indians, *Transplant Proc* 1989;21:3909-3912.
20. Kjellstrand CM. Age, sex, and race inequality in renal transplantation, *Arch Intern Med* 1988;148:1305-1309.
21. Held PJ, Pauly MV, Bovbjerg RR, Newmann J, Salvatierra Jr O. Access to kidney transplantation--has the United States eliminated income and racial differences? *Arch Intern Med* 1988;148:2594-2600.

22. Widmann FK. *Technical Manual of the American Association of Blood Banks*. Arlington, VA:1985:114.
23. Health Care Financing Administration. End stage renal disease program management and medical information system, update, 1989.
24. Milford EL, Ratner L, Yunis E. Will transplant immunogenetics lead to better graft survival in blacks?--Racial variability in the accuracy of tissue typing for organ donation: The fourth American workshop, *Transplant Proc* 1987;19(Suppl 2):30-32.
25. Johnson AH, Rosen-Bronson S, Hurley CK. Heterogeneity of the HLA-D region in American blacks, *Transplant Proc* 1989;21:3872-3873.
26. Bauer MP, Danilous JA. Population analysis of HLA-A, B, C, DR and other genetic markers, Terasaki PI, ed, *Histocompatibility Testing 1980*. Los Angeles, CA: UCLA Typing Laboratory, 1980;995-993.
27. Lazda VA, Blaesing ME. Is allocation of kidneys on basis of HLA match equitable in multiracial populations? *Transplant Proc* 1989;21:1415-1416.
28. Perez LM, Schulman B, Davis F, Olson L, Tellis VA, Matas AJ. Organ donation in three major American cities with large Latino and black populations, *Transplantation* 1988;46:553-557.
29. Salvatierra Jr O. Demographic and transplantation trends among minority groups, *Transplant Proc* 1989;21:3916-3917.
30. Greenstein SM, Schechner R, Senitzer D, Louis P, Veith FJ, Tellis VA. Does kidney distribution based upon HLA matching discriminate against blacks? *Transplant Proc* 1989;21:3874-3875.
31. Pollak R, Brusak BF, Wiberg CA, Mozes MF. Donor referral and organ procurement patterns in a large metropolitan area--a single center prospective study, *Transplant Proc* 1986;18:399-400.
32. The U.S. public attitudes toward organ transplants/organ donation. Source: 1987 Dow Chemical Company Survey conducted by the Gallop Organization.
33. The U.S. public attitudes toward organ transplants/organ donation. Source: 1985 Dow Chemical Company Survey conducted by the Gallop Organization.
34. Attitudes and opinions of the American public towards kidney donation. Prepared for the National Kidney Foundation, Inc., by the Gallup Organization, Inc., February 1983.
35. Callender CO, Bayton JA, Yeager C, Clark JE. Attitudes among blacks toward donating kidneys for transplantation: A pilot project, *J Natl Med Assoc* 1982;74:807-809.
36. Warren E, Hull AR, Prati RC, *et al*. Patient status in dialysis units, *Semin Nephrol* 1982;2:186-188.
37. John D, Callender CO, Flores J, *et al*. Renal transplantation in substance abusers revisited: The Howard University Hospital experience, *Transplant Proc* 1989;21:1422-1424.
38. *National Survey on Drug Abuse: Main Findings 1985*. National Institute on Drug Abuse, United States Department of Health and Human Services; Public Health Service; Alcohol, Drug Abuse and Mental Health Administration, DHHS Publication No. (ADM) 88-1586, p. 63, 1988.
39. Rovelli M, Palmeri D, Vossler E, Bartus S, Hull D, Schweizer R. Noncompliance in renal transplant recipients: Evaluation by socioeconomic groups, *Transplant Proc* 1989;21:3979-3981.
40. Laudicina SS: Medicaid coverage and payment policies for organ transplants: Findings of a National Survey. Washington, DC: Intergovernmental Healthy Policy Project--George Washington University, 1988.
41. Opelz G, Mickey MR, Terasaki PI. Influence of race on kidney transplant survival, *Transplant Proc* 1977;9:137-142.
42. Krakauer H, Spees EK, Vaughn WK, Grauman JS, Summe JP, Bailey RC. Assessment of prognostic factors and projection of outcomes in renal transplantation, *Transplantation* 1983;36:372-378.
43. Krakauer H, Grauman JS, McMullan MR, Creede CC. The recent U.S. experience in the treatment of end-stage renal disease by dialysis and transplantation, *N Engl J Med* 1983;308:1558-1563.
44. Opelz G, Pfarr E, Engelmann A, Keppel E. Kidney graft survival rates in black cyclosporine-treated recipients, *Transplant Proc* 1989;21:3918-3920.
45. Takemoto S, Terasaki PI. A comparison of kidney transplant survival in white and black recipients, *Transplant Proc* 1989;21:3865-3868.
46. Sanfilippo F, Vaughn WK, LeFor WM, Spees EK. Multivariate analysis of risk factors in cadaver donor kidney transplantation, *Transplantation* 1986;42:28-34.

47. Opelz G, Engelmann A. Effect of HLA matching in cyclosporine-treated black kidney transplant recipients, *Transplant Proc* 1989;21:3881-3883.
48. Perdue ST, Terasaki PI. Analysis of interracial variation in kidney transplant and patient survival, *Transplantation* 1982;34:75-77.
49. Knechtle SJ, Castle DC, Seigler HF, Bollinger RR. Renal transplantation in the American black, *Transplant Proc* 1989;21:3931-3933.
50. Vincenti F, Duca RM, Amend W, *et al.* Immunologic factors determining survival of cadaver-kidney transplants, *N Engl J Med* 1978;299:793-798.
51. Ward HJ, Koyle MA, Terasaki PI, Cecka JM. Outcome of renal transplantation in blacks, *Transplant Proc* 1987;19:1546-1548.
52. Sumrani NB, Hong JH, Hanson P, Butt KMH. Renal transplantation in blacks: impact of immunosuppressive regimens, *Transplant Proc* 1989;21:3943-3945.
53. Garvin PJ, Castaneda M, Codd JE, Mauller K. Recipient race as a risk factor in renal transplantation, *Arch Surg* 1983;118:1441-1444.
54. Diethelm AG, Blackstone EH, Naftel DC, *et al.* Important risk factors of allograft survival in cadaveric renal transplantation, *Ann Surg* 1988;207:538-548.
55. Pisch JD, Armbrust MJ, D'Alessandro AM, Sollinger HW, Kalayoglu M, Belzer FO. Kidney transplantation in blacks at the University of Wisconsin, *Transplant Proc* 1989;21:3926-3928.
56. Shapiro R, Tzakis AG, Hakala TR, Lopatin WB, Stieber AC, Starzl TE. Renal Transplantation in black recipients at the University of Pittsburgh, *Transplant Proc* 1989;21:3921-3925.
57. Dunn J, Vathsala A, Golden D, *et al.* Impact of race on the outcome of renal transplantation under cyclosporine-prednisone, *Transplant Proc* 1989;21:3946-3948.
58. Dawidson IJA, Coorpender L, Fisher D, *et al.* Impact of race on renal transplant outcome, *Transplantation* 1990;49:63-67.
59. Milgrom M, Gharagozloo H, Gomez C, *et al.* Results of renal transplantation in Miami analyzed by race, *Transplant Proc* 1989;21:3934-3936.
60. First MR, Schroeder TJ, Carey MA, Chavinson DS. Effect of race on transplant outcome and response to OKT3 monoclonal antibody therapy, *Transplant Proc* 1989;21:3949-3952.
61. Sommer BG, Sing DE, Henry ML, Ferguson RM. The influence of recipient race on renal allograft survival: A single institution analysis, *Transplant Proc* 1989;21:3929-3930.
62. Weller JM, Wu SC, Ferguson CW, Port FK. Influence of race of cadaveric kidney donor and recipient on graft survival: A multifactorial analysis, *Am J Kidney Dis* 1987;9:191-199.
63. Saunders PH, Banowsky LH, Reichert DF. Survival of cadaveric renal allografts in hispanic as compared with caucasian recipients, *Transplantation* 1984;37:359-362.
64. Iwaki Y, Kinukawa T, Schulman B, Smith R. Trans-Pacific Kidney Shipment, *Transplantation* 1983;35:506-508.
65. Sutherland DER, Moundry-Munns KC. Pancreas transplants in blacks and whites, *Transplant Proc* 1989;21:3968-3970.
66. Teperman L, Scantlebury V, Tzakis A, Staschak A, Todo S, Starzl TE. Liver transplantation in black recipients: Pittsburgh, *Transplant Proc* 1989;21:3963-3965.

SECTION 7

AGING

Chapter 44

Cases 7.0

Case 7.1: **THE INSISTENT NIECE**

An 85-year-old gentleman lived alone at home. He was doing well until one day when his niece found him unresponsive on the floor when she came by to check on him. She herself had health problems, the worst was arthritis in her knees that limited her own movement. But she found time during the week to see how her uncle was doing.

He was brought by ambulance to the hospital, where it quickly became apparent that he had suffered a very mild stroke. He also had pneumonia and congestive heart failure. No other problem was found except that his niece mentioned he was profoundly deaf. His deafness often interfered with his ability to understand and respond to questions.

Several months later, the general medicine service thought, with the appropriate consults, that he might be weaned from the respirator upon which he was put when he first entered. Eighty-five-year-old persons have a difficult time regaining their own breathing after so long a time, but he was considered "strong." His other problems had stabilized; his chest x-ray and blood gases were normal. But the service did not recommend putting him back on the respirator if his congestive heart failure returned, as it inevitably would, or should he get pneumonia again.

While he was in the process of being aggressively weaned in the ICU where he was transferred for this task, attempts were made to obtain his own wishes. He seemed unable to respond in any but the most elemental, pleasant way, by nodding his head. He was given a writing pad, but did not use it. He could squeeze a nurses' hand, but it quickly became clear that he always answered "yes," even when it was not appropriate.

He was successfully weaned, but was confined to his bed on the ward. Although he seemed to be improving, it was the opinion of the doctors that his generally weakened condition and the seriousness of his congestive heart failure would prevent him from getting out of bed again.

Throughout this process and later, his niece kept insisting that "everything possible be done to help my uncle." She was told repeatedly by the medical staff, and later by an ethics consultant on the case, that her uncle was in the final stages of his life. To put him on the respirator again would be to condemn him to die on that machine.

She could not accept this news. Her vision was that he would soon return home to his own apartment. He had been so independent up to now! So she refused to even consider not treating her uncle. She was appalled by the doctors' seeming unwillingness to do so.

Case 7.2: **MARIE'S LAST RESPONSE, ALMOST**

Seventy-nine-year-old Marie J. was found unresponsive on her nursing home bathroom floor. She had been having a succession of difficult health problems for the past five years. Initially her family, consisting of a sister in a city 100 miles away and a nephew in a nearby town, entered her in the nursing home for her progressive dementia, the cause being organic brain syndrome. She resisted this, and was bitter about it at the time.

Marie had had repeated bouts with tachycardia and anemia. No cause was found for the latter. Seven weeks prior to this event, she had returned from the hospital where she had had a colonoscopy. Most of the time since, she lay in a fetal position in her bed, but was able to get out and move around a little bit.

Like many other elderly persons in this state, she was just barely maintained on oral food and water, with recent aspiration pneumonias as a consequence.

The nursing home staff began CPR immediately, and summoned the ambulance. At the emergency room she was found to be severely dehydrated and in electrolytic imbalance. IV fluids and nutrition were begun to rehydrate her and restore her nutritional status. To this was added IV antibiotics for her pneumonia. A ventilator was placed to assist her in breathing, and she began on atropine and lidocaine before being transferred to an ICU bed under the care of a cardiologist. The picture is not yet clear about her cardiac status or the extent of any neurological damage from her heart attack.

The nursing home had been having its difficulties too. A large staff turnover meant that continuity of care had suffered. A telephone call has now been made to the hospital from the nursing home indicating that a DNR order had been in Marie's chart there. It had just been found.

The ICU staff are not sure that this order had been requested by Marie herself early upon admission, or had been placed subsequently by her geriatrician. He is unavailable at the moment. They are unable to reach the nephew.

Has Marie's autonomy been violated? Should the emergency room have gone "all out" to save her life in light of this development? Even if they knew she was "DNR" should they have tried to save her life? Now that the ICU staff know about the DNR order, what is their obligation to withdraw the respirator, antibiotics, IV fluids, and nutrition? Is there a different obligation for each of these technologies? Knowing the special legal status of IV fluids and nutrition, would it have been wiser not to institute them in the emergency room, given the advanced state of Marie's heart disease and her age?

Case 7.3: **FAMILY FEEDING**

Emma is an 82 year old woman who lived by herself, taking care of her eldest son. Her son was an alcoholic. Her two daughters and their husbands helped her care for her son. About a decade ago, she had a left mastectomy for cancer. The protocol included chemotherapy and follow-up. Emma had no recurrence. In addition, she had been treated for over 10 years for polycythemia vera eventually requiring periodic phlebotomies. Emma's children said that she often remarked that she wished her hands would be cut off because they hurt her so much.

The social worker in the outpatient center knew Emma well. She denied having any problems, so that no home care or other interventions were done. Her children, in their 60's, complained that she sometimes was not as clear about things as she should be. The son could not do much for his mother, being partially incapacitated by his alcoholism. However, from time to time he did go out for "Chinese." The daughters and their husbands, in turn, brought in lunch and dinner, and fed their mother and their brother. Each day, their mother would go with them to the store, although she needed considerable assistance to do so because she was getting frail. Nonetheless, both the social worker and the family members described her subsequently as being very independent and used to being in charge of all of them. Emma was widowed long ago.

On February 7, Emma was found at home unable to move her right side and unable to speak. Brought by the family to the emergency room, she was admitted immediately. Upon examination she demonstrated a dense right hemiparesis and global aphasia. Initially, her head and eyes were deviated to the left side and a right field defect was felt to be present. A CAT scan of her head demonstrated changes consistent with a severe stroke.

Following Emma's initial admission to the hematology service, she was transferred to the neurology service for treatment of her stroke. At that time, given her grave prognosis, the son and one daughter expressed their wish to limit attempts at resuscitation (no chest compressions, intubation, anti-arrythmics or ICU transfer), but to treat any infections and prevent any unnecessary discomfort. While her overall condition stabilized, Emma's neurological condition remained unchanged. The family would feed her small amounts of food and give her something to drink. This could be taken by Emma on the left side of her mouth, but only in minuscule amounts.

Emma's poor oral intake resulted in the administration of IV fluids. Several days later she developed a fever. An abnormal chest x-ray and urinalysis, indicating an infection, necessitated starting antibiotics. A swallowing study several days later revealed possible aspiration into the lungs; a feeing tube was placed. Emma would frequently pull out the feeding tube and the IV lines. Despite the need to replace the feeding tube a few times, the family insisted that Emma not be restrained. Because of her behavior and her eventual decline due to insufficient feeding, it became necessary to consider the placement of a percutaneous endoscopic gastrostomy tube directly into her stomach. Emma was transfused two units of blood in preparation for the operation. The day prior to the operation, the son and daughter elected to cancel. The reason for this cancellation had much to do with their continued attempts to feed their mother by mouth, and the worry that this operation would simply prolong her agony in this dependent and "undignified" condition.

Subsequently, an ethics consult meeting was held with the entire family, two ethicists, the social work service, the medical service, and the neurology service. The family tearfully expressed their mother's prior comments to them that she did not want any life-sustaining procedures to be performed. They had been in the process of looking into a Living Will for her, but this was never completed. The medical service told the family bluntly that since the patient was conscious and in stable condition, they could not "starve your mother to death." The service represented the unanimous opinion of all medical and nursing caregivers that it was "inappropriate to withhold nutrition, and that the placement of the feeding tube must proceed." Their argument was based on the view that the family's mother was not dying and that her wishes about this condition were not clear. However, one physician stated that he had no trouble with the family taking the patient home and allowing her to die, but as long as she remained in his care, he would override their wishes and have her fed the best way he knew how.

As a compromise, the social worker attempted to find a nursing home that might take the patient without a feeing tube in place, or a hospice program of some kind, although the consensus remained that the patient was not actually dying. Over the ensuing week, the patient's ability to increase her oral intake did not improve.

Consider the following questions:

1. Should the family have the right to make a decision concerning placement of the feeding tube for their mother?

2. Should the physicians allow the family's view of feeding their mother (with small amounts of food and water by mouth), to trump their medical judgement, leading

most certainly to the patient's death?

3. What are the rights and responsibilities of families in medical decision-making?

Case 7.4: **CONFUSION**

C.P., a 77-year-old widow, was admitted on October 28th because of a problem with aspiration. Her condition required intubation but she was extubated within days. Currently, her mental status is borderline. Her confusional states are episodic. However, she is now medically stable and ready to be discharged.

An ethics consult was requested on November 2. The medical staff believe that the patient should have round-the-clock custodial care because of the possibility of repeat aspiration. This is her second hospitalization for the same problem within the last six months. C.P. lives alone. A housekeeper provides coverage five days a week. On the weekend, her sister Louise, a woman in her early 1970s, stops by to check on C.P. and to provide her with meals. Contrary to the medical staff recommendation, Louise wants C.P. to be sent home. The medical staff are concerned that she will not receive the necessary care, especially on the weekends. The possibility of placing C.P. in a nursing home or intermediate care facility was suggested to Louise, but she insisted that she and the housekeeper can take care of Caroling at home.

A patient care conference was scheduled for November 7. Prior to the meeting, the ethics consultant spent twenty minutes talking with C.P. to informally assess her own competence to make decisions. She appeared anxious and somewhat confused. The consultant asked if she understood that the staff were concerned that if she went home she might choke again and not be able to get help. She said, "Yes." When the consultant asked what she would like to do when she leaves the hospital, she said, "Go home." She did not want to go to a nursing home. The ethics consultant asked if she could take care of herself and she replied, "I don't know." When asked if her sister could take care of her and she said, "No." Other attempts to engage her in conversation were met with, "I don't know."

The social worker, stopped by during this conversation and asked C.P. if she remembered what they had talked about earlier that morning. The patient said, "No." Their combined impression was that C.P. would not be able to take care of herself if she was alone when an emergency occurred. It is the opinion of medical staff and other members of the health care team that the patient is medically at risk if continual custodial care is not provided. The staff thought that legal action might need to be taken if Louise, the sister, did not indicate a willingness to provide supportive twenty-four-hour care.

A large interdisciplinary care conference was then held, lasting over one and one-half hours. The need for custodial care for C.P. because of the potential for repeat aspiration was explained to Louise. Louise said that C.P. would be fine at home and that there would be no problems providing care for her. When asked about weekend coverage, Louise said she would be there. However, Louise said she does not stay overnight, that she leaves to attend church, and that she goes out if she, "gets a call." At one point in the conversation, Louise said, "I have a son. I have my own home, my own life."

Although Louise claimed that everything has been going fine, this does not appear to be the case. For example, when the patient was admitted to the hospital she was severely hypothyroid, suggesting that she was not taking her prescribed medications. The home care nursing agency reported to the social worker that occasionally nurses have not been able to get into the house during the week because no one answers the door. When the social worker asked the patient if her sister took care of her, C.P. replied, "She doesn't want to."

At one point during the meeting, Louise said that her sister was admitted to the hospital because she "choked on a piece of bread." When the social worker asked if bread was on her diet, Louise minimalized the importance of the diet. The ethics consultant asked if Caroling was on a special diet and the medical staff noted that she was supposed to eat soft, "pureed", food. Louise said, "I wouldn't eat that stuff!"

Throughout the discussion Louise appeared defensive and accusatory and repeatedly said, "You don't think I'm good enough (to take care of my sister)." Louise could not give any assurances that she would be willing to provide twenty-four hour coverage for her sister on the weekend. The possibility of placement in a nursing home or other skilled care facility was suggested. Louise was adamantly opposed to placing her sister in a nursing facility. We asked what she thought about requesting additional help for the weekend. Louise again said, "You're telling me I'm not good enough." It was explained to her that we appreciated her concern for her sister and that the staff were as concerned for her welfare as she was. This made little or no impression on the sister.

The attending suggested that we would help her locate support services for weekend coverage. Louise rejected this offer. Exasperated, the attending physician then explained that if adequate around-the-clock care could not be provided on a continuing basis at home, she would be forced to take legal action to provide this necessary care.

If the sister continues to resist providing twenty-four-hour care for the patient,

1. Should the staff act only in the patient's best interests, ignoring the wishes of the sister/caretaker?

2. If so, are the best interests of the patient that she be properly fed at home?

3. Or are her best interests also to have a family member care for her?

4. Are you convinced that the patient cannot make an adequate decision in this case?

5. What strategies should be taken to continue to involve the sister?

6. How would the patient's autonomy and the sister's autonomy be overridden if the patient were to be sent to the nursing home?

Case 7.5: **REFUSAL OF ORDINARY TREATMENT**

The patient, N.G., is an 88-year-old white female with no known close relatives, who has been a patient at a nursing home over a three year period. The patient was originally admitted to the home with a diagnosis of chronic brain syndrome, secondary to generalized arteriosclerosis. She also had been known to have repeated urinary tract infections. On x-ray examination, she had two lesions in the chest which were located in the lower quadrants and probably represented either metastatic disease or non-infectious type of granulomas.

In the three year period following her admission to the nursing home, the patient was admitted to a hospital on five different occasions. These admissions followed the same general pattern. The patient usually refused to drink water except when forced to by the nurses and, over a period of several days, she would become dehydrated. Her blood urea nitrogen, which is a waste product characteristically found in elevated amounts in uremia, would gradually rise. The patient would become semi-comatose and would be admitted to the hospital for treatment with intravenous fluids. On each occasion, the patient would express a definite desire to die. On the last two admissions, these expressions became even more pronounced. On both of these occasions she told nurses and staff that she was going to quit drinking fluids because she wished to die and that she thought she could do this by halting her intake of fluids.

The patient had no known visitors during her hospital stays or at the nursing home. No one contacted the physicians regarding her status. The patient also told the physicians in the hospital that she did not wish to have intravenous fluids, that she wished to be left alone to die in peace.

N.G. was oriented to place but not to date. She had a poor memory for recent events and probably could be declared incompetent by a court, although there is some question whether all the physicians involved would testify to her complete incompetence.

The patient now has informed her nursing home attending physician once again that she is not going to drink fluids and wants to die in peace. Her attending physician, after much deliberation, enters an order on her chart that N.G. should not receive fluids forcefully, based upon her repeated requests. He also notes, "The nursing home opposes this action."

The case was submitted to the Nursing Home Ethics Committee, newly formed to consider just such a case. The physician assigned to the county nursing home came once a week and looked in on the patients. He also visited the inmates in the jail. He was, of course, a member of the committee, but was absent the day of deliberation. The rest of the committee was composed of a local minister, nurses, and an administrative aide. After discussing the patient's right of self-determination and the duties of health professionals to act in the best interests of the patient, the committee was divided about what to do in this case. Some members wanted to back the physician's order in the chart, but some nurses and the administrative aide opposed this action, saying that "this is tantamount to murdering the patient, since she is confused and cannot act in her own best interests." The committee meeting ended in disarray.

Questions raised in this case include:

1. Should the patient be again admitted to the hospital?

2. Should she be declared incompetent? By whom?

3. Does she have a right to die?

4. Who is responsible for her care?

5. What standards should a court develop for determining whether I.V. fluids should be discontinued?

Case 7.6: AGING AND PUBLIC POLICY

Mrs. Martha M., an 80-year-old widow whose only child died in the Korean War, was admitted to a Medical Center in January 1987, with fractures of the left femur and wrist, multiple contusions and bruises.

Mrs. M. had been living independently in an apartment complex for older persons. She has friends but no living family and she is dependent upon social security and a small pension for her support. She suffered her injuries while crossing a street carrying bags of groceries. She tripped and fell against the curb and sidewalk.

Examination on admission revealed that in addition to her fractures she had moderate generalized osteoporosis. Healing of the fractures, particularly of the femur, was delayed and her hospital stay prolonged. Mrs. M. became depressed, had episodes of confusion, and occasional urinary incontinence. A psychiatric consult established that Mrs. M. has no history of psychiatric problems, remains alert and oriented most of the time, but in extremely low spirits.

Because she exceeded the norm established under the DRG standard related to the fractures, her physician was asked to explain the "excessive" hospitalization. Mrs. M. was made aware of the inquiry by a hospital administrator. Her depression and occasional confusion continued.

When in late February her medical condition had reached a point at which her physician judged that she could be treated in a skilled nursing home, transfer was arranged, with some difficulty.

At this point, Mrs. M. had to surrender her apartment in order to make her meager resources available for payment of medical charges. With help from the hospital social worker, arrangements were made for some of her friends in her building to take temporary charge of personal papers, pictures, and other small items she wept about losing. Her furniture was sold.

In the nursing home, she progressed slowly. Being financially unable to return to independent living in an apartment, she remained in the nursing home for a period exceeding the coverage provided by Medicare. The nursing home wants to transfer her to a non-skilled facility.

Her nursing home physician is under pressure, and Mrs. M. as well, to find more financial resources for covering current charges. Failure will result in her being transferred to a facility which will accept her with coverage only through Medicaid plus her meager pension. Mrs. M's depression and anxiety have increased because of her lack of resources and her continuing weakness, though her fractures have now healed.

Both physicians continue to receive requests for justification of her treatment and length of stay, both in the hospital and in the skilled nursing facility. What is the right thing to do in this case?

Case 7.7: ALZHEIMER'S AND THE NURSING HOME

Dr. Thomas Corcoran is in private practice at a local community hospital.

The case concerns a 79-year-old patient of his with Alzheimer's Disease. His patient has never been married. He has no children. He has a brother in the mid-70's with cancer and he has a lady friend for the last five to six years with whom he is very close. Dr. Corcoran has known the patient between five and six years. About two to two and a half years ago, his patient started to deteriorate mentally and he was given a diagnosis of Alzheimer's Disease. In the last three years, his patient was in two different nursing homes. In one nursing home for one year and in the other nursing home for two years.

He has done relatively well until December 1, 1989. Prior to December he was able to recognize everyone around him, but at this point he became unable to. Also, he was ambulatory until last Thanksgiving. He has been bedridden since December. Dr. Corcoran says he will respond to any smiling face. On January 1, 1990, the patient became extremely dehydrated and developed pneumonia. Dr. Corcoran hospitalized him. He was hydrated and given antibiotics and the patient got better. In the last six months, the patient has become progressively sicker. He has lapsed into a near-vegetative state and within the last month he was barely able to eat. At this point Dr. Corcoran has not instituted any artificial feeding.

His problem is that he feels intense pressure to order fluids and nutrition (medically-delivered food and water) by the nursing staff at the nursing home. Recently he was called by three different nurses from the nursing home who said things to him like, "if you don't do something, he's going to die."

When his patient was first diagnosed with Alzheimer's Disease, Dr. Corcoran asked the brother if he had ever talked with the patient about a request that he may have made concerning his future health care. The brother said that no, he had not, but that he didn't think his brother would want to continue on life support indefinitely. The brother also indicated that he felt the doctor should follow his judgment in making decisions. The family would support him.

In January Dr. Corcoran suggested that his patient be given a DNR status and the brother was in agreement. Recently Dr. Corcoran suggested that no artificial feeding be initiated. The patient should not be given a feeding tube. The brother agreed.

Dr. Corcoran's primary dilemma is whether or not he is doing the right thing by resisting the initiation of artificial feeding in this case. Alzheimer's at this stage may or may not be considered a dying process. It depends on a point of view. The nurses are becoming more adamant.

Chapter 45

Life-Sustaining Interventions in Frail Elderly Persons -- Talking About Choices

F. Russell Kellogg, Madeleine Crain, June Corwin, and Philip W. Brickner

Control over the use of life-sustaining interventions is the subject of intense controversy. Participants in the ongoing debate include physicians who feel that they understand prognosis best, theorists who advocate for patient self-determination, and public policymakers concerned with growing costs of care. Most agree that involvement by elderly persons in making decisions about their own fate is appropriate.

Early communication with the elderly concerning advance directives has been recommended,[1] yet such discussion remains an uncommon practice.[2,3,4] Some physicians express concern that raising the subject may have adverse emotional effects, yet it has been found that patients expect physicians to initiate these discussions.[5,6] Talking with patients during routine visits allows for development of trust and understanding.[7] It also gives guidance to family members or others whose choices might not otherwise reflect patient wishes.[8,9,10] Timing is everything. When patients are acutely ill, consciousness is often clouded and the opportunity for participation in critical decisions is lost.[11]

We hypothesized that frail, elderly homebound persons have strong opinions regarding the use of these treatments and would welcome the opportunity to express these views to their physicians. We further hypothesized that, although frail, they desire control over their own lives and have substantial satisfaction with their quality of life. We also believed that discussion about the use of life supports would not result in depression or adverse emotional effects.

We studied the short-term impact of a physician-initiated, structured discussion with frail, homebound elderly patients concerning the use of urgent life-sustaining interventions. Effects of this discussion on their emotional health were evaluated, and we report the medical decisions made by this sample both initially and on follow-up 18 months later.

SUBJECTS AND METHODS

Subjects

Subjects were selected from the roster of one primary care physician (F.R.K.) in the long-term health care program for the frail elderly at St Vincent's Hospital and Medical Center in lower Manhattan. Of the 33 patients in his caseload, six were judged ineligible due to advanced dementia or language/communication problems. Of the remainders, the first 20 seen in the usual sequence of routine scheduled home visits were invited to participate. None had been involved in discussions of life-sustaining interventions within a year prior to the study. One of the 20 became unavailable due to hospitalization before completion of the

---

Source: Reprinted from *Archives of Internal Medicine*, Vol. 152, 1992, pp. 2317-2320, with permission from American Medical Association © Nov 1992.

study, and another tensed because he was mourning the recent loss of his wife. The final sample of 18 frail homebound patients included 15 women and three men with an average age of 81 years (range, 60 to 93 years); the two patients younger than 70 years had advanced multiple sclerosis. Three patients had mild senile dementia, and no patient was known to have a terminal illness at the time of the study. The average time in the profit for the 18 patients was 3 years; they had been under the direct care of the current physician for an average of 15.4 months (range, 2 to 50 months). Most of the patients suffered from multiple medical disorders, a characteristic of chronically ill, frail elderly persons. Patients selected were representative in age, health, functional status, and demographics of the total program.[12]

Procedure

Approximately 1 week prior to the planned physician visit in which life-support issues were to be discussed, a research assistant visited the patient and completed three rating scales after obtaining informed consent. Each of these instruments has been used in studies of elderly patients. The Zung Depression Scale[13] assesses self-rated depressive symptoms; Locus of Desired Control[14] measures the extent to which patients perceive themselves as having control over desired outcomes; and the Life Satisfaction Index A and Index B[15] measures perceived life satisfaction. Interview time averaged 30 to 60 minutes, and all patients agreed to repeat testing 6 weeks later. The physician-patient discussion took place in the patient's home immediately following a routine medical visit, using a standard format. The discussion included open-ended questions to identify the patient's personal values, hopes, fears, expectations, and treatment goals. Early participation in treatment planning was then invited, and the rationale was explained. The patient's knowledge of specific intensive care modalities, including cardiopulmonary resuscitation and intubation for mechanical ventilation and tube feeding, was then assessed. Information, including efficacy and associated risks, was provided.

Patients were next asked to express their wishes for or against each of these life-sustaining measures. If they were willing to receive emergency measures under certain circumstances, we sought clarification. The physician guided the discussion, answered questions, provided reassurance, and encouraged decision-making.

Throughout, patients were observed for quality of reasoning and comprehension of the subject. Corrected feedback was used to improve communication and understanding. Patients were then reassured regarding their current stable health status. The patient-physician discussion lasted an average of 30 minutes. All surviving subjects were reinterviewed 18 months subsequent to the initial dialogue to determine the durability of the decisions made.

The entire group's mean pre- and post-physician-patient discussion scores for each of the three instruments were evaluated by two-tailed *t* tests. The sample was then dividend into two groups based on initial internal and external focus of control scores. Prediscussion rating scale scores and postdiscussion rating scale scores in these subgroups were evaluated by mixed model analysis of variance.

RESULTS

Clinical Findings

Few patients expressed specific hopes, yet most placed some positive value on their day-to-day lives. Thirteen patients voiced no particular fears for the future. One patient expressed fear of the dying process, two of being placed in a nursing home, and two of becoming more disabled. On inquiry, 11 patients lacked a clear understanding of cardiopulmonary resuscitation and urgent intubation and five patients did not understand tube feeding. Clear preferences regarding use of each intervention usually emerged (Table 1). Most patients said that they were well prepared to accept death that would result from withholding life-support measures, and there was a near unanimous rejection of their use. On further inquiry, none of the patients reported the decisions to be disturbing or upsetting. All patients appeared to tolerate the discussion well, and many voiced appreciation for the opportunity to express their wishes. Eighteen months after the beginning of the pilot study, 16 of the 18 subjects remained alive and one of these 16 had been transferred to a nursing home. In both deaths, there was a change in decisions made during their final illness. One 75-year-old man, with end-stage emphysema and cor pulmonale, who initially requested use of all life supports needed for critical illness, ultimately refused the use of mechanical ventilation when he was informed that chronic ventilator dependency would most likely result. The second patient, a 91-year-old woman initially indecisive about the use of intubation and mechanical ventilation, was hospitalized with diabetes and sepis complicated by uremic coma. During her final days, the family consented to a palliative care approach based on the obvious futility of aggressive therapy.

Table 1 - Patient Expressed Choices

	Initial (n=18)			Follow-up (n=15)		
Choice	Yes	No	Defer	Yes	No	Defer
C.P.R.	1	17	0	4	10	1
Intubation	1	14	3	3	12	0
Tube feeding	0	18	0	1	13	1

Table 2 - Final Results of Patient's Expressed Choices

Choice	Yes	No	Defer
Cardiopulmonary resuscitation	1	12	2
Intubation	1	12	2
Tube feeding	0	13	2

Preferences obtained through research assistant reinterview of the 15 surviving mentally capable subjects at 18 month follow-up are presented in Table 1. Subjects whose responses appeared discordant to their original choices again underwent a physician-patient discussion for clarification. The discussions yielded preferences that were more similar to the original ones (Table 2).

For comparison, the clinical courses of 19 homebound patients, under the care of several program physicians, who were excluded from this study because of mental incapacity were reviewed retrospectively. Outpatient and inpatient medical charts as well as staff interviews were used. Of the 19, six patients have since died (three at-home and three in-hospital deaths). Four patients were admitted to nursing homes, and nine patients remain at home. Eleven patients had at least one hospital stay during the 18-month follow-up period. No documentation of prior discussions with patients or families was found in outpatient charts. Foreknowledge of patient wishes appeared to be generally lacking. In several instances during acute illness, defining limits to medical care was hampered due to lack of living relatives of six patients, psychiatric impairment and suspended patient abuse by a relative of one patient, and financial conflict of interest affecting decisions of another. Standard medical care including the use of life supports was carried out when medically indicated. Two demented patients underwent urgent intubation and mechanical ventilation for treatment of pneumonia, and each remained ventilator dependent for approximately 3 months in the hospital before death.

Table 3 - Rating Scale Results Before and After Physician-Initiated Discussion

				Initial Locus of Control				
	Whole Sample			Internal (n=9)		External (n=9)		
Rating Scale	Pre±SEM	Post±SEM	*t* Test	Pre	Post	Pre	Post	ANOVA Interaction
Zung Depression Scale	52.66±2.22	48.67±1.93	*t*(17)=-2.52;P=.038	50.89	46.11	53.22	51.22	P<1
Locus of Control	45.11±1.31	45.33±1.50	*t*<1	49.33	48.67	40.89	42.00	P<1
Life Satisfaction Index - A Scores	11.11±.754	11.44±.856	*t*<1	11.33	11.67	10.89	11.22	P<1
Life Satisfaction Index-B Scores	14.00±.997	15.56±.715	*t*(17)=1.60;P=.186	13.67	17.22	14.33	13.89	P(1,16)=5.32;P=.035

Rating Scales Data are summarized and statistics are presented in Table 3. Initially, Zung Depression Scale scores for the entire group were below the value for clinically significant depression and decreased slightly but significantly (P<.05) after the physician-patient discussion. The group perceiving themselves as being in control of life events (internal, n=9) scored above the mean (45.11), and the group lacking a sense of personal control (external, n=9) scored below the mean. Prediscussion and postdiscussion scores for the Zung and life satisfaction scales in the two groups were examined by mixed model analysis of variance. The locus of control group was the between-subject variable and time of testing (pro and post) was the within-subject variable. Results of these analyses showed that locus of control, endorsed life satisfaction, and depression scale scores did not change differentially within the two subgroups. There was no difference between groups on initial depression scale scores or in Life Satisfaction Index A or Index B scores. However, expressed Life Satisfaction Index B scores increased slightly but significantly (P<.05) after the physician-patient discussion in the subgroup having relatively internal locus of control; it was unchanged in the subgroup with external control beliefs.

Comment

We found that open consideration of critical care choices was welcomed by nearly all of this sample of homebound elderly, chronically ill persons and that it did not result in depression or despair. In fact, the entire group experienced a reduction in depression ratings, and those perceiving themselves in control of their lives reported increased life satisfaction scores 6 weeks later. Although patients have been surveyed regarding life-sustaining intervention in both an outpatient clinic,)[16] and in a hospital-based home care program,[17] we are unaware of any previous studies where: psychologic outcomes of these discussions have been systematically studied.

The subject of death arose frequently during discussions, and undue anxiety or fear was notably absent from patient responses. These aged persons seemed quite accepting of their own impending death, and the subject appeared to be a familiar one. This supports previous findings that death, for the elderly, is often neither welcomed nor feared but simply accepted as reality.[18] The findings of reduction of depressive symptoms in all subjects and increased life satisfaction scores in the group of patients with internal locus of control following the physician-patient discussion was unexpected. Others[19,20,21] have noted, however, that personal control over decisions is a major issue for the elderly and those feeling greater control are more likely to be positive in their attitudes and personal adjustment.

In our study, following a single physician-patient discussion, most of the patients were able to make preferences clear regarding cardiopulmonary resuscitation and urgent intubation. The remainder wished to consider choices further. If our findings are confirmed through more extensive prospective study, there may be significant ethical, legal, and economic implications. First, many frail elderly persons may not want to avail themselves of life-sustaining interventions if given the opportunity to choose; and second, if this is true, discussions of policy-level restriction on provision of such care may be unnecessary.[22,23,24]

Of significance was the lack of concordance in decisions made on reinterview by a research assistant 18 months after the initial discussion, following the same question format used by the physician in the initial dialogue. All changes in decisions made by four of the remaining 15 subjects were in the direction of more aggressive care. On subsequent discussion with the primary physician, who provided outcome-oriented information, three of these four individuals again decided to forego cardiopulmonary resuscitation and two deferred choices; two were undecided on intubation and tube feeding in the event of critical illness. None of these patients was obviously demented at this time. Final results are shown in Table 2. These findings indicate that the durability of decisions cannot be assumed and that subtle aspects of the framing of information may be crucial.

It is noteworthy that few of our patients had discussed life-sustaining interventions with significant others. Only one had made formal arrangements through a Living Will, and no one had previously raised the issue with a primary care physician. Although elderly persons, such as those in this sample, are perhaps assumed to have an expectation of physician paternalism, all welcomed the opportunity to make their own decisions.

This pilot study had several inherent limitations that hinder definitive conclusions. The study sample, while representative of our mentally intact long-term home health care patients, is modest in size and may not be representative of all homebound frail elderly. Also, durability of decisions cannot be assumed. Further, we cannot exclude the possibility that, some patients might suffer verse consequences after such a discussion or predict who they might be. Finally, the discussions were carried out by a single physician and the replicability of findings involving other physicians is yet to be determined.

Notes

1. Orentlicher D. Advance medical directives, *JAMA* 1990;263:2365-2367.
2. Gordon GH, Tolle S. Discussing life-sustaining treatment: A teaching program for residents, *Arch Intern Med* 1991;151:567-570.
3. Blackball LJ, Cobb J, Moskowitz MA. Discussions regarding aggressive care with critically ill patients, *J Gen Intern Med* 1989;4:399-402.
4. Gleeson K, Wise S. The Do-Not-Resuscitate order: Still too little too late, *Arch Intern Med* 1990:150:1057-1060.
5. Bedell SE, Delbanco TL. Choices about cardiopuimonary resuscitation in the hospital, *N Engl J Med* 1984;310:1089-1093.

6. Emanuel LL, Batty MJ, Stoekle JD, Ettelson LM, Emanuel E. Advance directives for medical care: A case for greater use, *N Engl J Med* 1991;324:889-895.
7. Kapp MB. Advance health care planning: Taking a 'medical future,' *South Med J* 1988;81:221-224.
8. Zweibel NR, Cassel CK. Treatment choices at the end of life: A comparison of decisions by older patients and their physician-selected proxies, *Gerontologist* 1989;5:615-621.
9. Seckler AF, Meier DE, Mulvihill M, Paris BE. Substituted judgment: How accurate are proxy predictions? *Ann Intern Med* 1991;115:92-98.
10. Stolman CJ, Gregory JJ, Dunn D, Levine JL. Evaluation of patient, physician, nurse, and family attitudes toward do not resuscitate orders, *Arch Intern Med* 1990;150:653-658.
11. Frankl D, Oye RK, Bellamy PE. Attitudes of hospitalized patients toward life support: A survey of 200 medical impatients, *Am J Med* 1989;86:645-648.
12. St Vincent's Hospital and Medical Center. *17 Years of Long Health Care at St Vincent's Hospital*. New York, NY: Dept of Comnunity Medicine, 1990.
13. Zung WWK. A self-rating depression scale, *Arch Gen Psychiatry* 1965;12:63-70.
14. Reid DW, Haas C, Hawlkings D. Locus of desired control and positive self concept of the elderly, *J Gerontol* 1977;32:441-450
15. Neugarten BL, Havighurst RJ, Tobin SS. The measurement of the satisfaction, *J Gerontol* 1961;16:134-143.
16. Finucane TE, Shumway JM, Powers RL, D'Alessandri RM. Planning with elderly outpatients for contingencies of severe illness: A survuy clinical trial, *J Gen Intern Med* 1988;3:322-325.
17. Havlir D, Brown L, Rousseau GK. Do-Not-Resuscitate discussions in hospital-based home care program, *J Am Geriatr Soc* 1989;37:52-54.
18. Bengtson VL, Cuellar JB, Ragan PK. Stratum contrasts and similarities in attitudes toward death, *J Gerontol* 1977;32:76-88.
19. Reid DW, Ziegler M. Validity and stability of a new desired control measure pertaining to psychological adjustment of the elderly, *J Gerontol* 1980;35:395-402.
20. Aldwin MM. Does age affect the stress and coping process? Implications of age differences in perceived control, *J Gerontol* 1991;46;174-180.
21. Reich JW, Zautra AJ. Dispositional control beliefs and the consequences of a control-enhancing intervention, *J Gerontol* 1991;46;174-180.
22. Bone RC, Elpern EH. Honoring patient preferences and rationing intensive care, *Arch Intern Med* 1991;151;1061-1063.
23. Hanson LC, Danis M. Use of life-sustaining care for the elderly. *J Am Geriatr Soc* 1991;39:772-777.
24. Callahan D. *Setting Limits: Medical Goals in an Aging Society*. New York, NY: Simon & Schuster, 1987.

Chapter 46

Decision-Making in the Incompetent Elderly: "The Daughter from California Syndrome"

David W. Molloy, Roger M. Clarnette, E. Ann Braun, Martin R Eisemann, and B. Shneiderman

Introduction

Decision-making regarding the care of the mentally incompetent patient is often complicated by legal,[1,2,3,4,5,6,7] economic[8,9,10,11,12] and ethical factors[13,14,15] that affect case management. The incompetent patient requires an advocate, a responsibility that generally falls upon the family. If a conflict over a patient arises within the family, the result may well be inimical to effective patient management.

On June 25th, 1990, the United States Supreme Court issued its decision in Cruzan v. Director, Missouri Department of Health, the first case in which the high court considered the termination of life-prolonging measures for incompetent patients. In a 5-4 decision, the Court upheld the decision by the Missouri Supreme Court that the feeding tube of Nancy Cruzan, a patient in a persistent vegetative state since 1983, could not be removed at the request of her parents. The reason was that there was no 'clear and convincing' evidence that the patient when competent had specifically indicated that she would not wish to be tube-fed if she ever became irreversibly unconscious.

The narrow import of the decision in Cruzan must be stressed. The Court ruled that it is constitutionally permissible for a state to require that life-prolonging measures for an incompetent patient remain in place unless the patient had left behind a clear directive excluding such measures in the event of a future state of incompetency. The Court did not rule that such a state rule is mandatory, but simply that a state may so rule if it chooses. The decision in Cruzan thus leaves intact the long line of cases beginning with, In the Matter of Karen Quinlan, in which state supreme courts have held that decisions to terminate life-prolonging treatment for incompetent patients should rest with the patient's family and physicians. The courts have further ruled that the court-room should be the forum of last resort for decision-making involving the termination of life-prolonging treatment for incompetent patients.

In the view of the judges, they have a role to play when there is in-family conflict that cannot be resolved in the health care setting. In that event, judicial action is called for, in which either the court makes the treatment decision or else vests that authority in a guardian appointed to act on the patient's behalf. (The trend in the more recent cases is to assign the decision to a guardian, not to the court itself.)

The "Daughter from California Syndrome" describes one such in-family predicament. In this case, an adult daughter, who had not seen her mother for five years, appeared on the scene when critical health care options were being considered for her incompetent mother.

Source: Reprinted from *The American Geriatrics Society*, Vol. 39, No. 4, 1991, pp. 396-399, with permission from American Geriatrics Society © 1991.

Upon being confronted with her mother's condition, the daughter responded with acute denial as well as anger and resentment directed against the medical staff. She refused to come to terms with her mother's condition, demanded inappropriate aggressive care, and impeded the management of the case. Health care directives[16,17,18,19,20,21] offer a possible solution to these problems by allowing competent individuals to choose their own health care before they become incompetent. We report this case because it illustrates many of the features of this syndrome.

Case Report

The patient, Mrs. M., was an 83-year-old widow with a five year history of Alzheimer's disease. She had been cared for by her 60-year-old daughter who never married and had taken an early retirement. Mrs. M. was admitted to a nursing home six months before her hospital admission because the daughter was no longer able to care for her at home. At that time, the patient was moderately demented, she no longer recognized her daughter, was incontinent of urine, and needed to be groomed, washed, and fed. Sometime later she fractured the neck of her left femur which necessitated surgical repair. Following surgery she refused to walk, was incontinent of urine and feces, and was a heavy two-person transfer.

After discussion with the daughter, a Do-Not-Resuscitate Order (DNR) was entered on the patient's chart and co-signed by her. Although the patient had not signed an advance directive, she had discussed termination of treatment issues with her daughter, who was confident that the DNR order would accord with her mother's wishes. The daughter further requested that we discontinue blood tests and provide palliative care in the event of a reversible or irreversible life-threatening illness. She also co-signed a request that medications be administered only for comfort and pain relief purposes.

When the second daughter arrived from California, it was quickly apparent that she had been unaware of her mother's recent deterioration. She was appalled at her mother's condition and she accused her sister of institutionalizing their mother for financial gain. She demanded that the DNR order be withdrawn and that the mother receive whatever treatment necessary to maintain life. She threatened to sue the hospital and all health care professionals treating her mother unless she was immediately transferred to the intensive care unit.

We arranged a meeting for the sisters with the medical staff. The daughter from California totally dominated the discussion. She took notes and threatened to sue everyone involved in her mother's care. There were follow-up meetings with the orthopedic surgeon, the internist, nurses, physiotherapists, occupational therapists, chaplains, and nutritionists. We spent considerable time with the daughter from California striving to deal with her denial, guilt, threats, and anger. She so intimidated her sister that the latter not only acquiesced in her demands, but also ceased to come to the hospital. We accordingly withdrew the DNR order and directed that the patient be treated aggressively in the event of further deterioration.

Soon thereafter the daughter from California returned home. Her sister resumed her visits to the patient, and at her written request, the DNR order and palliative care directions were reinstated. The patient Mrs. M. died two weeks later. The daughter from California did not attend the funeral.

Discussion

The care of the incompetent patient poses particularly complex problems for clinicians who must consider the wishes of the patient, family, and other health care workers. On occasion the wishes of the patient and/or family conflict with the mission statement of the institution or with the ethical principles of staff members.[22] Legal, economic, ethical, and religious factors may add to the complexity of the situation. Such issues arise more frequently in Geriatrics that in any other subspecialty. Indeed, few problem areas in medicine are more complex than decision-making for elderly incompetent patients.

Of course, the patient may have signed an instructional advance directive (i.e., Living Will) or a proxy advance directive (i.e., Durable Power of Attorney for health care). What if, however, the patient while competent, had not signed an advance directive or otherwise indicated treatment preferences to guide the decision-making process? Or what if there is an apparent conflict between the family's wishes and a living will direction or the views of a proxy nominated by the patient to make his/her health care decisions? In such cases, the hierarchy listed in Table I provides practical guidelines to facilitate decision-making for the incompetent patient.

The resolution of in-family conflict can be a difficult task. Resentment, grudges, rivalry or long standing animosity within the family can impair its ability to reach a consensus, sufficient to guide the incompetent patient's health care team. Denial, guilt, and anger among family members also impairs their ability to make rational decisions. In this case, the daughter from California was in an early stage of denial regarding her mother's illness. She may have hoped that her mother would recover to an extent enabling her to "make peace her" with her. The daughter's anger, guilt, and denial precipitated a crisis in management, disrupting a care plan that had been developed after considerable discussion and effort.

Strategies to deal with these situations include involving all those family members who wish to become involved in the discussions. It may be helpful to outline simply and exactly what decisions have to be made, and give a consistent description of the patient's condition. It is important to allow the family to make all the major treatment decisions.

Some of the strategies for dealing with the complex and time consuming issues that can arise when there is in-family conflict regarding the care of incompetent patients are listed on Table II.

In this case, interdisciplinary collaboration and support enabled the patient's health caregivers to defuse her anger and share the responsibility for dealing with this difficult, time consuming problem. The views of the daughter from California did not accord with the previously expressed wishes of the patient as reported by the daughter who had lived with and cared for the mother. It was the latter who knew the mother's feelings about terminal care and who sought to promote her best interests. She was thus the appropriate surrogate decision-maker for her mother, and in honoring her wishes for the DNR and palliative care only order, the medical staff was fulfilling its legal and moral responsibilities to the patient.

According to the President's Commission for the Study of Health Problems in Medicine, "A health care professional has an obligation to allow a patient to choose from among medically acceptable treatment options...or to reject all options."[23] Although physicians are not morally (or legally) bound to provide treatment they regard as "counter-therapeutic" or physiologically futile, it is nonetheless true that the threat of litigation (as in this case) cannot be taken lightly.[24] It is thus understandable that the medical staff complied with the daughter's demands for aggressive treatment.

This case illustrates the value of patient's advance directives. If the patient had, while competent, documented her views regarding a DNR order and a palliative care regimen, then the threats of the daughter from California could have been discounted. In other words, comprehensive health care directives completed by knowledgeable patients may serve to deflect conflict that can arise when the decision-making responsibility is laid upon family members. However, so long as incompetent patients have not left behind such directives, health care providers will be pressured into providing care against their better judgment because of the demands of family members like the daughter from California.

TABLE I

HIERARCHY OF DECISION-MAKING IN THE INCOMPETENT PATIENT

1. If the patient while competent had signed an advance directive, then his/her wishes must prevail -- even over the conflicting views of family members.

2. If the patient has left no directive, it is necessary to turn to the family. An in-family discussion of treatment options is called for, although as a general guideline actual decision-making authority should be allotted in accordance with the following priorized list: spouse, adult children, siblings, other family members. (The term spouse would include the patient's significant other.)

3. If there is unresolvable in-family conflict regarding case management of the patient, the court should be petitioned to appoint a guardian to act on the patient's behalf.

4. In the event that there is no one to speak for the patient, then the patient's health care providers should assume that role.

TABLE II

STRATEGIES FOR DEALING WITH THE DIFFICULT FAMILY

1. Convene a meeting with all family members who wish to play a role in the decision-making process for the incompetent patient. All health care professionals involved in the patient's care (e.g., family physician, specialists, nurses, physiotherapists, occupational therapists, social workers, nurses, and chaplains) should be invited to attend.

2. Provide the family with a consistent description in simple language of the patient's condition and prognosis. Use the same terms and responses because similar terms for the same condition may cause confusion and provoke the concern that there is disagreement within the medical team.

3. Outline in simple terms the areas wherein decision must be made, e.g.:
   a. treatment in the event of cardiac arrest;

   b. treatment in the event of acute reversible life-threatening illness (e.g. pneumonia);

   c. treatment in the event of acute irreversible life-threatening illness (e.g. stroke);

   d. nutrition -- special diets, nasogastric tubes, gastrostomy tubes, total parenteral nutrition; and

   e. routine blood work, and further investigations.

4. Give over control to the family: Advise the members that they must reach a consensus and then inform the health care team of their decision.

5. Nominate one family member to communicate with a team member (e.g. physician, head nurse, chaplain, or social worker).

6. Give the family a deadline to provide a decision, arrange follow up meetings for updates, provide a mechanism for the family to continue asking questions and to be kept informed of changes in the patient's condition.

7. If the family cannot arrive at a consensus, discuss their points of disagreement and follow-up with small group meetings to provide ongoing advice and information. If the family still cannot reach a consensus, then follow the wishes of the family members in accordance with the priorized list provided in Table I.

8. Finally, if all these measures fail, consult the Geriatric Service. Everyone else does.

Notes

1. Curran WJ, Hyg SM. Court involvement in right-to-die cases: Judicial inquiry in New York, *N Engl J Med* 1981;305:75.
2. Libow LS. The interface of clinical and ethical decisions in the care of the elderly, *M Sin Jour Med* 1981;48:480.
3. McClung JA, Kamer RS. Implications of New York's Do-Not-Resuscitate law, *N Engl J Med* 1990;323:270.
4. Glover JJ. The case of Ms. Nancy Cruzan and the care of the elderly, *JAGS* 1990;38:588.
5. Gasner MR. Cruzan vs. Harmon, and In the matter of O'Connor: Two anomalies, *JAGS* 1990;38:599.
6. Bopp J. Reconciling autonomy and the value of life, *JAGS* 1990;38:600.
7. Thomasma DC. Surrogate decisions at risk, the Cruzan case, *JAGS* 1990;38:603.
8. Yarborough MA, Kramer AM. The physician and resource allocation, *Clinics in Geriatric Medicine* 1986;2:465.
9. Scitovsky AA, Capron AM. Medical care at the end-of-life: The interaction of economics and ethics, *Ann. Rev. Public Health* 1986;7:59.
10. Bayer R, Callahan D, Fletcher J, *et al*. The care of the terminally ill: Mortality and economics, *N Engl J Med* 1983;309:1491.
11. Avorn J. Benefit and cost analysis in geriatric medicine, *N Engl J Med* 1984;310:1294.
12. Garber AM. Cost-containment and financing the long-term care of the elderly, *JAGS* 1988;36:355.
13. Lynn J. Conflicts of interest in medical decision-Making, *JAGS* 1988;36:945.
14. Hilfiker D. Allowing the debilitated to die, *N Engl J Med* 1983;308:716.
15. Callaghan D. *Setting Limits.Medical Goals in an Aging Society*. Simon and Schuster, 1987.
16. Lazaroff AE, Orr WF. Living wills and other advance directives, *Clinics in Geriatric Medicine* 1986;2:521.
17. Davidson KW, Moseley R. Advance directives in family practice, *The Journal of Family Practice* 1986;22:439.
18. Levenson SA, List ND, Zaw-Win B. Ethical considerations in critical and terminal illness in the elderly, *JAGS* 1981;XXIX:563.
19. Emanuel LL, Emanuel EJ. The medical directive, a new comprehensive advance care document, *JAMA* 1989;261:3288.
20. Eisendrath SJ, Jonsen AR. The living will, help or hindrance? *JAMA* 1983;249:2054.
21. Kelly JL, Elphick G, Mepham V, Molloy DW. *Let Me Decide*. McMaster University Press, 1989.
22. Miles SH, Singer PA, Seigler M. Conflicts between patient's wishes to forgo treatment and the policies of health care facilities, *N Engl J Med* 1989;321:48-50.

23. President's Commission for the study of Ethical Problems in Medicine and Biomedical and Behavioural Research. *Deciding to Forego Life-sustaining Treatment*. Washington, DC: US Government Printing Office, 1983.
24. The Appleton Consensus. *Suggested International Guidelines for Decisions to Forgo Medical Treatment*. Appleton, WI: Lawrence University Program in Biomedical Ethics,1988.

Chapter 47

Caring for Decisionally Incapacitated Elderly

Dallas M. High

Introduction

This paper will focus on the ethical aspects in caring for one of the most rapidly growing groups of special patients -- the decisionally incapacitated elderly. Even though most ethical issues regarding the elderly are similar to those in caring for younger patients, they arise with far greater frequency. However, the most difficult ethical issues occur when elderly patients are no longer capable of expressing their own wishes and participating in the health care decision process. These special people, once cognitively able, become decisionally helpless. A serious illness, stroke, mental as well as physical dependency, and various degrees of senile dementia, including Alzheimer's disease, are among the causes which may prevent a once capable older person from participating in decisions about his or her own health care. Often, long term institutional care is required.

Determining Decisional Incapacity

The health care professional's role in caring for elderly with questionable ability to make decisions becomes most complicated because the professional must determine at the outset whether a patient is capable of understanding his or her situation and making choices about it. It is not a case of determining whether capacity is an all or none category, and for that reason the professional should be alert to the varying degrees of decisional capacity and impairment evidenced by the patient. Further, the search for a clear definition of capacity/incapacity, together with a uniform set of criteria for making such determinations, has occasioned much dispute and controversy.[1] No one set of measurements has been agreed on nor is it likely that a single set would suffice, given the wide variety of cases and circumstances. Consequently, the professional must also weigh the gravity of any recommended protocol in the light of the patient's current ability to deliberate and consent or refuse. Accordingly, decisional incapacity is best understood as neither fixed in time nor determined by the age of the patient and/or the content of the decision. Capacities (and incapacities) to participate in care decisions are almost always decision specific, relative to specific tasks, and may fluctuate over time.

The professional's responsibility to determine whether a patient has decisional capacity is distinguishable from, often prior to, or even independent of, any judicial ruling on patient incompetency or disability. Of course, what the physician must make is a clinical determination. It is not a formal court declaration. It is often made with some urgency, and, in contrast with a judicial ruling, entails no privation of rights. Consequently, medical determinations of varying degrees of incapacity may coexist with the legal presumption of

Source: Reprinted from *Theoretical Medicine*, Vol. 10, 1989, pp. 83-96, with permission from Kluwer Academic Publishers © 1989.

competence or even a court determination of partial incompetency. For example, a patient may be fully able to handle her own financial affairs but not have decisional capacity to consent to renal dialysis due to temporary disorientation or confusion.

As a practical matter, the health care professional should assume, until there is contrary evidence, that an adult patient has decisional capacity. Advanced age of the patient is not warrant for a contrary presumption. At the same time, a professional should be alert to any evidence that a patient may lack capacity to comprehend information, communicate, or choose. Clues may emerge from conversations with the patient, from observation of behavior, or from discussions with family members or others. The task of the health care professional is basically to perform a functional assessment of the patient by using professional knowledge in formulating a judgment that would be understandable and intelligible to informed lay people ([3], p.172). A determination of patient incapacity should not be technically or medically esoteric.

The most useful approach is to ask whether a particular patient is or is not able to perform a specific decisional task. A functional assessment will include considerations of whether the patient[1] can take in and comprehend information regarding his or her specific medical situation,[2] can deliberate on accessible alternatives,[3] and can make a reasoned choice. Care must be taken not to confuse apparently irrational choices with a determination of inability to reason. Likewise, it should not be presumed that unusual beliefs held by a patient are evidence of decisional incapacity. Moreover, patient depression or anxiety should not be taken as *prima facie* evidence of decisional incapacity. The health care professional has the ethical duty to counter those effects as much as possible in order that a patient's capacity can be exercised as fully as possible. However, when it is determined that a particular elderly patient is decisionally incapacitated, the major ethical challenges for the professional just begin. Since an incapacitated patient, nevertheless, retains the rights of autonomy without the ability to act on those rights, the professional should respect those fights by assisting to facilitate proper surrogate decision-making and providing optimal beneficial care while guarding against undue paternalism.

Surrogate Decision-Making

When the elderly patient is decisionally incapacitated, it naturally follows that someone else must make decisions for the patient. But the simplicity of the ethical issues ends there. Complexity begins! Who should decide? What is the role of the family? What change, if any, occurs in the decisional role of the health care professional? What are the prior wishes and preferences of the patient? Can patient preferences be carried forward into a time of decisional incapacity? What standard for surrogate decision-making should prevail?

It is frequently presumed that, when the patient can no longer participate in care decisions, the physician must "take over." That presumption is well intended, since to abandon an incapacitated patient offends the moral senses of almost everyone, but it can evoke a professional zealousness and contravene patient autonomy. Such circumstances pose the problem of paternalism -- acting to override patient preferences for the patient's own benefit. But, at what time, if ever, is paternalistic behavior justifiable? Paternalistic behavior is not justifiable simply for the reason that the patient is decisionally incapacitated. In general, other conditions must be present to justify such behavior: (1) the intervention will provide more benefit than harm from nonintervention and (2) serious harm will likely result from nonintervention. It needs to be stressed that a decisionally incapacitated person does not lose the right to autonomy, including the right to consent to and refuse treatment, on the basis of the lack of capacity to exercise that right. For that reason the health care professional's role as the exclusive and preeminent decision-maker is best limited to emergency care. Beyond that the professional risks the danger of turning decision-making and consent into a vacuous process since the professional is also the very one who proposes and recommends treatment procedures. A similar danger arises if the professional does the selecting of the surrogate decision-maker. While the professional can be an advocate of the patient, extreme care must be exercised to ensure that surrogate selection is not based chiefly on who will most likely follow the professional's own treatment recommendations.

It is common practice to call on family members to serve as surrogate decision-makers in the event a patient is decisionally incapacitated. The family is a convenient choice because of ready availability. In addition, family members will likely be concerned about the good of the elderly patient, and often will be the best source of information regarding the patient's wishes, preferences and personal value history. Health care professionals should pay close attention to family members since the quality of surrogate decisions may best depend on an accurate reflection of the patient's own values and preferences. The moral warrant for family surrogate decision-making stems most importantly from the autonomy of the family as a primary social unit and from the fact that elderly patients usually prefer that family members should become their surrogates.[4]

Even though the moral warrant is clear and the practice of family surrogate decision-making is so widespread that it is unlikely to change, the legal authority of family surrogates has been disputed. Family members serving as court appointed guardians, of course, have surrogate/proxy authority. Moreover, in recent years in several states courts have ruled to authorize family members as surrogates.[5] Additionally, an increasing number of states have enacted statutes that support family involvement in decision-making, usually embedded in living will laws or informed consent statutes ([5], p.21). Some states have established a prioritized list of relatives authorized to make surrogate decisions even though the application of surrogate authority is limited ([6], p.41). Health care professionals should be well informed of case and statutory law in their own states regarding surrogate decision-making, since there is a lack of uniformity among the states on the issue. Nevertheless, it is reasonable to proceed on the premise that there is a rebuttable presumption in the law favoring family members for surrogate decision-making. The practice is workable -- even without further legal clarification -- provided there is unanimity among family members and the health professional. However, as evidenced by the current trend, it is expected that case law, as well as statutory law, will increasingly authorize family surrogate decision-making.

Dealing With Family Surrogates

Acknowledgment of the role of family members in surrogate decision-making does not absolve the health care professional of additional moral responsibilities within the dynamics of dealing with family members. For example, the ordinary hierarchy of surrogates, as expected by the elderly, is spouse, adult children, siblings, and other relatives.[4] Sensitivity to those dynamics within the family structure is important. It is advisable to ask relatives who have visited the patient whether other family members should be consulted. Every effort should be made to contact them to determine their agreement with decisions or willingness to accept decisions made by other family surrogates. Frequently families expect that group decision-making and consultation will be followed, and often that expectation coincides with the previously expressed wishes of the elderly patient. The health care professional may facilitate the surrogate decision-making by conferring with and making recommendations through an informally designated spokesperson for the family, but it should not be automatically presumed that the spokesperson is the oldest adult family member. Documentation of discussions with family surrogates, especially on crucial decisions, will prove essential.

In practice there is no substitute or short-cut for communication of clear and explicit information to surrogates. Equally important is the need for attentive listening to questions and responses, discerning signs of understanding and misunderstanding. Moreover, family surrogates are often the primary resource regarding prior expressed wishes of the decisionally incapacitated patient. But family surrogates should be viewed as persons who have special needs, too -- sometimes needs resulting from fear or anxiety -- at the time of a crisis involving a loved family member.

In the event that there is disagreement among family members about a particular decision or a disagreement between the health care professional and the family, the professional is obliged to make sure that these disagreements have not resulted from a lack of information, misunderstanding of information, or other forms of miscommunication. Steps should be taken to rectify any failures in the communication process. All possible avenues of informal resolution should be explored before turning to the courts. In any case the professional is obliged to weigh the interests of the patient with the interests and wishes of the family surrogates. The possibility of conflict of interest or other self-interested acts by family surrogates should be investigated. If there is well-grounded evidence that surrogate decisions are biased accordingly, then the best interests of patients ought to be decisive. In circumstances in which the previously expressed preferences of the patient are known, and there is strong evidence that the surrogate is acting in conflict of interest or on another bias, then the health professional ought to act to protect the preference of the patient.

Standards: Substituted Judgement Versus Best Interests

In recent years two different standards have evolved to guide surrogate decision-making: `substituted judgment' and `best interests' ([3], pp.177-181; [5], pp.10-16). Although these standards are now widely used in health care decisions, they are borrowed from the field of law. They originated in a different context, namely, decisions concerning control of the property of legal incompetents. Simply stated, the substituted judgment standard calls on family and caregivers to arrive at decisions which replicate decisions the patient would have made had the patient been capable of doing so. Under the best interests standard surrogate decisions are acceptable on the grounds that they benefit (and do not harm) the patient according to socially shared values of a hypothetical average person. By this standard, decisions may or may not reflect the patient's own preferences.

Substituted judgment attempts to follow a patient's interest on the basis of a right of self-determination and extend it to a time when the patient is incapable of self-directed exercise of that fight. In addition, a decision based on substituted judgment is one that is defined in accordance with the patient's own values and goals, subject to limitations by law or matters outside the discretion of a surrogate. For substituted judgment to be employed the patient's own views and preferences must be known, which can be derived from a variety of sources. The greater the discernment of the patient's views the more the surrogate's ability will be enhanced to decide in a way the patient would really have wanted.

Although it is rare that family members have no acquaintance with the views, values or goals of one of their elderly, the best interests of the patient must be considered when the views are unknown or lack sufficient clarity to enact them confidently. Surrogates are then obliged to focus on the patient's presumed interests as measured by the hypothetical average citizen or reasonable person concerning such objective factors as prolongation of life, pain and suffering, quality of life, success of treatment and restoration to normal functioning. However, an unambiguous assessment of these factors is often difficult given the fluidity of the medical condition of the patient and the fact that some factors may conflict with each other.

Because the substituted judgment standard approximates individual self-determination, legal scholars and various court jurisdictions have argued for the priority of this standard.[7] The medical profession, on the other hand, has remained more cautious since the incapacitated elderly are an especially dependent and vulnerable population.[8] However, professional fears of abandoning the incapacitated elderly to their own devices and preferences are probably exaggerated, especially when the health care professional puts forth extra effort to ascertain and comprehend the wishes, preferences and values of the patient. If patient preferences can be known and applied, substituted judgment is the most ethical course of action since it promotes personal autonomy more than the best interests standard does. As a practical matter, known patient preferences should be documented on the patient's chart.

Advance Directives

Substituted judgment is simpler to use and has greater reliability as a standard when the elderly patient, while capacitated, has provided directives regarding medical care in the event of decisional incapacity. The health care professional should be aware of the wide range of formal and informal advance directives that may be used and are, in fact, of interest to elderly patients. The following provides a topology of advance directives:

Instruction Directives

(1) Inferred communication: The desires and preferences of a person may be derived or deduced from the person's known sets of values, beliefs, tenets of personal religious practice or patterns of behavior. (2) Specific oral communication: Prior to incapacity, explicit desires and preferences may be expressed to family, friends, clergy, physician or attorney and may take the form of a statement about one's own self in reference to a possible or actual illness or a reaction to the medical treatment administered to another person. (3) Personal written instructions: Written statements or letters prior to incapacity assist to remove the uncertainty of relying on oral or inferred communications and can be used as a clear expression of the author's intentions and wishes if signed and dated. (4) Form letter or living will form: Model letter drafts, designed for widespread public use, may be signed, dated and witnessed and can serve to indicate some general intent of the author. Normally, these are limited to expressions concerning a terminal condition. (5) Statutory acts: Living Will laws: A properly executed advance directive document may be used to extend one's right by statute to control decisions regarding withholding or withdrawing life-sustaining treatment in the event of a terminal condition. Most states, not all, have living will laws.

Decision-making by Agent and/or Proxy

(1) Agent -- statutory priorities: Some states have established procedures for decision-making on behalf of incapacitated persons who have not executed any prior declaration. A list of persons (e.g., spouse, adult child, parent, etc.), by order of priority, is offered regarding who may serve as an agent. (2) Proxy -- durable power of attorney: To delegate another person, prior to incapacity, to act on one's behalf may be accomplished through the personal appointment of a proxy (e.g., relative, friend, etc.). The durable power of attorney can be designed to become effective only when the signer becomes decisionally incapacitated -- known legally as a `springing' durable power of attorney -- which is probably the preferred approach when formulated for health care decisions. Specific instructions and/or specific delegations of authority may be included.

Health care professionals cannot afford to ignore advance directives even when some practical objections are raised. Informal and formal directives are important sources of information about patient wishes and values. It is, therefore, part of the professional's duty to inquire whether an incapacitated elderly patient has prepared any advance directive (whatever its type) or spoken to anyone about treatment preferences, even though some instruction directives may lack specificity or can easily become outdated by the changing medical conditions of the patient. It is for these latter reasons that some professionals expressly prefer agent/proxy directives,[9] but those, too, are not without limitations -- e.g., the proxy may not know the incapacitated person's wishes.[10]

Since laws regarding instruction directives and durable powers of attorney are developing rapidly, the health professional should be informed of their legal status in one's own jurisdiction. Moreover, the health professional should be aware of the extent to which advance directives can be effectively used by the elderly in planning for future health care decisions. For example, it is possible in several states for a patient to do substantial planning by drawing up a letter of instruction and simultaneously using the durable power attorney to appoint a proxy decision-maker even though a statute has not been enacted explicitly extending a power of attorney to health care decision-making. Professionals, including but not limited to geriatricians, have a responsibility to make information on advance directives available to elderly patients and to encourage the principle that good planning for health care decisions is as important as preventive medicine. In fact, the professional should initiate discussions with elderly persons, while they are still capable, about preferences regarding life-sustaining treatment and other treatment preferences. Elderly patients usually welcome such open, candid, and caring discussions [[41], ([11], p. 1614)].

Advance directives cannot be viewed as a panacea for either professionals or elderly patients. While advance directives are useful, and there is a large measure of compatibility among the various instruments, conflicts can arise. If, for example, a patient has prestated his or her wishes in an informal letter and yet a surrogate decision-maker, such as a family member, does not wish to abide by the evidence contained in the letter, the professional should deal with the matter as a surrogate conflict of interest. On the other hand, if a state has enacted a living will law, and the patient has signed one, the wishes of the patient as expressed in the document are binding, even though it will be necessary for the health professional to interpret the applications in the light of the patient's condition. In all cases, patient preferences should be honored. The relative strength of the evidence of those preferences will be decisive in cases of dispute. Weak evidence in the form of inferred communication may be overridden by judgments promoting the best interests of the patient when both the surrogate decision-maker(s) and physician agree. Strong evidence, even strong corroborated oral evidence, generally should not be overridden. If a patient has written an instruction directive, a copy should be attached to the patient's chart.

The Frail Elderly and Do-Not-Resuscitate Order

Knowing an elderly patient's preferences in advance can and should have significant effect on determining the desirability of certain medical treatments. And there are few issues for which patient advance directives have a more important role than in decisions regarding cardiopulmonary resuscitation (CPR) or the issuance of a do-not-resuscitate order (DNR). The elderly are most frequently affected by these considerations because such decisions come toward the end of life when a person can no longer fully participate in the process. Moreover, not infrequently older patients are impaired by multiple medical disorders which contribute directly to the importance of DNR considerations.

The ethical grounds for a DNR order begin with the necessity of sound medical judgment that further treatment of the primary disease is futile. Although it is quite clear that health care professionals have no obligation to provide futile or useless treatment, arriving at a judgment that treatment is futile often involves considerable uncertainty. Consultation with other physicians may help establish an accurate prognosis.

Beyond that, any justification for a DNR order ought to include consideration of the following: (1) Is death from the primary disease imminent? (2) Is the patient irreversibly terminally ill and/or is there no reasonable prospect of restorative recovery for the patient? (The conventional designation of `terminal illness' is often inappropriate for the seriously ill elderly); (3) Is it anticipated that the patient will experience cardiac or respiratory failure? (4) Will suffering, pain, and the poor quality of life endured by the patient overwhelm the benefits of continued life?

Without a determination of the futility of medical treatment, cardiopulmonary resuscitation should be instituted and no DNR order should be given. Neglecting to determine the futility of medical treatment is not a warrant for the presumption favoring CPR. It is unethical for a professional to justify a bias toward CPR by simply ignoring the issue of whether treatment is futile. On the other hand, the factors of patient age, mental retardation, and chronic disease alone should not be taken as grounds for determining the medical futility of treatment or as justification for withholding CPR.

Any DNR order should, when possible, reflect the wishes of the patient even though sometimes it will be difficult to determine what those wishes are. On the other hand, many patients when able, will have stated their wishes through informal or formal means, including previous conversations with their physician and family members. The physician, in considering a DNR order, should always inquire concerning any evidence about the patients wishes. Often family members can be quite helpful in those circumstances. If the patient has never expressed wishes regarding DNR, then the physician should try to discover whether the patient had expressed preferences regarding who should act as a surrogate or proxy decision-maker and fully discuss the matter accordingly. In any case, when there are family members discussions should be initiated with those members.

Advance prospective discussions between the health care practitioner and the patient on such matters as CPR and DNR are well advised. Although such a practice is a cause for concern because it is considered awkward and painful, causing anxiety and depression or even suicide, there is little evidence confirming that patients are so affected ([12], p.1562). To the contrary, evidence suggests that elderly patients generally welcome such discussions, especially if it is initiated by the health care professional as a positive step in medical care planning.

If it is known that the patient, even if decisionally incapacitated, would have wished CPR, then no DNR order ought be written. If the family of an incapacitated patient disagree with the physician's judgment that a DNR order is indicated and a DNR judgment reflects the patient's wishes, then the DNR order should be postponed and discussion should be continued further in order to attempt to resolve the disagreement and clarify the patient's wishes. The family may not fully understand the medical circumstances or the wishes of the patient. If the family favors a DNR order and yet the patient wishes CPR or the physician does not judge that a DNR order is warranted, no DNR order should be written. The autonomy of the patient and sound medical judgment regarding the warrant of CPR hold priority over family wishes in this case.

Once the decision for a DNR order has been reached, it should be documented in the progress notes. This documentation should include notes on factors leading to the decision and a record of consultations and conversations with surrogate (e.g., family) decision-makers. The DNR order should be written explicitly in the order section of the chart. Everyone involved in the care of the patient should be informed. A DNR order should be regularly reviewed and reassessed by all parties concerned. The order may be rescinded at any time; once rescinded it can be reinstated.

Any decision to forego resuscitation should be clear, definite and well communicated. However, sometimes "slow," "partial," "limited," or "floor" codes, variously called, are considered. If such categories are employed to signify that less-than-full effort should be made, such as delaying the call for a full code or that only perfunctory CPR should be administered, then they are unjustified. Such informal orders often place nursing staff in an untenable position. If, however, these categories are used to make distinctions among CPR techniques and instruments, then strong justification of such a code should be provided and documented on a case by case basis. For example, a distinction may be drawn between the use of basic CPR and mechanical ventilation -- favoring the former while refraining from the latter. Such limited CPR may have justification, especially if the patient has provided advance wishes disfavoring mechanical ventilation. In no case, however, should "limited codes" be used to appease or reassure family that "everything possible was done."

It goes without saying that DNR orders ought to have no effect on the level of supportive and palliative care. DNR orders are in fact compatible with maximal supportive care. Unfortunately there is evidence to suggest that the DNR order, once written, does contribute to a reduction in attention to other forms of medical care for the patient ([13], p.811; [14], p.1168). Health care professionals must assiduously guard against that propensity for bias against supportive and palliative care of a frail elderly person for whom a DNR order has been written. Such discrimination is ethically untenable.

How decisions are best made about DNR orders for the frail elderly is only one among many important ethical issues which arise in care of the decisionally incapacitated elderly. There are other issues that are at least equally complex and difficult, including decisions about nutritional support, which in several ways parallels decisions about CPR. Moreover, new issues will likely emerge. In the final analysis ethics of care for the elderly patients who are highly vulnerable is at its worst when application of simple formulae is attempted. It is at its best when compassionate care involves full consideration of various points of view and diverse values, including their conflicts. Careful attention to a morally appropriate process of decision-making is a difficult but rewarding task when caring for a special and highly vulnerable class of fellow human beings.

Appendix: Bibliography

High's and Turner's essay[4] explores the preferences and expectations of the elderly regarding the role of family members in making health care decisions in the event of decisional incapacity. Findings are presented from in-depth studies of 40 men and women aged 67-91 years. The essay argues for more, rather than less, involvement of the family as surrogate decision-makers.

Legal and Ethical Aspects of Health Care for the Elderly[15] is an anthology, consisting mostly of original essays. This anthology is one of the few devoted entirely to legal and ethical issues in care of the elderly. The volume is useful and covers fights of long-term care residents, elderly decision-making in health care, financing of long term care, and legal issues facing long term care providers.

In the light of current ethical standards regarding the principle of autonomy and recent court decisions on "no code" orders Lee and Cassel[16] argue for establishing professional guidelines. A helpful stepwise approach to deciding not to resuscitate is presented.

Submitted in February 1984, as a "friend of the court" brief in the case known as, In re Claire C. Conroy, the document by Lynn[8] is an important expression of The American Geriatrics Society regarding the values and concerns in removing life-sustaining treatment of the elderly, especially nutrition and hydration. The document attempts to balance the value of patient well-being with the principle of following the known individual preferences of the patient.

The moral responsibilities of physicians caring for elderly with diminished competence are discussed in a paper by McCullough.[17] It is argued that decisional responsibilities should be grounded in the patient's past autonomy -- patient values and beliefs.

With the assistance of the patient's family, physicians should construct and record the patient's "value history."

Schneiderman, *et al.*[18] helpfully provide a discussion of the varieties of advance directives, including a comparison of instruction and proxy directives. The authors argue that physicians should regard it as a duty to counsel patients to express their wishes and preferences over future care in the event of incompetence.

Solnick,[5] a physician-attorney, discusses the determination of incompetence, standards of best interests, and substituted judgment, the legal authority of family surrogates/ proxies, and the developing legal/ethical roles of advance directives. An explicit procedure for proxy decision-making is proposed, including the establishment of proxy consent review committees in hospitals and nursing homes.

Use of the durable power of attorney for health care, with special reference to the California law, is concisely discussed in Steinbrook, *et al.*[9] The positive features of proxy decision-making laws, including legal immunity and removal of required familial consensus, as well as the unresolved legal issues, are considered.

In Wagner[19] results of a prospective survey of 163 female residents, aged 66 to 98 years, of a life contract residential home are presented regarding cardiopulmonary resuscitation (CPR). Seven percent wished CPR, 47% declined CPR, and 39% preferred the physician to choose at the time.

Notes

1. Roth LH, Meisel A, Lidz CW. Tests of competency to consent to treatment, *Am J Psychiatry* 1977;134:279-84.
2. Gutheil TG, Applebaum PS. *Clinical Handbook of Psychiatry and the Law*. New York, NY: McGraw-Hill, 1982.
3. President's Commission for the Study of Ethical Problems. *Medicine and Biomedical and Behavioral Research. Making Health Care Decisions*. Volume 1, Washington, DC: US Government Printing Office, 1982.
4. High DM, Turner HB. Surrogate decision-making: The elderly's familial expectations, *Theor Med* 1987;8:303-20.
5. Solnick PB. Proxy consent for incompetent non-terminally ill adult patients, *J Leg Med* 1985;6:1-49.
6. Society for the right to die, *The Physician and the Hopelessly Ill Patient*. New York, NY: Society for the Right to Die, 1985.
7. In the Matter of Claire C. Conroy, 486 A. 2d 1209 (N.J. 1985).
8. Lynn J. Brief and appendix for arnicus curiae: The American Geriatrics Society, *J Am Geriatr Soc* 1984;32:915-22.
9. Steinbrook R, Lo B. Decision-making for incompetent patients by designated proxy, *N Engl J Med* 1984;310:1598-1601.
10. High DM. Planning for decisional incapacity: A neglected area in ethics and aging, *J Am Geriatr Soc* 1987;35:814-20.
11. Lo B, McLeod GA, Saika G. Patient attitudes to discussing life-sustaining treatment, *Arch Intern Med* 1986;146:1613-5.
12. Lo B, Steinbrook RL. Deciding whether to resuscitate, *Arch Intern Med* 1983;143:1561-3.
13. Schwartz DA, Reilly P. The choice not to be resuscitated, *J Am Geriatr Soc* 1986;34:807-11.
14. Lipton HL. Do-not-resuscitate decisions in a community hospital, *JAMA* 1986;256:1164-9.
15. Kapp MB, Pies HE, Doudera AE, eds. *Legal and Ethical Aspects of Health Care for the Elderly*. Ann Arbor, MI: Health Administration Press, 1985.
16. Lee MA, Cassel CK. The ethical and legal framework for the decision not to resuscitate, *West J Med* 1984;140:117-22.
17. McCullough LB. Medical care for elderly patients with diminished competence: An ethical analysis, *J Am Geriatr Soc* 1984;32:150-3.

18. Schneiderman LJ, Arras JD. Counseling patients to counsel physicians on future care in the event of patient incompetence, *Ann Intern Med* 1985;102:693-8.
19. Wagner A. Cardiopulmonary resuscitation in the aged, *N Engl J Med* 1984;310:1129-30.

Chapter 48

The Use of Quality-of-Life Considerations in Medical Decision-Making

Robert A. Pearlman and Albert R. Jonsen

In recent months there has been considerable attention in the medical literature on life-sustaining treatments for chronically ill patients.[1,2,3,4,5,6,7,8,9] In several of these articles, the patient's quality-of-life is discussed as a factor affecting medical decisions.[5-9]

The traditional pressures in acute care facilities for aggressive treatment and the uncertainties of diagnosis and prognosis may make it difficult to predict the quality of a patient's life with or without treatment.[10,11] Other factors also may make quality-of-life difficult to predict. These include the physician's subjective values relative to the patient's characteristics, inadequate communication between physicians and patients, and problems with the measurement of quality-of-life.[5,10,12] The extent to which the patient's quality-of-life is considered in medical decisions and the variability in judgments among physicians have not been well defined in the literature.

This study was designed to provide a better understanding of physician consideration (mention) of patient quality-of-life in medical decisions. We studied the explicit mention of "quality-of-life" as an influential factor in a patient management problem (PMP) pertaining to the use of mechanical ventilation to sustain life. This paper presents the results of this research, defines quality-of-life, and provides guidelines for physician consideration of patient quality-of-life.

Methods

After the nature of the patient management problem was explained and informed consent was obtained, the patient management problem was presented to 205 physicians specializing in internal medicine or family medicine in King County, Washington. The physicians performed several tasks during this exercise, including: (1) indication of a treatment preference after the initial reading of the case description; (2) indication of the potential value of available (but unknown) case information; (3) selection of a limited amount of case information to acquire more detailed data about the clinical situation; (4) indication of a treatment decision as to whether to use intubation or current therapy without intubation after acquiring the additional ease knowledge; (5) explanation of the rationale for the treatment decision; and (6) prognostication regarding the patient's expected survival time. In a previous article, the precise details of the selection of subjects, the PMP, the management of case information, and the interview were presented.[13] In this paper we describe and discuss physicians' expressed consideration of the "patient's quality-of-life" as a reason for the treatment decision.

Source: Reprinted from *Journal of the American Geriatrics Society*, Vol. 33, No. 5, pp. 344-350, with permission from Williams & Wilkins © May, 1985.

Case Description
The patient management problem was modeled after American Board of Internal Medicine certification examination questions. It was developed to explore physicians' decisions to withhold mechanical ventilation.

The case presented a male patient with an acute exacerbation of his chronic obstructive pulmonary disease. The patient was an elderly-looking 69-year-old who lived in a nursing home, was easily incapacitated by shortness of breath, and had recently had a prolonged hospitalization (2 months) because of a similar episode. His forced expiratory volume in one second was 0.38 liters (12 percent), his forced expiratory volume in one second/vital capacity ratio was 0.22, and his forced expiratory flow (0.25-0.75 seconds) was 0.17 liters (9 percent). He had never expressed to his physician his view on conditions in which withholding therapy might be desirable, nor had he offered his own assessment of his quality-of-life. His physician had never inquired about these points. At this hospital admission he expressed concern about the possible need for intubation. However, a precise plan for dealing with worsening respiratory failure was not defined. Despite treatment with oxygen, antibiotics, bronchodilators, and steroids, the patient deteriorated into profound respiratory failure. This life-and-death situation forced the studied physicians to decide between intubation (life prolonging) and the currently administered drug regimen without intubation (allowing to die).

Additional information about the patient's physical and functional status while residing in the nursing home was available. However, the patient management problem required physicians to seek further information that was not provided initially in the case description. Available data about the patient's baseline, precrisis level of function included slight forgetfulness, mild depression, and inability to walk more than halfway across a room because of worsening shortness of breath. The questionnaire is available from the authors.

Data Analysis
Statistical analyses were accomplished with univariate and multivariate methods (SPSS).[14] Significance values are reported in the text with the name of the test statistic. Stepwise discriminant analysis was used to select and combine into an index a limited number of measures to best predict use of quality-of-life. The predictive ability of this index was validated by developing it on one-half of the data and using it to predict the use of quality-of-life in the other half of the data.

Results
Thirty-seven percent of all physicians justified their clinical decisions, at least in part, by explicit references to the "patient's quality-of-life." Forty-nine percent of those who decided not to withhold mechanical ventilation (nonintubators) volunteered quality-of-life as a rationale for their decision. In contrast, 29 percent of those who chose to intubate (intubators) mentioned quality-of-life as an influential factor affecting their treatment choice ($0.005 < p \leq 0.01$, unpaired *t*-test). Among nonintubators, approximately 87 percent indicated that the patient's quality-of-life positively supported their treatment decision. Among intubators, approximately 82 percent indicated that the patient's quality-of-life positively supported their treatment decision. This was determined by asking the physician how each factor affecting the therapeutic choice influenced their decision; that is, whether it supported, militated against, or had no impact. It is noteworthy that these divergent evaluations of an individual patient's quality-of-life were used to justify polar treatment decisions of clinical significance.

There was no appreciable difference in consideration of "quality-of-life" between specialties (39 percent for family medicine and 36 percent for internal medicine). However, residents in training programs considered quality-of-life more often than did attending physicians and private practitioners (47 percent for residents, 33 percent for attending physicians, 31 percent for private practitioners). The comparison between residents and other physicians was statistically significant, $0.025 < p \leq 0.05$ (X^2, 2 degrees of freedom). These data are presented in Table 1. Physicians who indicated that quality-of-life was a consideration thought it was an important factor. This was noted on a scale of increasing importance from 1 (unimportant) to 10 (very important).

Table 1. Quality-of-Life Rationale

	Physicians Mentioning Quality-of-life	Physicians Not Mentioning Quality-of-life
Treatment decision		
Intubators[1]	34 (20%)	85
Nonintubators[1]	42 (48%)	44
Specialty		
Internal medicine	48 (36%)	85
Family medicine	28 (39%)	44
Role		
Residents[2]	34 (47%)	38
Attending physicians[2]	18 (33%)	37
Private practitioners[2]	24 (31%)	54

1. $p \leq 0.01$.
2. $p \leq 0.05$ (residents versus others).

Physician consideration of "quality-of-life" as a factor influencing the treatment decision was associated with consideration of available specific case information and with several other volunteered explanations. Table 2 outlines the statistically significant correlates of quality-of-life consideration. Physicians who requested information either from the social worker or from the nurse at the nursing home and learned either that the family finances were depleted or that the patient was only able to walk halfway across the room, respectively, were more inclined to use quality-of-life as a justification for their treatment decisions ($p \leq 0.05$). Other expressed explanations, such as cost-benefit factors, the expected survival time (if intubated) for the patient, the patient's right to determine his own therapy, the physician's responsibility to sustain life, and the patient's prior hospital experience with respirator dependence, were significantly associated with the consideration of quality-of-life as a partial justification for the treatment decision ($p \leq 0.05$). Nonintubators cited the right of the patient to determine his own therapy and his prior hospital experience as a rationale along with consideration of quality-of-life ($p \leq 0.05$). On the other hand, intubators cited the patient's expected survival time and their own responsibility to sustain life ($p \leq 0.05$).

Physician consideration of quality-of-life was not associated with medical specialty (internal medicine or family medicine), religion, degree of faith, or estimates of the patient's survival time (if intubated). The relationship between quality-of-life consideration and a measure of moral judgment was also examined. Moral judgment was assessed by administering Robert Hogan's Survey of Ethical Attitudes to each physician.[13] This test explores the effects of the difference between an ethic of social responsibility and an ethic of personal conscience.[15,16,17,18] Use of quality-of-life as a factor in this treatment decision was not significantly associated with either ethical stance.

Table 2 shows a large number of variables that are significantly related to the consideration of quality-of-life as a justification for the treatment choice in this case management problem. One could predict, to some extent, use of quality-of-life by assessing any one of these measures. Using stepwise discriminant analysis, an index was developed that identified a limited number of measures that would best predict the mention or nonmention of quality-of-life. Table 3 reviews the important discriminate variables that were used in the stepwise analysis. The management of case information and other volunteered explanations appeared to significantly account for or explain the use of quality-of-life as a consideration in decision-making. The measures identified in Table 3 correctly predicted the consideration of quality-of-life in this therapeutic decision (justifying intubation or current therapy without intubation) with a probability greater than 80 percent.

Discussion

Consideration of "quality-of-life" in medical decision-making was systematically observed in a PMP. It was commonly voiced as a rationale for the medical decision by physicians inclined to withhold mechanical ventilation, physicians who considered the patient's survival time, and physicians who extensively focused on social information about the patient. However, the marked variation in perceptions of quality-of-life for a given patient gives rise to serious concerns about how physicians use this term.

The greater consideration of quality-of-life by residents may reflect several factors. The residents focus more on socioeconomic case information, which may, have influenced their consideration of quality-of-life. However, it is also possible that residents are more harshly judgmental about an older person's quality-of-life or more concerned with this issue than attending physicians or private practitioners. Whether this will change as the residents advance in their professional lives is unknown. Their consideration of quality-of-life may represent a cohort effect caused by recent changes in medical education or a temporary phenomenon due to their current age and experience.

The lack of association between consideration of quality-of-life and an ethical stance (based on Hogan's Survey of Ethical Attitudes) may reflect the ambiguous nature and the unprincipled use of the concept. If consideration of quality-of-life were a clearly defined professional responsibility, it might have correlated with the ethic of social responsibility. And if the consideration of quality-of-life represented attempts to avoid patient harm or promote patient well-being, it might have correlated with the ethic of personal conscience. However, as neither ethical stance appeared to be associated with consideration of quality-of-life, the principled rationale for such consideration is yet undefined.

The explicit consideration of quality-of-life in the case management of a nursing home patient with an acute exacerbation of chronic obstructive pulmonary disease reflects a more general and pervasive consideration of quality-of-life in health care decisions. In rheumatology, oncology, and geriatric medicine, quality-of-life is becoming a common measure of outcome and health status.[19,20,21,22] It would be extremely unusual for physicians not to be concerned about the quality of their patients' lives. Physicians, after all, work to diagnose and treat the medical causes of impaired quality-of-life in hopes of improving that quality. However, in recent years the term "quality-of-life" has taken on a more specific and problematic meaning in medicine.

Quality-of-life has come to serve as a criterion for the utility of intervention in many clinical situations, including those involving life-and-death decisions. However, there are some individuals who reject quality-of-life as an important determinant of the value of life. They consider life to have intrinsic worth and regard prolongation of life as the overriding determinant of the utility of an intervention.

TABLE 2. Correlates of Quality-of-Life Consideration

Reasons for Considering Quality-of-life	p Values
All subjects	
Preferencs for nonintubation	0.01
Residency status (role)	0.05
Valuation of physiologic information[1]	0.03
Valuation of professional information[1]	0.01
Valuation of socioeconomic information[1]	0.01
Consideration of the social worker's report[2]	0.001
Consideration of the nursing home report[2]	0.03
Consideration of general physiologic information[2]	0.04
Nonconsideration of general physiologic information[3]	0.04
Costs and benefits rationale[4]	0.04
Survival time rationale[4]	0.02
Patient's right to determine therapy rationale[4]	0.004
Physician responsibility to sustain life rationale[4]	0.04
Prior hospital experience rationale[4]	0.02
Nonintubators	
Valuation of general professional information[1]	0.04
Nonconsideration of th pulmonary function data[3]	0.006
Consideration of the social worker's report[2]	0.002
Patient's right to determine theraphy rationale[4]	0.02
Prior hospital experience rationale[4]	0.001
Intubators	
Valuation of general physiologic information[1]	0.02
Valuation of general socioeconomic information[1]	0.04
Nonconsideration of the repeat chest x-ray data[3]	0.03
Survival time rationale[4]	0.02
Physician responsibility to sustain life rationale[4]	0.04

1. Valuation refers to attributing a value to categories of information in terms of importance to the therapeutic choice.
2. Consideration here refers to selection of case information to obtain detailed data.
3. Nonconsideration refers to nonselection of detailed case information.
4. Rationale refers to a volunteered explanation.

TABLE 3. Significant Variables in a Discriminant[1]

Preference for nonintubation
Valuation of general professional information[2]
Consideration of the social worker's report[3]
Nonconsideration of complete blood chemistry data[4]
Nonconsideration of theophylline level report[4]
Survival time rationale[5]
Nonmention of rationale concerning the patient's soical attributes[5]

1. Split-sample analysis correctly predicted use of quality-of-life 80.9% of the time.
2. Valuation refers to attributing a value to categories of information in terms of importance to the therapeutic choice.
3. Consideration refers to selection of case information to obtain detailed data.
4. Nonconsideration refers to nonselection of detailed case information.
5. Rationale refers to volunteered explanations.

From this point of view, quality-of-life is a moot issue in clinical decision-making. In contrast, many individuals consider quality-of-life to be a vague complex of personal characteristics and social accidents and feel that medical interventions are worthwhile only to the extent that they can promote this beneficial state. In these situations, physicians actually may cite quality-of-life as their primary or one of several standards for treatment, as this study demonstrates. In situations in which quality-of-life connotes a vague set of attributes and conditions, the variability of perceptions of a patient's quality-of-life may be great, as this study suggests. The methods used in this study may have introduced other reasons for the variability in citing quality-of-life. These might include the limited amount of patient information given, the variability in the physicians' consideration of additional case information, and the possibility of idiosyncratic responses by physicians to a PMP that involves an open-ended interview.

Medicine abounds in clear and safe criteria for medical intervention -- for instance, a symptomatically low serum sugar concentration (hypoglycemia) indicates a need for administration of glucose, and severely elevated blood pressure indicates a need for administration of an antihypertensive regimen. When physicians move beyond these to such general criteria as quality-of-life, prudent use is required. Quality-of-life is a particularly imprecise criterion subject to misinterpretation and variable application. This does not imply that such a criterion is illegitimate; it does imply that its meaning should be as clear as possible and its use as responsible as can be.

Meaning

The term "quality-of-life" has no obvious meaning; it is not clear to which empirical states the term refers, nor is it manifest how any particular person will evaluate those states. A major result of this study is the demonstration that physician evaluation of a patient's quality-of-life is variable and can lead to diverse conclusions about treatment. A significant minority of the physicians studied considered the patient's quality-of-life sufficiently poor to withhold additional treatment, whereas other physicians considered it sufficiently good to justify implementing additional therapy. These results highlight the inherent ambiguity of the term "quality-of-life." Three possible definitions recently have been proposed to minimize the ambiguity in the term "quality-of-life."[19] Quality-of-life may reflect the subjective satisfaction by an individual with his or her own personal life (physical, mental, and social situation). Several authors who have written about quality-of-life in medical decisions have used this definition.[1,3,4,6,8,10] Another definition is that quality-of-life represents an evaluation by an onlooker of another's life situation. Two authors modified this definition for use with seriously ill, incompetent patients by recommending guidelines for considering patient quality-of-life. One author recommended judgment by "reasonable measures," whereas another author accepted the Canadian Law Reform Commission recommendation that evaluation of quality-of-life be made by competent patients of the same age and condition.[7,8] The third definition is that quality-of-life is the achievement of certain attributes highly valued in our society.

A common, clinical context in which the first definition occurs is when a patient presents a physician with a concern or complaint and the physician intervenes to diagnose and treat. In this situation, the most frequent paradigm of the physician/patient interaction, the patient has evaluated his or her own life and found it in some way unsatisfying.

The second definition finds common use in clinical settings when a physician or a patient's family member or friend makes an evaluative judgment about the patient's condition that reflects his or her own personal views about what the condition must be like. This often occurs in clinical discussions concerning the initiation or continuation of life-sustaining procedures for a patient incapable of making or expressing a personal evaluation. It may also occur when a seriously impaired patient could be queried about personal satisfaction but the reluctance or inhibition of others, including the physician, prevent this approach to the patient. Although these evaluations may be thoughtful and compassionate, they may not necessarily reflect the patient's own views on the condition. This second definition of quality-of-life may lead to inter-ratervariability because of differences in values. This operational definition probably was used by the physician respondents in this study.

The third definition is less obvious, but it is still influential in medical situations. Clinicians' perceptions of a patient's quality-of-life may be influenced by their perceptions of the difference between a patient's conditions and the achievement of certain attributes that the culture deems necessary or contributory to a life of good quality. Here, invidious prejudices may be hidden below the surface of apparently benign judgments. It has been demonstrated that these prejudices, often deeply buried, can strongly affect the treatment plans of physicians for these sorts of patients.[12,23,24,25,26]

Responsible Use

Responsible use of the inherently ambiguous concept of quality-of-life occurs when clinicians attune their interactions with patients to the values and goals of the patient. In these contexts, a patient's own evaluation of the quality of personal life may affect the nature of the clinician-patient relationship, the schedule for a diagnostic evaluation, the choice of a therapeutic intervention, and the determination of patient benefit or best interest. A common example in geriatric medicine is when a clinician recommends a walker rather than a nursing home for a patient with irreversible gait instability and the desire to remain independent. A less common example is when a clinician accepts a competent elderly patient's refusal of treatment because the proposed intervention will not improve the patient's overall quality-of-life in the patient's view. When consideration of a patient's quality-of-life is grounded in the patient's self-evaluation, it is important and relevant for good patient care. This use rarely poses an ethical concern. Ethical problems appear only when a patient's competency is in doubt or an incompetent patient's family proposes that the patient's quality-of-life does not justify a medical intervention.

The common use of quality-of-life as a factor in making a decision on withholding or withdrawing life-sustaining procedures represents a crucial ethical concern in patient care.[19] With an informed, competent patient who is able to communicate his or her feelings, respect for patient autonomy should foster respect for the patient's attitudes about the use of life-sustaining procedures. The underlying rationale is that this type of patient is able to determine what is beneficial for himself or herself (on the basis of his or her perceived current or future quality-of-life). This situation requires that a clinician's subjective evaluation of the patient's quality-of-life generally be relegated to the patient's opinions.[27] When a patient is unable to communicate his or her feelings about life-sustaining procedures, quality-of-life may be considered a decisive factor only if the patient's quality-of-life falls below a minimum standard and the intervention would only preserve this condition or maintain organic life.[19] One recommendation for minimal threshold is extreme physical debilitation and a complete loss of sensory and intellectual activity.[19] This threshold should be kept extremely low to ensure specificity. Only when the qualities common to human interaction have been irreversibly lost should the clinician's assessment of the patient's quality-of-life determine withholding of life-supporting therapy. Specificity is particularly important in avoiding the potential use of subjective judgments of poor quality-of-life based on socio-economic or other value-laden attributes ("false positives").

This minimum standard reflects respect for personal function, cerebration, and the essential qualities of being human.[28,29] This standard shows respect for the sanctity of human life and the need to safeguard this principle. These guidelines attempt to protect patient autonomy, to ensure justice by preventing capricious decision-making based on personal preferences, to promote beneficial results for patients, and to prevent doing harm.

In summary, in this study a PMP was used to demonstrate the use of quality-of-life considerations in medical decision-making. In clinical usage, quality-of-life is an ambiguous term. Quality-of-life may refer to a patient's subjective satisfaction with his or her life or a subjective evaluation by an observer of the patient's life. When quality-of-life is considered by the patient, responsible use of this evaluation helps clarify the "best interests" of the patient was well as what is beneficial for that patient. An ethical problem arises in situations in which clinicians consider withholding or withdrawing life-sustaining procedures without knowledge of the patient's preferences. In this context, it is responsible to include consideration of a patient's quality-of-life in medical decision-making only under the following conditions: the qualities of human interaction must be lacking, the patient must be unable to express his preferences, and the situation must be such that life-sustaining procedures serve only to prolong a life that is only biologically functional.

There are no current guarantees that the subjective evaluation by a clinician of a patient's quality-of-life will result in the evaluation's ethically responsible use. Responsible use occurs when a clinician's subjective evaluation (projection) concerning a patient's quality-of-life assists him or her in communicating with the patient and in giving compassionate care. Responsible use also occurs when clinicians analyze their own values to prevent personally biased judgments. As Fletcher has written, "A person's values, therefore, are the key to his or her ethical position. Failure to state one's values whether through dishonest camouflage or lack of self knowledge is a source of much more heat than light in ethical discourse."[28]

See Authors for Questionnaire: Case Description and Procedures for Patient Management

Notes

1. Bayer R, Callahan D, Fletcher J, *et al.* The care of the terminally ill: Morality and economics, *N Engl J Med* 1983;309:1490.
2. Wanzer SH, Adelstein SJ, Cranford RE, *et al.* The physician's responsibility toward hopelessly ill patients, *N Engl J Med* 1984;310:955.
3. Bedell SE, Delbanco TL. Choices about cardiopulmonary resuscitation in the hospital: When do physicians talk with patients? *N Engl J Med* 1984;310:1089.
4. Wagner A. Cardiopulmonary resuscitation in the aged, *N Engl J Med* 1984;310:1129.
5. Avorn J. Benefit and cost analysis in geriatric care: Turning age discrimination into health policy, *N Engl J Med* 1984;310:1294.
6. Watts DT, Cassel CK. Extraordinary nutritional support: A case study and ethical analysis, *J Am Geriatr Soc* 1984;32:237.
7. Besdine RW. Decisions to withhold treatment from nursing home residents, *J Am Geriatr Soc* 1983;31:602.
8. Thomasma DC. Ethical judgments of quality of life in the care of the aged, *J Am Geriatr Soc* 1984;32:525.
9. Stollerman GH. Quality of life treatment decisions and the third alternative, *J Am Geriatr Soc* 1984;32:483.
10. Pearlman RA, Speer JB. Quality of life considerations in geriatric care, *J Am Geriatr Soc* 1983;31:113.
11. Thibault GE, Mulley AG, Barnett GO, *et al.* Medical intensive care: Indications, interventions and outcomes, *N Engl J Med* 1980;302:938.
12. Eisenberg JM. Sociological influences on decision-making by clinicians, *Ann Intern Med* 1979;90:957.
13. Pearlman RA, Inui TS, Carter WB. Variability in physician nonethical decision-making: A case study of euthanasia, *Ann Intern Med* 1982;97:420.
14. Nie NH, Hull CH, Jenkins JG, *et al. SPSS: Statistical Package for the Social Sciences*. New York, NY: McGraw-Hill, 1975.

15. Hogan R. A dimension of moral judgment, *J Consult Clin Psychol* 1970;36:205.
16. Hogan R, Johnson J, Emler N. A socioanalytic theory of moral development, *New Directions for Child Development* 1978;2:1.
17. Hogan R, Dickstein E. Moral judgment and perceptions of injustice, *J Pers Soc Psychol* 1972;23:409.
18. Lorr M, Zea R. Moral judgment and liberal-conservative attitude, *Psychol Rep* 1977;40:627.
19. Jonsen AR, Siegler M, Winslade WJ. *Clinical Ethics*. New York, NY: Macmillan, 1982:109-38.
20. Spitzer WO, Dobson AJ, Hall J, *et al*. Measuring the quality of life of cancer patients, *J Chronic Dis* 1981;34:585.
21. Oliver H, Blum MH, Roskin G. The psychiatrist as advocate for post surgical "quality of life," *Psychosomatics* 1976;27:157.
22. Poe WD. The physician's dilemma: When to let go, *Forum Med* 1980;3:163.
23. Crane D. *The Sanctity of Social Life: Physicians' Treatment of Critically Ill Patients*. New York, NY: Russell Sage Foundation, 1975.
24. Sudnow D. *Passing On*. Englewood Cliffs, NJ: Prentice-Hall, 1967.
25. Uhlmann RF, McDonald WJ. An empiric study of nonresuscitation, *Clin Res* 1982;30:45A.
26. Shaw A, Randolph JG, Manard B. Ethical issues in pediatric surgery: A national survey of pediatricians and pediatric surgeons, *Pediatrics* 1977;60:588.
27. President's Commission for the Study of Ethical Problems in Medicine and Biomedical and Behavioral Research. *Making Health Care Decisions: The Ethical and Legal Implications of Informed Consent in the Patient-Practitioner Relationship*. Washington, DC: Library of Congress, 1982:38.
28. Fletcher J. *Humanhood: Essays in Biomedical Ethics*. Buffalo, NY: Prometheus Books, 1979:122.
29. Fletcher J. Four indicators of humanhood: The enquiry matures, *Hastings Cent Rep* 1974;4:4.

Chapter 49

Access to Health Care for the Elderly

David C. Thomasma

Salus Aegroti Suprema Lex

Let's face it. Although a national consensus is building for reform of the health care system, it still remains a very complex political, public policy, and ethical issue. With good reason. Virtually alone among advanced countries, the United States does not yet consider it a right for all citizens to have equal access to health care. Nothing less than a social transformation is required in order to properly develop a just health care delivery system. This is especially true regarding the aged. Indeed, one is tempted to use the term "social revolution" when contemplating the vast scale of changes needed in our sense of community in order to do the elderly justice.

Even the best of the arguments about rationing health care for the elderly require such a social transformation. This equity is grounded in the nature of health care itself, as a social good, and not in the State or Federal Government. Health care is a good essential for civil society. Health care is not jut another service or commodity; it involves a unique melding of beneficence and business. In the main, then, the social transformation of which I speak involves equity for all citizens with respect to health care provision.

Individual states are committing to this notion. Hawaii has a well-respected system that covers everyone in its Prepaid Health Care Act and its State Health Insurance Plan. The former requires coverage for anyone working more than 19 hours a week, and the latter provides coverage for those who fall into the gap between Medicare and Medicaid and the employer mandated insurance. While everything in Hawaii is more expensive than on the mainland, its health care costs are typically twenty-five percent lower than on the mainland.[1] Colorado will try to cover all its citizens by providing coverage from two or three insurance carriers, essentially modeling its care on the Canadian efforts.[2] Minnesota is known for its coverage under HMO's. Almost eighty-five percent of its citizens are covered. Oregon's extensive effort at establishing the basis for rationing in order to cover more of its citizens on Medicaid has gone for naught at present, but will surely be refined and be re-presented to the Federal Government.

The issue of access to care lay largely confined to academic discussion until voters in Pennsylvania made their concerns known by overwhelming Richard Thornburgh's 1991 Senatorial race through a surprise election of Harris Wofford. Fifty percent of those who voted for Wofford said that the top issue for them was national health insurance, that Wofford supported and Thornburgh did not.[3] In 1992, Presidential candidates touted their own version of such reform, as did senators and congressmen and women. In the midst of the politics it is too easy to forget that health care is a good and a service prerequisite for the

---

Source: Reprinted from *Business and Professional Ethics Journal*, Vol. 12, No. 2, pp. 3-18, with permission from © Business and Professional Ethics Journal.

well-being of all human beings. In earlier times, the essential moral quality of health care was embedded in the professional codes of the caregivers themselves, largely physicians and nurses. With the rise of modern, corporate, technology-based health care, the former one-on-one relationship between doctor and patient became institutionalized. Hospitals were no longer like a hotel where physicians signed their patients in and out at will. Suddenly, with escalating costs and the subsequent social and political monitoring, the doctor-patient relation became a provider-patient one, with government, third-party payers, institutions themselves, and a myriad of other specialists and ancillary caregivers counted as well. All of these players have complementary and sometimes competing interests in the reform of the health system as well.

Besides the problem of expanding services and concomitant cost control, there is the familiar litany of lack of coverage for those without health insurance. People without insurance, for example, experience delays that contribute to four times the hospitalization rate than people with insurance for problems that could have been treated earlier from a visit to the doctor.[4] Other problems with the system make it creak and groan in comparison with those delivery systems in other countries. At the very least, coverage for basic health care for all is a desirable goal of any decent human society, though we have difficulty determining what that basic care might entail. It is not just unfortunate that millions of us have no access to health care, and that the middle class often can no longer afford it. Rather it is unjust, since not providing it has been an act of political choice.

Reform, Cutting Costs, and Justice

There are many causes of the continued upward spiral of costs that contribute to the sense of crisis about our health care system. As the costs continue to rise at twice the inflation rate, every one of us suffers from decreased access, losses of jobs due to lack of competitively-priced products, increased co-payments in insurance plans, and the like. Industry in the U.S. is spending almost half of its profits on health care, compared with 7 percent in 1960.[5] Unions are cast in the role of protesting cuts in benefits because they thought they contracted for lifetime health care benefits.[6]

As part of the coming social transformation, Americans will begin husbanding their resources with much more care than they did in the past. Greater efficiency alone will save enormous sums of money, against which the malpractice problem is a red herring. Indeed, a series in *Consumer Reports* in the July and August 1992 issues points out that twenty percent of the $817 billion spent in the U.S. on health care in 1991, about $200 billion is spent on unnecessary and harmful treatment, bureaucratic waste, and errors.[7] Computer programs have been developed to help companies cut costs of health care, since these have gone up seventy-five percent in the last five years. In one bill of $105,000.00 the computer program found $25,000.00 in billing errors.[8]

Some of these cost-contributing causes are impervious to straightforward political resolution. Rather, the causes are driven by the inherent value-system of medicine and health care technology. Good examples are the proliferation of institutionalization of health care since the 1950s and the expansion of concomitant subspecialties. Another is the intrinsic law of technological development that suggests constant improvement and progress rather than stability as a fundamental value. As a result, pictures in promotional literature, magazines and newspapers tend to show happy specialists and administrators outside the newest 7-ton magnet for the MRI rather than happy home-care nurses helping an elderly citizen live a partially-independent life in her own environment. The latter is too stable and time-tested to catch our eye. The former is sexy and exciting! And costly.

Yet reform is coming, since economic self-interest will always win the day. Before we begin any flag-waving about reforms, however, we should recognize that desire to reform stems from two major competing interests. Some support for reform arises from high-minded principles of justice while other support stems from a desire to control costs. Admittedly, cost control itself may stem from a sense of justice, that some costs -- e.g., those covering the last few months of people's lives -- are out of proportion to the real needs individuals have for day-to-day health care. Nonetheless, the primary incentive for cutting costs is the economic one driven by competition and the need for jobs, and not one based principally on one or another vision of justice.

Many countries have been able to combine both interests in reasonable plans, but it is difficult. How may we simultaneously provide greater coverage at less cost? If we do not succeed, our products become even less competitive on the world market and our access for all citizen diminishes at an even greater pace than today.

Even granting one or the other of the two competing interests, there is widespread disagreement among parties within each of these opposing camps. Consider the different notions of justice that drive alternate proposals for rationing and/or access by many of our colleagues. Or think of the schemes for controlling costs that clash with one another: cut benefits, cut bureaucracy, eliminate government from the doctor-patient relationship, establish more governmental control of costs, provide chits for private purchase of insurance, and so on. These conflicting views lead to a need to consider the nature of justice itself. Will conflicts always be inevitable?

The Virtue of Justice

The virtue of justice is the strict habit of rendering what is due to others. Embodied in this brief definition, however, is one of the most complex of all the virtues. One reason for its complexity is that it has no mean, unlike all the other virtues. Since all persons are assumed to possess fundamental dignity, and human affairs being less than perfect even in the best of circumstances, it is impossible to be "too just." Clearly, on the other hand, defects in rendering what is due to individuals and societies are only too abundant throughout human history.

There are three major elements of the virtue of justice: distributive, commutative, and rectificatory. Aristotle had expanded on earlier notions of the Greek philosophers that justice was the habit of giving another his or her due. He saw that a difference lay between giving one's due on grounds of the common good (distributive justice) and on grounds of one's own individual good (rectificatory and commutative).[9] This insight enabled Aristotle to expand on another social virtue, friendship, arguing that it is right and good to love other persons for their own intrinsic goodness.[10] Later, St. Thomas Aquinas developed the virtue of justice further, and took from it insights about the social virtues and friendship which applied to the theological virtue of charity.[11] From this perspective, the social virtues acquired an additional impetus towards altruism not even present in classical, Greek thought. Somehow the ends of a good society dovetailed into a loving community in which the ultimate good for all citizens could be at least partially realized.

Seen not as a virtue, but as a principle, justice is the most complex of the standard four principles of autonomy, beneficence, non-maleficence, and justice. It is the only one that is simultaneously a virtue and a principle. As a virtue, it is a character trait, a habitual disposition to render to each what is due him. As a principle, it ordains that we act in such fashion that we render to each what is due her and that we treat like cases alike. There is, thus, an element of justice in each of the other principles since we owe it to humans not to harm them, to respect their autonomy, and to do good when we can. Justice, therefore, has a certain prior status in determining the right and the good. In this sense, it limits the exercise of our own autonomy and our obligation to respect the autonomy of others. A good example is requests by patients for medically contraindicated treatment, medically futile treatment, or unreasonable requests. But these are a matter of another paper. Suffice it to note that justice sets limits on the absolutization of autonomy to which the autonomy-based models of the doctor-patient relationship tend.

Much of the difficulty arising in public discussions about commutative or distributive justice can be anchored in this reality of justice and its lack of a mean. It is not obvious to anyone, the way it might be with regard to intemperance or pusillanimity, or some of the extremes that are regulated by other virtues, what the proper balance due individuals and groups might be. As a result, long, torturous, bitter political disputes result. How does one pay recompense to those whose ancestors were slaves? How does one right the inequities in a system that is constantly evolving? How much should be paid in awards to a person who now suffers as a consequence of a doctor's ineptitude?

These discussions, including the important issue of access and rationing of health care, are always public ones, since they involve the common good. For this reason it is easy to forget that, at root, justice is a virtue about giving another individual, albeit a member of society, his or her due.

The determination to resolve international inequities, right the wrongs done to the environment, care for future generations, foster peace, are all part of the virtue of justice, whose voice, in Aquinas' view, is the altruism of agapeistic ethics.[12] Human rightness can never be sufficient. It is a far cry from the ideal community at any time in human history. St. Thomas, in his commentary on Job, puts the matter beautifully:

> Since their legislators cannot extend them to all singular cases, human laws are concerned with universal matters and with what occurs in most cases. How general human statutes are to be applied to individual deeds must be left to the prudence of the agent. As a result, man is open to many instances in which he falls short of rectitude, even though he does not run counter to human positive law.[13]

In other words, human society will always be insufficiently just. "The poor you have always with you." All we can hope to accomplish is an asymptotic effort towards greater justice to all.

The Virtue of Justice and Rationing Health care

My proposal is a secular, agapeistic, altruistic ethics grounded in the healing task. It cannot make sense in medicine, even to cure, if one is not aimed at healing the patient. Healing the patient requires exquisite attention to the medical good, and to the patient's value system in which the good to be done is negotiated. Edmund Pellegrino and I have called this, beneficence-in-trust, since it holds in trust the values of the patient during the negotiation about the actions to be done.[14] In my view, then, the only defensible ethical position is to base rationing solely on medical need.

The effort to do justice to the individual is both intelligent and a struggle. It requires intelligence to continually adjust to changing situations, and in them, keep the other's needs and goods in view. As James Drane says:

> It is one thing to cultivate the urge for fairness; another to know what fairness is. All virtue involves the use of prudence and intelligence because virtues are refinements of human persons who cannot help but be in the world in an intelligent way. There is no such thing as blind virtue or ignorant virtue or unconscious virtue.[15]

Doing justice to individuals means that any system of rationing, or better put, access control, must involve clinical flexibility, so that physicians and patients may negotiate the good to be accomplished in the interaction, based not only on the medical good just cited, but also on the patients' value hierarchies.

This clinical adjustment requires practical intelligence. Hence, the virtue of justice involves a struggle. It is often a painful task to constantly adjust and balance conflicting needs and goods, especially if they are under our voluntary care. The task of equalizing or of being fair is one that takes constant vigilance and monitoring. Calabresi and Bobbitt argue that despite any efforts made, human society inevitably creates tragic choices because the resources are always scarce, and, in their words, "no general discussion can anticipate the various associations, connotative and emotive, which the members of a society may attach to a particular good; hearts are different from livers."[16]

Duties Based on the Virtue of Justice

Current theories of justice, like the principle of beneficence itself, are transformed by a theory of the virtues. The notion of justice in contemporary theories is ultimately practical and prudential. We owe others their due because we want them to give us our due, and because we want to protect ourselves from the unjust claims of others. Justice is a requirement for a peaceable society and the protection of legitimate self-interests. If we practice justice, we can thereby assure happiness for all. Justice, on this view, is a claim we have on the community -- compliance with which is an obligation of communal living. In its highest expressions, it might be justified as owed to humans because they are worthy of respect and dignity.

On the view of the virtues, however, justice has its deepest roots in love; it is an extension of the charity we should show to others.[17] Not to do justice would be to relapse into self-interest, to turn from love of the other to love of self. Love testifies that the claims of others upon us are the claims of our brothers and sisters in a community of compassion and care. By that fact, individuals are entitled to be loved especially in health care settings.

Love generates and transmutes justice. As St. Augustine held, justice is the concern and love that individuals in a community must show to others. Charity is for him "...the root of all good."[18] It truly is the "vis a tergo" moving us to justice. Justice energized by love transcends the legalistic justice of a chess game approach to our duties to one another. Justice therefore expresses special concern for those in pain, the poor, the troubled, the oppressed, and the outcast. Justice transformed by communal concern is expressed in concrete acts of beneficence towards specific persons. Justice therefore is not only conformity with abstract principles. Such justice does not focus on strict interpretations of what is owed in accordance with some calculus of claims and counter-claims. Instead, it offers the way of love illuminated by a medical commitment to others. Medically-driven justice does not rest solely on the virtue of justice itself, but modulates and illuminates it by a principle of a very different sort, the principle of beneficence-in-trust, and sometimes by a religious commitment to care for vulnerable individuals in a religious health care setting.[19]

Is Rationing Care for the Elderly Morally Possible?

In a pluralistic society it is necessary to establish standards through political and legislative action, develop and polish them through constant discussion, and interpret them in the courts. These standards should be seen, however, as minimum requirements to give others their due. The reason for this is that there are the already alluded to limitations on human wisdom, the limits of benevolence, and conflicting claims and interpretations of the good. Precisely because we are conscious individuals acting with others in society, we must be committed, as Rawls claimed, to act justly in concert about the common good.[20]

This is important, especially for the debate about access and rationing with regard to the elderly. Sometimes I am appalled by arguments that attempt to elevate to the maximum a minimalist understanding of human society and the social virtues. This minimalist move to the maximum occurs whenever proposals are made to develop health care rationing or access on the basis of lesser goods than medical need, or on the basis of theories of the common good that neglect the individual good. As already argued, the roots of justice lie in the conjunction of the individual and common good, not in the promotion of one to the detriment of the other.

The struggle for justice, then, involves trying to treat equal persons equally and unequal persons unequally. Fairness treats persons who have equal standing and needs equally, but those who do not have such equal standing and need require additional attention. If persons arrive in this life having good health, access to primary care and preventive medicine, but limited public funding for access to interventionist medicine might make sense. But not everyone emerges from the womb with this kind of equality. Some individuals are damaged by either genetic makeup or trauma at birth that requires them to enter a more interventionist scheme of medicine to "equalize" them with those of us who were born in good health. These persons are "unequal" compared to the healthy at the starting gate. Their individual good is different from more healthy individuals at this point, and the common good of all suggests righting this imbalance at the start.

It is in this context of balancing individual and social good that the problem of intergenerational justice should be formulated. Could it not be argued against the view that older people use too much of our health care resources that the hard work of the elderly throughout their life entitles them to some recompense during old age? After all, they built the roads and bridges, symphonies and schools we now enjoy. Why add to their burdens in later life by requiring additional sacrifices?

While the elderly may gobble up inordinate relative amounts of health care dollars, while doing so they are not using other resources of society, such as the parks, roads and bridges, etc., that the rest of us are enjoying. It seems to me that general resource use balances out in the end. What about justice as equity? Can there be an egalitarian theory of justice when we ask one group, the elderly, to bear disproportionate burdens (relative to a response to their health care needs, not the amount of care they currently obtain)? What would be the source of obligations to sacrifice for younger generations? Since they have raised children and grandchildren already, haven't they already discharged such obligations? In my view, the principle of intergenerational justice cuts both ways to such an extent that it is not helpful in developing an equitable formula for limiting access to care for the elderly on the basis of age.

If rationing of care for the elderly is to occur within any national plan, it is important to understand how the current crisis came about. It is insufficient to cite failures in public health or preventive medicine. The very successes of modern medicine have also caused disruptions. Failures as well as successes have caused the loss of institutional identity. Consider the problem of the gerification of society. This problem is almost directly caused by the successes of control of infectious disease, and the suppression of the effects of high blood pressure. Major interventions such as open-heart surgery, insulin treatment, and cancer chemotherapy are also aids in helping people live longer.

But as gerification continues, disruptions are caused in the community. Some, like Daniel Callahan, argue that society must cut off its high technology medicine past a certain age;[21] other leading authorities write: "There is no hope of carrying the burden of old age that the future has in store without assistance from the family and neighbors at least equal to that given at the present time."[22] This burden will require a rethinking of the goals of human life (e.g., not retirement in Florida, but taking care of elderly parents in a mother-in-law wing on one's house in Chicago). It also challenges us to re-develop our conception of the community, the community of healers.

Access by Care Categories

Modern health care is a unique melding of charity and business, of compassion and attention to fiscal responsibility. Incentives to hold down costs and to increase the quality of care should be built into whatever national plan emerges from our public debate. But so too should incentives to provide care to those in need based upon that very need. In a previous paper,[23] I have argued that the only moral method of rationing care must be one based upon objective categories of need that I called Functional Status Care Categories. Briefly, these categories provide objective standards for allocating health care to individuals, based on medical need and the impact of illness on their bodies. I can only note at this point that these categories provide criteria for rationing care on the basis of the following principles so far adumbrated. These now serve to summarize my argument:

1) **Rationing must be based on medical need.** No other schema, including that of providing "basic care," satisfies the demands of the kind of justice I have propounded.

This is the problem with any scheme -- like the Oregon plan -- that propounds rationing on the basis of primary or basic care. If "basic care" is to be provided, what would not be covered? This is not just a strategic question. It represents the moral center of the enterprise that is health care delivery. Robert Veatch has argued very clearly that "The assumption that care that is basic in the sense of being simple, low tech, primary, inexpensive and/or preventive, will be cost-effective and therefore will be basic in the sense of deserving priority is suspect."[24] Veatch holds, rather, that one should speak of a "morally appropriate level of care," and leave the determination of this to public discussion.

2) **Flexibility within the categories of care is essential.** The flexibility requirement stems from the nature of doing justice to individuals within the realm of the common good. In this regard, coupling individual advance directives with thoroughly discussed therapeutic plans can help define the likely outcomes and their impact on the patients' lifeplans. This is especially helpful when treating the elderly who, more often than the young, have developed clear goals for their lives and defined the role of health care provisions within those goals.

3) **Nonetheless, control over provision of care should be decided in advance, on the basis of functional status.** The radical transformation of the original doctor-patient relationship into one that includes many other interests creates a sense of chaos and loss of control, especially over essential values in caring for elderly individuals in our society. There are ways of providing care to all persons without asking any of them to give up essential goods and services. Indeed, Arthur Caplan notes that, although the near-unanimous response of bioethicists to the crisis in health care has been to counsel explicit discussion of rationing plans,[25] the Minnesota HealthRight plan avoids this approach entirely: "While inequities remain under HealthRight, no individual or group is required to give up important or life-preserving benefits."[26] Caplan calls this a form of "tweaking the ethicist's tail."

Conclusion

There are important ethical considerations in formulating any national health program. The first must be that the elderly are not marginalized by a youth-oriented culture.[27] Second, what is "due" to the elderly includes recompense for their many sacrifices throughout their life, so that the principle of intergenerational justice cuts both ways. Third, there must be a check and balance on inappropriate deployment of medical technologies. The Care Categories I have proposed can do this. Fourth, patients ought to be able to have control over their care, so that they do not experience difficulties and delays in obtaining appropriate and approved treatment. The fifth point is that the moral character of the institutions of health delivery and the practitioners of health care should not be betrayed through bureaucratic requirements. The sixth ethical consideration is that, since some form of rationing will be required regarding specific treatments to be made available, the national health program itself should be designed to be as efficient as possible. This means that greater effort must be made than heretofore to put available monies in patient-care rather than in administrative overhead costs. Seventh, the quality of human judgement and flexibility for treating individual differences should be maintained as far as possible, so that formulaic responses to human pain and misery are avoided. Otherwise treating people with respect will diminish.

If a "winner" Federal plan ever does emerge it will probably have features of each of the state initiatives mentioned at the outset, as well as a few others. A good example is Clinton's plan. He predicts savings of $700 billion by century's end. The plan would couple universal insurance coverage by requiring all businesses to insure their workers, but hold costs down to the rate of inflation by capping them and by giving tax credits to small businesses. Other pieces of the plan include a requirement that insurance companies take anyone and a reduction in overhead costs. The cost-control features are the most controversial, since they would limit the amounts physicians and hospitals would receive for care of the patients.[28] Individuals could choose their own doctor or plan. The latter would be evaluated and a quality-assessment would be given the consumers each year to aid their choices. The poor would be covered by the government. Medicaid would be phased out, and Medicare altered to reflect these changes. Universal coverage would then be insured, as well as choice.[29]

These are all good ideas that emerge quite readily from our national debate. But how does one control costs by holding them at the rate of inflation? Health-costs now increase at about 10 percent a year. The obvious answer is to establish state boards that set doctors' fees and pre-pay the health care needs to health care networks. The incentives to save money would then be their responsibility, much the same way the DRG's work now. Those who save could re-invest the money, and the savings for the Federal Government would be used to pay coverage for some of those now uninsured who do not have jobs. A national health care board would set the annual budget.

Plans like this one seem to have all the right components, with the proper balance between government control and responsibility and private incentives and problem-solving. Because they are offered during election years, though, the details are rosier than reality might suggest. I have suggested an additional feature of such plans, one that relies upon objective standards of viability or function by which certain treatments are judged ahead of time to be appropriately discussed, and others are not. This status category method of controlling access and cost would enhance other features of what might be called multiple control national health plans.

Notes

1. Worthington R. Hawaii tries health coverage for all. *Chicago Tribune* 1992 Sep. 8:Sec. 1, 23.
2. Governor Roy Romer outlines Coloradocare reform plan. *American Hospital Association: Convention Daily* 1992 July 29:1.
3. Iglehart J. From the editor, *Health Affairs* 1991;10(4):5-6.
4. Neus E. Delay in care aggravates health woes of uninsured. *Chicago Sun-Times* 1992 Sept. 21: Sec. 1, 17.
5. Study: Industry spends almost half of profits on health care: A report on "Future of Corporate Health Benefits: A National Report," conducted by researchers at Loyola. *Loyola World* 1992 Aug. 27:9.
6. Unions protest navistar bid to cut health benefits. *Chicago Tribune* 1992 Aug. 12:Sec. 3, 3.
7. Healthcare in crisis, *Consumer Reports* 1992;57:519-531.
8. Software ferrets out billing errors. *Chicago Sun-Times* 1992 Sept. 21:34.
9. Aristotle. *Nicomachean Ethics* 1-7:1129a1-1135a14.
10. *Ibid.*, VIII-IX:1155a1-1172a15.
11. Aquinas T. *Summa Theologiae* II-II:57-80.
12. Phelan GB. Justice and friendship, *The Thomist: The Maritain Volume, Dedicated to Jacques Maritain on the Occasion of His Sixteenth Anniversary*. New York, NY: Sheed & Ward, 1943:153-170.
13. Aquinas T. *Exp. in Job*, c. 11, lect. 1;Parm., XIV, 49; Cf. In: Bourke V. Foundations of justice, *Proceedings of the American Catholic Philosophical Association* 1962;36:19-28.
14. Pellegrino ED, Thomasma DC. *For the Patient's Good.* New York, NY: Oxford University Press, 1988.
15. Drane J. *Becoming a Good Doctor: The Place of Virtue and Character in Medical Ethics.* Kansas City, MO: Sheed & Ward and the Catholic Health Association, 1988:106.
16. Calabresi G, Bobbitt P. *Tragic Choices: The Conflicts Society Confronts in the Allocation of Tragically Scarce Resources.* New York, NY: W.W. Norton & Co., 1978:150.

17. See Pellegrino ED, Thomasma DC. *The Christian Virtues in Medicine* (In preparation).
18. St. Augustine, *Fathers of the Church* (Sermon 73.4), as cited by Walsh WJ, Langan JP, Patristic social consciousness -- The church and the poor, In: Haughey JC, ed. *The Faith that Does Justice*. New York , NY: Paulist Press, 1977.
19. The question about the continuity or discontinuity of the supernatural and the natural virtues is still an intriguing one. Robert Sokolowski has examined this relationship in a brilliant monograph, illuminating both kinds of virtue. See his *The God of Faith and Reason.* Notre Dame, IN: University of Notre Dame Press, 1982.
20. Rawls J. *A Theory of Justice.*Cambridge, MA: Belknap Press of Harvard University Press, 1971.
21. Callahan D. *Setting Limits.* New York, NY: Simon & Schuster, 1987.
22. Sheldon JH. *British Medical Journal* 1950;1:319.
23. Thomasma D. Functional status care categories and national health policy, *Journal of the American Geriatrics Society* 1993;41(4):437-443.
24. Veatch RM. Should basic care get priority? Doubts about the Oregon way, *Kennedy Institute of Ethics Journal* 1991;1(3):187-203, quote from 203.
25. Caplan A. *If I Were A Rich Man, Could I Buy a Pancreas?* Bloomington, IN: Indiana University Press, 1992.
26. Caplan A, Priester R. For better or for worse? The moral and policy lessons of Minnesota's HealthRight legislation, *Kennedy Institute of Ethics Journal* 1992;2(3):201-217, quote from 214.
27. Binstock RH, Post SG, eds. *Too Old for Health Care? Controversies in Medicine, Law, Economics and Ethics*. Baltimore, MD: Johns Hopkins University Press, 1991.
28. Locin M. Clinton touts health plan savings: Candidate predicts $700 billion benefit by century's end. *Chicago Tribune* 1992 Sept. 25:Sec. 1, 5.
29. McNulty T. First look at health plan: Doctor choice, universal coverage included. *Chicago Tribune* 1993 April 10:Sec. 1, 1,4.

Chapter 50

Ethical Dilemmas in Long-Term Health Care

Lawrence R. LaPalio

Almost two million Americans live in nursing homes and the number is expected to grow for another forty years. Ethical dilemmas of medical-decision making are generally the same for nursing home residents as they are for the elderly living in different environments. However, living in a nursing home introduces special circumstances which must be considered. When a patient enters a nursing home, they intrinsically represent a population of patients that are at high risk from mortal events due to their underlying health status and age which in part a poor prognosis.

Before going any further, let me first define five major principles of medical ethics. ***Beneficence*** is the obligation to do good and act in the best interests of your patients. When the time honored principles of medical ethics is to alleviate pain and suffering. ***Non-maleficence*** is the obligation to avoid harm. This principle of medical ethics goes back to the earliest written record of ancient times. First, do no harm. ***Autonomy*** is respect for a person's right of self determination. Individuals have the right to choose health care options including those at the end of life and we, as health care providers, have the responsibility to elicit patient preferences about treatment decisions. ***Justice*** is the duty to treat individuals fairly and without discrimination and to distribute resources in a non-arbitrary and fair manner. ***Infidelity*** is the duty to keep the promises. Unpleasant information should not be withheld from patients simply because it is unpleasant. The provision of information, even if unpleasant, allows the patient to make informed choices. These informed choices form the basis of the Doctor/Patient relationship.

Most decisions to withhold treatment in the nursing home emerge from three distinct categories:

1. **"DO-NOT-RESUSCITATE" (DNR)**
2. **"DO-NOT-HOSPITALIZE" (DNH)**
3. **"DO-NOT-TREAT" (DNT)**

"DO-NOT-RESUSCITATE" decisions were first considered an acute care hospital in the middle 1970's. It has become a standard medical practice in all care facilities to institute resuscitative measures unless there is a contrary order in the chart. Cardial pulmonary resuscitation was first designed to resuscitate patients in acute care hospitals during a witnessed cardiac arrest. In nursing homes, most deaths are not witnessed and patients do

Source: Reprinted from *Ethical Dilemmas*, pp. 7-10, with permission from University Press of American © May 1994.

not suffer from acute cardiac events alone. They usually have other complex complicating diseases that do not respond to cardial pulmonary resuscitation. Even witnessed cardiac arrests in nursing homes lack the sophisticated life support machinery, drugs, and professionals that permits the survival of resuscitated patients in spite of catastrophic damage to numerous vital functions. When we look at the outcomes of CPR, in acute care hospitals, 60% of patients who are resuscitated survive the acute event but only 20 to 25% ever leave the hospital. In nursing homes, less than 1% of the patients survive.

"DO-NOT-HOSPITALIZE" and "DO-NOT-TREAT" orders are much more difficult to deal with. Decisions to withhold treatments should be done prospectively in a nonemergency situation whenever possible. All too often we find ourselves making these very difficult decisions during a crisis. I hope today to present an algorhythm to follow that will help avoid confusion and aid in these very difficult decisions. The first and foremost issue is to have the correct diagnosis with a reasonable prognosis. If you don't know the disease that we're dealing with and we don't know the natural history of the disease process, then how can we make decisions about proper care. The decision to tube feed a patient with an acute stroke must be based upon our ability to judge whether the patient will recover in a reasonable period of time. The diagnosis and prognosis are extremely important in any decision to limit treatments.

The second important aspect of medical decision-making has to do with patient preferences. In medicine there are often multiple equally afficatious treatments for the same disease process and the patient must tell us which treatment best suits their needs. For example, if I were to ask three different people how to get to McCormick Place from the western suburbs of Chicago, the first may say, "Take the Eisenhower Expressway to Lake Shore Drive, go south and get off at the proper exit." The second may say, "Go east on I-55 to Lake Shore Drive and go north to the proper exit." The third may say, "Take 22nd Street straight down until you reach McCormick Place". The real answer is that it depends. It depends upon the day of the week, the traffic, the weather, the kind of car you drive, etc. This is true for many medical decisions, that the proper treatment depends upon patient preferences.

One of the major obstacles that we face in long term care is that the patient often does not have the decision-making capacity to let his preferences be known. We deal with many patients with dementing illnesses. When this occasion arises, it is our responsibility to try to ascertain what the patient would have wanted if the patient could make their own decisions. The way we deal with this is to ask the people who know the patient best and that usually is a family member.

The best way to ascertain what a patient wants is to ask that patient directly and the time to ask that question is when the patient is cognitively intact and able to make their own decisions. In Illinois, there are two legal documents that we can ask the patients to sign where they can make their preferences known. The Durable Power of Attorney for Health Care and the Living Will. These advanced directives are written documents that patients may sign to authorize another person to make health care decisions for them in the event that they can no longer make them themselves. This will allow us to make decisions that are consistent with the patient's wishes. The Durable Power of Attorney for Health Care can authorize someone called an agent to make any and all health care decisions in the event that a patient is unable to do so for themselves. It can also contain health care instructions that they want the agent to follow and the document can start or stop at any time they choose. It can be revoked or changed and agents may be changed if a patient desires. The Living Will is a much more limiting document designed to limit medical treatments but more specifically states that death should not be artificially postponed. This document states that if you have an incurable or irreversible injury or illness judged to be terminal by your attending physician and that you are going to die soon, you direct that medical treatments be withdraw or withheld as determined by your attending physicians.

The differences between a Durable Power of Attorney and a Living Will are that in the Durable Power of Attorney you direct an agent or a person you know and trust to make decisions for you. In the Living Will you are allowing your doctor to make these decisions. The Durable Power of Attorney may be in effect for months or years whereas the Living Will generally only takes effect within the last few weeks of your life. In Illinois, if the patient does not have an advanced directive, when the patient meets certain criteria the physician may appoint a surrogate who can legally make health care decisions.

The last issue that needs to be dealt with is something that we call "Quality-of-Life." Quality-of-life is a value that can only be judged by the individuals whose lives are being affected by the decisions that we make. Quality-of-life is a very nebulous term and it is important for us to remember that we should not impose our individual values on our patients to determine the definition of quality. Again, we must try to ascertain what the patient's definition is and what the patients want or would have wanted for themselves if they could make the decisions.

It is my belief that we should be proactive in dealing with these ethical decisions in medicine and that the best way to make these decisions is not to sweep them under the carpet but to put the issues on the table and discuss the possible outcomes in a responsible manner. It is my belief that the best way to deal with these issues is for each individual nursing home or group of nursing homes develop ethics committees with members from many professions and different walks of life to help create and guide institutional policies to deal with these issues.

Chapter 51

Accepting Death Without Artificial Nutrition or Hydration

Robert J. Sullivan, Jr.

Many nursing facilities throughout the United States provide daily support services for incompetent and semi-comatose residents being kept alive through the use of feeding tubes. For most such individuals, recovery is impossible. For some residents, ethical and legal concerns of their caregivers preclude withdrawing support under any circumstance. For others, sustenance is provided out of fear that death by dehydration and starvation will cause pain and suffering.[1,2,3,4,5,6,7,8,9] Those involved in assisting families with decisions regarding tube feeding can attest to the emotional turmoil this choice engenders.

Tube feeding has recently come to be viewed as medical therapy rather than simply providing sustenance.[10,11,12] Accordingly, physicians, patients, and caregivers need to understand it's efficacy in each situation for which it is considered. To prolong life, feeding by any route is invaluable. To relieve pain and suffering at life's end, its usefulness is less clear.

Most individuals kept alive by tube feeding in the waning days of life cannot express their feelings about their treatment.[13] Those able to communicate complain of physical and emotional discomfort caused by the presence of a nasogastric or gastrostomy tube. Semi-conscious individuals commonly require restraints to prevent them from pulling tubes out.[13,14,15,16,17] Tube feeding via either nasogastric, gastrostomy or parenteral placement can produce significant medical complications, including agitation, epistaxis, nasal alarnecrosis, aspiration pneumonia, airway obstruction, pneumothorax, hydrothorax, nasopharyngitis, eustachitis, esophagitis, esophageal stricture, leakage, infection at insertion site, weight loss, metabolic disturbances, and anemia.[13,18,19,20,21,22,23,24,25,26]

Less well understood are the physical and emotional effects of dehydration and starvation. Does tube feeding provide relief that outweighs any discomfort and medical risk entailed? Stimulated by an experience with a competent and alert individual who accepted death without nutrition or hydration, I undertook a review of the literature was undertaken focused upon the implications of food and water deprivation.

Case Report

A 78-year-old female developed vaginal bleeding. Endometrial biopsy established a diagnosis of adenocarcinoma and a hysterectomy with bilateral salpingo-oophorectomy and local node resection was performed. Pathologic examination confirmed widespread metastatic disease. Papanicolaou smears of peritoneal washings were positive for malignant cells. External abdominal radiation and P^{32} instillation were administered and the patient was discharged.

Source: Reprinted from *Journal of General Internal Medicine*, Vol. 8, 1993, with permission from Hanley and Belfus, Inc. © April 1993.

A second course of radiation was administered to the vaginal area following tumor recurrence.

Eight months later, the patient developed a small bowel obstruction that resolved with nasogastric suction. Within a month the obstruction reoccurred. Surgical exploration revealed a severe radiation fibrosis with numerous adhesions. A jejunal stricture was resected and bowel integrity re-established. No tumor was found and peritoneal washings were negative for malignant cells. The patient returned home where she regained strength and function. Three months later her abdomen again became distended and she developed massive edema of her legs. She was hospitalized and underwent paracentesis which revealed a clear yellow effusion that was free from malignant cells. X-ray studies of her chest, and a CT of her head failed to find any evidence of metastatic disease. Her situation changed for the worse when she began to vomit fecal-smelling material. Abdomen films revealed a small bowel obstruction. The patient was offered surgery to alleviate her intestinal blockage, but refused when the surgeon could not guarantee freedom from obstruction recurrence or promise that a colostomy could be avoided. Thereafter she consistently refused medical therapy for her condition.

The patient had no family to advise her or the hospital staff in regard to the wisdom of her decision. She was discharged to a nursing facility for support and comfort after confirmation in the hospital that her resolve was immutable, that her decision was made with consideration of available alternatives, that she was in her right mind and that she was not depressed. The ethical issues surrounding her decision have been described elsewhere.[27]

The patient's death was inevitable since food and fluid intake was impossible due to complete bowel obstruction. Although obstructed, there appeared to be no bowel necrosis. She was free from pain, but troubled by repeated vomiting. Nasogastric suction was instituted as a means to alleviate retching. Two liters of fluid were withdrawn from her stomach, and she immediately felt better. Continuous gastric drainage was provided hereafter, and intravenous fluids were administered to maintain hydration. She settled into a period of stability that persisted for 13 days while she awaited death. During this time she repeatedly complained about discomfort and inconvenience caused by the IV infusion, and questioned its value. On the 14th day she became increasingly exasperated because she had not died, and ordered the intravenous fluids discontinued. She refused oral fluids and kept her mouth moist with glycerine swabs.

Thirty-three days following the initiation of her gastric suction, and twenty days after discontinuing intravenous fluids, she began to accept ice chips to moisten her mouth. She did this only after being convinced by the staff that all oral intake was promptly removed by the stomach suction and would not prolong her life. Throughout this period she remained lucid, and actively participated in her program of personal daily care.

Throughout her entire course, she was free from pain. She repeatedly requested that she be relieved of life by injection of a lethal dose of morphine. This request was respectfully declined by her physician who did offer to relieve any pain or discomfort. Two weeks following the initiation of her fast, she explored with her physician how she might go about receiving a regular "therapeutic" dose of narcotic to relieve boredom, and help with sleep. She offered to feign abdominal pain to justify treatment. Her request for a narcotic was endorsed by the nursing staff, who were ambivalent about her decision and uncertain about how to make her comfortable as death approached. Morphine was thereafter administered intramuscularly on request initially at the rate of 8 mg every four hours. She found this comforting, and gradually increased the frequency of requests until she received 56 mg/day on days 25 to 28 of her fast. Thereafter her morphine requests declined steadily. She readily acknowledged to her physician that this medication was not for pain relief, but for narcosis. She refused benzodiazepines because she perceived that they provided only sleep, and cause depression.

Her urinary output averaged 200 ml/day following discontinuation of intravenous fluids. Nasogastric tube drainage was between 100 and 200 ml daily with a slight increase when ice chip were consumed on days 33 through 41 of her fast.

Throughout the entire episode, a substantial effort was made by the nursing staff to assure her comfort. Attention was given to documenting the volume of her intake and output, but all diagnostic maneuvers were halted. When she continued to live far beyond her expectations and those of the staff, a blood specimen was obtained with her consent on day 25 of her fast (day 12 of her dehydration). Her sodium, which was 135mmol/L at the onset of her obstruction, had risen to 157mmol/L and her chloride had risen from a baseline of 103 to a level of 112 mmol/L, her blood urea nitrogen was 18 to 21 mg/dl, and her creatinine was 1.0 to 1.5 mg/dl. Her uric acid increased from 5.5 to 6.8 mg/dl. All other laboratory parameters were remarkably normal.

At no time in her final illness, despite her dehydration and starvation, did she complain of discomfort. She received visits from friends, and wrote numerous letters. During her final month of life she was offered surgical relief of her intestinal obstruction on several occasions. However, she remained steadfast in her resolve to decline therapy until her death. Her friends visiting during this period uniformly confirmed that she was a woman who knew her own mind, and had the courage of her convictions. At no time was she known to be mentally ill nor did she ever receive psychotherapy. Throughout her life she was always mildly obese, and had no history of depression, bulemia or anorexia. On the 41st day after the onset of obstruction she drifted into a semiconscious state, followed by a coma. She died peacefully on the forty-second day of her fast, and the twenty-ninth day of dehydration.

Review of the Literature

Reports of death associated with dehydration and starvation are uncommon in a medical literature that focuses primarily on methods of successfully avoiding such outcomes. However, there exists a remarkable body of information relevant to the clinical aspects of fluid and food abstinence.

Although dehydration is not a part of standard medical therapy, it is commonly encountered in a number of clinical situations and thus its impact is fairly well understood. Following the cessation of fluid intake, hypernatremia develops slowly and induces few neurologic symptoms initially.[28] Worsening hypernatremia causes confusion, weakness and lethargy which eventually progresses to obtundation and coma.[29,30,31,32] Inferences about the clinical course of dehydration can be drawn from studies of hyperosmolar conditions suffered by individuals who undergo osmotic diuresis and dehydration due to elevated glucose levels. Experience suggests that they slowly sink into unconsciousness over a period of days without complaint of pain or discomfort.[33] Anecdotal reports of cancer patients in their final hours of life suggest an improved sense of well-being follows cessation of fluid therapy with reductions in secretions and coughing, nausea and vomiting, urinations, pulmonary and peripheral edema, and diarrhea.[34,35] One recurring physical complaint related to the absence of oral fluid intake is a dry mouth which can be relieved with swabs, sips of fluid or sucking on ice chips.[35,36,37,38] Thus, from the available data, it appears that systemic dehydration induces little pain or discomfort provided the mouth is kept moist.

Starvation is variously characterized in the medical and lay literature as an adverse event, a religious experience, and a therapeutic modality. Beginning with biblical references, prolonged fasting has been used as a means of seeking inspiration.[39] Christ is said to have spent forty days in the wilderness without food.[40,41] The medical impact of a modern-day religious fast of 36 days was documented by Kerndt and colleagues.[42] Of particular note in the Kerndt report was the absence of discomfort experienced by the subject who continued a rigorous schedule of daily meetings, conferences, and worship while maintaining a detailed journal of activities.

At the turn of the century there was considerable interest in fasting for health.[43,44] A number of "professional fasters" enjoyed public attention, and some were subjected to various levels of scientific study. Benedict's report of Mr. Levanzin's 31 day fast in 1915 revealed that total abstinence was tolerated without apparent physical discomfort.[45]

Starvation to achieve weight reduction has been advocated dating from the early 20th century.[46] Bloom's studies in the 1950s initiated the modern era of fasting to achieve therapeutic weight loss. He reported that his subjects experienced an absence of hunger and a sense of well being.[47] Research by Duncan *et al.* confirmed these findings and suggested the anorectic effect was due to ketonemia provoked by the fast.[48] Laboratory studies confirmed this fact[49] and showed that hunger rapidly reappears when ketosis is relieved by ingesting small amounts of carbohydrate.[50,51,52,53] A controlled investigation by Keys *et al.*, duplicating famine conditions, revealed that hunger disappears with total starvation while semi-starvation makes food an omnipresent obsession.[54] This may help explain the depravity in human behavior observed during times of natural disaster and war when individuals are forced to rely upon meager and inconsistent food resources.[55]

Laboratory studies have shown that urinary nitrogen excretion diminishes progressively with prolonged starvation.[56] With a reduced ureaload, there is little need for obligatory water excretion and urine volume may fall to 200 mL per day. Indeed, a fasting individual may have fluid requirements almost fully met by water produced through fat metabolism.[56]

Some remarkably long fasts were reported during the era of starvation for weight loss including 117 days, 249 days, and 382 days.[57,58,59] A common theme among the weight-loss studies was the ability of the subjects to function well without food for prolonged periods. Reports of death due to cardiac arrhythmia and myocardial damage induced by starvation brought an end to this mode of therapy for obesity.[60,61,62] Semi-starvation diets using protein supplements to "protect essential organs" also have proven hazardous.[63,64]

In contrast to the intense discomfort associated with semi-starvation, total starvation is associated with euphoria.[42,47,51,59,65,66] Instead of pain, food deprivation may induce analgesia.[67,68,69] Mental function is maintained throughout a fast[45,47,70] with lethargy, apathy, and irritability encountered only in the terminal phases.[54,71]

During starvation the body shifts its metabolic processes to rely upon energy reserves in adipose tissue presumably to preserve protein integrity as long as possible.[70] Hunger strikers in Northern Ireland are thought to have died after fasts of 74 and 76 days when they depleted their fat stores.[72,73] Mohandas Gandhi avoided death by limiting his 14 lifetime fasts each to a maximum of 21 days,[74] which presumably stayed within his adipose tissue reserves.

In situations of extreme dehydration and starvation, several mechanisms are postulated to cause death. Neutropenia[75] and a reduction in white cell function[76] associated with protein deficit permits the development of sepsis leading to death. Arrhythmias related to myocardial degeneration[61] or to electrolyte imbalance[62,64,76] cause cardiac arrest. Weakness from muscle protein catabolism leads to inadequate clearing of chest secretions and subsequent pneumonia.[51] Clouding of consciousness due to a hyperosmolar state leads to depressed respiration with aspiration and pneumonia. While discomfort is possible in each situation mentioned, none of these events is known to be associated with significant pain or prolonged suffering.

Discussion

Based upon the case presented and upon the available literature, it is possible to predict with some assurance the clinical course of an individual dying with dehydration and starvation. The majority of persons who embark on this course will be debilitated from an underlying illness that has robbed them of bodily fat reserves and thus reduced their ability to survive. Even then, death may not come quickly. By utilizing water generated in the metabolism of remaining adipose tissue they may sustain circulatory function for a remarkable period of time. When significant adipose stores are present and renal function is well preserved, as can be encountered in healthy individuals who suffer a massive stroke, survival without food or water can continue for weeks.

Fasting individuals will not likely experience pain induced by fluid or food abstinence. Indeed, mild euphoria can be anticipated, accompanied by an increased tolerance for pain. Absence of oral fluid intake will produce a dry mouth which can be relieved with ice chips or swabs. Problems with excessive secretions, edema, or incontinence may be alleviated.

Worthy of particular attention is the potential for inadvertent induction of discomfort through amelioration of ketonemia. The administration of even small amounts of carbohydrate can block ketone production and rekindle hunger. Intravenous mixtures of 5% Dextrose and water provide ample carbohydrate to cause this metabolic shift.[53] It is senseless to continue fluids after a decision has been made to discontinue food. If any sustenance is provided by vein or by feeding tube, it should be tailored to the full nutritional requirements of the patient and constantly monitored in perpetuity to assure comfort.

In the setting of dehydration and starvation, death can occur from a multitude of causes. Arrhythmia, infection, and circulatory collapse due to volume depletion are common terminal events. The clinical course of each should be rapid and, ideally, not associated with perceived discomfort by the patient.

Based on this clinical report and a review of the literature, it is likely that prolonged dehydration and starvation induce no pain and only limited discomfort from a dry mouth which can be controlled. For individuals carrying an intolerable burden of illness and disability, or those who have no hope of ever again enjoying meaningful human interaction, the withdrawal of food and fluid may be considered without concern that it will add to the misery.

Notes

1. Steinbock B. The removal of Mr. Herbert's feeding tube, *Hastings Cent Rep* 1983;13:13-6.
2. Brahams D. The right to be allowed to die: Self-induced starvation and the right to die without undue misery, *Med Leg J* 1984;52:113-6.
3. Dresser RS. Ethics law and nutritional support, *Arch Intern Med* 1985;145:122-4.
4. Micetich KC, Steinecker PH, Thomasma DC. Are intravenous fluids morally required for a dying patient? *Arch Intern Med* 1983;143:975-8.
5. Olins NJ. Feeding decisions for incompetent patients, *J Am Geriatr Soc*1986;34:313-7.
6. Conroy, 486A. 2d 1209 (NJ1985).
7. Steinbrook R, Lo B. Artificial feeding: Solid ground, not a slippery slope, *N Engl J Med* 1988;318:286-90.
8. Meyers DW. Legal aspects of withdrawing nourishment from an incurably ill patient, *Arch Intern Med* 1985;145:125-8.
9. Callahan D. On feeding the dying, *Hastings Cent Rep* 1983;13:22.
10. *Deciding to Forego Life-Sustaining Treatment: A Report on the Ethical, Medical and Legal Issues in Treatment Decisions*. Washington, DC: President's Commission for the Study of Ethical Problems in Medicine and Biomedical and Behavioral Research, 1983.
11. American College of Physicians Ethics Manual, *Ann Intern Med* 1989;111:333.
12. *Current Opinions of the Council on Ethical and Judicial Affairs of the American Medical Association-1989: Witholding or Withdrawing Life-Prolonging Treatment*. Chicago, IL: American Medical Association, 1989.
13. Ciocon JO, Silverstone FA, Graver LM, Foley CJ. Tube feedings in elderly patients: Indications, benefits, and complications, *Arc Intern Med* 1988;148:429-33.

14. Quill TE. Utilization of nasogastric feeding tubes in a group of chronically ill, elderly patients in a community hospital, *Arch Intern Med* 1989;149:1937-41.
15. Champlin L. Compassionate witholding of feeding: Are physicians protected? *Geriatrics* 1987;42:37-42.
16. Lo B, Dornbrand L. Guiding the hand that feeds, *N Engl J Med* 1984;311:402-4.
17. Lo B, Dornbrand L. Understanding the benefits and burdens of tube feedings, *Arch Intern Med* 1989;149:1925-26.
18. May M, Nellis KJ. Nasogastric intubation: Avoiding complications, *Resident Staff Phys* 1984;30:60-2.
19. Lipman TO, Kessler T, Arabian A. Nasopulmonary intubation with feeding tubes: Case reports and review of the literature, *J Parenteral Enteral Nutr* 1985;9:618-20.
20. Boscoe MJ, Rosin MD. Finebore enteral feeding and pulmonary aspiration, *Br Med J* 1984;289:1421-22.
21. Miller SK, Tomlinson JR, Sahn SA. Pleuropulmonary complications of enteral tube feedings, *Chest* 1985;88:230-3.
22. Schorlemmer GR, Battaglini JW. An unusual complication of nasoenteral feeding with small diameter feeding tube, *Ann Surg* 1984;199:104-6.
23. McCredie JA, McDowell RFC. Esophageal stricture following intubation in a case of hiatus hernia, *Br J Surg* 1958;46:260-1.
24. Douglas KW. Esophageal strictures associated with gastroduodenal intubation, *Br J Surg* 1955;43:404-9.
25. Hafner CD, Wylie JH, Brush BE. Complications of gastrointestinal intubation, *Arch Surg* 1961;83:147-60,
26. Rombeau JL, Barot LR. Enteral nutrition therapy, *Surg Clin North Am* 1981;61:605-20.
27. Sullivan R. When your patient decides to die, *North Carolina Med J* 1987;48:223-4.
28. Kastin AJ, Lipsett MB, Ommaya AK, Moser JM. Asymptomatic hypernatremia, *Am J Med* 1965;38:306-12.
29. Nadal JW, Pedersen S, Maddock WG. A comparison between dehydration from salt loss and from water deprivation, *J Clin Invest* 1941;20:691-703.
30. Billings JA. Comfort measures for the terminally ill: Is dehydration painful? *J Amer Geriatr Soc* 1985;33:808-10.
31. Rose BD. Hyperosmolar states -- hypernatremia, In: *Clinical Physiology of Acid-Base and Electrolyte Disorders*, 3rd Ed. New York, NY: McGraw Hill Book Co, 1989:639.
32. Arieff AI, Guisado R. Effects on the central nervous system of hypernatremic and hyponatremic states, *Kidney Int* 1976;10:104-8.
33. Cahill GF. Hyperglycemic Hyperosmolar Coma: A syndrome almost unique to the elderly, *J Amer Geriatr Soc* 1983;31:103-5.
34. Terminal Dehydration, (Editorial) *Lancet* 1986;1:306.
35. Zerwekh JV. The dehydration question, *Nursing* 1983;83:47-51.
36. Baines MJ. Control of other symptoms. In: Saunders CM, ed. *The Management of Terminal Illness*. Chicago, IL: Year Book Medical Publishers, 1978.
37. Lamerton R. *Care of the Dying*. New York, NY: Penguin Books, 1980.
38. Billings JA. *Outpatient Management of Advanced Cancer: Symptom Control, Support and Hospice-in-the-Home*. Philadelphia, PA: J.B. Lippincott, 1985.
39. Arbesmann R. Fasting and prophecy in pagan and Christian antiquity, *Traditio* 1951;7:1-71.
40. Luke. 4:1-2.
41. Matthew. 4:3-3.
42. Kerndt PR, Naughton JL, Driscoll CE, Loxterkamp DA. Fasting: The history, pathophysiology and complications, *West J Med* 1982;137:379-99.
43. Sinclair U. *The Fasting Cure*. New York, NY: Mitchell Kennerley, 1911.
44. Haskel CC. *Perfect Health -- How to Get It and How to Keep It*. London: LN Fowler, 1901.
45. Benedict FG. *A Study of Prolonged Fasting*. Washington, DC: Carnegie Institution of Washington, 1915.
46. Folin O, Denis W. On starvation and obesity, with special reference to acidosis, *J Biol Chem* 1915;21:183-92.

47. Bloom WL. Fasting as an introduction to the treatment of obesity, *Metabolism* 1959;8:214-20.
48. Duncan GG, Jenson WK, Cristofori FC, Schless GL. Intermittent fasts in the correction and control of intractable obesity, *Am J Med Sci* 1963;245:515-20.
49. Owen OE, Caprio S, Reichard GA, Mozzoli MA, Boden G, Owen RS. Ketosis of starvation: A revisit and new perspectives, *Clinics in Endocrinology and Metabolism* 1983;12:357-79.
50. Stunkard AF, Rush J. Dieting and depression reexamined: A critical review of reports of untoward responses during weight reduction for obesity, *Ann Intern Med* 1974;81:526-33.
51. Saudek CD, Felig F. The metabolic events of starvation, *Am J Med* 1976;60:117-26.
52. Felig P, Owen OE, Wahren J, Cahill GF. Amino acid metababolism during prolonged starvation, *J Clin Invest* 1969;48:584-94.
53. Aoki TT, Muller WA, Brennan MF, Cahill GF. Metabolic effects of glucose in brief and prolonged fasted man, *Am J Clin Nutr* 1975;28:507-11.
54. Keys A, Brozek J, Henschel A, Mickelsen, Taylor HL. *The Biology of Human Starvation.* Minneapolis, MN: The University of Minnesota Press, 1950.
55. Zimmer R, Weill J, Dubois M. The nutritional situation in the camps of the unoccupied zone of France in 1941 and 1942 and its consequences, *N Engl J Med* 1944;230:303-14.
56. Cahill GF. Starvation in man, *N Engl J Med* 1970;282:668-75.
57. Drenick EJ, Swenseid ME, Blahd WH, Tuttle SG. Prolonged starvation as treatment for severe obesity, *JAMA* 1964;187:100-5.
58. Thomson JT, Runcie J, Miler V. Treatment of obesity by total fasting for up to 249 days, *Lancet* 1966;2:992-6.
59. Stewart WK, Fleming LW. Features of a successful therapeutic fast of 382 days duration, *Postrad Med J* 1973;49:203-9.
60. Spencer IOB. Death during therapeutic starvation for obesity, *Lancet* 1968;1:1288-90.
61. Garnett ES, Barnard DL, Ford J, Goodbody RA, Woodehouse MA. Gross fragmentation of cardiac myofibrils after therapeutic starvation for obesity, *Lancet* 1969;1:914-16.
62. Runcie J, Thomson TJ. Prolonged starvation -- A dangerous procedure? *Br Med J* 1970;3:432-35.
63. Fisler JS, Drenick EJ. Starvation and semistarvation diets in the management of obesity, *Annu Rev Nutr* 1987;7:465-84.
64. Michiel RR, Sheider JS, Dickstein RA, Hayman H, Eich RH. Sudden death in a patient on a liquid protein diet, *N Engl J Med* 1978;298:1005-7.
65. Vertes V, Genuth SM, Hazelton IM. Supplemented fasting as a large-scale outpatient program., *JAMA* 1977;238:2151-3.
66. Baird IM, Parsons RL, Howard AN. Clinical and metabolic studies of chemically defined diets in the management of obesity, *Metabolism* 1974;23:645-57.
67. Hamm RJ, Lyeth BG. Nociceptive thresholds following food restriction and return to free-feeding, *Physiology & Behavior* 1984;33:499-501.
68. Hamm RJ, Knisely JS, Watson A, Lyeth BG, Bossut FB. Hormonal mediation of the analgesia produced by food deprivation, *Physiology and Behavior* 1985;35:879-82.
69. Bodner RJ, Kelly DD, Spiaggia A, Glusman M. Biphasic alterations of nociceptive thresholds induced by deprivation, *Physiol Psychol* 1978;6:391-5.
70. Cahill GF. Starvation in Man, *Clin Endocrinol Metabol* 1976;5:397-415.
71. Fliederbaum J. Clinical aspects of hunger disease in adults, In: Winick M, ed. *Hunger disease -- Studies by the Jewish Physicians in the Warsaw Ghetto*. New York, NY: John Wiley & Sons, 1979:11-36.
72. Korock M. Hunger strikers may have died of fat, not protein loss, *JAMA* 1981;246:1878-9.
73. Leiter LA, Marliss EB. Survival during fasting may depend on fat as well as protein stores, *JAMA* 1982;248:2306-7.
74. Jack HA. *Gandhi Reader: A Source Book of His Life and Writings*. New York, NY: AMS Press, 1965.
75. Drenick EJ, Fisler JL, Dennin HF. The effect of allopurinol on the hyper-uricemia of fasting, *Clin Pharmacol Ther* 1971;12:68-72.
76. Silber T. Anorexia nervosa: Morbidity and mortality, *Pediatr Ann* 1984;13:851-9.

SECTION 8

DYING

Chapter 52

Cases 8.0

Case 8.1: ***"PLEASE, PLEASE KILL ME"***

Jamie Lou Martin was a vivacious and happy 26-year-old who worked as a waitress. Driving home from work one evening, she suddenly lost control of her car, veered across seven lanes of traffic and flipped over. She awoke after two months in a coma to find herself paralyzed from the lips down. Jamie needed a feeding tube, a respirator, a catheter, and a special mattress to regulate her body temperature. Worse, she was in constant, excruciating pain, and the doctors told her they didn't expect it to go away. Because they didn't want her to become addicted, the doctors prescribed only mild painkillers on a four-hour schedule. She had an ulcer, a hernia, blood clots in her legs, even an impacted tooth that no one could fix because her jaw couldn't be pried open. She could think and reason, but she was unable to speak so she had to communicate by blinking her eyelids. Tediously, with the help of an alphabet board, she told her family repeatedly that she didn't want to live like this. Sometimes she would blink out the words, "Please kill me." Other times it was, "Pull the plug," or, merely, "Die." The family steadfastly refused to honor these requests. They insisted that God must have spared her life for a purpose.

Thirteen months after the accident, Jamie was released from the hospital and went "home" to a fully-equipped long-term-care wing that had been added to the house by the insurance company. Homecoming did not cheer Jamie up as expected. She continued to repeat her request to die over and over.

Gary Weidner, a next-door neighbor in his fifties, had a habit of "hanging around" Jamie's home even before her accident, but now he spent far more time with her than with his wife and two children next door. He intensively explored rehabilitation possibilities and outfitted his van to accommodate her special wheelchair so he could take her on occasional outings. She persuaded him to contact a lawyer on her behalf who arranged for her to execute a living will. Since she was unable to move her hands, Weidner signed it in her name.

When she tried to refuse her food tube on the basis of the living will, the family would not allow this. Finally, she asked Weidner: "Will you help me die?" He finally agreed and devised a plan to kill both her and himself the first time they were left alone by cutting their wrists and throats.

He succeeded in killing Jamie, but he survived and was charged with first-degree murder. The situation has torn the family apart. Jamie's sister devoted herself actively to Weidner's defense (and eventually moved in with him); Jamie's grandmother wrote a letter to the judge asking for a lenient sentence for Weidner; Jamie's parents remain bitterly angry at him for his act.[1]

Questions

1. Do you think a physician should have helped by offering assisted suicide?

2. If not, do you think Weidner deserves to be tried and convicted of murder?

3. Are some kinds of killing morally acceptable?

4. If so, are the most acceptable those kinds in which persons request their own death?

5. Does it matter that the person be suffering to make this request? Do they have to be dying?

Case 8.2: **M.I.'S DIABETES**

M.I. was an 81-year-old diabetic woman who had been in fairly good health until she came to her family physician of 20 years with complaints of fatigue, loss of appetite, vomiting after meals, and "aching all over." She was a strong woman otherwise, a "young" elderly person who cared for other family members and was involved in their lives. Her husband had died 15 years before from what she described as "a horrible debilitating cancer."

She was hospitalized, during which time extensive tests were performed to attempt to diagnose her problems. They included bone scans, CAT scans, colonoscopies with the accompanying dreaded bowel preps, gallium scans, x-rays, and biopsies. Also included were the routine blood draws, intravenous lines, rectal examinations, and all the other importunities of hospitalization. The patient was grouchy about all this, but cooperated with these procedures.

After nearly one month of hospitalization her symptoms had not noticeably improved. Her complaints remained a mystery. Evidence of an early cancerous polyp in her descending colon was found, however. She was reluctant to even consider surgery for it, which would have been a partial colon resection with ileostomy. "I have friends," she said, "who have had that bag and it's horrible." Her nausea and vomiting continued despite numerous medications. The diabetes, too, was difficult to control. Each day she became more aggravated and impatient, saying, "When are you going to let me out of here? I'm not getting any better."

One day she said: "I am old, have lived a long life, and accomplished what I wanted to in life. I hope I just die suddenly of a heart attack or something; I'd like to go quickly without all this pain. I can't take any more of these tests and the shots. I'm in pain. I hope you'll let me go if something happens. No respirator stuff." This was said in the presence of her family doctor and the hospital staff. The family doctor encouraged her to "hang in there." He emphasized that she was a tough and young 81-year-old.

Later that day she suffered a cardiac arrest. While one doctor argued that they should not intervene, others had already started CPR. Should this be discontinued?[2]

Case 8.3: **MR. S.'S STROKE AND ANTIBIOTICS**

The neurologists and nurses assembled to discuss treatment for Mr. S. following his massive stroke. His wife, her son and daughter were also present, as was the ethics consultant.

Mr. S. was a very active man. He had been a union organizer in a major industrial city. It was clear from the way his wife and his children talked about him that he was a powerful, independent person, accustomed to always being in the "command module." Although he was 82-years-old, he had never really "retired" from his involvement with union affairs. He had been painting the ceiling of the living room in his home where he lived for over 40 years when he had his stroke. According to his wife, all he said was: "I feel faint. Help!" He has been bedridden and semi-comatose ever since.

It has now been six weeks after the stroke. His stroke was so extensive that none of the physicians managing his care thought he would survive. Now, however, they note that his heart seems strong enough that he may continue for some time "in this state." His family all insist that "he would not have wanted to live like this." He has no Living Will, Durable Power of Attorney, or other form of advance directive. But he did make his wishes known informally.

Mr S., the neurologist explains, has 3 major problems impeding recovery: 1) his advanced age; 2) CVA, massive with paralysis; and 3) loss of swallow reflex. He is fed by nasogastric tube. The patient also is aphasic. He will continue to develop pneumonias. This was presented to the family, and summarized as a very poor prognosis. Since the patient is now DNR, the discussion focused on antibiotic interventions. The family noted that the patient was very practical and strong and often said he would not want to linger while dying. His wife had had a moderate stroke three years ago, but recovered. She thought that would mean that he was familiar with the disease.

The neurologist recommended, that although the patient was not now "dying," antibiotic therapy either be withdrawn or withheld in the future. The family asked to think about his and promised to let caregivers know their decision. The recommendation was made on the basis of the following ethical principles:

1. The previous expressed wishes of the patient.

2. Taking responsibility for our technology.

3. The benefits/burdens calculus (The patient will continue to decline despite any antibiotic interventions).

4. As the prognosis becomes grim, the status of everyday interventions like antibiotics becomes more problematic.

Are these reasons sufficient to justify withholding life-prolonging treatment from a patient who is now in a stable condition? Are quality-of-life judgments being made in this case? Are the patient's best interests being served by the doctors and family? How does withdrawing and withholding antibiotics differ from active, direct euthanasia?

Case 8.4: CONSCIOUSNESS AND SUFFERING

Mrs. King lived a long and useful life. She was active and involved in the community. Near the end of this life, she lived with her daughter, who herself was a widow with three children, in a well-to-do section of a major city. For about six years, she practiced Mary Baker Eddy's principles of Christian Scientist, but took them with a grain of salt. She taught her daughter and grandchildren that there was a higher power in life, and that all human beings have access to that power.

Seven months before her 95th birthday, she suffered a massive stroke. She was brought to the regional medical center, just one block from her home. No one thought she would survive. Eventually however, she was weaned off the respirator, recovered from infections, and was sent home to 24 hour a day care in her old room. She is now paralyzed on the left side, profoundly deaf even if hearing aids, and can apparently see only out of the right eye. Otherwise she is alert. She is lifted out of bed each day to use the toilet (she is still not incontinent), and will give specific directions about what she wants to eat (e.g., ice cream, but "small portion please.") Usually she must read questions and write responses because of her deafness. Sometimes long questions escape her.

Since returning home, she has repeatedly asked to be helped to die. Each member of the family has given her permission to do so. The room she is in is decorated with pictures of her life, and large paper butterflies to symbolize the transformation of life. Further Mrs. King has told of two near-death experiences. In both she describes a beautiful crystal room, filled with light, in which many of her friends were present, though other people she did not know. One friend in particular talked to her, but told her she had to go back. The family since then has prayed out loud with her for her friend to come and take her.

When asked why she wants to die, Mrs. King answers that the pain in her back is one reason. The second is that she hates just lying in bed and "doing nothing." She has been consistent in her wishes, cooperative about her care, and shows no signs of depression. Her family regards her wishes as consistent with her lifestyle and values. All of these preferences were repeated in the presence of her physician, an ethicist, her daughter, and her nurse, on several occasions.

Her heart and other functions are strong.

Her physician has been prescribing medication for her pain. In large doses its only effect is to make her constipated, and causes her more pain.

It occurs to her that until this time, she has been trying to treat Mrs. King's pain. What if she begins to treat Mrs. King's consciousness as the source of the patient's suffering? Higher doses of pain medication could be used to let her drift off to sleep. She would waste away rather rapidly.

Is this a valid form of euthanasia?

Drafted and used with permission of William Andereck, M.D.

Case 8.5: FOOD AND WATER FOR A DYING COMATOSE PATIENT

A 73-year-old white female was referred to the Oncology Service because of pain in the thoracic spine. Six months previously (at age 72) she had had a resection of a poorly differentiated squamous cell carcinoma of the soft palate followed by radiotherapy. Work-up documented metastatic bone disease. Narcotic analgesia and chemotherapy with methotrexate were instituted with transient benefit. Two months after an initial response, the bone pain worsened. Escalation of narcotic doses led to somnolence and worsening mental status and the patient was admitted.

In the three months prior to admission, the performance status of the patient declined from being fully ambulatory to being confined in bed. There had been a 25 pound weight loss due to her disease process and dysphagia as a result of increasing doses of narcotic resulted in respiratory depression and hypotension. Radiotherapy to the thoracic spine and chemotherapy with cisplatinum were begun with palliative intent. The cancer is not curable.

On the fifteenth hospital day, the patient was found without vital signs. Resuscitation resulted in restoration of sinus cardiac rhythm. Vasopressors and a respirator were instituted. Later, vasopressors were weaned but the patient remained in deep coma with no response to painful stimuli and no spontaneous triggering of the respirator.

After discussion with the family, the decision was made to allow the patient to die without any further diagnostic or therapeutic interventions. Three days later the patient remains in deep coma. After further discussion with the family, the I.V. is intentionally discontinued but the respirator is maintained.

Death will occur in 5 to 7 days from cardiovascular collapse secondary to dehydration. The patient cannot survive the current hospitalizations even if aggressive treatment were performed.

This case is an example of attempting to control intense pain, with the knowledge ahead of time that such control in these dosages may induce death as well. Furthermore, the nursing staff was indignant about the decision made in this case. They lined the walls in the patient's room while the discussion with the husband occurred. Some cried. Others objected in the hallways. The ethicist and managing physician in this case had to "put out a lot of fires" in this case. A nursing supervisor was so angry that she later resigned her position, and entered law school to pursue a degree in law.

Questions:

1. Is this a case of euthanasia?

2. Once a patient's death is judged to be imminent, what are the responsibilities of the treating physician?

3. In this case, at the time the patient was found to be without vital signs, could the physician have unilaterally decided to withhold resuscitation? Who should be consulted in the decision?

Case 8.6: THE TRANSFUSED CAT

A 76-year-old widow is in a near brain-dead condition after suffering respiratory arrest on a ventilator. Nine months ago she required open-heart surgery. Since that time she has never left the Medical Intensive Care Unit (MICU) of an acute care facility, suffering one crisis after another due to her underlying atherosclerosis and diabetes. Throughout this stormy course, her only and unmarried daughter, a very obsessive kind of matron, has kept copious notes of what the doctors said, nursing the hurts, angers, and occasional errors. Everyone associated with the widow's care is certain that a lawsuit is pending.

The daughter refuses any discussion of a Do-Not-Resuscitate status for her mother. Besides suspected reasons of not wanting to "let go," which accompany her personality, she articulates a family tradition of "fighting to the bitter end." This tradition was exemplified during the death of an aunt and the death of her father. The daughter consulted with her mother's oldest sister (age 94), who encouraged her not to give up. "Even our cat got transfusions when it was dying," she says. She has missed only one day of being at her mother's bedside, when she herself was sick.

Her mother has never asked not to be kept alive in this condition. In fact, she has requested throughout her treatment that "everything possible be done." She was alert, but suffering, until one week ago when she suffered the respiratory arrest. The family is wealthy and can pay for the care. The neurologist consultant, and all other physicians, nurses, patient relations coordinators, social workers, and ethicists on the case think it is time to stop prolonging the patient's dying.

Case 8.7: MR. MCINTYRE'S LAST-MINUTE REQUEST

James McIntyre, a 28-year-old diabetic, had been on renal dialysis at the Medical Center for a number of years. He was legally blind and could not walk because of progressive neuropathy. He had become increasingly disenchanted because of the stress on both his family's finances and his lifestyle created by his need for hemodialysis three times a week. Because of his despair and anger, his wife had ceased to be supportive and did not want to continue to transport him back and forth to the Medical Center and to attend to his needs between dialysis sessions. Mr. McIntyre came to the conclusion that continued dialysis was unacceptable for him, and, after numerous discussions with his nephrologist, Robert Lincoln, and other members of the nephrology unit and dialysis staff, he decided to discontinue dialysis. He was fully aware that this would inevitably result in his death. His only concern was that he be kept as comfortable as possible until then. Dr. Lincoln and Mr. McIntyre's family accepted his request, feeling that he had made the decision freely and with full awareness of its implications.

Before Mr. McIntyre was taken off dialysis, he and Dr. Lincoln arrived at an agreement about the way in which his final hours would be handled. They decided that Mr. McIntyre would be admitted to the hospital to receive medication, probably morphine sulfate, as needed to control any symptoms that he suffered during this period. In addition, Dr. Lincoln promised to remain with Mr. McIntyre when he returned to the hospital after discontinuing dialysis. Dr. Lincoln also promised that he would, himself, administer the necessary medication to keep Mr. McIntyre comfortable. Further, he agreed not to put Mr. McIntyre back on dialysis should Mr. McIntyre request it under the influence of uremia, morphine sulfate, and ketoacidosis (the last resulting from the cessation of insulin). Mrs. McIntyre concurred with her husband's and Dr. Lincoln's decision.

Mr. McIntyre terminated his dialysis as well as his insulin and was admitted to the hospital some time later in a uremic state.

He had begun to suffer cramps and severe itching, and requested medication which he was given according to the previous agreement. He slept most of the evening and that night, periodically awakening to request more medication. Dr. Lincoln and Mrs. McIntyre were with him throughout. At approximately 3:00 A.M. that morning, Mr. McIntyre awoke complaining of pain and, at that point, asked Dr. Lincoln to put him back on dialysis. Dr. Lincoln and Mrs. McIntyre considered this request, but ultimately decided to abide by the original agreement with Mr. McIntyre.

Dr. Lincoln gave him another injection of morphine sulfate. Mr. McIntyre died in his sleep at approximately 7:00 A.M.

Case 8.8: **MR. B.'S LEFT LEG**

Mr. B's left leg has been amputated due to a serious infection. He is currently sedated and on a respirator.

He is 31-years-old, and a railroad worker. Apparently he scratched his leg when he feel one day after tripping over a railroad tie. He thought nothing of the scratch or the subsequent infection until it entered his system. He became febrile and difficult to control. At that time, he was brought to the emergency room, and evaluated. None of the systemic antibiotic treatments worked, and Mr. B. eventually had to sign for the surgical removal of the left leg before the infection took his life. Nonetheless, his condition, although stable, is extremely serious.

Mrs. B. requested a family and staff meeting, along with an ethics consult, to discuss her husband's condition and further treatment. A meeting was held with the respiratory service, emergency service, medical service, infectious disease service, psychiatry, clinical nurse specialists in trauma, nurses, the chaplain who had been working with Mrs. B., her sister Sharon, and the clinical ethicist.

Mrs. B. had many questions e.g., Why are so many physicians involved in the case; why did the infection occur on the leg; how far was it going to spread; were she and her children at risk for the infection; was her husband at risk for AIDS because of his many transfusions. The doctors present tried to answer her questions and explain Mr. B.'s poor prognosis. Mrs. B. expressed great concern about her husband's future quality of life and she was unsure about what to tell her children regarding his hospitalization. The psychiatrist offered to speak with Mr. B. and the children (Cassandra age 7, Abigail age 4, Jordan age 2).

The perception of everyone at the meeting was that Mrs. B. was bravely trying to endure a situation that had devastated her young family. Primarily she was torn between honoring the wishes of her husband, as she tried to conceive of them, and honoring his best interests. The former led her to consider continued treatment, while the latter would lead to her request no further treatment. Mr. B., though on a respirator, was still capable of some discussion, although he had to write his answers and often was either too tired or lapsing into a coma from the infection.

Normally, the underlying ethical principle in a case like this is respect for patient autonomy in medical decision-making. Since at this time Mr. B. is unable to speak for himself we must rely on the "substituted judgment" of his wife. Mr. B. said that several weeks ago she and her husband were discussing the problems of a friend with cancer who underwent a mastectomy. She asked her husband what he would do if faced with a health crisis -- he said "fight." She believes this is the attitude he would take in making decisions about his treatment now. Mrs. B. appears to be respecting her husband's expressed wishes concerning his will to live and his willingness to accept a life that would be physically compromised. Nonetheless the physicians involved think that they have done everything they can, and that Mr. B. is slowly slipping toward death.

Questions:

1. Should Mr. B. be made DNR without the wife's consent, based on his poor prognosis only?

2. If shortly physicians consider him to be dying, how are decisions to continue treatment in the face of medical futility to be handled?

3. Can physicians act in the best interests of patients without their consent, since the wife is not automatically a legal guardian unless appointed by a court?

4. How can the health care team deal with the anxiety and guilt either a decision to continue or one not to continue will create in this young family? Should the likelihood of guilt be foreseen, how should this probable outcome be factored into the ethical decision to be made?

Case 8.9: THE QUADRIPLEGIC NURSING HOME PATIENT: REFUSAL OF ARTIFICIAL FEEDING

Mr. Smith is quadriplegic as a result of a spinal cord injury suffered in an accident. He has lived in Spring Hills, a residential longterm care facility, for one year. Mr. Smith is sixty years old; he is married with two grown sons. However, he has not lived at home for 17 years. His

35-year-old son lives with his mother, Mr. Smith's wife; his 31-year-old son lives down the block from his mother and brother.

When the spinal cord injury occurred, Mr. Smith made his wife durable power of attorney for health care. At that time he told his wife and sons that he did not want to be kept alive indefinitely by artificial means.

Three weeks ago, Mr. Smith fell and since that time his condition has deteriorated. He is unable to swallow; he receives nutritional support through a gastrostomy tube. Two days previously, Mr. Smith refused artificial feedings. He told his physician that he "was ready to die." His decision upset other residents and many of the nursing staff. Some of the staff did not think it was appropriate to withhold feeding from him. Other staff had been devoted caretakers for him and they were confused about his decision. Mr. Smith was not terminally ill. Although he may have experienced the recent fall as a "set back," the staff believed that his condition would be stabilized relatively soon.

Mr. Smith's doctor was frustrated with his behavior. She knew that he could be a difficult patient. At the rehabilitation institute where he was first treated, Mr. Smith was known to have "fired" a physician with whom he disagreed. Currently, Mr. Smith's physician was concerned about his competency. A psychiatric consultation conducted six months ago revealed that Mr. Smith had a narcissistic personality. A psychiatric evaluation conducted one month ago indicated that Mr. Smith was depressed. Although anti-depressants were prescribed, Mr. Smith was noncompliant with his medications. When Mr. Smith refused tube feeding, his physician recommended another psychiatric consultation to ascertain competency. At first Mr. Smith refused, but then agreed. Mr. Smith was determined to be mentally competent.

The Spring Hill facility has a policy that requires patients to be terminally ill or death imminent before allowing life sustaining treatment to be withheld. Because Mr. Smith was not terminally ill, nor was death imminent, the staff at Spring Hill were attempting to transfer Mr. Smith to another facility where his request could be honored.

In the meantime, Mr. Smith continued to refuse tube feeding. He also insisted that he did not want to be transferred to another facility. In the course of attempting to resolve the situation, the physician learned some disturbing news. Some of the staff caring for Mr. Smith believed that his family was being coercive. For example, one nurse said that when his wife was not there, Mr. Smith would take additional fluids. Also, the younger son told Mr. Smith's physician that his father "did not really want to die." To confuse matters even more, Mr. Smith said that he would be willing to go home to die, but several staff overheard his wife say that she did not want him to come home. Staff believed that Mr. Smith's wife was pressuring him to refuse feeding because their medical insurance coverage for the nursing home was going to end soon.

Consider the following questions:

1. If a patient is mentally competent, must his wishes always be respected?

2. What should a physician do when a patient appears to be influenced by a "coercive" family?

3. If the patient is competent, even if he is being unduly influenced, must his wishes be respected?

4. What factors influence considerations of the limits and extent of patient rights? For example, do you think the patient is trying to commit suicide?

5. What are the obligations of the institution in this case? Should it take into account the feelings and concerns of the other residents? If so, how should others with whom one is living "shape" decisions to be made about an individual? If the institution agrees with the patient, is it assisting in his suicide?

6. How "durable" should a power of attorney be? For example, should it last only a short while before having to be renewed?

Notes

1. Migler R. Please, please kill me! *Good Housekeeping* 1988:160, 274-277.
2. Based on a case submitted to the Medical Humanities Program by Karen Judy a 1989 Third-year medical student, Loyola University of Chicago Stritch School of Medicine, Chicago, Il.

Chapter 53

When Self-Determination Runs Amok

Daniel Callahan

The euthanasia debate is not just another moral debate, one in a long list of arguments in our pluralistic society. It is profoundly emblematic of three important turning points in Western thought. The first is that of the legitimate conditions under which one person can kill another. The acceptance of voluntary active euthanasia would morally sanction what can only be called "consenting adult killing." By that term I mean the killing of one person by another in the name of their mutual right to be killer and killed if they freely agree to play those roles. This turn flies in the face of a longstanding effort to limit the circumstances under which one person can take the life of another, from efforts to control the free flow of gum and arms, to abolish capital punishment, and to more tightly control warfare. Euthanasia would add a whole new category of killing to a society that already has too many excuses to indulge itself in that way.

The second turning point lies in the meaning and limits of self-determination. The acceptance of euthanasia would sanction a view of autonomy holding that individuals may, in the name of their own private, idiosyncratic view of the good life, call upon others, including such institutions as medicine, to help them pursue that life, even at the risk of harm to the common good. This works against the idea that the meaning and scope of our own right to lead our own lives must be conditioned by, and be compatible with, the good of the community, which is more than an aggregate of self-directing individuals.

The third turning point is to be found in the claim being made upon medicine: it should be prepared to make its skills available to individuals to help them achieve their private vision of the good life. This puts medicine in the business of promoting the individualistic pursuit of general human happiness and well-being. It would overturn the traditional belief that medicine should limit its domain to promoting and preserving human health, redirecting it instead to the relief of that suffering which stems from life itself, not merely from a sick body.

I believe that, at each of these three turning points, proponents of euthanasia push us in the wrong direction. Arguments in favor of euthanasia fall into four general categories, which I win take up in turn: (1) the moral claim of individual self-determination and well-being; (2) the moral irrelevance of the difference between killing and allowing to die; (3) the supposed paucity of evidence to show likely harmful consequences of legalized euthanasia; and (4) the compatibility of euthanasia and medical practice.

Self-Determination

Central to most arguments for euthanasia is the principle of self-determination. People are presumed to have an interest in deciding for themselves, according to their own beliefs about

---

Source: Reprinted from *The Hastings Center Report*, March-April 1992, pp. 52-55, with permission from University Press of America © March-April 1992.

what makes life good, how they will conduct their lives. That is an important value, but the question in the euthanasia context is, "What does it mean and how far should it extend?" If it were a question of suicide, where a person takes her own life without assistance from another, that principle might be pertinent, at least for debate. But euthanasia is not that limited a matter. The self-determination in that case can only be effected by the moral and physical assistance of another. Euthanasia is thus no longer a matter only of self-determination, but of a mutual, social decision between two people, the one to be killed and the other to do the killing.

How are we to make the moral move from my right of self-determination to some doctor's right to kill me -- from my right to his right? Where does the doctor's moral warrant to kill come from? Ought doctors to be able to kill anyone they want as long as permission is given by competent persons? Is our right to life just like a piece of property, to be given away or alienated if the price (happiness, relief of suffering) is right, and then to be destroyed with our permission once alienated?

In answer to all those questions, I will say this: I have yet to hear a plausible argument why it should be permissible for us to put this kind of power in the hands of another, whether a doctor or anyone else. The idea that we can waive our right to life, and then give to another the power to take that life, requires a justification yet to be provided by anyone.

Slavery was long ago outlawed on the ground that one person should not have the right to own another, even with the other's permission. Why? Because it is a fundamental moral wrong for one person to give over his life and fate to another, whatever the good consequences, and no less a wrong for another person to have that kind of total, final power. Like slavery, dueling was long ago banned on similar grounds: even free, competent individuals should not have the power to kill each other, whatever their motives, whatever the circumstances. Consenting adult killing, like consenting adult slavery or degradation, is a strange route to human dignity.

There is another problem as well. If doctors, once sanctioned to carry out euthanasia, are to be themselves responsible moral agents -- not simply hired hands with lethal injections at the ready -- then they must have their own independent moral grounds to kill those who request such services. What do I mean? As those who favor euthanasia are quick to point out, some people want it because their life has become so burdensome it no longer seems worth living.

The doctor will have a difficulty at this point. The degree and intensity to which people suffer from their diseases and their dying, and whether they find life more of a burden than a benefit, has very little directly to do with the nature or extent of their actual physical condition. Three people can have the same condition, but only one will find the suffering unbearable. People suffer, but suffering is as much a function of the values of individuals as it is of the physical causes of that suffering. Inevitably in that circumstance, the doctor will in effect be wearing the patient's values. To be responsible, the doctor would have to share those values. The doctor would have to decide, on her own, whether the patient's life was "no longer worth living."

But how could a doctor possibly know that or make such a judgment? Just because the patient said so? I raise this question because, while in Holland at the euthanasia conference reported by Maurice de Wachter elsewhere in this issue, the doctors present agreed that there is no objective way of measuring or judging the claims of patients that their suffering is unbearable. And if it is difficult to measure suffering, how much more difficult to determine the value of a patient's statement that her life is not worth living?

However one might want to answer such questions, the very need to ask them, to inquire into the physician's responsibility and grounds for medical and moral judgment, points out the social nature of the decision. Euthanasia is not a private matter of self-determination. It is an act that requires two people to make it possible, and a complicit society to make it acceptable.

Killing and Allowing to Die

Against common opinion, the argument is sometimes made that there is no moral difference between stopping life-sustaining treatment and more active forms of killing, such as lethal injection. Instead I would contend that the notion that there is no morally significant difference between omission and commission is just wrong. Consider in its broad implications what the eradication of the distinction implies: that death from disease has been banished, leaving only the actions of physicians in terminating treatment as the cause of death. Biology, which used to bring about death, has apparently been displaced by human agency. Doctors have finally, I suppose, thus genuinely become gods, now doing what nature and the deities once did.

What is the mistake here? It lies in confusing causality, and culpability, and in failing to note the way in which human societies have overlaid natural causes with moral rules and interpretations. Causality, (by which I mean the direct physical causes of death) and culpability (by which I mean our attribution of moral responsibility to human actions) are confused under three circumstances.

They are confused, first, when the action of a physician in stopping treatment of a patient with an underlying lethal disease is construed as causing death. On the contrary, the physician's omission can only bring about death on the condition that the patient's disease will kill him in the absence of treatment. We may hold the physician morally responsible for the death, if we have morally judged such actions wrongful omissions. But it confuses reality and moral judgment to see an omitted action as having the same causal status as one that directly kills. A lethal injection will kill both a healthy person and a sick person. A physician's omitted treatment will have no effect on a healthy person. Turn off the machine on me, a healthy person, and nothing will happen. It will only, in contrast, bring the life of a sick person to an end because of an underlying fatal disease.

Causality and culpability are confused, second, when we fail to note that judgments of moral responsibility and culpability are human constructs. By that I mean that we human beings, after moral reflection, have decided to call some actions right or wrong, and to devise moral rules to deal with them. When physicians could do nothing to stop death, they were not held responsible for it. When, with medical progress, they began to have some power over death -- but only its timing and circumstances, not its ultimate inevitability -- moral rules were devised to set forth their obligations. Natural causes of death were not thereby banished. They were, instead, overlaid with a medical ethics designed to determine moral culpability in deploying medical power.

To confuse the judgments of this ethics with the physical causes of death -- which is the connotation of the word kill -- is to confuse nature and human action. People will, one way or another, die of some disease; death will have dominion over all of us. To say that a doctor "kills" a patient by allowing this to happen should only be understood as a moral judgment about the licitness of his omission, nothing more. We can, as a fashion of speech only, talk about a doctor killing a patient by omitting treatment he should have provided. It is a fashion of speech precisely because it is the underlying disease that brings death when treatment is omitted; that is its cause, not the physician's omission. It is a misuse of the word killing to use it when a doctor stops a treatment he believes will no longer benefit the patient -- when, that is, he steps aside to allow an eventually inevitable death to occur now rather than later. The only deaths that human beings invented are those that come from direct killing -- when, with a lethal injection, we both cause death and are morally responsible for it. In the case of omissions, we do not cause death even if we may be judged morally responsible for it.

This difference between causality and culpability also helps us see why a doctor who has omitted a treatment he should have provided has "killed" that patient while another doctor -- performing precisely the same act of omission on another patient in different circumstances does not kill her, but only allows her to die. The difference is that we have come, by moral convention and conviction, to classify unauthorized or illegitimate omissions as acts of "killing." We call them "killing" in the expanded sense of the term: A culpable action that permits the real cause of death, the underlying disease, to proceed to its lethal conclusion. By contrast, the doctor who, at the patient's request, omits or terminates unwanted treatment does not kill at all. Her underlying disease, not his action, is the physical cause of death; and we have agreed to consider actions of that kind to be morally licit. He thus can truly be said to have "allowed" her to die.

If we fail to maintain the distinction between killing and allowing to die, moreover, there are some disturbing possibilities. The first would be to confirm many physicians in their already too-powerful belief that, when patients die or when physicians stop treatment because of the futility of continuing it, they are somehow both morally and physically responsible for the deaths that follow. That notion needs to be abolished, not strengthened. It needlessly and wrongly burdens the physician, to whom should not be attributed the powers of the gods. The second possibility would be that, in every case where a doctor judges medical treatment no longer effective in prolonging life, a quick and direct killing of the patient would be seen as the next, most reasonable step, on grounds of both humaneness and economics. I do not see how that logic could easily be rejected.

Calculating the Consequences

When concerns about the adverse social consequences of permitting euthanasia are raised, its advocates tend to dismiss them as unfounded and overly speculative. On the contrary, recent data about the Dutch experience suggests that such concerns are right on target. From my own discussions in Holland, and from the articles on that subject, I believe we can now fully see most of the likely consequences of legal euthanasia.

Three consequences seem almost certain, in this or any other country: the inevitability of some abuse of the law; the difficulty of precisely writing, and then enforcing, the law; and the inherent slipperiness of the moral reasons for legalizing euthanasia in the first place.

Why is abuse inevitable? One reason is that almost all laws on delicate, controversial matters are to some extent abused. This happens because not everyone will agree with the law as written and will bend it, or ignore it, if they can get away with it. From explicit admissions to me by Dutch proponents of euthanasia, and from the corroborating information provided by the Remmelink Report and the outside studies of Carlos Gomez and John Keown, I am convinced that in the Netherlands there are a substantial number of cases of nonvoluntary euthanasia, that is, euthanasia undertaken without the explicit permission of the person being killed. The other reason abuse is inevitable is that the law is likely to have a low enforcement priority in the criminal justice system. Like other laws of similar status, unless there is an unrelenting and harsh willingness to pursue abuse, violations will ordinarily be tolerated. The worst thing to me about my experience in Holland was the casual, seemingly indifferent attitude toward abuse. I think that would happen everywhere.

Why would it be hard to precisely write, and then enforce, the law? The Dutch speak about the requirement of "unbearable" suffering, but admit that such a term is just about indefinable, a highly subjective matter admitting of no objective standards. A requirement for outside opinion is nice, but it is easy to find complaisant colleagues. A requirement that a medical condition be "terminal" will run aground on the notorious difficulties of knowing when an illness is actually terminal.

Apart from those technical problems there is a more profound worry. I see no way, even in principle, to write or enforce a meaningful law that can guarantee effective procedural safeguards. The reason is obvious yet almost always overlooked. The euthanasia transaction will ordinarily take place within the boundaries of the private and confidential doctor-patient relationship. No one can possibly know what takes place in that context unless the doctor chooses to reveal it. In Holland, less than 10 percent of the physicians report their acts of euthanasia and do so with almost complete legal impunity. There is no reason why the situation should be any better elsewhere. Doctors will have their own reasons for keeping euthanasia secret, and some patients will have no less a motive for wanting it concealed.

I would mention, finally, that the moral logic of the motives for euthanasia contain within them the ingredients of abuse. The two standard motives for euthanasia and assisted suicide are said to be our fight of self-determination, and our claim upon the mercy of others, especially doctors, to relieve our suffering. These two motives are typically spliced together and presented as a single justification. Yet if they are considered independently -- and there is no inherent reason why they must be linked -- they reveal serious problems. It is said that a competent, adult person should have a right to euthanasia for the relief of suffering. But why must the person be suffering? Does not that stipulation already compromise the principle of self-determination? How can self-determination have any limits? Whatever the persons motives may be, why are they not sufficient?

Consider next the person who is suffering but not competent, who is perhaps demented or mentally retarded. The standard argument would deny euthanasia to that person. But why? If a person is suffering but not competent, then it would seem grossly unfair to deny relief solely on the grounds of incompetence. Are the incompetent less entitled to relief from suffering than the competent? Will it only be affluent, middle-class people, mentally fit and savvy about working the medical system, who can qualify? Do the incompetent suffer less because of their incompetence?

Considered from these angles, there are no good moral reasons to limit euthanasia once the principle of taking life for that purpose has been legitimated. If we really believe in self-determination, then any competent person should have a right to be killed by a doctor for any reason that suits him. If we believe in the relief of suffering, then it seems cruel and capricious to deny it to the incompetent. There is, in short, no reasonable or logical stopping point once the turn has been made down the road to euthanasia, which could soon turn into a convenient and commodious expressway.

Euthanasia and Medical Practice

A fourth kind of argument one often hears both in the Netherlands and in this country is that euthanasia and assisted suicide are perfectly compatible with the aims of medicine. I would note at the very outset that a physician who participates in another person's suicide already abuses medicine. Apart from depression (the main statistical cause of suicide), people commit suicide because they find life empty, oppressive, or meaningless. Their judgment is a judgment about the value of continued life, not only about health (even if they are sick). Are doctors now to be given the right to make judgments about the kinds of life worth living and to give their blessing to suicide for those they judge wanting? What conceivable competence, technical or moral, could doctors claim to play such a role? Are we to medicalize suicide, turning judgments about its worth and value into one more clinical issue? Yes, those are rhetorical questions.

Yet they bring us to the core of the problem of euthanasia and medicine. The great temptation of modern medicine, not always resisted, is to move beyond the promotion and preservation of health into the boundless realm of general human happiness and well-being. The root problem of illness and mortality is both medical and philosophical or religious. "Why must I die?" can be asked as a technical, biological question, or as a question about the meaning of life. When medicine tries to respond to the latter, which it is always under pressure to do, it moves beyond its proper role.

It is not medicine's place to lift from us the burden of that suffering which turns on the meaning we assign to the decay of the body and its eventual death. It is not medicine's place to determine when lives are not worth living or when the burden of life is too great to be borne. Doctors have no conceivable way of evaluating such claims on the part of patients, and they should have no right to act in response to them. Medicine should try to relieve human suffering, but only that suffering which is brought on by illness and dying as biological phenomena, not that suffering which comes from anguish or despair at the human condition.

Doctors ought to relieve those forms of suffering that medically accompany serious illness and the threat of death. They should relieve pain, do what they can to allay anxiety and uncertainty, and be a comforting presence. As sensitive human beings, doctors should be prepared to respond to patients who ask why they must die, or die in pain. But here the doctor and the patient are at the same level. The doctor may have no better an answer to those old questions than anyone else; and certainly no special insight from his training as a physician. It would be terrible for physicians to forget this, and to think that in a swift, lethal injection, medicine has found its own answer to the riddle of life. It would be a false answer, given by the wrong people. It would be no less a false answer for patients. They should neither ask medicine to put its own vocation at risk to serve their private interests, nor think that the answer to suffering is to be killed by another. The problem is precisely that, too often in human history, killing has seemed the quick, efficient way to put aside that which burdens us. It rarely helps, and too often simply adds to one evil still another. That is what I believe euthanasia would accomplish. It is self-determination run amok.

Chapter 54

Family Consent to Orders Not to Resuscitate: Reconsidering Hospital Policy

J. Chris Hackler and F. Charles Hiller

Hospital policies typically require that resuscitation be initiated for every cardiopulmonary arrest unless a Do-Not-Resuscitate (DNR) order has been written, and further, that patient or family permission be obtained before the order is written. Thus, it is possible for family members to block a DNR order for patients who will not benefit from the procedure and whose suffering may be prolonged or increased, as the following cases illustrate.

Report of Cases

Case 1

An 18-year-old woman with a diagnosis of choriocarcinoma with extensive pulmonary metastases was transferred to the intensive care unit because of difficulty in breathing. Shortly after admission to the hospital, she required intubation and mechanical ventilation. After a two-week period of gradual improvement with chemotherapy, her condition began to worsen, with the development of adult respiratory distress syndrome. Two chest tubes were inserted for bilateral pneumothoraxes, and a tracheostomy was performed, but ventilation became progressively more difficult, requiring very high ventilating pressure and oxygen concentration. Seven weeks after admission, the patient's mother indicated a desire to move the patient to a hospital managed by a religious order, but she was unable to find an ambulance service willing to transport the patient in such a fragile condition. The mother's native language was not English, so that communication and development of good physician-family rapport was difficult.

The patient's condition deteriorated progressively despite continued intensive management and support. The family was approached regarding the possibility of a DNR order. Despite the obvious hopelessness of the situation, the mother refused permission. After a long and relentless downhill course despite full support, the patient went into cardiac arrest ten weeks after admission, and vigorous efforts at resuscitation failed.

Case 2

A six-year-old girl, who had undergone an abdominal exploration and appendectomy at another hospital one month earlier, presented with apparent severe abdominal sepsis and underwent surgery immediately. Post-operatively she developed a duodenal fistula for which a gastrostomy was performed, along with an ileostomy, a serosal patch, and closure of a colonic fistula as well as the duodenal fistula. Shortly after these procedures, she suffered a stroke with resultant severe brain damage. Soon thereafter the physician began cautiously to

Source: Reprinted from *The Journal of the American Medical Association*, Vol. 264, No. 10, pp. 1281-1283, with permission from American Medical Association © Sep. 1990.

broach the possibility of a DNR order with the girl's mother but met firm resistance. The patient was taken back to the operating room six weeks after admission for abdominal exploration and underwent multiple repairs and resections. Chronic drainage from a recurrent fistula continued to be a problem. Three months after admission, a central venous line was placed.

The physician began confronting the mother more aggressively and in several long sessions explained that her daughter was going to die and that the treatment she was receiving was painful to her. Hospital policy required approval by the next of kin for DNR status, but the mother refused to consider any limitation of treatment. Several more operations were performed four and six months after admission. By this time her abdomen had multiple fistulas from all parts of the small bowel and large amounts of drainage. Multiple infections were treated with intravenous antibiotics, and she was resuscitated several times. During her final resuscitation she was asystolic for 30 to 45 minutes. Her mother was called during the course of resuscitation but would not allow it to be stopped. The patient lay in deep coma for four days. When the physician flatly refused any longer to be a part of the patient's care, the mother, after considerable delay, relented. The expiration summary noted that "the ventilator was turned off, as the patient's condition appeared hopeless." She died ten months after admission.

Comment

The requirement of family permission to withhold treatment reflects a fundamental principle of medical ethics; that patients have a right to participate in decisions about their care. Surrogacy preserves a measure of patient autonomy beyond a point at which it would otherwise be lost. It succeeds in this purpose to the extent that surrogates choose as the patient would have chosen. When there is no evidence of patient preference, the rationale for family surrogacy is different: promoting patients' best interests by choosing advocates who are most concerned with their welfare, or respecting the integrity of the family as a social unit.[1]

Hospital policies which recognize the authority of family members to speak for the patient should be encouraged and supported for all the above reasons. It is important, however, that those policies also recognize appropriate limits to that authority. Some limits are already generally accepted. Surrogates may not reject life-sustaining treatment when there is no evidence of patient preference and it is clear to others that the treatment is in the best interest of the patient. Parents cannot refuse necessary transfusions or operations for their children or deny them pain medication based on their own religious beliefs or values. In like manner, surrogates should not be able to demand treatment that is futile or that adds to the patient's suffering when there is no indication the patient wants it and it is clearly not in the patient's best interest.

Both patients discussed above received treatment, including cardiopulmonary resuscitation (CPR), that was useless or which needlessly prolonged a painful dying. In neither case was the surrogate attempting to determine either the preference or the best interests of the patient. The patients were resuscitated because hospital policy seemed to leave no option. Cardiopulmonary resuscitation had to be performed in the absence of a DNR order, and such an order could be written only with family consent. These are typical features of hospital policies across the country, and we believe they should be changed in the following manner: (1) Do not require discussion with patient or family of CPR as an option if it is clearly futile, as defined below. (2) If it is not clearly futile, then require discussion of CPR with patient or family, but do not require family agreement to the treatment plan in every case.

Proposal 1

Do not require that futile CPR be offered to patients or families. A procedure is futile in the strict sense that we intend when there is no possibility that it will accomplish its intended physiological effect. Cardiopulmonary resuscitation would be futile when it would not successfully reestablish cardiopulmonary function. The justification for any medical intervention is that it offers the possibility of benefits which outweigh its burdens. Thus, there can be no medical or ethical justification for treatment which is clearly futile, offering no hope of any medical benefit. There seems to be general agreement that there is no obligation to provide futile treatment. For example, the Council on Ethical and Judicial Affairs of the American Medical Association recommended to the Association's House of Delegates in 1987 that a patient's or family's choice for resuscitation should be honored "unless it would be futile." Moreover, the Council has held that "physicians should not provide, prescribe, or seek compensation for services that are known to be unnecessary or worthless."[2] Since there is no obligation to provide pointless CPR and arguably even an obligation not to provide it, patients and families cannot justifiably demand it. Therefore, policy should not require family assent to a DNR order under such circumstances.

When CPR is clearly useless, physicians should not be required to discuss it as an option. Respect for patient autonomy does not require that the physician initiate discussion of medically pointless procedures. If there is no case to be made for a procedure, there should be no need to make one against it. Useless CPR should be no different from useless tonsillectomy in this respect.

Moreover, most families are not accustomed to being offered a treatment with the suggestion that it be refused. Some will assume that if care is offered it must have some benefit and will interpret refusal as giving up or abandoning the patient. No matter how clearly the medical case against CPR is made, some families will find the decision to forgo it emotionally or ethically difficult, and some will find it impossible. There is no point in making families agonize over the matter and worry that they are breaking faith with their loved ones. To do so may create unnecessary suffering, strife, or guilt and may produce deadlock with an unsophisticated, death-denying, or guilt-ridden family.

To summarize, there is no obligation to provide useless treatments, patients or families have no right to demand them, and physician integrity may prohibit offering them; patient autonomy does not require discussion of useless treatments, and compassion for struggling families may in some cases argue against it. Thus hospital policy should allow physicians to write DNR orders without family consent or discussion, if CPR would be futile.

Considerable care will be required in drafting such a policy, since the term "futile" is not a precise or well-defined clinical term. Its "categorical ring," as Youngner[3] pointed out, "masks a more subtle complexity." In addition to physiological inefficacy, "futility" may refer to inability to postpone death, to prolong life for a certain (variable) period, or to maintain an acceptable quality of life. It may also refer to a very low probability of achieving any one of the above goals.[3,4] Simple statements of futility are inherently incomplete, being ambiguous with respect to the goals of treatment and vague with respect to the probability of success. Thus, any policy concerning futile treatment must be explicit about the meaning that it attaches to the term. That a treatment is futile in the strict sense -- there is no possibility that it would be effective or would postpone death -- is a medical judgment that physicians may make without regard for patient or family values, so that such treatment need not be discussed with patient or family.[3,5] That a treatment would be futile in any broader sense -- that it would preserve a life of insufficient length or quality, or that the chance of success is too low to justify the effort, suffering or cost -- would involve value judgments that properly belong to the patient or surrogate (though the next proposal is that surrogate authority should not be absolute).

Proposal 2
Do not require family consent to DNR status in every case. When resuscitation provides any benefit, it should be discussed with the patient or an appropriate surrogate. Even if the physician feels strongly that resuscitation is not advisable because the burdens outweigh the benefits, the patient or surrogate should have the opportunity to assess the chances of success and the desirability of any extension of life, and their wishes should almost always be followed. Resuscitation obviously should be undertaken if a patient with decision-making capacity requests it. The matter is a bit more complicated, however, when the request is from a surrogate.

The moral authority, and in some jurisdictions the legal authority, of surrogates is broad, but it is not unlimited. As noted earlier, it is widely accepted that surrogates must follow one of two decision-making criteria. To the extent that there is reliable evidence what the patient would choose, the surrogate must express the patient's own presumed choice. As evidence for the patient's preference grows weaker, the surrogate should attempt to ascertain the patient's best interests. The surrogate's judgment in this regard may not be purely idiosyncratic, based upon the surrogate's own unusual set of values. It must satisfy a general test of reasonableness, taking into account such things as relief of suffering, restoration of functioning, and quality and extent of life sustained.[1] Although the majority of surrogates function responsibly within these limits, some do not. Out of respect for the family as a social unit and concern for the feelings of its members, physicians are properly patient and sympathetic with families as they struggle with the stressful burden of surrogacy. At a certain point, however, respect for the family must give way to concern for the patient. Hospital policy should not force physicians to inflict additional suffering on their patients when surrogates insist upon burdensome treatment for unacceptable reasons. It is wrong to inflict pain on one person without chance of significant benefit to satisfy another person, or out of slavish adherence to an occasionally misdirected procedural principle.

We are not suggesting that physicians should ignore the needs of family. Aggressive support of dying patients may be necessary to give families time to accept the inevitable or to allow a relative time to arrive at the bedside. But family needs should be clear and compelling to justify additional suffering by the patient.

We are not suggesting that the proper role of surrogates be reduced. Reasonable people applying similar criteria of suffering, quality-of-life, and so on may disagree about the patient's best interests. In such cases physicians should defer to the opinion of the family. But when the family does not and will not deliberate in an appropriate manner, or when their views about suffering and quality of life differ substantially from those of most reasonable people (and there is no indication that the patient shared such views), then physicians should not be forced by hospital policy to adhere to family preference.

Finally, we are not suggesting that physicians act precipitously or unilaterally. Seemingly irreconcilable differences can sometimes be mediated by introduction of a facilitator such as a chaplain, an ethicist, a social worker, or a nurse skilled in conflict resolution. Intransigent disagreements may be taken to an institutional ethics committee for discussion. Hospital policy may require formal review by some such group when there is an ultimate disagreement between family and physician. We maintain only that the review process should include an examination of the surrogate's reasoning to determine if appropriate criteria are being followed, and if they are not being followed, cessation of treatment should be possible (though of course not mandatory).

To summarize our second proposal, even if CPR would not be clearly futile, physicians should be able to write a DNR order without family consent if: (1) the patient is unable to consent; (2) the burdens of the procedure would clearly outweigh the benefits; (3) the surrogate does not provide an adequate reason for refusing consent; and (4) the physician has made appropriate attempts at mediation (as established by hospital policy).

Conclusion

It is difficult to believe that a hospital or a physician who discontinued treatment would have legal difficulties if a review panel agreed that surrogate reasoning was improper and that the best interests of the patient excluded CPR. There are several reasons for this. First, the legal duty of the physician and the hospital is to the patient only; there is no duty to the surrogate. The surrogate's role is to assist the physician in determining what the physician's duty to the patient is. If the physician acts in the best interest of the patient and not contrary to the patient's wishes (as they may be known or inferred), then that duty to the patient has been fulfilled. Second, the authority of surrogates is limited, as previously noted; even the decisions of legal guardians are subject to review. The courts increasingly are using a so-called reasonable person standard to assess medical decisions. Applying this standard to surrogate choices would discredit uninformed or irrational preferences. Third, it is unlikely that a lawsuit would ever be brought. The purpose of medical malpractice lawsuits is to recover damages for harm to the patient, but the treatment is being withheld in this case precisely to avoid harming the patient. The patient's representative would have to refute the physician's contention, sustained by peer review, that the treatment itself would have harmed the patient and thus prove that withholding treatment caused the patient to suffer more than administering it or that the treatment could have restored the patient to some degree of health. Finally, courts generally wish to protect the integrity of the medical profession and are loathe to force physicians to practice what they consider bad or unethical medicine.

The last point is especially important. Courts tend to defer to the ethical judgment of the profession when they know what it is. For example, the opinion of the Council on Ethical and Judicial Affairs of the American Medical Association has been influential in recent decisions concerning the withdrawal of feeding tubes. Similar statements by organized medicine on the present matter would help set authoritative professional standards to which physicians and hospitals could appeal in justifying their actions or policies.

We thank Anne Owings Wilson, J.D., for her contribution to the "Conclusion" section.

Notes

1. *Making Health Care Decisions*. Washington, DC: President's Commission for the Study of Ethical Problems in Medicine and Biomedical and Behavioral Research, 1982:Chap 9.
2. *Current Opinions of the Council on Ethical and Judicial Affairs of the American Medical Association*, 1986:Sec 2.17.
3. Youngner SJ. Who defines futility? *JAMA* 1988;260:2094-2095.
4. Lantos JD, Singer PA, Walker RM, *et al*. The illusion of futility in clinical practice, *Am J Med* 1989;87:81-84.
5. Tomlinson T, Brody H. Ethics and communication in do-not-resuscitate orders, *N Engl J Med* 1988;318:43-46.

Chapter 55

Understanding the Benefits and Burdens of Tube Feedings

Bernard Lo and Laurie Dornbrand

Tube feedings for patients with severe dementia, metastatic cancer, or stroke present controversial management decisions. Artificial feedings might benefit patients by reversing malnutrition or dehydration and prolonging life in patients who are unable to take adequate nutrition by mouth. But Quill's[1] careful empirical study shows that feeding tubes may not accomplish these goals and may impose significant burdens on patients with severe, irreversible illness.

Technology should benefit the patient.
Philosophers have asserted that medicine should benefit the patient, according to the patient's definition of benefit.[2] Feeding tubes can benefit patients when they provide time to treat underlying medical problems or clarify prognosis or when prolongation of life is feasible and desirable. But Quill found that feeding tubes seldom gained time for underlying reversible conditions to be successfully treated. In only two cases were feeding tubes removed because patients improved. It is questionable whether feeding tubes prolonged life in any clinically meaningful way, since 64% of the patients died in the hospital.

The goal of care was patient comfort in 38% of the cases studied. But there was disturbing evidence that feeding tubes may actually cause patient distress rather than enhance comfort. Restraints were applied in over 50% of patients to prevent them from pulling out their feeding tubes. It is hard to argue that treatment which requires patients to be restrained makes them more comfortable, particularly when they cannot appreciate how the feeding tube will help them.[3] Instead, such restraints seem undignified, humiliating, or even cruel. Sedation or "chemical restraints" to prevent patients from pulling out their tubes might seem more acceptable aesthetically but are equally undignified and also have significant side effects. Previous studies have also documented other important adverse effects of tube feedings. The incidence of aspiration pneumonia has been reported to be 47%.[4]

Quill's study was unable to determine whether the quality-of-life of these patients was improved. Competent patients should be asked whether they feel less hungry, stronger, or improved in any other way. For incompetent patients, physicians (and nurses and family members) need to decide how to assess whether feeding tubes enhance quality of life, particularly when the goal of care is patient comfort. It is hard to justify tying down patients for the sake of speculative and unobservable benefits. Quill's study also did not assess whether feeding tubes led to biomedical improvement, such as increased serum albumin levels or increased muscle mass. While improvement in such parameters is possible, improved laboratory results per se are not necessarily the goal of care.

Source: Reprinted from *Archives of Internal Medicine*, Vol. 149, Sep 1989, pp. 1925-1926, with permission from University Press of America © Sep. 1989.

Tube feedings should not be considered "ordinary" care.
Some physicians believe that tube feedings are basic, humane care that must always be provided, just like a clean bed. But the distinction between "extraordinary" and "ordinary" care has been rejected by most writings on medical ethics and almost all court decisions regarding artificial feedings.[5,6] Rather than trying to label a technology as "extraordinary" or "ordinary" care, we should look at the individual patient and his or her clinical situation.[6] The issue is not the nature of the technology, but whether the benefits of the technology outweigh the burdens for the individual patient. Quill provides dramatic evidence that tube feedings may impose significant burdens or harms, with little demonstrable benefit.

Informed consent should be obtained for tube feedings.
Quill's suggestion that physicians obtain informed consent for feeding tubes is reasonable. Like other treatments, feeding tubes should be used only when they can achieve the goals of care and when patients or surrogates agree to their use. Courts have ruled that treatment without the consent of the patient may constitute malpractice.[7] Because decisions about tube feedings often concern incompetent patients, physicians should anticipate these decisions and encourage competent patients to indicate their preferences. In addition, doctors can recommend completing a durable power of attorney for health care, which allows patients to appoint a surrogate to make decisions for them if they become incompetent.[8] Such surrogates should follow the previously explained wishes of the patient.

Consent by the patient or permission by a surrogate for feeding tubes was rarely documented in this study. Not only did patients not *consent* to feeding tubes, but they often did not even *assent*. Quill suggests that pulling out a feeding tube is a "nonverbal expression that the patient wants the tube out." Many observers might disagree with this inference, since removing the tube may be a reflex rather than a purposeful action. But we should all agree that pulling out a feeding tube is not an indication for restraints; instead, physicians should reconsider whether tube feedings are appropriate. If they are, patients may be less likely to pull out gastrostomy or jejunostomy tubes that nasogastric tubes.

Quill's findings should be read by judges as well as by physicians, patients, and families. In several landmark decisions involving feeding tubes in demented patients, courts have not appreciated the burdens feeding tubes may impose. In the Conroy case,[9,10] a severely demented elderly woman repeatedly pulled out her nasogastric tube. The court ruled that a feeding tube could be discontinued if the patient would have refused it or if it was not in her best interest. But the court required more evidence that Ms Conroy's repeatedly pulling out her tube to conclude that tube feedings were not in her best interest. What further evidence would be reasonable to require? As a dissenting judge pointed out, there must be a point at which we would be ready to say "Enough." If we cannot answer this question, we may be requiring many patients with dementia or metastatic cancer to have a feeding tube or restraints in place before they are allowed to die.

Notes

1. Quill TE. Utilization of nasogastric feeding tubes in a group of chronically ill, elderly patients in a community hospital, *Arch Intern Med* 1989;149:1937-1941.
2. Pellegrino ED, Thomasma DG. *For the Patient's Good: The Restoration of Beneficence in Health Care*. New York, NY: Oxford University Press, 1988.
3. Lo B, Dornbrand L. Guiding the hand that feeds: Caring for the demented elderly, *N Engl J Med* 1984;311:402-4.
4. Ciocon JO, Silverstone FA, Graver LM, Foley CJ. Tube feedings in elderly patients, *Arch Intern Med* 1988;148:429-43.

5. Steinbrook R, Lo B. Artificial feedings: Solid ground, not slippery slope, *N Engl J Med* 1988;318:286-90.
6. *Deciding to Forego Life-Sustaining Treatment: A Report on the Ethical, Medical, and Legal Issues in Treatment Decisions*. Washington, DC: President's Commission for the Study of Ethical Problems in Medicine and Biomedical and Behavioral Research, 1983.
7. Appelbaum PS, Lidz CW, Meisel A. *Informed Consent: Legal Theory and Clinical Practice*. New York, NY: Oxford University Press, 1987.
8. Steinbrook R, Lo B. Decision making for incompetent patients by designated proxy, *N Engl J Med* 1984;310:1598-1601.
9. *In re* Conroy, 98 NJ 321, 486A2d 1209 (NJ 1985).
10. Lo B, Dornbrand L. The case of Claire Conroy: Will administrative review safeguard incompetent patients? *Ann Intern Med* 1986;104:869-73.

Chapter 56

Helga Wanglie Revisited: Medical Futility and the Limits of Autonomy

David H. Johnson

There is little to indicate from her circumstances that events would propel Helga Wanglie, an 86-year-old Minneapolis woman, into the center of public controversy.[1] We know little of her life prior to the events that removed her from the world of conscious, sentient beings. By the time of her death on 4 July 1991, Mrs. Wanglie had become the focus of a nationwide public and professional debate on the fights of a patient in a persistent vegetative state (PVS) to receive aggressive medical treatment when such treatment is felt by the patient's doctors not to be in the patient's best interests.

Superficially, the Wanglie case appears to be the latest in a line of cases involving the issue of whether to continue life support in a patient in a persistent vegetative state. In this sense, Helga Wanglie resembled Karen Quinlan and Nancy Cruzan. In the Wanglie case, however, the roles of the family and the physicians were reversed, with the family, rather than the physicians, insisting on continuing treatment. This reversal of roles reflects significant changes in the way that society in general and the medical profession in particular view decision-making at the end of life.

The fact that Mrs. Wanglie was in a persistent vegetative state was the key element that convinced many of her careproviders that life support should be discontinued. Her respirator became the symbol of life-sustaining care in the ensuing discussion around the question of withdrawal of aggressive care. The respirator was actually just one aspect of the entire "package" of aggressive care measures she was receiving. Her care providers, in fact, appeared to be saying that she should not be treated in the ICU at all regardless of whether she required a respirator.

Yet, it was the respirator that acquired great symbolic significance for the staff, the family, and the public. To the staff it was mechanical, intrusive, expensive, and ultimately futile. To Mrs. Wanglie's family, such arguments were irrelevant and incorrect. The respirator was not futile; it was keeping her alive, the outcome they desired. The respirator was the one element of Helga Wanglie's care that, when removed, would quickly result in her death.

Although virtually all commentators on the case mentioned that her husband, Oliver Wanglie, was an attorney, there has been little, if any, discussion of the impact this may have had on the decisions made by hospital administrators and physicians. A significant part of the reluctance of Mrs. Wanglie's care providers to act against Mr. Wanglie's wishes may have stemmed from their fear of a law suit. Fear of litigation may have been as significant a factor in the refusal of physicians outside HCMC to accept Helga Wanglie as a transfer patient as was any consensus that in her case aggressive care was outside the limits of medicine.

Source: Reprinted from *Cambridge Quarterly of Healthcare Ethics*, Vol. 2, 1993, pp. 161-170, with permission from Cambridge University Press © 1993.

Patient Autonomy

During the past two decades, a gradual public consensus has evolved that patients are entitled to make their own medical decisions. Within the bioethics and medical communities, this consensus is reflected in the primacy of patient autonomy over physician autonomy and beneficence.

Applied to the Wanglie case, the principle of patient autonomy dictates: 1) that Oliver Wanglie, acting as his wife's surrogate decision-maker, possessed the authority to decide whether his wife would have wished continued aggressive care; and 2) that her physicians should abide by his decision. This primacy of patient autonomy in end-of-life decisions was emphasized by both Ackerman and Anger in their analyses of the Wanglie case.

Ackerman, an academic ethicist, argued that the principal issue in Wanglie is whether her life was worth prolonging.[2] This, she stated, is not a medical issue, but a question of values, and there is no reason to think that physicians are more qualified to render judgments about this than anyone else. She also based her opinion on the fallibility of medical diagnoses and her assumption that the members of the health maintenance organization (HMO), whose premiums paid for Mrs. Wanglie's care, "by being members of this plan committed themselves to a practice of medicine that does not take cost into account."[3]

These last two assertions are questionable. Even if the diagnosis of PVS was wrong and Mrs. Wanglie regained consciousness, she could well have been worse off. She would still be attached to a respirator and would still have irreversible pulmonary disease as well as being severely disabled neurologically. Second, Ackerman presented no evidence that the members of the HMO would support paying higher premiums to underwrite the care of patients like Mrs. Wanglie. Polls have shown that a great majority of Americans would not wish to be kept alive under circumstances like Mrs. Wanglie's. Why should we suppose that others would be willing to pay for the cost of her care when they would not choose that care for themselves?

Angell, the editor of the New England Journal of Medicine, also applied the autonomy principle to support the court's decision to make Oliver Wanglie his wife's guardian. "Any other decision," she wrote, "would be inimical to patient autonomy and would have undermined the consensus on the right-to-die that has been carefully crafted since the Quinlan case."[4]

I do not agree with Angell's statement that a decision supporting the hospital and Mrs. Wanglie's physicians would endanger the right-to-die consensus. Legally, the doctrine of patient autonomy and the right to die are predicated on a patient's liberty interest in rejecting unwanted medical treatment and exist in dependently of any right of access to treatment. This principle was expressed as early as 1914 by Judge Cardozo in his assertion that "every human being of adult years and sound mind has a right to determine what shall be done with his own body..."[5] As Tomlinson and Brody and Veatch and Spicer noted, it does not follow that the existence of a right to reject unwanted treatment implies a similar right to receive desired treatment.[6,7]

There has been a fundamental dissatisfaction among many physicians with the view that the role of medicine is to provide treatment as long as the possibility of extending biologic life remains. It is out of this disaffection, in part, that many physicians have endorsed the principle of patient autonomy, viewing it as supporting the limiting of treatment when further treatment would only prolong the process of dying. Such was the case with Quinlan, Cruzan, and numerous other patients who faced an "existence" of dependence on tube feedings and respirators without possibility of recovery.

The Wanglie case represented a significant turning point. From the clinicians' perspective, adherence to patient autonomy no longer yielded the desired result when patients requested treatment considered by the clinician to be of no benefit. Beleaguered physicians, in attempting to resolve the conflict between patient autonomy and their belief in the necessity of limiting treatment in selected cases, embraced the concept of medical futility. They believed it could offer an effective and equitable resolution to questions of limiting treatment at the margins of life.

Medical Futility and the Appropriateness of Care

The conflict between Mrs. Wanglie's physicians and her family echoed current discussion within the medical profession concerning the issue of medical futility and the limits of care. This discourse centers around the question of whether physicians have a responsibility to provide care they consider to be "futile," "non beneficial," or "medically inappropriate." The corollary to this question is whether patients or their surrogates have a fight to demand such treatment.

Arguments in favor of granting physicians authority to limit care in cases where continued treatment is thought to be futile are similar in many respects to earlier arguments in favor of physician autonomy. Common to each is the assumption that physicians are agents whose moral authority both authorizes and obligates them to make decisions based on their perceptions of their patients' best interest. To ascertain whether a proposed treatment will help or hurt a patient, the physician must evaluate both means and ends. Is treatment X likely to accomplish its goal? Is goal Y within the realm of appropriate medical goals? If either the treatment (means) or its goal (ends) is found to be inappropriate, then the physician has no obligation to offer that treatment. Fundamental to this point of view is the assumption that physicians owe no duty to assist patients or families in at training nonmedical goals.

The courts have traditionally accorded the medical profession the authority to determine its own standards of practice. This principle is recognized as part of the basic law of medical malpractice. The standard by which an individual physician is judged is based on the practice of other physicians.

At present, there is no universally recognized standard of medical practice regarding the treatment of patients like Helga Wanglie. Until relatively recently, PVS patients like Helga Wanglie usually died quickly of complications of their multiple medical problems. Patients like Nancy Cruzan were cared for at home or in chronic care facilities. They rarely occupied ICU beds. Patients like Helga Wanglie, however, are increasingly common as the capacity of medicine and technology to stretch the limits of life continues to expand and consume health care resources.

In response to the dilemmas posed by caring for hopelessly ill patients, organized medicine has formulated a series of consensus reports. Often these efforts have come from societies representing specialty areas within medicine. For example, the report from the Society of Critical Care Medicine states:

> Treatments that offer no benefit and serve to prolong the dying process should not be employed. In light of a hopeless prognosis, the indefinite maintenance of patients reliably diagnosed as being in a persistent vegetative state (PVS) raises serious ethical concerns both for the dignity of the patient and for the diversion of limited medical and nursing resources from alternative applications that could offer medical and nursing benefit to others. The PVS patient should be removed from the ICU unless it is not possible otherwise to meet the patient's nursing care needs. A PVS patient should not be maintained in the ICU to the exclusion of a patient who can derive benefit from ICU care.[8]

The effect of such reports has been to foster the beginnings of a consensus within the medical profession on the appropriate care of patients for whom aggressive medical treatment is felt to offer no benefit. Reports like that of the Society of Critical Care Medicine are based on the principles of physician autonomy and beneficence. However, they add to the moral basis of their argument the concept, rooted in classical Greek medicine, that a physician owes no duty to provide futile care.[9]

The reluctance of Helga Wanglie's doctors to continue aggressive treatment stemmed from their belief that such treatment was "futile" and not in her best interests. In their estimation, further intensive care offered no hope of either improvement in her medical condition or in the quality of her life, and therefore did not serve an appropriate medical purpose. As her physicians, they considered that they were uniquely qualified to determine whether continued treatment was warranted.

The Wanglie family, however, believed that continued treatment was not futile because it would prolong Mrs. Wanglie's life. In addition, irrespective of questions of futility, the family maintained that only they had authority to discontinue treatment.

Oliver Wanglie's refusal to accede to his wife's physicians created a problem for the hospital and medical staff. They felt that they could not ethically use physician prerogative to override his refusal to terminate treatment nor could they invoke such authority based upon their right to act in Mrs. Wanglie's "best interests." Instead, the hospital administrators and her physicians argued that continued aggressive care was "inappropriate medical treatment"[10] and "non-beneficial in that it could not heal her lungs, palliate her suffering, or enable this unconscious and permanently respirator-dependent woman to experience the benefit of the life afforded by respirator-support."[11] Because the hospital anticipated that others would argue that the respirator was effective in keeping her alive by enabling her lungs to perform their respiratory function, it chose not to characterize the respirator as futile.[12]

Much of the discussion on futility and the limits of care has focused on finding a clinically useful definition of futility that would be broadly supported within the medical profession. The differing perspectives of Mrs. Wanglie's family and physicians on the definition of futility are critical because there is currently no clear agreement on just what constitutes futile medical treatment. To be useful to physicians, a definition of futility must be applicable not only in situations like the Wanglie case, about which there was relative consensus, but also in relation to more ambiguous cases, which are more common and do not lie at such an extreme along the futility continuum. For example, is a respirator futile treatment for an 86-year-old person with severe, irreversible pulmonary disease who develops pneumonia that might be successfully treated?[13]

One of the principal reasons that futility is difficult to define is that a treatment can only be futile in relation to a specific goal. Consequently, discussions about futility must inevitably become discussions about the appropriateness of goals as well. For example, Oliver Wanglie's assertion that his wife's respirator was not futile treatment was not irrational. From his perspective the respirator accomplished its job of keeping his wife alive. He simply differed with her physicians about the goals of using the respirator.

In an article on futility in clinical practice, Lantos and colleagues acknowledged the difficulty of defining futility, which they described as "simply the end of a spectrum of low-efficacy therapies."[14] In many circumstances, physicians are unable to reach agreement that a particular therapy is futile and thus not worth pursuing.[15]

Lantos *et al.* found two principal sources for this disagreement: 1) physicians may reasonably differ over the chance of a treatment success, and 2) they may not concur as to the goals of the therapy. A significant source of disagreement among physicians or among patients, their families, and their physicians may be because they value outcomes, including symbolic outcomes, differently.[16] Furthermore, both social and psychological factors may interfere with the physician's estimation of the likelihood of success or assessment of the goals of therapy.[17,18]

The same factors may also interfere with a patient's or family's estimation of the probability of success or their interpretation of the goals of therapy. The Wanglies obviously disagreed with the physicians with regard to both the likelihood of success (they believed a miracle might happen) and the goals of therapy (any state of life is worth preserving at all costs).

Schneiderman, who is both a physician and ethicist, and his colleagues also used probability of success in relation to treatment goals as the cornerstone of an analysis of medical futility.[19] They argued that futility can be expressed in either quantitative or qualitative terms. A treatment can be said to be futile in a quantitative sense when the expectation of success is "so unlikely that its exact probability is incalculable."[20] In practice, they suggested that if a treatment has been useless in the previous 100 cases as determined by the physician's own experience or that of colleagues or as documented in the medical literature, then it can be said to be futile.

Schneiderman's approach is open to criticism. First, one must ask whose goals the treatment is useless in relation to -- the patient's or the physician's? Furthermore, because they value outcomes differently, physicians may disagree over whether a treatment is useless. Second, in considering the probability of success of treatment, most physicians operate at an impressionistic level. Few physicians can count 100 cases within their own experience with enough similarity to the case at hand to yield a useful comparison. Even fewer have the time to do the research that would be required to make such an outcome assessment. Schneiderman's method of assessing quantitative futility is simply impractical.

The goal of treatment, according to Schneiderman *et al.*, should be "improvement of the patient's prognosis, comfort, well-being, or general state of health."[21] Treatment that is futile in a qualitative sense is, therefore, one that "merely preserves permanent unconsciousness or that fails to end total dependence on intensive medical care."[22] Any treatment that fails to meet either the quantitative or qualitative standard is considered futile or non-beneficial and physicians are not required to provide that treatment. Continuing to provide aggressive care to Helga Wanglie clearly meets Schneiderman *et al.*'s criterion for qualitative futility.

This definition of qualitative futility, however, ignores the fact that some patients and families might elect treatment that preserves permanent unconsciousness or total dependence on ICU care, particularly when the alternative is death. Qualitative futility as presented by Schneiderman *et al.*'s justified by an appeal to the principles of physician autonomy and beneficence. Although their proposal may make sense from a health policy perspective, policies involving limiting care to PVS patients should be based on public and professional consensus. They presented no evidence, however, that such a consensus exists.

The concept of medical futility has been criticized from the perspective of both the principle of patient autonomy and the tenets of the right-to-life movement because it relies excessively on the physician's value judgments, which may or may not be in accord with the patient's values. Tomlinson and Brody, in their discussion of futility in the context of cardiopulmonary resuscitation, readily acknowledged that futility judgments inevitably involve value judgments as well.[23] They asserted that the everyday practice of medicine involves frequent value judgments that lead physicians to recommend one treatment over another.

Physicians, they argued, must have the authority to evaluate the goals of treatment to fulfill their obligations to patients. Professional responsibility requires that physicians have the discretion to decide when the treatment offers no benefit to the patient or is likely to do more harm than good.[24] In either case, the physician has no obligation to offer the treatment. From this perspective, the measurement of benefit, harm, and good is ultimately part of the physician's duty to the patient.

Several recent articles have emphasized the inherent limitations of basing medical decisions on futility arguments.[25] Common to each of them is the understanding that, with the exception of those treatments that cannot possibly achieve their desired outcomes, judgments about medical futility are ultimately subjective. They depend upon assessments not only of the achievability of a goal, but also of the appropriateness of the goal as viewed by the physician.

Given that patient autonomy may dictate that physicians provide to PVS patients care that they deem inappropriate, the authors have sought to establish a rationale for withholding treatment for PVS patients that is independent of both patient autonomy and medical futility arguments. Although acknowledging the importance of autonomy in medical ethics, Truog *et al.*, Veatch and Spicer and Brody each emphasized that the dictates of patient autonomy must be balanced against the competing claims of equitable allocation of resources and respect for the integrity of the health care professions.

Truog and his colleagues, all of whom are physicians, created what are, in effect, guidelines for clinicians who are faced with treatment requests that they feel should not be honored from patients or surrogates. When confronted with such a conflict, Truog *et al.* suggested that initial efforts be focused on clarification of the issues and improvement of communication. If these efforts fail and the patient's request represents a conflict with professional ethics, then the physician should either transfer the patient to another provider[26] or bring the conflict into a public forum, such as a hospital ethics committee or the courts.[27]

Truog *et al.*, however, did not address the issue of how an ethics committee should approach the issue nor did they tell us how a physician should respond to the committee's suggestions. If, for example, the committee should endorse withholding further care, is the physician then free to do so?

Veatch and Spicer pointed out that autonomy is a liberty fight, and although it unequivocally confers the fight to reject unwanted treatment, it does not imply a corresponding fight to access to care. In general, Veatch and Spicer proposed that life-prolonging care desired by a competent patient should always be provided, the sole exception being those cases in which care imposes an inequitable burden on society or third parties.[28] However, in such cases it is society, rather than the clinician, that must decide to terminate care. This would be effected through a societal decision not to pay for such care.[29]

This suggestion yields little comfort to the clinician faced with this situation because it is precisely the clinician who must give the order to "cut the patient off." Simply because society or an insurance company will not pay for a specific type of care does not mean the physician's or the hospital's duty to the patient is terminated. Indeed, recent case law suggests that when patients require a specific treatment, physicians may have a duty to contest the insurer's decision.[30]

Like Truog *et al.* and Veatch and Spicer and Brody rejected futility-based arguments as sufficient reason to limit care for PVS patients, in part because he argued that the prolongation of life is an intrinsic goal of medicine. Brody suggested that PVS patients should instead be accorded a lower priority for care, based on society's need to ensure a rational and equitable allocation of its scarce health care resources.[31] Rationing care to PVS patients is justified because they "are not persons in any plausible account of personhood."[32] Unlike Veatch and Spicer, Brody argued that individual physicians have a role in decisions to allocate care. Although acknowledging that to do so might represent a conflict with a physician's duty to the patient, he pointed out that in the practice of medicine a physician must inevitably deal with competing claims involving patients, society, family, and profession. The physician's goal is to achieve a fair balance among these claims rather than to emphasize only one of them.[33]

Taking the Wanglie Case to Court

There is disagreement among commentators on the Wanglie case regarding the appropriateness of the hospital's legal strategy. Schwartz and Mishkin, both of whom are attorneys, suggested that the hospital chose to litigate the wrong issue. By focusing on the appointment of an independent conservator for Helga Wang lie, the hospital's legal strategy failed when it did not achieve the goal of having the court appoint a third party as Mrs. Wanglie's conservator. Given Minnesota law, the court may well have had no recourse other than to appoint Oliver Wang lie as his wife's guardian.[34] The district court thus did not have the opportunity to address the fundamental issues of the Wanglie case. Had the hospital instead pursued a court order allowing it to terminate the respirator, then the court would have had to directly address the issue of whether Mrs. Wanglie's physicians could lawfully cease life support based on their determination that continued aggressive treatment would not provide her medical benefit.

Callahan, however, argued that the decision to go to court was premature. Because there is at present no public consensus regarding the issues presented by the Wanglie case, to move toward a judicial determination before that consensus has developed risks unfairness to the Wanglies as well as the possibility that a judge might decide that PVS patients have an absolute fight to aggressive care irrespective of futility or lack of medical benefit. Callahan urged caution in proceeding toward judicial solutions until physicians and the lay public are able to develop appropriate standards.[35]

Callahan's analysis, however, ignored the role that judicial proceedings have in the development of a public and professional consensus. Until the hospital went to court, Helga Wanglie was simply another patient in the Hennepin County Medical Center ICU. The ensuing discussion of the issues raised by the Wanglie case in the press and professional literature occurred precisely because the hospital attempted a judicial resolution. The act of going to court focused public attention on Mrs. Wanglie.

The same argument can be applied to the development of the right-to-die consensus over the past two decades. That consensus exists today in part because the parents of Karen Quinlan and Nancy Cruzan sought judicial relief. Adjudication is appropriate in cases like Helga Wanglie's because it brings into focus the contending arguments and stimulates public and professional discussion of the critical issues.

The Courts should not be invoked in all end-of-life decisions. The court is not a substitute for empathic and reasoned discussions between physicians and patients and families. Nor does the court supplant the role of hospital ethics committees. As Schwartz noted, ethics committees can provide a valuable service by helping the court to focus upon the fundamental issues involving withdrawal of care in cases when that care is beyond the limits of medicine.[36] Rather, the courts have an important role in the social and political processes that underlie the creation of consensus.

Looking to the Future

Decisions to limit care for PVS patients should not be made by physicians alone. Rather, a broad consensus representing informed medical, legal, ethical, and lay opinion is required. Attempts at achieving consensus must ultimately address the question of what are the limits of autonomy. Does a patient's unequivocal right to reject unwanted care extend to a right of access to desired care? If the care is capable of achieving the ends desired by the patient and is technically feasible to deliver, does the physician have a duty to provide that care? Do patients have a special fight to life-sustaining care?

Initially, efforts to answer these questions should be limited to patients in a persistent vegetative state, in part because there already exists within the medical community the basis for a consensus regarding their care. In addition, the focus should be on withholding intensive and hospital-based care rather than on withholding all care. Limiting the discussion in this fashion is in keeping with the principle of equitable allocation of resources as the ethical basis for withholding care.

Consensus building should focus upon three basic questions. First, do clinicians have an ethical responsibility to provide on request hospital-based care to PVS patients? This question should be addressed by hospital ethics committees, professional groups, public policy groups, and community organizations.

Second, do clinicians have a legal duty to provide such care when requested? This is a matter for the legislatures and the courts. Assuming that it is determined that no duty exists, then either statutory or common law protection must be extended in the form of a "hold harmless" policy to those clinicians who, in good faith, withhold requested care.

Third, should insurers pay for hospital-based care for PVS patients? Efforts to achieve consensus on this issue are properly directed to legislatures and administrative agencies as well as commercial insurers. If it is determined that neither an ethical nor a legal duty to provide such care exists, then, as a matter of public policy, it is proper that insurers should not pay for such care.

Although this consensus is developing, we must continue to address these issues forthrightly, one case at a time. Unless we do so, physicians will continue to "err on the side of caution" and, on demand, provide treatments of question able benefit to patients like Mrs. Wanglie. As Stephen Miles noted, this would represent the "ultimate irony in a country that does not recognize a universal right to beneficial therapies."[37]

Notes

1. For the facts of the Wanglie case I have relied on two sources. Miles SH. Informed demand for "non-beneficial" medical treatment, *New England Journal of Medicine* 1991;325:512. Cranford RE. Helga Wanglie's ventilator, *Hastings Center Report* 1991;21(4):23.
2. Ackerman F. The significance of a wish, *Hastings Center Report* 1991;21(4):27-28.
3. See note 2. Ackerman. 1991;21(4):29.
4. Angell M. The case of Helga Wanglie, *New England Journal of Medicine* 1991;325:511.
5. *Schloendorff v. New York Hospital*, 1914:211 NY 125.
6. Tomlinson T, Brody H. Futility and the ethics of resuscitation, *Journal of the American Medical Association* 1990;264:1276-9.
7. Veatch RM, Spicer CM. Medically futile care: The role of the physician in setting limits, *American Journal of Law and Medicine* 1992;18:15-23.
8. Task Force on Ethics of the Society of Critical Care Medicine. Consensus report on the ethics of foregoing life-sustaining treatments of the critically ill, *Critical Care Medicine* 1990;18:1437. Quoted In: Rie MA. The limits of a wish, *Hastings Center Report* 1991;21(4):24-25.
9. Lantos JD, Singer JD, Walker RM, *et al.* The illusion of futility in clinical practice, *American Journal of Medicine* 1989;87:81.
10. See note 1. Cranford. 1991;21(4):23.
11. See note 1. Miles. 1991;325:513.
12. See note 1. Miles. 1991;325:513.
13. This was Helga Wanglie's statement at the beginning of her saga.
14. See note 9. Lantos *et al.* 1989;87:81.
15. See note 9. Lantos *et al.* 1989;87:82.
16. See note 9. Lantos *et al.* 1989;87:83.
17. See note 9. Lantos *et al.* 1989;87:82.
18. For a comprehensive review of the pitfalls of decision-making under conditions of uncertainty, see Tversky A, Kahneman D. Judgment under uncertainty: Heuristics and biases, *Science* 1974;185:1124.
19. Schneiderman LJ, Jecker NS, Jonsen AR. Medical futility: Its meaning and ethical implications, *Annals of Internal Medicine* 1990;112:950.
20. See note 19. Schneiderman *et al.* 1990;112:950.
21. See note 19. Schneiderman *et al.* 1990;112:950.

22. See note 19. Schneiderman *et al.* 1990;112:950.
23. See note 6. Tomlinson, Brody. 1990;264:1277.
24. See note 6. Tomlinson, Brody. 1990;264:1277.
25. Truog RD, Brett AS, Frader J. The problem with futility, *New England Journal of Medicine* 1992;326:1560-4. See note 7. Veatch, Spicer. 1992;18:15. Brody B. Special ethical issues in the management of PVS patients, *Law, Medicine and Health Care* 1992;20:104.
26. Physicians chose this route out of their ethical conflict in the Baby L case. See Paris JJ, Krone, RK, Reardon F. Physicians' refusal of requested treatment, *New England Journal of Medicine* 1990;322:1012.
27. See note 25. Truog *et al.* 1992;326:1563.
28. See note 7. Veatch, Spicer. 1992;18:23.
29. See note 7. Veatch, Spicer. 1992;18:29.
30. *Wickline v. State of California*, 228 Cal. Rptr. 661 (Cal. App. 2 Dist. 1986).
31. See note 25. Brody. 1992;20:113.
32. See note 25. Brody. 1992;20:104.
33. See note 25. Brody. 1992;20:113.
34. Schwartz R. Autonomy, futility, and the limits of medicine, *Cambridge Quarterly of Healthcare Ethics* 1992;1:159-64.
35. Callahan D. Medical futility, medical necessity, *Hastings Center Report* 1991;21(4):30, 34.
36. See note 34. Schwartz. 1992;1:163.
37. Miles SH. Legal procedures in Wanglie: A two-step, not a sidestep, *Journal of Clinical Ethics* 1991;2:285-6.

Chapter 57

What Does Life Support Support?

Albert R. Jonsen

The question "What does life support support?" is a daunting one. Given the awesome dimensions of the concept "life," it is difficult to know what sources of evidence to draw upon or what manner of analysis to employ. In the absence of clear directions, the ancient style adopted by preachers (although this essay is not a sermon) might be appropriate: cite a text, relate a parable, and then expatiate somewhat on the meaning of text and parable for human life. Unlike the sermon, whose text and parable preachers select from their Scriptures, the text for this essay comes from a very contemporary source, the *New York Times*; the parable is a story from the most up-to-date critical care unit. The text is a brief letter that appeared as a comment on a piece written several weeks earlier by Judge Irving R. Kaufman of New York:[1]

> As a physician and particularly as a director of a hemodialysis unit, I applaud Judge Irving R. Kaufman's effort to bring the issue of the technological prolongation of life of the terminally ill from the isolation of ethical contemplation to the public arena with a plea for society to institutionalize its moral verdicts by legislation... [B]oth physicians and families must daily face Judge Kaufman's question: "Under what circumstances may life sustaining therapies be withheld from a severely deformed or terminally ill person?"[2]

The writer, Robert L. Scheer, then makes a rather peculiar statement; this statement is the text for this essay:

> In the absence of a clearly stated instruction from the patient, I cannot stop artificial kidney treatments, regardless of how useless such treatments may have become in saving the patient's life. And, contrary to popular belief, the family of such a patient cannot tell us to stop dialysis or do anything but attest to their knowledge of the patient's previously expressed desires...

An answer is urgently needed.

Is it not strange that a physician writes that he feels obliged to continue a treatment "regardless of how useless such treatments may have become?" Is it not strange for anyone to feel obliged to perform the useless? Yet, these words are a striking expression of the paradoxes we presently face in using the technologies generally described as "life support." This paradoxical remark of the letter writer stands, then, as the text for this essay.

Source: Reprinted from *The Pharos*, Winter 1987, pp. 4-7, with permission from Alpha Omega Alpha Honor Medical Society © 1987.

A parable is defined as "a short fictitious story used to illustrate a religious or moral lesson." The following parable is short and will illustrate a moral point but is real rather than fictitious. Two years ago, in Moffitt/Long Hospital, University of California at San Francisco, a young woman lay for sixty-four days in the intensive care unit. She was legally dead from the moment of her admission. She had been legally dead from the time she left the referring hospital in Northern California. Yet for sixty-four days, her bodily processes were maintained in order to bring to viability the fetus in her womb. When she died as the result of a cerebral accident, she was pregnant with a twenty-two-week fetus. At the plea of her husband, and with the agreement of physicians, she was intubated and immediately brought to our hospital, where the most refined and sophisticated techniques were applied to maintain her vital processes until her baby could be safely delivered. A healthy baby, slightly premature, was delivered from a cadaver. The woman who had conceived the infant was not in persistent vegetative condition. She was not in permanent coma. She was literally brain dead, meaning that there was clear neurological evidence that she had lost irreversibly all functions of the brain, including those of the brain stem. That is the legal definition of brain death in the state of California and most states in the union. This is the parable for a moral lesson.

All the medical techniques used to accomplish that feat are the techniques casually referred to as "life support." The ventilator, hemodialysis, intravenous alimentation, and hydration are commonly applied to the living to support life. In this case, for most of the time those techniques were used, they were applied to a cadaver. It seems rather inaccurate to talk about life support of a cadaver. The parable obviously illustrates an extreme case. Yet it points out again, just as the text does, some of the paradoxes posed by contemporary technological means of the support of vital processes. In moving from text and parable toward an answer to the question that titles this essay, a brief review of medical history will reveal how this paradoxical situation arose. Each step in the development has been an important and positive one in itself. Yet, taken together, they create a difficult medical and moral problem.

A few readers may recall the Drinker Tank; perhaps a few wise, white-headed physicians actually used one. Such mechanical behemoths lie shrouded in dust in the basement of a hospital here and there. At the beginning of the history of modern life support techniques is the Drinker Tank. This device, more commonly known as the "iron lung," was a time-cycled negative pressure ventilator: an iron cylinder that enclosed the patient up to the neck. By applying a rhythmic cycle of subatmospheric pressure in phase with inspiration, it created a rebound effect that facilitated expiration. This clumsy ancestor of all life support systems was invented by Philip Drinker and Louis Shaw in 1928 to deal with the devastating polio epidemics of that era. At the height of these epidemics in the late 1940s, close to 4,000 patients were treated in this manner annually. Improved understanding of the disease process and of respiratory physiology led to a high rate of success. In a study of 500 acute poliomyelitic respiratory patients, 73 percent of the patients became free of the respirator within two years of treatment. Of those, 83 percent became respirator free within six months.[3]

In 1953, John H. Gibbon, Jr., performed heart surgery during which the life of the patient was supported entirely by the blood oxygenator that he had painfully developed over the previous quarter century. This heart-lung machine made possible the age of cardiac surgery.[4] During the 1960s much more efficient and sophisticated positive pressure ventilators came into use, giving rise to the modern intensive care unit. At the same time, renal dialysis, which had been pioneered by Willem J. Kolff in the 1940s, became possible on an ongoing basis, due to Belding H. Scribner's invention of the arteriovenous access shunt.[5] During the 1970s great progress was made in perfecting techniques for intravenous alimentation and for hyperalimentation.

Finally, the opening years of the eighties saw the first clinical use of implanted mechanical circulatory supports, both the totally implantable artificial heart and the left ventricular device, either of them being used on a temporary or permanent basis.[6]

This very sketchy history, which could have included other devices and other events, shows that when we speak of life support, we describe a technical-physiological interface that enables the delivery of nutrients that are essential for metabolism, allows the elimination of wastes, and provides the mechanical and electrochemical energy to sustain vital activities. Each of these techniques, in and of itself, sustains, or substitutes for, an organ vital to integration of the organism. That is precisely what was done in the case of the young mother at Moffitt/Long Hospital. A chain of machines was put together to provide a technological interface with a physiological process. Each particular process was integrated with other processes, delivering nutrients, eliminating wastes, and providing necessary stimulus for energy.

All of this is marvelous. Patients are alive today, in intensive care and cardiac care and neonatal intensive care units, whose lives are being supported precisely by these means. Many of those patients will not leave the hospital. Many more will leave the hospital and succumb within a fairly short period of time, as recent studies on the mortality and morbidity of patients who have gone through intensive care demonstrate.[7] Many will return home healthy and well. Clearly, these developments are extraordinarily beneficial to many human beings. Why, then, is there a problem? Why does the writer of our opening text have a problem? Why does Judge Kaufman have a problem? And why do we call it an ethical problem?

There are certainly plenty of technical problems with life support. Most of the major techniques have their limitations and their adverse effects. The recent history of the artificial heart demonstrates the range of technical problems that have to be overcome to provide an effective and efficient mechanical circulatory support system. Each implantation shows some new problem that is not precisely anticipated. The problem of emboli, for example, resulting primarily from the structure of the valves in those hearts, was not anticipated in the animal studies, which had suggested that the major problem would be hemolysis. Yet, each clinical experience teaches its lessons. And so it has been with the other major technologies; ventilators advanced from negative to positive pressures, hemodialysis found more efficient routes of access, etc.

So each new technology presents new clinical and technological problems; continual improvement and refinement goes on with all of them. But we say that these technologies also pose ethical problems. Indeed, it is commonly suggested that the concern about ethical problems in medicine is stimulated primarily by the advances in medical technology. So, there is a general impression that this enormously positive and quite beneficial development creates ethical problems. It may be useful to be more precise about the nature of these problems: In our civilization, we have gotten very good at defining technical problems and remain fairly primitive in defining ethical ones.

Two features of life support or, better, organ support technology give rise to the ethical question. Both are features not so much of the technology but of its historical development. One is that the technical developments have moved from partial support to total support. We speak of a "support system." The Drinker Tank was a mechanical device able to exert mechanical pressure sufficient to substitute for the loss of the intercostal musculature. It performed one function only: it moved air in and out. But, as technologies for support of other organs were invented, machine came to be added to machine in tandem. It does little good, for example, to be able to deal with respiratory failure if there is no way to eliminate wastes, should kidneys fail. To the ventilatory support is added dialysis and to these, hyperalimentation; the elements of total system, getting essential nutrients in and wastes out, are being assembled. This, in effect, was done in the parable of the cadaver mother.

It is relatively rare that patients end up on total system, although some patients get fairly close to it. Yet, as the steps toward total system are taken in an intensive care unit, signs of concern appear among those responsible for the care of the patient. Intubation is almost routine. When dialysis needs to be added, some questions are raised, and when the need for hyperalimentation arises, people begin to argue. As steps are taken toward total system, the suspicion appears that an ethical problem is brewing. Of course, we must recognize that the total system is not really total. It is only quasi-total. And here we glimpse one of the genuine reasons why we have an ethical problem. The system is quasi-total because we have no direct brain support system. The brain can be perfused by supporting ventilatory and circulatory systems, but that is indirect brain support. When the central nervous system is seriously damaged, particularly in its higher cognitive functions, we have no direct intervention. Thus we confront the sort of patient about whom ethical questions are most frequently raised: one whose heart and lungs and kidneys and circulatory system are being supported but whose cognitive functions are profoundly and permanently destroyed.

The parable of the cadaver mother illustrates this most vividly: it is very obvious that she is no longer a person in the world. Her fetus is being nurtured in a cadaver; had it not been for that intrauterine life, she would have been consigned to the grave. The situation can be slightly changed: a pregnant woman has lost cerebral functions and fits the criteria for persistent vegetative condition. Such a person is not in fact dead, but such a person will never feel any consciousness, will never experience the joy of being a new mother, will never see her child grow. The most famous case of life support in recent times, Karen Ann Quinlan, exemplified the support of a life without consciousness; many of the cases now under review by the courts are of this sort. These are the cases that troubled Judge Kaufman and Dr. Scheer. They should trouble us all. Thus, the fact of quasi-total life support is the first facet of the ethical problem.

The second reason we worry about life support arises from the move from temporary support systems to permanent support systems. The ancients who remember the Drinker Tank might recall that it was intended for temporary use, although for many unfortunate patients it turned permanent. When we see old photos of vast wards with twenty and thirty people permanently in iron lungs, we forget that its inventors and users hoped that it would supply for temporary loss of muscular power; if respite could be given, the power would, it was hoped, be restored. In fact, by the mid 1950s, only 13 percent of patients remained dependent two years after initiation of treatment; half of these needed support only at night.[3] The intent to devise a technique for permanent use does not appear until the development of chronic hemodialysis (if we exclude the internal cardiac pacemaker). Now there is mechanical circulatory support, which can be used either on a permanent or temporary basis. It is interesting that the temporary use of the circulatory support devices was almost bypassed to jump into the permanent use. It is almost as if the temporary adjunct to nature has been forgotten in the enthusiasm to build a technological person.

We are now seeing the move from temporary to permanent systems in many situations, such as the use of the ventilator for patients with chronic lung disease or for young people with muscular dystrophy who are put on ventilators permanently at the age of fourteen or fifteen. Once again, however, as in the partial to total move, we recognize that we are not dealing with permanent in the genuine sense, but only of the quasi-permanent. No matter how long support can be provided, a time comes when death conquers even the power of the machine. Yet, with artificial hearts, with ventilators, with other sorts of implanted systems, permanent support to the end of persons' lives seems to many a desirable objective. They will live out those lives with a machine as an intimate part of themselves. We know little about how humans will tolerate the technology-personal interface. Obviously, we have two decades of experience with renal dialysis. Obviously, people will, as they always do, react in unique fashion. Still, I believe we here encounter another reason to think of life support as an ethical problem: we face the fact that there will be people living who are not entirely themselves.

Indeed, both in the dimensions of time and space, persons whose lives are supported in this fashion, may not be "themselves."

We talk about the maintenance of life; we don't often talk about the maintenance of personhood. It interests me little, indeed, not at all, to be alive as an organism. In such a state, I have no interests. It is enormously interesting for me to be a person. With my history, with my place in life, doing the things I enjoy doing, loving those I love, causing the problems that I like to cause, I live my life. It is the perpetuation of my personhood that interests me; indeed, it is, probably, my major and, perhaps, my sole real interest. Life support development or organ support development, however, has led us to the situation in which personhood seems either totally or partially lost, while organic life is maintained. This is, of course, a profound philosophical problem: the very nature of human life and personhood.

The profound philosophical problem, which has been pondered by savants since the beginnings of our culture, need not be answered in full in order to reach some acceptable resolutions of particular problems. During the past decade, many of the perplexing questions about foregoing life support have been addressed by physicians, philosophers, and by the law. The work of the President's Commission for the Study of Ethical Problems in Medicine and Biomedical and Behavioral Research (1979,1982) drew the scholarly speculation and the practical suggestions into policy formulations that met widespread approval. Two reports of the commission, in particular, advanced the understanding of ethical issues surrounding life support, Defining Death (1981)[8] and Deciding to Forego Life-Sustaining Treatment (1983).[9]

Defining Death reviewed the scientific, philosophical, theological, and legal considerations that underlie the determination that death has occurred. The report clarified the criteria for declaring a person dead on the evidence that all functions of the brain had irreversibly ceased. A Uniform Definition of Death Statute was proposed, which has been adopted into law in the majority of states. This action has eliminated the widespread confusion about the term "brain death," which to some meant permanent loss of consciousness and to others loss of intrinsic organic unity. The Uniform Statute selects the latter as the most appropriate concept for public policy and clinical decision making.[8]

Deciding to Forego Life-Sustaining Treatment reviewed the principles and values involved in the application of various technological means of supporting life. The appropriate use of cardiopulmonary resuscitation and the conditions under which life-sustaining technology might be withheld or withdrawn were examined in detail. In general, the principle of "proportionality" should govern these decisions: the benefits deriving from any intervention should, in the eyes of the patient or those responsible for the patient's well-being, balance the burdens that the patient may have to bear as a result of the treatment. The report analyzed certain clinical situations in the light of this general treatment and concluded that sound justification could support the decision to forego life support. The clearest of those situations are the ones in which intervention would be medically futile, or when a competent patient has refused treatment, or when a patient is deemed to be in a persistent vegetative state.[9]

Nonetheless, despite notable advances in understanding the ethics of life support, the ancient philosophical problem remains. It is not impossible to appreciate that the support of organic life alone, as in the case of brain death, or the support of life in which all signs of consciousness are extinguished imposes no moral obligation. It makes sense, within the values of our culture, to respect the choice of a competent person who dismisses the further attendance of physicians, even if death will result. Yet, the problems posed by the capability of technological support pass beyond these cases. Often, the consciousness of the patient is not extinguished but is diminished or has never matured. Often, the physical experiences of such a patient appear to others to be painful or, at best, uncomfortable, despite solicitous care. Such patients are those about whom we ask the questions raised above: Is quasi-total or quasi-permanent support of continued life an obligation that can be demonstrated to fall on physicians and others responsible for the patient? If life cannot be lived in a fashion that the person, even with profound limitations, finds tolerable, must anyone with technological skills strive to support that life?

The meaning of life is a perennial philosophical question and will not be answered any better by modern bioethicists than by the Greeks, the Medievals or the Enlightenment savants. We do have, however, a dimension of the problem that they did not, namely, life totally or quasi-totally, and permanently, or quasi-permanently, supported by machine. The philosophers may ponder this problem. Yet, we will always return to the intuition that life is supported, not by any machines, however wonderful, but by the personal perception of one's history, by the love of one's family and friends, by engagement, however simple, in the ongoing currents of the social and natural world. Unless our life-support technology can support such life, it is empty of human significance. The bodies of those ravaged by disease must be supported so that they can awake to signs of the human world.

Notes

1. Kaufman IR. Life-and-death decisions. *New York Times* 1985 Oct 6.
2. Scheer RL. Decisions of life and death require our judges' guidance, letter to the editor. *New York Times* 1985 Oct 19:26.
3. Affeldt JE, Bower AG, Dail CW, *et al*. Prognosis for respiratory recovery in severe poliomyelitis, *Arch Phys Med Rehab* 1957;38:290-95.
4. Comroe JH Jr. *Exploring the Heart: Discoveries in Heart Disease and High Blood Pressure*. New York, NY: W.W. Norton & Co., 1983.
5. Scribner BH, Blagg CR. Maintenance dialysis, In: Rapaport FT, Dausset J, eds. *Human Transplantation*. New York, NY: Grune & Stratton, 1968:80-99.
6. Shaw MW, ed. *After Barney Clark: Reflections on the Utah Artificial Heart Program*. Austin, TX: University of Texas Press, 1984.
7. Myers LP, Shroeder SA, Chapman SA, *et al*. What's so special about special care? *Inquiry* 1984;21:113-27.
8. President's Commission for the Study of Ethical Problems in Medicine and Biomedical and Behavioral Research. *Defining Death: A Report on the Medical, Legal and Ethical sues in Determination of Death*. Washington, DC: U.S. Government Printing Office, 1981.
9. President's Commission for the Study of Ethical Problems in Medicine and Biomedical and Behavioral Research. *Deciding to Forego Life-Sustaining Treatment: A Report on the Ethical, Medical, and Legal Issues in Treatment Decisions*. Washington, DC: U.S. Government Printing Office, 1983:6089.

Chapter 58

The Sorcerer's Broom -- Medicine's Rampant Technology

Eric J. Cassell

Like the broom in "The Sorcerer's Apprentice," technologies take on a life of their own. To bring them under control, doctors must learn to tolerate ambiguity, resist the lure of the immediate, cease fearing uncertainty, and rechannel their response to wonder.

Major changes are contemplated for health care in the United States, motivated by economic forces and maldistribution of health services. Technology, a thing unique unto itself, however, will confound most any attempt to change the health care system or redirect its fundamental goals. Further, if there is one thing that can be singled out as the engine of the medical economic inflation now occurring everywhere in the world, it is the seemingly irresistible spread of technology into every level of medicine irresistible to doctors, patients, and nations alike. Evidence that technology is a problem is everywhere in medicine. In intensive care units the world over, the technology of monitoring, organ support, and resuscitation is used where it is appropriate -- related to the aims and purposes of the sick person. It is also used where it is inappropriate, defined by the capabilities of the technology and the consequent expertise of physicians rather than -- or even contrary to -- the good of the sick person.

Like the broom in *The Sorcerer's Apprentice*, technologies come to have a life of their own, not only because of their own properties but also because of certain universal human traits. Technologies come into being to serve the purposes of their users, but ultimately their users redefine their own goals in terms of the technology. As a class, technologies are reductive, oversimplifying, impatient, intolerant of ambiguity, and democratic. They spread much more quickly than the ideas that inform them. Democracy has only gradually spread over the world: the transistor radio did it in a decade.

It is not necessary or useful to revisit the long history of the debate about the wonders or dangers of technology except to acknowledge its existence and the literature it has engendered, from Goethe's, *Faust* to Huxley's, *Brave New World*. On the other hand, systematic concern about technology is largely a child of the second half of the twentieth century. (The famous 1911 edition of the Encyclopedia Britannica has no entry on technology, while the 1974 edition devotes thirty pages to it.) This is not an antitechnology essay. In medicine, one can no more be antitechnology than antiscience. There is no going back to a prescientific or nontechnological medicine -- who would want to? The issue is how to solve the difficulty epitomized by Emerson's observation, "Things are in the saddle and ride mankind." Technology is not the problem; it is the relationship to it of those who employ it that is problematic. If this is not solvable, our entire project is a waste of time.

The definition of technology presents problems for which dictionaries are no help,

---

Source: Reprinted from *Hastings Center Report*, Nov-Dec, 1993, pp. 32-39, with permsision from The Hastings Center © 1993.

because the term can be used in a manner so broad as to defeat understanding. Thus, any tool employed in a craft could be said to be that craft's technology. In this discussion, I want to limit the term to the modalities and instrumentalities that greedy extend the power of human action, sensation, or thought in ways that are independent of the particular user. In addition to the instruments and devices usually considered as technology, we should include, for the sake of understanding, high-power medications -- cardiac, antimicrobial, psychotropic, or whatever -- that greatly extend our therapeutic power. It is our power that technology expands.

Technology is not science. They are frequency lumped together-as in "sci-tech" -- but they are distinct. Science is not my topic. The topic is to see what there is about PET scanners, MRI, angioplasty, endoscopy, automated chemistry machines, and so on -- the whole wondrous parade, not the science that spawned them -- that poses problems for medicine.

Technologies are reductive and oversimplifying. Much of their hold on medicine, however, is a result of two prior reductive steps in the history of medicine. The first step was reducing the problem of human illness -- with all its intricate physical, social, emotional, and cultural aspects -- to the biological problem of disease. Diseases were initially defined as physical entities with unique anatomical (later biochemical) characteristics and unique causes. These two unique characteristics permitted precise definitions. Precise definitions, in addition to anatomically (or biochemically) discernable characteristics, finally permitted the productive entrance of science into medicine. The second reductive step follows from the scientific investigation of diseases. Here the findings of science become the accepted picture of the disease, further oversimplifying the problem. The scientific discovery of the disease agent completes the simplification as the agent, for example, the tubercle bacillus, becomes the virtual equivalent of the disease, tuberculosis. These definitions, identifiable characteristics, scientific investigations, and consequent technologies perpetuated the oversimplification of human illness. There is, however, a certain circularity whose presence should be acknowledged. Disease definitions permit the entrance of science. Science increases knowledge of the disease by employing technologies and promoting the development of further technology. These technologies come about became of the scientific understanding of the disease and reinforce the original picture of disease that started the cycle. This circle also contains the values that direct the technologies toward the facts that support the values. Breaking out of such a circle is one of our tasks, but not an easy one.

What I have just noted may be the way technology entered medicine, but knowing this will not end its almost autonomous grog. We will not solve the problem of technology without providing other solutions or defenses against the human characteristics that lead to our difficulty. I will discuss five such characteristics: wonder and wonderment, the lure of the immediate, unambiguous values, the avoidance of uncertainty, and the human desire for power.

Wonder

The first hold that technology has on us I call wonder and wonderment. When I lecture at unfamiliar institutions, I'm frequency taken on a tour of the place. Once, in Pittsburgh, I was shown their new cardiac cath labs -- four of them! Why? Did they think I'd never seen a cath unit? Why didn't they take me by somebody's office (whispering, so as not to disturb) and say, "There's one of our smartest doctors?" Because everybody loves the new and the shiny, especially when it does fantastic or seemingly inexplicable things that enthrall us. Wonder is a state that throws animals out of equilibrium -- not just human animals, but also quizzical dogs. Make a funny sound at the dog and it tilts its head: what's this? Children get wide-eyed. The wonderment must be reduced to bring the world back into order. So people (and dogs, I guess) have to figure out what the wondrous thing is and how it works. And, of course, how to control it. I could demonstrate this in a minute to any audience of American physicians. If I were to put on a table a funny-looking device that had a screen and strange keyboard, people would soon start poking at it, manipulating the keys to see if they could bring up the control system, find out what it is and how it works. Wonder is not easily put aside and is quickly reawakened-one taste leads to a desire for more.

Wonder and wonderment cause physicians to use and overuse their technology. They like to see it in action -- and they want a new model as soon as possible. Wonder may seem a childish motivation in a very serious pursuit. It is childish; that is one of its attractions. It helps solve the problems of boredom, absence of meaning, and loss of motivation. But it needs to be kept in check. The human body is wondrous and so is the psyche, which is why some doctors love to take the body apart and others love to pry into the psyche. Yet surgeons are socialized, as are psychiatrists, never to cut into the body or mess in the mind unless it is for the patient's good. We know that curiosity -- an aspect of wonder -- is not easily held in check, but much time in medical education is spent successfully socializing doctors to hold their curiosity in check. This says it can be done.

The Lure of the Immediate

The second reason for technology's hold on physicians is that it roots us in the immediate, the now of its presence. The numbers of the readout, images on film, dexterity required for its deployment, technical complexities, tubes, wires, plugs, valves, needles, gauges, mirrors, focusing devices, and on and on exist in the here and now -- the immediate moment. But these things are immediate in another related, but perhaps more important sense: They are unmediated by our own reasoning. The technological output is a thing in and of itself. Computer jargon even has a name for it, WYSIWYG, What You See Is What You Get The user doesn't have to reason from one output to another; each is distinct.

How different from the patient A bundle of large questions, a life that exists only in the most fragmentary sense in the here and now. Look at a patient, see only the here and now, and you have missed the truth of a sick person. Any one moment of life -- in an intensive care unit or a nursing home -- contains only one bit of the importance of something much larger. A human life is a trajectory through time, the historic route of a society of complex parts, as Whitehead explained. Sick persons, all persons, are difficult to understand. The doctor in attendance is also a society of complex parts pursuing a historic route that interacts with the patient.

It is not that doctors are lazy; it's just that they have come to accept these technologies and their output as the equivalent of the thing being tested.

God bless the immediate -- no need to get caught up in all that complex sick person stuff. That is why, given a complicated human question in the care of the sick, we doctors love to start talking about physiologic parameters, calling up diseases or planning some tests. For example, the attending physician and medical students stood outside the room of a dying patient whose suffering could not be controlled. Did they speak about her suffering, or what to tell her or do for her? No, they were reading her test results and x-ray films -- irrelevant to her present problem but much simpler and more immediate.

Why isn't the examining hand on the abdomen just as immediate as looking at a readout or computer-generated image? Because it isn't just a hand, or sensations in the fingers, it is a doctor feeling responsible for the approximation to an unseen reality of what fingers tell -- and what it means. Why isn't the same thing true of the image on the film? It can be true, it should be true. The physician viewing the image should be reasoning about what must have come before and what will follow from the information contained in the image. And then how that information fits in with what he or she knows of the patient and the patient's interests, desires, purposes, fears, and concerns. But as the technology gets better it becomes more autonomous, it tells you directly what it means in immediate terms -- like the computer-generated EKG interpretations. Or a specialist, whose sole job is to interpret the image, tells you what it means in unmediated terms. As we all know, physicians less often read their own x-rays (even with the interpretation in hand), or go to the pathology department when the biopsy is being read, or question the precision, accuracy, or validity of the automated chemistry report. It is not that doctors are lazy; it's just that they have come to accept these technologies and their output as the equivalent of the thing being tested.

There are specialties in medicine that have always lived more in the immediate than others -- surgeons are the best example. The open wound, flowing blood, and exposed viscera are more immediate than the evolution of a drawnout illness. The special attraction of the immediate is one of the reasons that surgeons are different from internists (or the other way around).

The systems of angers that we teach physicians about diseases are ill suited to frame the longer term, larger questions raised by the sickness of the person to whom the monitors are connected. Science has ruled out of court the information from values and aesthetics by which we live our lives, allowing only brute facts. One of the advantages of the immediate is that it provides answers -- information -- when more relevant understanding would require deeper reasoning and greater involvement from doctors as persons. Understanding cannot operate separately from the resorter, as can the computer. Immediacy and its lesser requirement for reason facilitates a detachment from the suffering of a patient. Thus we are held in thrall by technology as much by the seeming advantage of the immediate as we are by its wonder.

The Lure of the Unambiguous

The third aspect of technology, unambiguous values, keeps it employed sometimes even when it is inappropriate. Watch the movie of a coronary arteriogram. It's like a Western, where you can quickly tell the good guys from the bad guys. The values are clear and unambiguous. With adequate dye in the vessels, a good coronary arteriogram is anatomically clear. You can compare it to those taken previously and subsequently. A good coronary artery is open and a bad one is obstructed, although there are criteria for degrees of good and bad. A good obstruction is short, with adequate runoff, and not so tight that an angioplasty balloon won't get through it or that it cannot be bypassed. Although they may disagree with one another about details, cardiologists are absolutely clear and straightforward about such things. When they are not, they make new criteria to remove ambiguity.

Virtually all technology is marked by similarly unambiguous values. In fact, lack of ambiguity is essential to good medical science. If cardiologists at Cornell cannot speak the same language and mean the same thing by technical terms as those at Stanford, Oxford, and the Hôtel de Dieu, then international research is impossible and progress in medical science will be impeded. So, on the face of it, the unambiguous seems reasonable -- except that we physicians do not generally know how or when to abandon it. Many, in fact most, of life's simple pleasures are also unambiguous. We generally know what is good and bad behavior -- food, wine, and sex. On the other hand, the development of sophistication in nontechnological pursuits involves appreciation of complexity and ambiguity. Sophistication in technology, I believe, goes in the other direction. More sophisticated means less ambiguous; the better the piece of equipment, the clearer the values.

But good or bad as measured by technology is not necessarily the same thing as good or bad for patients. Coronary artery disease and its technologies are a case in point. Imagine an instance, common enough, where a middle-aged man without symptoms wants to join an exercise program. He is required to have a treadmill exercise test. His test results (following the usual Bruce protocol, which approximates no exercise you have overdone) are positive by published criteria. He is advised that these unambiguous criteria often indicate coronary artery disease and should be followed by a thallium stress test. The test (in this case) is also positive and he is advised that he should have a coronary arteriogram. (In many instances the thallium scan is considered redundant -- the patient goes directly to the arteriogram.) The arteriogram shows (in this instance) significant obstruction of a coronary artery. Subsequently, a coronary artery angioplasty is done to reduce the obstruction. This little scenario is extremely common in the United States -- and increasingly so elsewhere. There is no quality evidence that the outcome of this chain of events makes a positive difference in the life of such a patient -- that asymptomatic patients with a positive test who go to angioplasty or bypass surgery do better than patients who are not so treated. The relationship between what is considered good and bad in the results of the tests and what is best for the patient is at the very least obscure and at the worst, just plain wrong.

What has happened is that because available technology permits visualizing the major coronary arteries, atherosclerosis of these vessels, which can be demonstrated unambiguously, has come to be taken definitionally as the equivalent of coronary heart disease. Coronary heart disease is a more complex entity than merely atherosclerosis of the major coronaries, although the two are often associated. For example, at autopsy one will commonly see old people whose coronary arteries are so flied with the calcium deposits characteristic of advanced atherosclerosis that one wonders how blood ever gets through them. Why did they have coronary artery disease but show no evidence during life of loss of everyday function due to heart disease? Because they did not have heart disease. Unfortunately, physicians infrequently attend autopsies nowadays and thus are not exposed to this common phenomenon. Conversely, sometimes one sees a patient with clear-cut signs of coronary heart disease, but little evidence of obstructed coronary arteries.

The second demonstration of the absence of the disease but the presence of a marker that technology has elevated disproportionately is the person captured on the treadmill whom I described a moment ago. If persons like this have hearts with good pumping function -- normal ejection fraction -- they do very well with their operations or angioplasties. They ought to. They don't have heart disease.[1]

As I suggested previously, human sophistication is marked by tolerance for ambiguity, whereas sophisticated technology removes ambiguities. It does this by narrowing down the field of difference between what is good and what is bad, so that ultimately one test result is taken to be good and another result bad. And that is how the state of the coronary arteries became accepted as the equivalent of a disease of the heart itself in the circumstances I have described. This is Whitehead's fallacy of misplaced concreteness writ large.

We must not forget that technological measures of value, even as they achieve a life of their own, are derived from human values. When medicine's priorities (another word for values) are too simplistic, they will be represented by a technology that also exemplifies simple values. For example, giving a part priority over the whole allows you to sustain an organ but lose sight of what is best for the whole person. We value the preservation of structure over the preservation of function. We value the body over the person, we value survival over maximum function, and length of life over quality of life.

The development of technology is not an event but a process. Technology is invented to solve problems arising out of the pursuit of medical values. Technological values, however, foster medical values that are intolerate of ambiguity, which subsequently leads to a new stage of technology. As a result, the sophistication necessary for physicians to tolerate the ambiguity inevitably following on attempts to break out of the circle is stifled. The odd thing is that if one faulted modern physicians for lack of sophistication they would most likely dismiss the criticism by pointing to the sophisticated equipment they use.

So, to wonderment and the lure of the immediate, we add unambiguous values as a reason why technology runs doctors rather than vice versa.

The Pursuit of Certainty

The central problem that physicians confront is uncertainty, which is the next reason for the dominance of technology. It is doubt that grays hair. Many years ago Renée Fox wrote an essay called "Training for Uncertainty" that appeared in *The Student Physician*, a book about the socialization of medical students based on studies of the class of 1954 at Cornell.[2] She identified two reasons for uncertainty. First, defects in the knowledge of the individual physician, and second, the inadequacies of the profession's knowledge. Even if I, impossibility granted, knew everything medicine knew, I would not know everything. There would still be uncertainties. But in an ideal world of complete knowledge, in this view, we could be certain. Unfortunately, as Sam Gorovitz and Alasdair MacIntyre pointed out years ago at a meeting at The Hastings Center, there are two other roots of uncertainty that can never be removed.[3] The first is that every decision, small or large, is made about the future, and the future is ineluctably uncertain. All medical decisions are about the future, since the future starts an instant from the present Second, uncertainty can never go away because all of science, medical science or any other, is about generalities. But every patient is a particular individual and necessarily different in some respect from the general. Thus, clinical judgments are always uncertain, and medical knowledge necessarily involves uncertainties. In clinical medicine as elsewhere, the more important the knowledge required by the decision, the less tolerable is the uncertainty. Since physicians commonly make decisions that have profound implications for the lives of others, uncertainty is a constantly disturbing factor in medical practice. Patients have the same uncertainties as physicians, or worse. They commonly solve them, ultimately by trust-trust in the physician -- which increases the burden of the doctors' uncertainties. Physicians follow the same path as they trust their consultants and their technology.

There are a number of strategies to reduce uncertainty, and technology can play a part in each of them. The first strategy is to shrink the clinical problem until it is not that of a particular sick person, but of an organ. For example, a patient complains of pains in the chest that are of an unusual type. The pain does not seem to be related to exercise, position, or food, yet it has been persistent. The question of heart disease is raised, yet one test for heart disease after another is shown to be normal. The patient is reassured that the pain does not represent heart disease because the tests are negative. This may in fact be correct, but the pain, not the presence or absence of heart disease, is the problem. The positive or negative certainty of each test provides an answer to the redefined problem and reduces the physician's uncertainty. Perhaps the patient will also be reassured, but perhaps not. The physician's statement, "Your problem is not..." is not nearly as good a response as a positive answer to the question raised by the symptom: "Your chest pain is a result of..." Further, the question of chest pain has been changed to the question of coronary heart disease, which is changed to the question of coronary artery disease. And, as I have noted, changing the question is a result of available technology.

Redefinition of the problem in terms of a technological answer is often employed in the case of back pain. Here, the questions of cause and treatment with regard to the patient's pain become a question about the pathological anatomy of the spine, which can be answered by consulting a picture of it. As we know, the cost of this picture has risen steadily over the last decade as the initial simple x-rays of the spine have been superseded by computerized tomography and most recently by magnetic resonance imaging. The image on the film -- with its implication of objective certainty -- comes to stand for the patient's back pain, to the point where greater weight is given to the image on the film than to the patient's pain.

Problems such as chest or back pain were previously addressed by taking the patient's history and doing a physical examination. But these diagnostic methods were fraught with uncertainty and were particularly dependent on the skill of the individual physician. These techniques had the further disadvantage of forcing the physician to confront an intractable source of uncertainty: the individuality of the patient. Technological methods move the evidence employed in diagnosis away from the patient and reduce the impact of the patient's particularity on the physician. In using them, physicians mistakenly believe they can reduce uncertainty by changing the patients problem to one for which there is a technological answer. They then reduce the problem from that of the patient to that of an organ or body part for which a technology exists, and they distance themselves from the patient by employing that technology. On the therapeutic side, technologies may reduce uncertainties by providing treatments that, although of unquestionable value in some situations, are employed in situations where they have no utility.

Technology would not produce problems in relation to uncertainty if it did not, in fact, frequently reduce uncertainty, sometimes dramatically. Probably because of the change produced by effective technologies, I believe that doctors are no longer trained in the management of uncertainty in the fashion first described by Fox. As a consequence, they tend to utilize any diagnostic or therapeutic technique that promises to reduce uncertainty. This leads to a sort of Gresham's law of technology: whatever technique promises greatest certainty, even if inappropriate, will diminish the use of techniques associated with greater uncertainty. It is the case that hard facts drive soft facts into hiding, which in turn drive softer facts into oblivion. Technologies produce hard facts.

All the wonder, dislike of ambiguity, and fear of uncertainty that afflict doctors are present among patients. And the stakes are highest for them. In the current medical world of the United States, patients have a significant voice in the choice of diagnostic strategies and treatment. They are generally knowledgeable to an unprecedented degree. Not surprisingly, their knowledge is greatest about new technologies and treatments, details of which fill the pages of newspapers, magazines, and health promotion newsletters. It is fair to say that many patients believe that it is the test rather than the physician that makes the diagnosis, and the drug rather than the physician that effects the cure. (If a CAT scan shows a lung minor, did it make the diagnosis? A physician chose a CAT scan rather than, say a plain film of the chest and decided to image the chest rather than, say, the abdomen. The CAT scan was employed in the diagnosis.) Consequently, patients have been an active force in the increasing deployment and dominance of technology.

Technology Is Self-Perpetuating

Employing one technology frequently leads to the use of another. This is most easily demonstrated by the function of computers in neonatal intensive care units. Commonly, each "bed" in a neonatal unit has its own computer to analyze and display the physiological state of the infant. The requirement of computers for digital information encourages the proliferation of instrumentation that produces such data. Similarly, when automated blood chemistry machines make redundant the manual skills of technicians, other automated laboratory examinations become necessary because technicians no longer do the tests by hand. The results consequent on the use of one technology frequently raise questions that can apparently only be answered by other technologies. Computerized tomographic images of the central nervous system may introduce doubt that only magnetic resonance imaging can resolve. General expectations have been created among physicians about levels of accuracy, certainty, and lack of ambiguity that can only be met by other technologies -- even if such accuracy, certainty, and lack of ambiguity are not important in a particular instance.

Doctors who have mastered a technology tend to use it as often as possible -- not necessarily for reasons of profit, but because they love their skills and technologies. As noted earlier, problems tend to be redefined so that a technology, becomes appropriate when it might otherwise not be.

A saying that makes the point has become popular among physicians, "To the man with a hammer, everything is a nail."

Power

The final reason for the inappropriate use of technology is the power it confers on physicians and their institutions. While the meaning of power seems self-evident, some further explication is required. The power to act is basic to human existence and is employed to control or influence events. In its absence we feel powerless, which is a self-destructive state. We exist for ourselves and for others in our actions; when we act, we simultaneously create ourselves and our world. The scope and effectiveness of our actions in both self-creation and influence on the world are determined by the degree of our power. Since we are social beings, virtually all of our actions take place in a world of others, and our power is relative to the power of others.

Thus, my ability to act among others is partly dependent upon permission to exercise my power by those more powerful or my desire to exercise my power in relation to those less powerful. Frequently the word "hierarchy" is used to refer to social ranking according to power. Power does not reside in us only as individuals but also by virtue of our acknowledged place in society -- in our social status. Thus, hierarchy may be role dependent rather than the result of self-generated power. Power relationships -- which also exist among and between animal groups -- are dynamic. It is difficult to exaggerate the importance of the exercise and experience of power.

In using technological methods, physicians mistakenly believe they can reduce uncertainty by changing the patient's problem to one for which there is a technological answer.

Even in sophisticated societies, the ability to do things better than others do them confers power. Possessions confer power because they bestow status -- material wealth is the most obvious example -- but so does access to objects of superior efficacy. In fact, changes in one's access to things containing superior efficacy in themselves may alter one's status. A well-known ethnographic example involves a culture in which the only available axes, made of stone, were in the possession of the tribal elders. These axes were not only used to cut wood, but were also a measure of status and a factor in barter among tribes. Western missionaries came to the tribe and offered steel axes as incentives for conversion to their religious beliefs. Wide distribution of these powerful objects -- both totemic and effective -- dramatically altered hierarchical and status relations within the tribe and its associations with its neighbors.

Technology, as noted earlier, is employed in this discussion to refer to modalities and instrumentalities that gratify extend the power of human action, sensation, or thought and that have this efficacy independent of the particular user. There is little doubt that one of the attractions of technology is its ability to confer status and rank on individuals. Medical power is demonstrated when a plastic surgeon makes someone look younger, when infection is treated, blood pressure is lowered, or pain relieved. Every therapeutic and diagnostic act is a demonstration of efficacy and thus of power. The therapeutic effectiveness of the relationship between patient and doctor is dependent in part on a belief in the physician's individual and institutional power over the forces of nature. In previous epochs, the physician's power came not only from his or her shared knowledge of the body and disease, but also from the personal development of knowledge about the sick and sickness and demonstrated effectiveness in the diagnosis and treatment of patients. Personal power of this sort takes many years to develop and is inevitably a result of the ripening of the medical self. Technology confers power on individual doctors with much less personal involvement. The modern tendency toward specialization encourages this more easily gotten power because it narrows the amount of knowledge necessary to exercise it.

Technology also gathers to itself personnel and space that exhibit power and tend to be self-perpetuating. Intensive care units are the perfect examples, as are transplant units. In medicine as elsewhere, technology engenders special training, which furthers the world view of technology, which further increases political power. Employing or having access to technology also garners social power or status from laypersons, the press, the university, or the hospital trustees. In like manner, technology confers status on hospitals and other medical institutions. The example I gave earlier about being shown around shiny cardiac cath labs when I visited a Pittsburgh hospital can also be used to exemplify a hospital showing off its power.

Technology would not confer power on doctors and the profession of medicine if it were not seen by the larger society as having power in itself. It erroneously appears to free the patient from the necessity of depending on the individuality and individual skills of the physician. Uniform fee schedules that pay for a particular act -- office visit, surgery, etc. -- reflect the falsehood that doctors dispense a uniform technology rather than a personal individual service. It is not a surprise, in view of this widespread public belief in the independent power of technology, that physicians, who are influenced by the public they serve, depend increasingly on technology regardless of whether its use is appropriate.

Knowledge at a Distance

In our daily lives we are accustomed to confronting much of our world in its representation, rather than in itself -- in photographs, recordings, radio, movies, and television. This has produced the widened perspective and scope of knowledge about things distant and dose to us with which we are all familiar but which, especially for doctors, cause problems. Technology represents a kind of knowledge. In fact, it epitomizes the twentieth century ideal of knowledge -- scientific, objective, and existing seemingly separate from humankind. In medicine, the scientific knowledge and subsequent technology developed in response to the challenge posed by sickness and suffering has assumed an actuality more convincing than the reality of sick persons themselves. Consider this common situation. A patient has severe pain in the hip, and the doctors can find no evidence of disease. With each negative test, increasing doubt is raised about whether the patient is truly in pain. Then a radionuclide bone scan is done, showing cancer in the hip bone. The patient will now be believed. Why is the celluloid rectangle with fuzzy black dots more believable than the patient's pain? The usual answer, that the pain is subjective, won't hold water. The pain may be subjective, but the report of pain is a thing that can be evaluated. Further, we are of a piece. We cannot have severe pain without its being reflected in other aspects of our physical, social, and psychological selves.

A person with severe pain moves, acts, thinks, feels, displays emotion, and relates to others differently from the same person pain free. All of these features are apparent to others or can be evoked -- they are objective.

Objectivity alone isn't the issue. The way we would know that the man really has pain does not meet the ideal of medical scientific knowledge developed over the last 150 years. Scientific. knowledge, surely not the only way to know things, has come to be accepted as more actual than patients or their pain or suffering. Medicine's technology also produces representations of patients' original reality that are another reality in themselves. For example, EKGs, x-ray machines, monitors, CAT scanners, magnetic resonance imaging machines, and PET scanners are all imaging devices that distance physicians from the sick person. Their focus of interest is inevitably drawn away from the patient and onto the part or the disease -- out of the context of the whole patient and the patient's lived world?[4] Realizing this, physicians and commentators and critics of medicine have largely depended on moral injunctions to return medicine's focus to the sick person. It is an uphill struggle because the problem is based, in part, on the nature of medical knowledge itself and is firmly embedded in the mindset of the late twentieth century.

The Counterspell for the Sorcerer's Broom

Technology holds sway over medicine and its public because of its self-perpetuating character and its enhancement of power, as well as its capacity to induce wonder, root us in the immediate, remove ambiguity, and increase certainty. Since this is not well understood, it is hardly surprising that technology, by itself inert and useless (although beckoning for attention through its inherent purposes), should be blamed for the troubles it brings. The real culprits, however, are the doctors who use it, the public that loves it, and the narrow knowledge on which it is based. Medical technology's form and character arise from medicine's focus on disease and pathophysiology as the arena in which the origins and solutions to human sickness are to be found. The values on which it is based come primarily from the spectrum of pathophysiological and anatomical criteria for disease and normality, now largely defined and perpetuated by the technology. Our task, it seems to me, is to stop blaming, regulating, and complaining about technology -- without which modern medicine is unthinkable -- and start working toward a solution based on understanding, as we have done with so many others. The search for new goals of medicine now going on at The Hastings Center can be one step in such a task. I believe the new goals will turn out to be old ones, that we should be trying to return medicine and doctors toward a focus on persons sick and well and on their suffering.

Conversely, no change in the ends and purposes of medicine is possible without bringing technology under control. Toward this end we must learn how to teach doctors, who are in themselves the primary instruments of diagnosis and treatment, to tolerate uncertainty, accept ambiguity, deal with the complex, and turn away from mere wonder. Accepting these assignments and redirected goals and following them as far as they lead will be a sufficient task for decades.

Notes

1. Because this essay is about technology, I have simplified the discussion of coronary heart disease and its relation to coronary artery disease. A thorough analysis of the issue and the evidence that bears on it does support the same conclusions.
2. Fox RC. Training for uncertainty, In: Merton RK, *et al.*, ed. *The Student Physician: Introductory Studies in the Sociology of Medical Education.* Cambridge, MA: Harvard University Press, 1957:20741.
3. Gorovitz S, Maclntyre A. Toward a theory of medical fallibility, *Hastings Center Report* 1975;5(6):13-23.
4. Toombs K. *The Meaning of Illness.* Boston, MA: Kluwer Academic Publishers, 1992:Chap. 2.

Chapter 59

The Ethics of Letting Go

David C. Thomasma

"Of course we can't withdraw the respirator. He's not brain dead." How often have your heard those words? How often have you thought that this simple statement governs the care of the chronically ill or dying patient? Unfortunately it does not. But its very simplicity can lull today's physician into an ethical somnolence. It can too easily substitute for the difficult reasoning at the bedside demanded by the patient's condition and the value hierarchy that appears in each individual case.

Arguably the leading cause for such ethical somnolence is the intense pressure on physicians to prolong life at all costs. It is natural to hang on to patients and to hold out hope for distressed families. Physicians are often attacked for their insensitivity when they prolong life and hold out hope against the odds. Quite the contrary. I suggest that it is often not insensitivity, but rather exquisite sensitivity that leads physicians to these behaviors.

Prolonging Life at all Cost

Chosen for medical school in part for their altruism and in part for their love of science, the challenge of protecting life looms large in every physician's value system. Formed by constant and insistent interventionist training, those same physicians have had daily, even hourly, reinforcement of their proclivities to respect life by prolonging it. Patients laud their doctors when they are successful in this all-important venture: "My doctor is a whiz. No one knew what to do. But she saved my life!"

In addition to these natural tendencies and the educational and experiential reinforcements of protecting human life in practice, society itself supports intervention rather than restraint. Most of our cultural and even legal assumptions are that physicians will act always to protect and foster human life, not destroy it. For this reason some states have a 48 hour rule, whereby pediatricians can take over the care of children whom they suspect of being victims of child abuse for 48 hours while they contact the court for a more permanent arrangement. It is assumed, often wrongly, that in the absence of other directives, individuals must be resuscitated. Once again a mark of respect for the value of human life. The "Good Samaritan" laws cover physicians who intervene to save the lives of strangers who are not their own patients. Again an example of society's support for life-prolonging activities.

Thus, physicians who act to preserve life do so from a sensitive effort to do what they perceive is right and good, to establish their own borders of a struggle with disease and death. That struggle was not much discussed in medical school. Yet it formed the warp and woof of a physician's commitment to life and to the patient's good.

Source: Reprinted from the *Journal of Critical Care*, Vol. 8, No. 3, pp. 170-176, with permission from W.B. Saunders Company © 1993.

Distress, Confusion, Social Change

Since the days of medical school, enormous stress cracks have formed on and below the surface of medicine. For starters, rampaging medical technology has driven up the cost of health care far beyond annual inflation percentages. Businesses and the government itself constantly attempt to hold down health care costs by controlling the usages of these technologies, ironically at the very time that they are advancing the state of the art of medicine. The way to control the technologies is to control the reimbursement to health care institutions and to doctors themselves. So one social change is a letup of the insistence that everything possible be done to preserve life. Yet this occurs in the context of a general lack of restraint in American society, that tends to move upward and onward without limits.

Second, as this technological intervention is applied to chronically ill and dying patients, the disease from which they suffer advances far beyond its extent in the old days. In the old days, families did not bring their loved ones to the hospital to die. They died at home, without IV fluids and nutrition, without shunts, without antibiotics, without respirators. No one would dispute the benefit of these latter advances in medicine when applied properly and with judiciousness and balance. But when they have been applied even with these qualities, and persons have advanced in their chronic or terminal disease to a point of real suffering and pain, then are physicians not responsible for this technology? Many argue that they are, to the point of offering their patients active, direct euthanasia as a way out near the end.

In fact, this is one of the most powerful arguments for direct euthanasia. If we have individuals in an advanced state of severe pain and suffering because we gave them a better quality of life for a time, then is it not human and humane to help them exit with the least amount of further suffering? I have argued together with co-author Glenn Graber that sometimes death is a good for patients, and that the very essence of being a moral person is to bring about the good.[1] Indeed, the basis of Natural Law ethics is the dictum: "Do good and avoid evil."

Additionally, by focusing on control over dying, the argument that persons have a right to die is strengthened. A more vigorous assertion is created. It is expressed, for example, by Joseph Fletcher, an early, continuous, and strong proponent of a right to die. Fletcher says: "Death control...is a matter of human dignity. Without it persons become puppets. To perceive this is to grasp the error lurking in the notion that life, as such, is the highest good."[2] In order for individuals to control the circumstances of their own dying, it is argued, they must be empowered to request active, direct euthanasia. They have a "right to die." This right creates duties in caregivers and others to assist in a good death. Thus Sidney Wanzer argues that in an era of intensive efforts to help patients back to good health a counterbalancing intensive intervention is necessary on behalf of the patient for whom life is truly not worth living. This action supports their control in terminal illness.[3] Physician- assisted suicide in this view is seen as distinct from euthanasia, since the patient performs the life-terminating act (like Janet Adkins did with Dr. Kevorkian's machine, when he assisted in the his first suicide).

But is direct euthanasia required by an argument that we must take responsibility for technology or respect the right to die? A counterargument comes from physicians' concerns about either the perceptions of the community about physicians being involved in voluntary active euthanasia,[4] or more profound arguments about traditional commitments to the value of human life. Thus Leon Kass presents a thoughtful articulation of what is owed a dying patient by the physician. He argues that humanity is owed humanity, not just "humaneness," (i.e., being merciful by killing the patient). Kass argues that the very reason we are compelled to put animals out of their misery is that they are *not* human and thus demand from us some measure of humaneness. By contrast human beings demand from us our humanity itself. This thesis, in turn, rests on the relationship "between the healer and the ill" as constituted, essentially, "even if only tacitly, around the desire of both to promote the wholeness of the one who is ailing."[5] This is still a majority view among physicians, perhaps as many as 75%.

Studies have shown that physicians do not evaluate whether a patient is dying solely on the basis of biomedical data. They also take into account the important features of human interaction, and the proportion between therapeutically available interventions and the possible outcome.[6] Such interactive concerns tend to present counterpressures to a straightforward honoring of patient wishes with respect for euthanasia requests. Needless to say, fears about litigation also contribute to reluctance to honor patient requests, even for increases in pain control medication.

In light of these considerations, it is important to keep in mind that what are called "life-prolonging technologies" applied inappropriately to the dying may in fact be "death-delaying technologies." Managing the dying person's death is the most important role for the physician in the modern era of high technology medicine. This is a skill that requires extremely important value-sensitivity, as well as extensive medical and interpersonal skills. Without these qualities, professional distress can be the only result.

Preserving Human Function

Most Americans are sympathetic with persons who must die a slow, lingering, painful death due to severe terminal illness. We can understand how, even when pain is controlled, the suffering that accompanies dying must also be addressed. For this reason a good argument can be made that doctors should assist in dying, in bringing about a good death, in the face of burgeoning medical technology.[7] For the most part this can be accomplished by what is called passive euthanasia, by withholding or even withdrawing medical technology at the patient's request.[8] Withholding and withdrawing are forms of taking responsibility for our technology, as I pointed out above.[9] Keeping it out of the dying process at the request of the patient and family is a way of honoring the primacy of human life and human values over the mere brute existence of machines.

Another form of improperly prolonging life is to prolong suffering in conditions of hopeless injury to life. "Hopeless injury" as Braithwaite and I defined it, is:

> A condition in which there is no potential for growth or repair; no observable pleasure or happiness from living...and a total absence of one or more of the following attributes of quality of life: cognition or recognition, motor activity, memory or awareness of time, consciousness, and language or other intelligent means of communicating thoughts or wishes.[10]

Daily life is full of interactions with "things" -- non-human and fundamentally incomprehensible to most persons. We sometimes get so used to technological processes that we behave as though they are substitutes for human and compassionate care. Eating for many elderly and dying patients has been replaced by tubes; participating in the spiritual and material values of human life has been replaced by "merely surviving," as a being subjugated to the very products of human imagination. As Illich observes:

> Medical civilization is planned and organized to kill pain, to eliminate sickness, and to abolish the need for acts of suffering and dying[11]...The new experience that has replaced dignified suffering is artificially prolonged, opaque, depersonalized maintenance.[12]

Such "beings" on depersonalized maintenance may no longer be as human as the rest of us, precisely because of this subjugation. This is no way to respect the value of human life. Is a permanently unconscious being without any ability to relate to its environment a "person?" Jonsen wonders just what exactly life support supports: "We talk about the maintenance of life; we don't often talk about the maintenance of personhood." "It interests me little," he says, "indeed, not at all, to be alive as an organism. In such a state I have no interests. It is enormously interesting for me to be a person...it is the perpetuation of my personhood that interests me; indeed, it is probably my major and perhaps my sole real interest."[13]

Many technologies developed for specific groups of patients are now used for other patient populations where their effect has yet to be evaluated. Because the equipment makes the provider feel better, it is used. When technologies become more accessible, e.g., dialysis, cardio-pulmonary resuscitation, there is less of an imperative to justify their use. When ICU beds are plentiful, dying patients are tucked into them.

The effect of overuse of technology without evaluation of its efficacy and, frequently, without patient involvement, is to increase patient and family suffering. It may prolong the suffering of dying, and it provides social suffering by wasting resources that might benefit those with potentially reversible diseases.

The ICU is a prime illustration of both the effective use and the misuse of technology in our society. The cost of an ICU bed is approximately $2,000-$3,000 a day. Other hospital beds cost about one-half that amount. Seventy to eighty percent of patients leave the ICU alive. Many of these are post-operative patients. But of thosc who are critically ill with chronic disease or major medical or surgical problems, the mortality rate is 40-60%.[14] A case in point comes from treatment of AIDS. According to NIH statistics, the mortality rate in ICUs for ventilated AIDS patients is at least 85%. Those with first incidence of pneumonia often benefit from the ICU. But the weak or chronically ill will almost certainly die tethered to their machines.[15]

In a society such as ours, with its problems of poverty, homelessness, gaining access to health care, and denigration of the weak, we need to maintain constant vigilance about protecting persons from both undertreatment and abandonment and inappropriate overtreatment. In both instances, we will be shepherding our technology to good human aims.

The Goal of Medicine

Thus, the most volatile ethical issue confronting medical practice today is euthanasia because it is based on the "rights" model of resolving ethical concerns, rather than upon a more interactive and personal model favored by physicians.

Against the backdrop of reports about active euthanasia from the Netherlands and concomitant reports from the United States, the medical profession's official position remains solidly that of its traditional repugnance for directly causing or intending death. Reviews of gradual changes in attitude among physicians themselves, or among traditionally strong interventionist services like emergency medicine, demonstrate a growing acceptance of passive and even active, direct euthanasia.[16]

The American Medical Association published its Judicial Council guidelines on withholding and withdrawing life sustaining treatment in 1986. There the AMA stated: "The social commitment of the physician is to sustain life and relieve suffering. Where the performance of one duty conflicts with the other, the choice of the patient should prevail."[17]

This view seems to represent an endorsement of double-effect euthanasia, in which one action, control of pain, made lead to another effect, the death of the patient. The AMA has endorsed letting the patient decide in such a matter.

Dramatic advances have occurred in underlining the rights of patients not only to determine the treatments they desire and do not desire during the dying process, but also the development of the rights to choose treatments at any time during life, not just while dying.[18] The efforts of patient advocacy groups in sponsoring and supporting legislation and court deliberations have been outstanding. The Living Will and Advance Directives, including the Durable Power of Attorney, all point to eventual further clarification of these rights. What is important to note is that the underlying motivation for the development of such instruments is the prevention of suffering.[19,20] It would make sense to extend these rights to even greater control over the dying process.

Joan Beck noted in her column about the Nancy Cruzan case, that people need to get on the record early about their wishes regarding life-prolonging technology. Noting the usefulness of

Living Wills and the Durable Power of Attorney, she says:

> Unfortunately, living wills are not always honored by hospitals and the courts to which right-to-die cases may be referred...The court's ruling makes it even more imperative to push legislatures in every state to enact clear and merciful rules to protect people from being trapped in a limbo of dying and to give their loved ones the means and legal protections to come to their rescue.[21]

It is ironic that life-prolonging technology can also prolong dying. At the apogee of our technological capacity to promote the good of prolonging life we are faced with the truly terrifying consequences of that technology, what Beck calls "the limbo of dying." Most people are not afraid of death. Death can be seen as a release from a body that has increasingly betrayed us. But we are afraid of prolonged dying and the attendant suffering. Many lay people, discussing the Janet Adkins case that occurred in Michigan, suggested that "there ought to be some way out" when suffering becomes too much for a person.

Indeed the very goal of medicine should be to help patients advance their life-plans by providing either a cure or healing. Most often this is possible. But eventually it is not. It may be no longer possible for individuals in advanced stages of dementia, or persons with severe neurological damage, or persons with advanced cancer and heart disease, and so on. Consequently to continue to treat them, to provide fluids and nutrition or other medical interventions, is not to honor them as persons, but to continuously subjugate them to their disease. Withholding and withdrawing care can be done, not on the basis of whether they are brain-dead, but on the basis of their values and their life-plans.

Letting Go

The heart of a massive public discussion about "letting go" of patients, ought to include the question about what sort of society we ought to be. Have we become so disjointed as a society that people feel the need to dispatch themselves early in a chronic disease rather than trust others to care for them? Christine Cassel, M.D. is very worried that elderly persons, in light of the Cruzan decision, will want to commit suicide rather than subject themselves to possible violations of their values in nursing homes and hospitals after they become senile.[22] Evidence exists that there is a growing trend in elder suicide.[23] Will people increasingly feel threatened by high-technology hospitals where they are stripped of their values at the same time they are stripped of their clothing and put into the beds? Do we have to carry all sorts of lengthy legal documents on our person about our wishes regarding medical technology should we become ill or get in an accident?

Social parsimony may lead to increased pressures to euthanize those citizens who no longer are capable of a minimal quality of life. This action may be justified on the basis of advance directives (pure autonomy arguments), the benefits/burdens calculus (social benefit argument), or pure utilitarianism (the greatest good for the greatest number).

Based on these concerns, letting go of patients must also factor-in their vulnerability. In a previous work Edmund D. Pellegrino and I derived an axiom of vulnerability from the nature of medicine as a special kind of human activity.[24] We held that to attain the goal of the medical encounter -- a right and good healing action for a particular patient -- several axioms were necessary, the violation of any one of which imperil the goal. Observing the vulnerability principle was one of these necessary axioms.

The principle of vulnerability can be stated this way: In human relations generally, if there are inequities of power, knowledge, or material means, the obligation is upon the stronger to respect and protect the vulnerability of the other and not exploit the less-advantaged party. This is a principle of general ethics, applicable to all sorts of human relationships. It generates an obligation of altruism, i.e., taking others into account in our use of power, knowledge, or other possessions. This taking of vulnerability into account is a bilateral or multilateral affair when more than two persons are involved.

Goodin, in his *Protecting the Vulnerable,* analyzes important cases regarding the vulnerable in contracts, business relations, professional ethics, family relations, among friends, and with respect to benefactors.[25] He builds an inexorable case in social justice that society bears specific responsibilities towards those who, in any particular relationship, are more vulnerable to exploitation or harm. The heart of his argument is that we usually assume that the basis for special responsibilities to protect the vulnerable from harm come from self-assumed duties and obligations, often self-assumed through contracts, implied or explicit. A good example of the former might be the obligation of families to provide for their children first, over caring for others in society,[26] or the obligation of a health professional for his or her own patient over other needy persons in society, as Veatch argues.[27,28]

This assumption is probably wrong, according to Goodin. Rather than obligations grounded in contracts by which we voluntarily commit ourselves to a limited range of persons (as the Libertarians would have it), the obligation is grounded in the vulnerability of the persons themselves: Examining several cases closely, however, suggests it is the *vulnerability* of the beneficiary rather than any voluntary commitment per se on the part of the benefactor which generates these special responsibilities.[29]

Consider the issue of expendability. Expendability is a judgment regarding the balance between the quality of life of vulnerable individuals and the needs and wants of society itself. From a purely utilitarian standpoint, those who contribute nothing to society, and drain its resources, are expendable. Drs. Binding and Hoche, Nazi party euthanasia theorists, called such persons "ballast existence." In their view, when economic times are prosperous, society does not ask questions about caring for expendable individuals. When times get difficult, then such "ballast existence" must be eliminated.

Concerns about vulnerability of patients have led many thinkers to counter an emphasis on autonomy with the need for beneficence as well.[30,31] The implications of conflicts about medical ethics and ethical theory for active euthanasia include the increased role of the health provider's values in caring for the dying patient, greater attention to the *relation* between physician and patient, rather than exclusive focus on the needs and wants of the individual patient alone, and questions about the kind of society we ought to be. James Bopp, general counsel of the National Right to Life committee, commenting on the Cruzan case, argues for example that society cannot establish a general rule that third parties can end the lives of persons in permanent vegetative states.[32] While I disagree precisely on this point, the issue does focus on the importance of maintaining compassionate respect for human life in our society.

For the U.S. today the danger of euthanizing the vulnerable exists in the economic sphere.[33] Will it be easier to use a simple method of dispatching those persons whose care costs too much, or who are now considered to be a burden on society, like the aged and the poor, than to address their suffering, which sometimes is overwhelming even for the most dedicated caregivers? As Joseph Cardinal Bernardin noted in an address on Euthanasia at the University of Chicago Hospital, "We cannot accept a policy that would open the door to euthanasia by creating categories of patients whose lives can be considered of no value merely because they are not conscious."[34]

The technological fix of injecting dying patients is not only easier to conceptualize and implement than the more difficult processes of human engagement, but is also "suggested" by technology itself. The training and skills of modern health professionals are overwhelmingly nurtured within a bath of technological fixes. By instinct and proclivity, all persons in a modern civilization are tempted by technical rather than personal solutions to problems. This is the real issue for Cardinal Bernardin, for example, who poses this question:

What would we be suggesting to one another and to our society, if, seemingly with the

> best of motives, we were to say that those who are sick, infirm, or unconscious may be killed? How could we allege that such actions would not affect us individually and collectively?[35]

Such actions are a form of "privatizing life," denying its social and communal dimensions as both a private and public good.

Therefore the concerns of disvaluing human life through technical responses to human suffering should not be dismissed as hopelessly conservative and neurotic. The overbearing experience of the 20th Century is one in which persons have been put at the mercy of technology. Caution about this reversal of the creative process, wherein persons are now subject to their own creations, is not only justified, but important in developing any social policy and legislative process.

Notes

1. Thomasma DC, Graber GC. *Euthanasia: Toward an Ethical Social Policy*. New York, NY: Continuum, 1990.
2. Fletcher JF. Indicators of humanhood: A tentative profile of man, *Hastings Ctr Rep* 1972;2:1-4.
3. Wanzer SH. Maintaining control in terminal illness: Assisted suicide and euthanasia, *Humane Medicine* 1990;6(3):186-88.
4. Gaylin W, Kass L, Pellegrino ED, Siegler M. Commentaries: Doctors must not kill, *JAMA* 1988;259:2139-40.
5. Kass L. Arguments against active euthanasia by doctors found at medicine's core, *Kennedy Inst of Ethics Newslett* 1989;3:1-3,6.
6. Muller J, Koenig B. On the boundary of life and death: The definition of dying by medical residents, In: Lock M, Gordon D, eds, *Biomedicine Examined*. Dordrecht/Boston: Kluwer Academic Publishers, 1988:351-374.
7. Cerne F. Mercy or murder? Physician's role in suicide spurs debate, *AHA News* 1990;26:1,5.
8. Stanley JM, ed. The Appleton consensus: suggested international guidelines for decisions to forgo medical treatment, *J Danish Med Assoc* (Ugeskr Laeger) 1989;151:700-706; reprinted in, *J Medical Ethics* 1989;15:129-136.
9. Cranford RE, Weir RF, Lo B, Meisel A, Childress JF, Cassel CK, Dresser RS, Robertson JA. The care of the dying: A symposium on the case of Betty Wright, *Law, Medicine and Health Care* 1989;17: 205-268.
10. Braithwaite S, Thomasma DC. New guidelines on foregoing life-sustaining treatment in incompetent patients: An anti-cruelty policy, *Ann Int Med* 1986;104:711-15.
11. Illich I. *Medical Nemesis: The Expropriation of Health*. New York, NY: Pantheon, 1976:106.
12. Illich, p 154.
13. Jonsen A. What does life support support? In: Winslade W, ed. *Personal Choices and Public Commitments: Perspectives on the Humanities*. Galveston, TX: Institute for the Medical Humanities, 1988:61-69, quote 66-67.
14. Raffin TA, Shurkin JN, Sinkler W III. *Intensive Care: Facing the Critical Issues*. New York, NY: W. H. Freeman & Co., 1988:185.
15. Raffin, p 175.
16. Sprung CL. Changing attitudes and practices in forgoing life-sustaining treatments, *JAMA* 1990;263:2211-2215.
17. American Medical Association Council on Ethical and Judicial Affairs. Withholding and withdrawing life-prolonging medical treatment, In: *Current Opinions of the Council on Ethical and Judicial Affairs of the American Medical Association.* Chicago, IL: AMA, 1986:12-13.
18. The Times Mirror Center for the People and the Press. *Survey: Reflections of the Times: The Right to Die*. Washington, DC: Times Mirror Center for the People and the Press, 1990.
19. Mehling A. Living wills: Preventing suffering or a deadly contract? *New York State Government News* 1988:14-15.

20. Mehling A, Neitlich S. *Right-to-die backgrounder*. New York, NY: News from the Society for the Right to Die, 1989:3 pages.
21. Beck J. Life or death? Put your views on the record early. *Chicago Tribune* 1990, July 12:Sec 1, 23.
22. Thomasma D. The Cruzan decision and medical practice, *Arch Int Med* 1991;151:853-854.
23. Conwell Y, Rotenberg M, Caine ED. Completed suicide at age 50 and over, *J Am Geriatr Soc* 1990;38:640-644.
24. Pellegrino ED, Thomasma DC. *A Philosophical Basis of Medical Practice*. New York, NY: Oxford University Press, 1981:119-154.
25. Goodin RE. *Protecting the Vulnerable*. Chicago, IL: University of Chicago Press, 1985.
26. Goodin, pp 4-5. As he points out, sociobiologists claim that our genetic makeup itself may dictate that we confine "reciprocal altruism" rather narrowly to our family.
27. Veatch RM. *The Foundations of Justice*. New York, NY: Oxford University Press, 1986.
28. Veatch RM. *A Theory of Medical Ethics*. New York, NY: Basic Books, 1981:324-330.
29. Goodin RE. pp. xi, 42-108.
30. Pellegrino ED, Thomasma DC. *For the Patient's Good: The Restoration of Beneficence in Health Care*. New York, NY: Oxford University Press, 1988.
31. Loewy E. The restoration of beneficence, *Hastings Ctr Rep* 1989;19:4.
32. Weinstein M. US supreme court to hear first case involving right-to-die, *ACP Observ* 1989;9:9.
33. Scitovsky AA, Capron AM. Medical care at the end of life: The interaction of economics and ethics, *Ann Rev Pub Health* 1986;7:59-75.
34. Bernardin J. *Euthanasia: Ethical and legal challenge*. Address to the Center for Clinical Medical Ethics, University of Chicago Hospital, 1988:16.
35. See note 34:14.

Chapter 60

Physician Refusal of Requests for Futile or Ineffective Interventions

John J. Paris and Frank E. Reardon

Several recent articles raise an issue long unaddressed in the medical literature: physician compliance with patient or family requests for futile or ineffective therapy.[1,2,3,4,5] Although they agree philosophically that such treatment ought not be given, most physicians have followed the course described by Stanley Fiel, in which a young patient dying of cystic fibrosis was accepted "for evaluation" by a transplant center even though he had already passed the threshold of viability as a candidate for a heart-lung transplant.[6] Dr. Fiel reported this action was taken not in the hope of doing the transplant but so that the family could assure themselves they had done "everything possible." The patient, after a long and stressful cross-country flight, arrived at the hospital in respiratory failure. He died soon thereafter far from home and familiar surroundings.

How do we respond to families and physicians who seek refuge from unwanted painful reality in "futile end-stage gestures?" In an essay on the futility of attempted resuscitation of end-stage terminally ill patients, the authors noted that until recently, that question took a back seat to patient autonomy in discussions of medical ethics.[7] In the ethics and legal literature, if the patient judged the treatment ineffective it could be withheld or withdrawn. But if treatment were demanded by the patient, even against the physician's recommendation, autonomy, not futility, carried the moral weight.

That mind set is starkly present in Susan Wolf's insistence that the patient, even if near death, or the family should have full decision-making authority concerning life-support systems; "the decision belongs to the patient."[8] Dr. Edmund Pellegrino, one of the nation's most respected and sensitive ethicists and the director of Georgetown University's Center for the Advanced Study of Ethics, concurred with that view when he wrote of the dying AIDS patient that although the patient or surrogate can decide to withhold or withdraw treatment, the physician cannot independently arrive at such a judgment; "the physician is, neither morally employed or qualified to make decisions about the quality of life of another person."[9]

The outer reaches of granting patient (or family) requests -- no matter how bizarre or unreasonable they may seem -- were explored in one article in which the authors insisted that "even the irrational choices of a competent patient must be respected if the patient cannot be persuaded to change them."[10] This philosophy was written into public policy when the state of New York enacted a statute (on the recommendation of the New York State Task Force on Life and the Law) that requires physicians to obtain the informed consent of a competent patient or the family of a decisionally incapable patient before they may legally write a Do-Not-Resuscitate (DNR) order. Results of such action can be perverse.[11]

Source: Reprinted from *Cambridge Quarterly of Healthcare Ethics*, Vol. 2, 1992, pp. 127-134, with permission from Cambridge University Press © 1992.

When asked at a medical meeting if this policy meant a physician would be required to undertake what was believed to be a futile attempt at cardiopulmonary resuscitation (CPR) if requested to do so by a competent patient (or presumably by the family of an incompetent terminally ill patient), the New York Health Commissioner, Dr. David Axelrod, replied: "There is a fight to CPR so I think the patient has to get it." "But," he continued, "that is pretty rare. How often does that happen?" The responses from the assembled physicians were "Often," "Everyday," and "All the time."[12]

With an approach that places near total control in the hands of the patient, no moral legitimacy is given to a physician's refusal of requested treatment. The physician is reduced from moral agent -- one with professional responsibilities and limits on what may legitimately be done -- and transformed into an extension of the patient's (or family's) whim, fantasy, or unrealizable hopes and desires. Such a relationship not only distorts the physician's role, it destroys the very autonomy it was designed to enhance. If patient's rights to demand medical intervention are left unchecked, physicians could be unwilling partners in harmful, self-mutilating, and even self-destructive patient actions.

Participation in harm to the patient has never been within the description of the patient-physician relationship. From the time of Hippocrates, the first principle of medicine has been "do no harm." Individuals approach a physician because they perceive a problem they believe the doctor can help relieve or overcome. Physicians examine the patient, and on the basis of medical training, knowledge, experience, and expertise, they assess the issue and, within the limits of available resources, make a judgment on whether there is a medically effective response to the problem.

Even in the time of Hippocrates, however, physicians recognized that sometimes the patient's condition was beyond their influence or that the patient might out of ignorance ask for that which is "deceitful" or not helpful. In such cases, the prudent Greek physician had no obligation to attempt to treat the patient.[13]

In today's shared decision-making, the physician makes a diagnosis of the problem and an assessment of the potential efficacy of medical interventions. The patient then weighs the possible alternatives and outcomes and, on the basis of personal values, accepts or rejects the recommended procedure. This process of selecting the best intervention for a particular patient is thus a joint venture of the physician and the patient. The patient is not bound to accept the recommended procedure and may engage the physician in further discussion of alternative responses to the problem. Should none prove acceptable, the patient is free to withdraw from the medical relationship, seek nontraditional or home remedies, or to forgo treatment altogether.

None of this, however, implies that the patient, if dissatisfied with the physician's proposals, may compel the physician to undertake patient-proposed interventions. There are legitimate constraints to patients' "right to treatment:" "Health care professionals or institutions may decline to provide a particular option because that choice would violate their conscience or professional judgment, though, in doing so they may not abandon a patient."[14]

Constraints may also be imposed to allocate resources more effectively or equitably. We will discuss only the first issue: physician refusal based on professional judgment of ineffectiveness or futility. The larger, more complex issues of cost-containment and allocation of limited resources, although of pressing public interest, are beyond the scope of this paper.

As of 1990, the literature on physician refusal of requested treatment was sparse.[15] The few published reports were restricted to relatively uncontroversial issues in primary care such as refusal of antibiotics for viral infections or CAT scans for routine headaches. Since 1990, there has been a burst of interest in the topic, including such issues as heart-lung transplantation,[16] surgery on patients in a persistent vegetative condition,[17] allocation of limited resources,[18] and maternal-fetal conflict.[19]

The debate has centered primarily on CPR and the requirement of patient or family consent for DNR orders.[20,21,22] The futility of attempting CPR in certain cases was first documented in a 1983 study that revealed 98-100% mortality in patients with metastatic disease, acute strokes, sepsis, renal failure, and pneumonia.[23] The same statistics applied to those for whom resuscitation took longer than 30 minutes. In such cases "the issue of patient autonomy is irrelevant."[24]

Tomlinson and Brody distinguished three rationales for a DNR order: no medical benefit, poor quality of life after CPR, and poor quality of life before CPR. They adopted Blackhall's position that "Physicians have no obligation to provide, and patients and families have no fight to demand, medical treatment that is of no demonstrable benefit."[25] In such cases, the patient's or family's desire for CPR is irrelevant. The decision is entirely within the physician's technical expertise. The most physicians should do when CPR is believed futile is to communicate that information to the patient or family so that they will understand the reason for making the decision not to intervene.

Only when the patient declines CPR because of present or anticipated quality of life factors do the patient's values or desires determine the decision. In such instances, personal values, not physician preferences, prevail.

Similar thinking was applied to the issue of resuscitation in the elderly.[26] The data showed that resuscitation is successful (success was defined as survival to discharge) in only 3.8% of the cases and never for arrests of elderly patients that are unwitnessed or that occur outside the hospital. Resuscitation is likewise unavailing even in witnessed hospital events in elderly patients with nonventricular arrhythmias.

The same situation prevails for cardiac arrests during the first 72 hours of life in very low birth-weight babies. In one study, none of the 488 babies who received CPR in the first 3 days of life survived, indicating that in such instances CPR is "innovative" or "nonvalidated" therapy and as such need not be provided or, if offered, should be presented to the family as an experimental procedure.[27]

These studies of CPR showed that an emphasis on the process of patient involvement rather than on the purpose and restricted effectiveness of CPR distorts the focus and shifts the debate from futility to the issue of patient autonomy. Younger[28] tried to move the emphasis back to an understanding of futility with comments on an article in which the author observed that CPR is "rarely effective and in many cases futile" in the setting of a long-term care facility.[29] Younger questioned how we define futility. Does futility signify absolute impossibility? Is it purely physiological? Does it include the ability to revive heartbeat but not achieve discharge from the hospital? How much quality of life and social value does the term embrace?

John Lantos and colleagues joined the debate and challenged the clinical usage of futility, arguing that there is no consensus among physicians as to the meaning.[30] Physicians disagree on both the chances of success and on the goals of the therapy. Some invoke futility only if the success rate is 0%, whereas others declare a treatment futile with a success rate as high as 18%. Further social and psychological factors may cloud a physician's estimate of success. Some consider liver transplantation futile for an alcoholic patient because of the likelihood of recidivism. Others consider a treatment futile if all it can provide is a chance for a couple of days or weeks in an intensive care unit. Yet, "Such a goal can be of supreme value to a dying patient."[31]

Even if a physician believes that a therapy will not be beneficial or that the chance of success is low, when the alternative is death the presumption should favor a request for treatment. The goals of the patient and the family, not the physician's assessment of the efficacy of treatment, determine medical futility and thus control decision-making.

Futility can be distinguished from the logically impossible, the implausible, the unusual, the rare, or the hopeless.[32] Futility can refer to "any effort to achieve a result that is possible but that reasoning or experience suggests is highly improbable and that cannot be systematically produced."[33]

As a practical example, if in the last 100 cases a medical treatment has been useless, it should be regarded as futile. The same would be true if all the intervention did was preserve patients in a persistent vegetative condition or sustain them in a dependency on the high-technology of the ICU. These ideas echoing Moore's challenge to the propriety of instituting "desperate remedies for desperate patients, desperately hopeless from the outset."[34] For Moore, patients must be offered more than pain, suffering, and cost; the use of a procedure must be justified by a realistic expectation of prolonged benefit.

This insistence that the physician has a positive obligation to refuse a requested intervention that cannot restore health or functioning to a desperately hopeless patient is not new. It is found in the writings of both Hippocrates and Plato. Hippocrates admonished physicians to acknowledge when efforts will probably fail: "Whenever therefore a man suffers from an ill which is too strong for the means at the disposal of medicine, he surely must not even expect that it can be overcome by medicine." He further warned the physician in words perhaps too strong for modern taste that to attempt futile treatment is to display an ignorance that "is allied to madness."[35]

In *The Republic*, Plato noted that medicine that "pampers" the disease was not used by the Asdepian physicians: "For those whose bodies were always in a state of inner sickness he did not attempt to prescribe a regime...to make their life a prolonged misery...Medicine was not intended for them and they should not be treated even if they were richer than Midas."[36]

A similar approach is found in the Vatican's 1980, "Declaration on Euthanasia" where the medical decision-making involves not only patient requests but a strong emphasis on physician judgment.[37]

But for such a decision to be made, account will have to be taken of the reasonable wishes of the patient and the patient's family, as also of the advice of the doctors who are specially competent in the matter. The latter may in particular judge that the investment in instruments and personnel is disproportionate to the results foreseen; they may also judge that the techniques applied impose on the patient strain or suffering out of proportion with the benefits which he or she may gain from such techniques.

Physicians' ethical obligation to act as moral agents, to exercise independent judgment on the extent to which their ministration could help or harm the patient, was the basis for our essay on "Baby L, " a case in which physicians at a major pediatric hospital refused a mother's request to institute what was thought to be a life-prolonging procedure.[38] To our knowledge, the medical team's refusal to put a severely compromised, blind, deaf, and neurologically devastated infant -- who had spent all of her 23 months of existence dependent on intensive care treatment -- on a ventilator marked the first time physicians had refused a request for potentially life-prolonging treatment for a patient in acute crisis.

The refusal was not based on cost concerns nor allocation worries because Baby L's medical expenses, though well in excess of $1 million, were covered by third-party payments. The refusal was based on the medical team's assessment that unless a reversal or amelioration of the underlying condition could be expected, painful interventions would be futile and inhumane. The medical team judged that no intervention could produce a reversal of the infant's condition.

No other facility or physician could be located who was willing to care for the infant as the mother directed. When the case was brought to court by the mother, who wanted "everything possible" to prolong the life of the child, the physicians informed the court that they would decline to participate in an action that would violate their ethical obligation to "do no harm" to their patient. As support, they cited the recent ruling of the Massachusetts

Supreme Judicial Court in Brophy v. New England Sinai Hospital that there is nothing in the law "which would justify compelling medical professionals...to take active measures which are contrary to their view of their ethical duty toward their patients."[39] That ruling provided the legal basis for the moral stand taken by the physicians. Further challenge to their position ended when the court found a physician who was willing to care for the child as the mother directed.

The controversy over futility did not end with Baby L. We were subsequently involved in the case of E.T., where the neonatologists at a Chicago hospital sought a court order to terminate ventilator support on a 4-month-old, very low birthweight, early gestational infant whose grade IV intercranial bleed had eroded most of its cerebral cortex. Despite a bleak prognosis with no possibility of recovery and certain demise in the NICU, the mother would not consider any lessening of intensive therapy. With unanimity among the health care team, the ethics consultation service, the pediatric ethics committee, legal counsel, and the hospital administration, a court order was sought to transfer guardianship and withdraw the ventilator. The infant died before the issue of withdrawal could be argued.

The issue of the futility and the requirement of family consent for orders not to attempt further life-prolonging measures in desperately ill dying patients was the subject of two important essays and an accompanying editorial in a recent issue of *JAMA*.[40,41,42] Hackler and Hiller report on two cases that resemble that of E.T. in which physicians under parental pressure utilized measures and resuscitation contrary to their medical judgment on utterly hopeless cases. In one case an 18-year-old and in the other a 6-year-old died despite prolonged intensive management. In the case of the 6-year-old, the physicians were so exasperated after final resuscitation, during which the patient was asystolic for 30-45 minutes while the mother refused to allow them to stop, that they flatly refused any longer to be a part of the patient's care.

The authors propose that it is a mistake to believe that CPR must be offered and refused in all cases. As they note, "respect for patient autonomy does not require that the physician initiate decisions of medically pointless procedures."[43] Useless CPR, they observe, is no different in this regard from useless tonsillectomy. If it is not indicated, it ought not be discussed.

Further, they note, it is a strange way of proceeding "to offer a treatment with the suggestion it be refused." If a treatment is being offered, the expectation is that there is a benefit perceived by the one who does the proffering. To decline the offer might make the patient or family seem ungrateful or callous. Because there is no need to offer or even discuss a decision to withhold useless treatments, Hackler and Hiller conclude that "Hospital policy should allow physicians to write DNR orders without family consent or discussion, if CPR would be futile."[44]

If, as Fiel's case report describes, a family insists on treatments the physician believes inappropriate, these authors believe the physician must focus on the best interest of the patient. In their words "It is wrong to inflict pain on one person without chance of significant benefit to satisfy another person out of a slavish adherence to an occasionally misdirected procedural principle."[45]

Tomlinson and Brody provide a sound philosophical basis for not seeking patient (or family) authorization for omitting futile procedures. Far from undermining autonomy, they argue that the mixed messages inherent in requesting patient consent to withhold futile therapy serves to undermine, not enhance, autonomous choice. Mixed messages give false hope, provide unrealizable expectations, and enhance the incentive for harmful misadventure. Further, they believe attempts to confine futility to the physiologically impossible misstate by overstating the issue. Medical assessments are based on human moral judgments, not metaphysical certitude.

In every case, "reasonable certainty" will mean "reasonable probability," not "absolute certainty."

If so, the question is not whether but which value judgments physicians may use in deciding whether to meet patient demands. This question signals a turn away from individual conceptions toward social conceptions of reasonable and worthwhile nature of the goals of medical procedures. A challenge to an individual request is made only with the background assumption that no reasonable-person would want medical interventions in such circumstances. That, claim Tomlinson and Brody, "is a social judgment of 'reasonableness,' not an individual one." It does not suspend judgment about what ends are worth pursuing nor does it locate all value within the individual. Only within the context of social judgments of the range of rational conceptions of the goal may the individual legitimately expect his or her wishes to be followed. Unlike Hackler and Hiller, Tomlinson and Brody believe that the patient and family should be informed-not asked-about the decision to omit resuscitation so that families will more fully understand and accept that all that could be done for the patient had been done.

To overcome the potential for abuse of physician discretion, the decision to omit a requested medical treatment ought not be made on the personal predilections of the practitioner but on well-established medical criteria and more broadly based social warrant that, in turn, must be shared with the patient. The safeguard against professional arrogance and arbitrariness, as Tomlinson and Brody note, is not patient arbitrariness but an effective patient-physician dialogue.

The practice of medicine has shifted from a purely physician determination of what can and should be done to one in which the patient is fully involved in the decision-making process. In the course of that shift, the emphasis on patient rights, integrity, and autonomy has led some to believe that the patient not only participates fully in the decision-making process but has the final say on what is to be done.

The untoward consequences of that approach are evident in the hospital policies that require utterly useless attempts be made at resuscitating end-stage terminally ill patients. Rather than respecting patient autonomy, policies that insist on doing "whatever the patient wants" may undermine true respect for the patient' s dignity.

Physicians as moral agents should exercise professional judgment in assessing patient requests. If the request goes beyond well-established criteria of reasonableness, the physician ought not feel obliged to provide it. Physician refusal of requests for futile or ineffective treatments is not an abandonment of the patient; it is an assertion of professional responsibility.

Notes

1. Paris JJ, Crone RK, Reardon F. Physicians' refusal of requested treatment: The case of Baby L, *New England Journal of Medicine* 1990;322:1012-5.
2. Hackler JC, Hiller FC. Family consent to orders not to resuscitate, *Journal of the American Medical Association* 1990;264:1281-3.
3. Hackler JC, Hiller FC. Family consent to orders not to resuscitate: Reconsidering hospital policy, *Journal of the American Medical Association* 1990;264:1281-3.
4. Fiel SB. Heart-lung transplantation for patients with cystic fibrosis, *Archives of Internal Medicine* 1991;151:870-2.
5. Tresch DD, Sims FH, Duthie EH, *et al*. Clinical characteristics of patients in the persistent vegetative state, *Archives of Internal Medicine* 1991;151:930-2.
6. Fiel S. Heart-lung transplantation for patients with cystic fibrosis, *Archives of Internal Medicine* 1991;151:870-2.

7. Tomlinson T, Brody H. Futility and the ethics of resuscitation, *Journal of the American Medical Association* 1990;264:1276-80.
8. Wolf SM. "Near death"--in the moment of decision, *New England Journal of Medicine* 1990;322:208-10, See p. 209.
9. Pellegrino E. Ethics in AIDS treatment decisions, *Origins* 1990;19:539-44.
10. Brock DW, Wartman SA. When competent patients make irrational choices, *New England Journal of Medicine* 1990;322:1595-9.
11. New York State Task Force on Life and the Law. *Do Not Resuscitate Orders: The Proposed Legislation and Report of the New York State Task Force on Life and the Law*. Albany, NY: The Task Force, 1986.
12. Rosenthal E. Rules on reviving the dying bring undue suffering, doctors contend. *New York Times* 1990 Oct 4:A1.
13. Amundsen DW. The physician's obligation to prolong life: A medical duty without classical roots, *Hastings Center Report* 1978;8:23-30.
14. *Deciding To Forego Life-Sustaining Treatment: A Report on the Ethical, Medical and Legal Issues in Treatment Decisions*. Washington, DC: President's Commission for the Study of Ethical Problems in Medicine and Biomedical and Behavioral Research, 1983:3.
15. Paris JJ, Crone RK, Reardon F. Physicians' refusal of requested treatment: The case of Baby L, *New England Journal of Medicine* 1990;322:1012-5.
16. Fiel S. Heart-lung transplantation for patients with cystic fibrosis, *Archives of Internal Medicine* 1991;151:870-2.
17. Tresch DD, Sims FH, Duthie EH, *et al.* Clinical characteristics of patients in the persistent vegetative state, *Archives of Internal Medicine* 1991;151:930-2.
18. Hadore DC. Setting health care priorities in Oregon. Cost-effectiveness meets the rule of rescue, *Journal of the American Medical Association* 1991;265:2218-25.
19. Chervenak FA, McCullough LB. Justified limits on refusing intervention, *Hastings Center Report* 1991;21:12-8.
20. Younger SJ. Who defines futility? *Journal of the American Medical Association* 1990;260:2094-5.
21. Tomlinson T, Brody H. Futility and the ethics of resuscitation, *Journal of the American Medical Association* 1990;264:1276-80.
22. Tomlinson T, Brody H. Futility and the ethics of resuscitation, *Journal of the American Medical Association* 1990;264:1276-80.
23. Bedell SF, Delbanco TL, Cook EF, *et al.* Survival after cardiopulmonary resuscitation in the hospital, *New England Journal of Medicine* 1983;309:569-76.
24. Blackhall LJ. Must we always use CPR? *New England Journal of Medicine* 1987;317:1281-4, See p. 1281.
25. Tomlinson T, Brody H. Ethics and communication in do-not-resuscitate orders, *New England Journal of Medicine* 1988;318:43-6, See p. 43.
26. Murphy DJ. Do-not-resuscitate orders: Time for reappraisal in long-term care institutions, *Journal of the American Medical Association* 1989;260:2098-2101.
27. Lantos JD, Miles SM, Silverstein MD, *et al.* Survival after cardiopulmonary resuscitation in babies of very, low birth weight: Is CPR futile therapy? *New England Journal of Medicine* 1988;318:91-5.
28. Younger SJ. Who defines futility? *Journal of the American Medical Association* 1990;260:2094-5.
29. Murphy DJ. Do-Not-Resuscitate orders: Time for reappraisal in long-term care institutions, *Journal of the American Medical Association* 1989;260:2098-2101.
30. Lantos JD, Singer PA, Walker RM, *et al.* The illusion of futility in clinical practice, *The American Journal of Medicine* 1989;87:814.
31. See note 30. Lantos *et al.* 1989;87:83.
32. Schneiderman LJ, Jecker NS, Jonsen AR. Medical futility: Its meaning and ethical implications, *Annals of Internal Medicine* 1990;112:949-54.
33. See note 32. Schneiderman *et al.* 1990;112:950.
34. Moore FD. The desperate case: CARE (costs, applicability, research, ethics), *Journal of the American Medical Association* 1991;261:1483-4, See p. 1483.

35. Selection from the Hippocratic Corpus: "The Art" (circa 5th-4th century B.C.). In: Reiser SJ, Dyck AJ, Curran WJ, eds. *Ethics in Medicine: Historical Perspectives and Contemporary Concertos*. Cambridge, MA: MIT Press, 1977:6-7.
36. Plato. *The Republic*. Translated by GMA Grube. Indianapolis, IN: Hackett Publishing Co., 1974.
37. Vatican. Declaration on euthanasia, the sacred congregation for the doctrines of the faith, In: *Deciding to Forego Life-Sustaining Treatment: A Report on the Ethical, Medical, and Legal Issues in Treatment Decisions*. Washington, DC: President's Commission for the Study of Ethical Problems in Medicine and Biomedical and Behavioral Research, 1983:300-6, See p. 306.
38. Paris JJ, Crone RK, Reardon F. Physicians' refusal of requested treatment: The case of Baby L, *New England Journal of Medicine* 1990;322:1012-5.
39. *Brophy v. New England Sinai Hospital* 398 Mass., 417, 497 N.E. 2d 626 (1986).
40. Hackler JC, Hiller FC. Family consent to orders not to resuscitate: Reconsidering hospital policy, *Journal of the American Medical Association* 1990;264:1281-3.
41. Tomlinson T, Brody H. Futility and the ethics of resuscitation, *Journal of the American Medical Association* 1990;264:1276-80.
42. Younger SJ. Futility in context, *Journal of the American Medical Association* 1990;264:1295-6.
43. Hackler JC, Hiller FC. Family consent to orders not to resuscitate: Reconsidering hospital policy, *Journal of the American Medical Association* 1990;264:1281-3.
44. See note 3. Hackler and Hiller. 1990;264:1282.
45. See note 3. Hackler and Hiller. 1990;264:1283.

Chapter 61

Medical Futility: The Duty Not to Treat

Nancy S. Jecker and Lawrence J. Schneiderman

Partly because physicians can "never say never," partly because of the seduction of modern technology, and partly out of misplaced fear of litigation, physicians have increasingly shown a tendency to undertake treatments that have no realistic expectation of success, For this reason, we have articulated common sense criteria for medical futility.[1] If a treatment can be shown not to have worked in the last 100 cases, we propose that it be regarded as medically futile. Also, if the treatment fails to restore consciousness or alleviate total dependence on intensive care, we propose such treatment be judged futile, This definition provides clear end points and encourages the profession to review data from the past and perform prospective clinical studies that not only report treatments that work but also treatments that do not work, We have also argued that, in a variety of settings, physicians have no ordinary ethical obligation to offer futile interventions (Schneiderman *et al.*, unpublished).[2,3,4,5,6] Although physicians should inform and discuss all decisions to withhold or withdraw medical treatments with patients, they need not obtain the patient's permission to desist from futile interventions.

In this paper, we examine in closer detail the ethical implications of medical futility. Section one introduces an illustrative case involving a dearly futile medical treatment, Section two outlines three contrasting positions regarding the ethical responsibility of physicians involved in the case. These positions hold that the physician is: 1) allowed; 2) encouraged; or 3) required to refrain from using a futile therapy. We clarify the reasons supporting each viewpoint but urge acceptance of the third, and strongest, ethical stance. The concluding sections of the paper describe an emerging consensus in this area and review objections to our position.

The Case

Arthur Archer (not his real name) was a 66-year-old man who was admitted for treatment of metastatic carcinoma of the lung, Upon admission to the hospital, he was informed of his fights under the Patient Self-Determination Act to refuse any unwanted treatments. Prior to beginning chemotherapy, Mr. Archer was informed by Dr. Foster (not her real name) of the anticipated toxicity of the treatment and of the limited chance of sustained and qualitatively good response to treatment. Furthermore, Dr. Foster told Mr. Archer that in the event of a cardiac arrest during his treatment program, she would not attempt cardiopulmonary resuscitation (CPR). She explained that in patients with metastatic cancer, CPR had a negligible chance of success and an almost certain chance of prolonging his suffering before dying in the intensive care unit (ICU).

Source: Reprinted from *Cambridge Quarterly of Healthcare Ethics*, Vol. 2, 1993, pp. 151-159, with permission from Cambridge University Press © 1993.

In other words, CPR would be futile. Mr. Archer accepted Dr. Foster's decision and a do-not-attempt resuscitation order was written.

The night after chemotherapy was started, Mr. Archer developed an acute myocardial infarction with periods of irregular heartbeat. The physician on duty that night, Dr. Wilmot (also not his real name), told Mr. Archer that CPR would probably be necessary and obtained Mr. Archer's consent. Shortly thereafter, Mr. Archer underwent a cardiac arrest, and Dr. Wilmot immediately instituted efforts at CPR. These efforts failed, however, and the patient died. The next day at case conference, Dr. Wilmot and Dr. Foster, as well as several other physicians, engaged in a heated debate over whether CPR should have been attempted. A conference was arranged, and an ethics consultant was asked to join the group. During this conference, the physicians referred to an empirical study that summarized the experience at several medical centers. This study reported that when CPR was required and attempted in a total of 147 patients with metastatic cancer, not one patient survived to hospital discharge. The author of the report concluded that such treatment was futile and should not be attempted. The question was raised, therefore, "should CPR have been attempted in Mr. Archer?" But the debate then turned to the larger question: What are the ethical options and duties of physicians when treatment is shown to be of so little likelihood of success? In the discussion that followed, several views were aired, most notably the following:

1. Dr. Wilmot was ethically permitted to refrain from attempting CPR, but he was also ethically permitted to perform it.

2. Dr. Wilmot should have been encouraged not to perform CPR on Mr. Archer. That is, the conclusion of the study and the recommendation by the study's author might be considered an ethical guideline that physicians are urged, but not required, to follow.

3. Finally, some argued that once a treatment is shown to be futile, Dr. Wilmot was ethically required, as a matter of professional duty, to refrain from attempting it.

In the first instance, allowing Dr. Wilmot to make an individual decision about attempting CPR on a patient with metastatic cancer would be ethically analogous to allowing an obstetrics and gynecology physician to decide whether or not to meet a woman's request to perform therapeutic abortion. The medical profession, although accepting abortion as a legal choice for all women, takes an ethically neutral stance and allows individual physicians to opt out of performing the procedure as a matter of personal conscience. Therefore, the physician is not ethically wrong to refuse to comply with a patient's demands for this particular treatment.

In the second instance, encouraging but not requiring Dr. Wilmot to refrain from attempting CPR is ethically analogous to a physician's decision to support life in patients in persistent vegetative state. Several professional societies recommend against maintaining patients in a persistent vegetative state.[7,8,9] Yet, physicians are neither ethically nor legally bound to pursue these advisory recommendations. Similarly, Dr. Wilmot may be ethically free to attempt CPR on Mr. Archer; however, refraining from CPR would be an ethically preferable course.

In the third instance, the ethical equivalent of a duty to omit futile therapies is the duty to treat patients with HIV infection. The medical profession has clearly mandated that it is the duty of all physicians not to discriminate against patients on the basis of their HIV status. Therefore, a physician who refuses to treat a patient simply because the patient has this condition would be regarded as violating an ethical duty. Similarly then, attempting CPR in patients with metastatic cancer may be considered *prima facie* wrong for all physicians by virtue of violating professional standards against applying futile treatments. Furthermore, this effort would be wrong even if Mr. Archer had not only consented to, but had emphatically demanded, CPR, because physicians are generally bound by the standards of their profession.

The Ethical Viewpoints

Having sketched three viewpoints regarding a physician's duty to cease futile interventions, we now proceed stepwise. First, we show the reasons why physicians should ordinarily be allowed to refrain from offering or continuing futile treatment. Then we will indicate arguments defending a stronger point: physicians should generally be encouraged to omit futile therapies. Finally, we will present the still stronger case that physicians should generally be required to decline the use of futile interventions. Throughout, our arguments draw on historical traditions of medicine and relate these to contemporary critical medicine settings.

The Weakest Ethical Stance

A central aim of the profession of medicine is to use the art and science of medicine for the purpose of helping the patient. In Mr. Archer's case, overwhelming odds exist that CPR would not benefit him. Physicians who offer futile interventions under such circumstances are in fact deceiving their patients and compromising professional standards of medicine. Through offering a treatment to a patient, a physician conveys that the treatment represents a medically acceptable alternative. But if the treatment actually is almost certain to fail, what value is it to the patient? If the patient is misled into believing in the treatment's efficacy, then the physician has violated the patient's trust. If the physician informs the patient that the treatment is futile and offers it anyway, the physician conveys a confusing double message.[10] In short, physicians who prescribe treatments that they are reasonably confident will not improve patients' conditions break trust with patients and denigrate the practice of medicine. Their conduct allies medicine with quackery and physicians with charlatans.

The provision of futile treatment is additionally objectionable when the act violates a physician's personal ethical convictions. In this case, a refusal to allow the physician to withhold or withdraw futile interventions does not take seriously the physician's own ethical autonomy and agency. It would be akin to mandating that physicians who oppose abortions perform them. In these cases, requiring the use of futile interventions wrongly signals that physicians are merely tools for enacting others' (patients') goals and do not possess, as individuals and as members of a profession, independent ethical standards and ends.

A Moderate Ethical Stance

Suppose that, on the above grounds, we agree that Dr. Wilmot was free to withhold CPR on Mr. Archer. Dr. Wilmot might reasonably conclude that, therefore, he was as free to use futile interventions as he was to withhold them. Either way, his actions would be beyond reproach.

The difficulty this proposal encounters is that pounding on the chests of patients, such as Mr. Archer, in a futile attempt to get the heart started is not an ethically neutral act. Ribs can be broken, the trachea damaged, and not uncommonly the brain never completely recovers from oxygen deprivation. Moreover, in Mr. Archer's and many other cases, CPR only instills false hope that the patient will somehow pull through, that a miracle will happen. The truth is that even if Mr. Archer had survived the cardiac arrest, he would most likely have to endure the prolonged pain, discomfort, and suffering associated with the dying process, and almost certainly he would never have survived to hospital discharge. This violates one of the oldest ethics of the medical profession: omit whatever is injurious to patients.

Even when futile interventions do not exact such a heavy toll, physicians should be encouraged to withhold and withdraw them because the profession of medicine was never intended to practice non-beneficial medical care. Rather, medicine's aim has always been to help the sick. Affirming this age-old ethic, the President's Commission for the Study of Ethical Problems in Medicine and Biomedical and Behavioral Research stated in 1983 that "the care available from health professionals is generally limited to what is consistent with role-related professional standards and conscientiously held personal beliefs."[11] It is ironic that in no other profession but medicine are members asked to transgress professional and personal standards to satisfy a client's wishes. Thus, it is never expected that accountants will perform audits and prepare financial statements in ways that run counter to generally accepted accounting principles to improve a client's chances of obtaining a bank loan. Nor is it ever imagined that architects will design buildings that violate building codes simply because customers want structures built from materials that appeal to them yet are unsafe. Only in medicine do patients sometimes claim entitlement to receive whatever medical treatment they wish, regardless of the likelihood of success and regardless of the quality of outcome to be achieved. This expectation must be revisited or the integrity of the medical profession will not remain intact.

A final reason why physicians should be encouraged to avoid non-beneficial treatment is that applying such treatment leads physicians to neglect their positive duties to help dying patients. In the care of dying patients, the physician's primary duty is to comfort the patient by relieving pain and responding to the patient's situation in an empathic and caring way. The use of futile treatments distracts physicians from these goals by focusing their attention on debating useless interventions. Thus, at a time when the physician's greatest offering is to alleviate the patient's pain and suffering to help the patient achieve as good a death as possible, the focal topic of conversation among the medical team becomes whether or not to attempt aggressive technological interventions. Meanwhile, scant attention may be given to the patient's physical, emotional, and spiritual needs.

A Strong Ethical Stance

So far we have defended two progressively stronger claims concerning the ethical responsibility of physicians under futile circumstances. The weak claim held that physicians are free to withhold or discontinue futile therapies. The moderate stance maintained that physicians should also be encouraged to do so. We now make the still stronger case that physicians are ordinarily required to forego futile interventions.

The bases for this stronger claim are threefold. First, in the absence of a general professional ethic affirming the scope and limits of physicians' obligations, the meaning and ethical implications of futility fall prey to abuse. For example, if Dr. Foster and Dr. Wilmot were free to use "futility" to mean whatever they wish, then their debate over whether or not to attempt CPR on Mr. Archer may have had multiple, hidden subtexts. Did Dr. Foster think Mr. Archer too old to be receiving such expensive medical treatment? Was she subconsciously withholding CPR because the patient was not as pleasant or interesting or grateful as other patients under her care? Perhaps the second physician, Dr. Wilmot, did not experience this, having known Mr. Archer so briefly. Did Dr. Foster find her time taken away from other patients whom she thought had greater need for her and better chances of a successful outcome? All these factors could incline physicians to invoke the term "futility" as a subterfuge for rationing, cost containment, or refusals to treat vulnerable patients. In other words, the absence of a profession-wide standard governing the use of futile treatments invites abuse by allowing ethical standards to be tailored to suit outside ends. We can expect that whichever ethical claims about futility support the financial, legal, or other purposes of individual physicians or their institutions will be invoked. To avoid such abuse, the profession of medicine must not only encourage physicians to omit futile treatments but must endorse a general ethical position opposing the use of futile methods. Only then can abuses be recognized for what they are. Only then are patients promised some reprieve from economic and legal considerations that thwart patient advocacy.

A second reason for assigning an obligation to refrain from futile treatment to all physicians is that the public tightly looks to the medical profession to set general standards for appropriate medical treatment. Physicians in our society practice medicine as part of a publicly sanctioned profession: society grants the profession authority to certify individual practitioners as competent to act in the best interests of patients. By virtue of receiving such authority, the profession receives the public's trust, just as other professions are entrusted to address spiritual needs or educate the populace. To be worthy of the public's trust, a profession is obliged to set ethical guidelines for its members. In medicine, leaving standards for beneficial and non-beneficial medical practice to individual clinicians abdicates the profession's responsibility to the society.

Finally, physicians are ethically obligated to avoid futile medicine because its use exploits the public's fear of death and feeds inflated ideas about what medicine and science can achieve. Contemporary physicians bear special obligations in this area because they practice in a society that extols, even worships, science and technology and clings tenaciously to exaggerated ideas about what these methods can accomplish. To counter this tendency, the profession of medicine should take a firm and public stand stating the limits of what their profession can and will do. In the absence of such a commitment, society will continue to assign Godlike responsibilities to physicians, and individuals and families will continue to hold physicians and hospitals hostage by insisting that clinicians achieve miraculous feats.

An Emerging Consensus

There are signs that professional medical and biomedical organizations are rising to the challenge of affirming medicine's limits. Thus, as early as 1983 the President's Commission wrote that "A health care professional has ah obligation to allow a patient to choose from among medically acceptable treatment options...or to reject all options. No one, however, has an obligation to provide interventions that would, in his or her judgment, be counter-therapeutic."[12] In 1987, the Hastings Center claimed in its Guidelines on the Termination of LifeSustaining Treatment and the Care of the Dying[13] that "if a treatment is dearly futile...there is no obligation to provide the treatment."

Other medical organizations have begun to follow suit. In 1991, the American Medical Association's Council on Ethical and Judicial Affairs published "Guidelines for the Appropriate Use of Do-Not-Resuscitate Orders." The Council held that CPR may be withheld, even if previously requested by the patient, "when efforts to resuscitate a patient are judged by the treating physician to be futile."[14] In the same year, the American Thoracic Society (an organization of the American Lung Association) took a similar stand and claimed that "Forcing physicians to provide medical interventions that are clearly futile would undermine the ethical integrity of the medical profession."[15] During the same period, the Task Force on Ethics of the Society for Critical Care Medicine published a consensus report stating that, "Treatments that offer no benefit and serve to prolong the dying process should not be employed."[16]

Answering Objections

On what bases might someone dissent from the emerging consensus we have described? On what grounds might someone take issue with the strong ethical position that we have defended? In what follows, we summarize and answer a series of possible objections to our proposal.

A first objection insists that the patient, rather than the profession of medicine, should be allowed to decide whether or not the quality of outcome achieved by an intervention is acceptable. In other words, qualitatively poor results should at least be presented to the patient or surrogate as an option.[17] We believe a distinction is in order. The quality of outcome associated with an intervention falls along continuum, ranging from good to borderline to poor. Thus, at one end are outcomes where quality of life is seriously compromised, yet important life goals can still be accomplished and life itself can still be appreciated by the patient. Treatments to maintain a patient in such a condition are well above the threshold of medical futility, and the decision of whether to receive or forego therapy properly rests with the patient (or surrogate). For instance, outcomes requiring frequent hospitalization, confinement to a nursing home, or severe physical or mental handicaps are not futile, and any decision to pursue them should be decided by the patient. At the other end of the continuum are qualitatively poor results that are clearly futile and need not be offered to patients. This category includes, for example, therapies intended to continue patients in a persistent vegetative state, or treatments that result in overwhelming suffering for a predictably brief period of time. Finally, still other outcomes fall between these two end points and represent borderline cases. In these cases, ample disagreement exists among the medical profession concerning the quality of outcome associated with an intervention. Under such circumstances, futility is not confidently established and the decision to receive or decline treatment should be the patient's (or surrogate's).

A second objection with which our proposal may be met holds that the determination of medical futility is a value judgment, and attempts to render a valuefree account of futility are unsuccessful.[18] Physicians are no better equipped than laypeople are to render value judgments. In response, we agree with and underscore the point that the determination of both quantitative and qualitative futility entail value decisions. Likewise, affirming a duty to define futile interventions "constitutes a value commitment. Thus, we object to physicians claiming authority to render futility judgments under the guise of purely "scientific", or "technical" expertise. Instead, the proper basis for assigning physicians authority to set standards for the practice of medicine is that an ethical dimension is an integral component of the historical and contemporary role of the profession in society. The fact that society shuns those who practice medicine solely to make a profit, wield power, or achieve status reveals that we expect physicians to employ their skills to help the sick and promote the good of the society. This expectation is justified, so long as the profession of medicine continues to espouse principles of service and its members persist in putting themselves forward as advocates for patients.

Another objection that may be mounted against our proposal holds that requiring physicians to refrain from futile treatments sometimes constitutes an unfair violation of patients' religious or other convictions. In particular, declining to sustain a patient in a persistent vegetative state may be at odds with the religious or other values of those who hold that life itself is sacred and thus worth preserving even in an unconscious state.[19] The answer to this objection is, first, that religious teachings are extraordinarily difficult to interpret and apply to specific medical contexts.[20] Second, our society's division of church and state limits the reach of religious views in public policy formation. The profession of medicine gains authority and sanction from the entire society it serves. Thus, its standards should incorporate diverse religious and other perspectives, rather than reflecting the creed of any single religious or other group. When the profession articulates standards that embody a reasoned synthesis of Community values, then particular individuals and groups will still object. However, practitioners of medicine should not succumb to dissenters' wishes under these circumstances. They should instead indicate that medicine is properly governed by values and commitments of the profession.

A quite different objection to our proposal holds that to grant the medical profession authority to define medical futility and set ethical standards in this area is to embark on a perilous and slippery slope that will inevitably yield excessive medical paternalism or, worse, a medical profession guided by invidious racial and other stereotypes. Just as physicians who practiced under Germany's Third Reich applied invidious discrimination in assessing patients' quality of life, so too physicians today may institutionalize prejudices that are legion in the larger society. They may extend an initial authority to refrain from clearly futile interventions to other cases in which the quality of life associated with an intervention is impaired, but remains well worth living.

It is important not to dismiss such concerns lightly. Abuses of futility can produce devastating consequences, and physicians cannot be expected to be immune from prejudices that are widely accepted in society. Nonetheless, the best way to stem possible abuses is to make explicit and public policies regarding the definition and ethical implications of medical futility. Only with explicit policies in place can individuals recognize abuses for what they are. In the absence of clear public standards in this area, futility judgments will still be made; they will simply be made in inconsistent and sometimes insensitive ways. In contrast to explicit criteria and standards, implicit attitudes are not thought through, not applied consistently, not accountable to the public, and not insulated from arbitrary and unfair manipulation.

In addition, physicians who desist from futile interventions remain obligated to communicate with patients and family members and to continue to offer palliative and comfort measures to the patient. We agree with those who hold that the objective of discussions at this point is not to obtain the patient's or family's permission to desist from futile therapies but to enhance their information and understanding of the medical situation.[21]

A final concern that might be expressed in response to our proposal is indicated by the view that talk about futility is in reality a convenient "code" for talking about rationing and cost containment. If so, then it is manipulative and unethical to disguise economic matters in this fashion. In reply it can be said that rationing, cost containment, and futility display distinct meanings and ethical norms.[22] Rationing always indicates a choice about the distribution of medical treatment to one patient versus another. Futility has no explicit distributive meaning but refers instead to a specific cause-and-effect relationship in a particular patient. In addition, rationing can be distinguished from futility because the circumstances of rationing always presuppose scarcity, whereas an intervention may be futile even when it is abundant and readily available. The ethical implications of rationing and futility are also distinct. Rationing is evaluated as just or unjust by reference to theories of distributive justice. Yet the ethical implications of futility are judged by reference to a consensus reached within the profession and sanctioned in the larger society.

Cost containment also differs in its meaning and ethical implications from futility. Whereas the goal of cost containment is to reduce overall medical expenditures, the point of identifying interventions as futile is to determine that they are not beneficial to the patient. Thus, futile interventions remain futile even if they are relatively inexpensive so that omitting them does not significantly reduce health expenditures. In contrast to futility, cost containment is ethically evaluated according to justice principles and theories.

Conclusion

Physicians are ordinarily required to refrain from using futile interventions. This general ethical stance should be publicly endorsed by the medical profession and embodied in institutional policies at all levels. In the absence of a clear and consistent ethical standard, ethical choices will continue to be made regarding the use of futile therapies, but they will be subject to various abuses. Explicitly stated criteria and values hold out the promise of more consistent and ethical standards for medical practice.

Notes

1. Schneiderman LJ, Jecker NS, Jonsen AR. Medical futility: Its meaning and ethical implications, *Annals of Internal Medicine* 1990;112:949-54.
2. Jecker NS. Knowing when to stop: The limits of medicine, *Hastings Center Report* 1991;21(3):5-8.
3. Jecker NS, Schneiderman LJ. Futility and rationing, *American Journal of Medicine* 1992;92:189-96.
4. Jecker NS, Pearlman RA. Medical futility: Who decides? *Archives of Internal Medicine* 1992;152:1140-4.
5. Jecker NS, Schneiderman LJ. Ceasing futile resuscitation in the field: Ethical considerations, *Archives of Internal Medicine* 1992;152:2392-2397.
6. Schneiderman LJ, Jecker NS. Futility in practice, *Archives of Internal Medicine* [in press].
7. Task Force on Ethics of the Society of Critical Care Medicine. Consensus report on the ethics of foregoing life-sustaining treatments in the critically ill, *Critical Cam Medicine* 1990;18:1435-9.
8. American Thoracic Society, Bioethics Task Force. Withholding and withdrawing life-sustaining therapy, *Annals of Internal Medicine* 1991;115:478-85.
9. President's Commission for the Study of Ethical Problems in Medicine and Biomedical and Behavioral Research. *Deciding to ForegoLife-Sustaining Treatments*. Washington, DC : Government Printing Office, 1983.
10. Brody H, Tomlinson T. Futility and the ethics of resuscitation, *Journal of the American Medical Association* 1990;264:1276-80.
11. See note 9. President's Commission. 1983:44.
12. See note 9. President's Commission. 1983:44.
13. The Hastings Center. *Guidelines on the Termination of Life-Sustaining Treatment and the Care of the Dying*. Indianapolis, IN: Indiana University Press, 1987:19.
14. American Medical Association, Council on Ethical and Judicial Affairs. Guidelines on the appropriate use of do-not-resuscitate orders, *Journal of the American Medical Association* 1991;265:1868-71, at 1870.
15. See note 8. American Thoracic Society. 1991;115:481.
16. See note 7. Society of Critical Care Medicine. 1990;18:1436.
17. Veatch RM, Spicer CM. Medically futile care: The role of the physician in setting limits, *American Journal of Law and Medicine* 1992;18:15-36.
18. Truog RD, Brett AS, Frader J. The problem with futility, *New England Journal of Medicine* 1992;326:1560-4.
19. Angell M. The case of Helga Wanglie: A new kind of "fight to die" case, *New England Journal of Medicine* 1991;325:511-2.
20. Jecker NS, Pearlman RA. Medical futility, reply to Letter to the Editor, *Archives of Internal Medicine* [in press].
21. Tomlinson T, Brody H. Ethics and communication in do-not-resuscitate orders, *New England Journal of Medicine* 1988;318:43-6.
22. See note 3. Jecker, Schneiderman. 1992;92:189-96.

Chapter 62

The Negotiation of Death: Clinical Decision-Making at the End of Life

Jacquelyn Slomka

Introduction

The emphasis on ethical decision-making in health care today has been attributed in part to the extensive use of technology that has led to situations in which an individual's life, as defined in the physical or biological sense, can be prolonged past the point of "natural" death. In today's hospital intensive care unit, the terminally ill patient caught in the web of medical technology can escape through death in two ways: the physical organism reaches its breaking point and the body can no longer function, even with technological coercion; or the physician, patient, and family decide to withdraw various life-sustaining technologies and allow death to occur.[1] The occurrence of death by a process of withdrawing or withholding life-supporting technological interventions involves deliberations among physicians, patients, and families in a process that has been characterized as the negotiation of death.[2]

Although the exact frequency of occurrence of treatment withdrawal that results in death is not known, some studies indicate that approximately 70% of patients who die in hospital have "Do-Not-Resuscitate" status, a designation that often leads to a less intensive level of care for the patient that includes the negotiation of the withholding or withdrawal of therapies.[3] The ethics of end-of-life decision-making and the appropriate use of life-supporting therapy often is discussed theoretically in the medical and bioethics literature. Issues such as informed consent, the need for effective communication, advance directives, surrogate decision-making, patient autonomy, definitions of life and death, legal uncertainties, and the appropriate use of 'do-not-resuscitate' orders have been addressed. (See, for example,[4,5,6,7]) Empirical studies of limiting treatment have focused on the incidence of and family/patient involvement in "Do-Not-Resuscitate" (DNR) status, characteristics of patients with DNR orders, the intensity of therapy after DNR designation, the reasons for and manner of treatment withdrawal and cost savings associated with treatment limitation.[3,8,9,10,11,12]

Although the bioethics literature extensively discusses the ethics of decision-making in the forgoing of life-sustaining therapy, little information is available about the actual decision-making process that occurs in the clinical setting. Ethical decision-making is often guided by an analysis of ethical principles or values. Frequently-cited ethical principles include autonomy (freedom of self-determination), beneficence (doing good), non-maleficence (doing no harm), and justice (fairness).[13] The tension between values of respecting a person's right to autonomous choice and the obligation to do good to that person is seen as a basic paradigm for analysis that can lead to the clarification of moral quandaries in medicine ([14],p.99). Difficulty arises, however, because abstract moral principles cannot be universally

---

Source: Reprinted from *Social Science and Medicine*, Vol. 35, No. 3, pp. 251-259, with permission from Elsevier Science Ltd., Pergamon Imprint © 1992.

and uniformly applied to the complexities of the clinical setting. Recently, a trend has emerged in bioethics in which the focus for ethical decision-making is less on the application of abstract principles and more on the meaning of particular facts of specific cases as interpreted and experienced by the participants.[15] This paper reflects the latter trend in its focus on a particular case and on the eventual sharing of meanings that occurred through negotiation in the decision-making process.[16]

In the clinical situation the negotiation of treatment withdrawal that results in death may involve different views, different "realities," which must be reconciled. According to Rosen,[17] bargaining for or negotiating reality is a process in which actors, each with a different view of what is true about a situation, attempt to make their view of the situation prevail. Because the situation must be defined and resolved, each person's concept of reality is subject to negotiation. In the intensive care unit, two levels of meaning may require negotiation. On one level the meaning of the overall situation may need to be resolved: Is the patient's condition hopeless or is there a chance for recovery? On another level, the meanings of individual technologies may have to be negotiated when physicians, patients, and families attribute various and often conflicting meanings to medical technologies. Cardiopulmonary resuscitation (CPR) for example, may be viewed by either physician or family as one last desperate hope or as an assault upon a dying patient.[18]

Rosen also notes that as each person involved in the negotiation of the reality of the situation puts forth his/her own viewpoint, success in negotiation will depend on the position of relative power each person can claim in the context ([17],p.574). Physicians are likely to maintain control of clinical decision-making because society confers on medicine a scientific, economic, political, linguistic and symbolic power and authority. But physician control also occurs specifically at the level of patient/family/physician interaction. Following Scheff,[19] physicians can exert control if the patient or family relinquishes control to them: 1) because of their authority as medical experts; 2) because of their skill in controlling the meaning of the patient's prognosis through a subjective presentation of the "facts" of the situation; and 3) because the physicians control access to medical treatment. On the other hand, the patient or family can challenge medical authority if they are assertive, if they are sophisticated about medicine and health care, or if they present an implied threat of legal action.

In the following case of differing views between family and physicians, the reality of the situation that eventually prevailed had to be negotiated and defined. The patient's demise became a negotiated death, a bargaining over how far medical technology should go in prolonging life or in prolonging death. I suggest that in its present form, decision-making in the forgoing of life-sustaining therapy often is less a question of the application of traditional ethical values than one of a "cascade" of decisions, which occurs in the context of differential power relations among professionals and patients and families, and which imparts a symbolic value to the negotiation process.

Case Example

Mr. John Ortello (a fictitious name) was a 66-year-old married male whose diagnoses included sepsis, emphysema with respiratory failure, and recurrent ventricular tachycardia (a potentially fatal heart arrhythmia) that was controlled by an implanted automatic defibrillator. He was semi-comatose and respirator-dependent. Attempts to "wean" him from the respirator (i.e., enable him to breathe on his own without a machine) had failed. After obtaining consent from his family, a "Do-Not-Resuscitate" (DNR) order was written. That is, if the patient's heart should stop, he would not undergo cardiopulmonary resuscitation. He was being treated with antibiotics and total parenteral nutrition ("TPN" -- a type of artificial nutrition that is administered directly into a large vein).

A proposal to administer amphotericin B, a potent antifungal medication, was based on the physicians' judgment that if the patient's fungal infection could be cured, his lungs might regain their function. Because of the patient's poor prognosis and the uncomfortable and potentially dangerous side effects of this medicine, the physicians consulted the patient's wife, two sons, and daughter. The family believed they reflected the patient's wishes in refusing the medication on his behalf.

Two days later, after discussion with the family, the doctors turned off Mr. Ortello's implanted defibrillator. The expectation that the patient would die fairly soon (because the device had been firing often) did not occur. Four days later there was consternation among the health care team because the patient's TPN had been stopped when the defibrillator was discontinued with the expectation of rapid demise, and now Mr. Ortello was not receiving nutrition. The doctors decided to attempt to wean the patient from the respirator with the understanding that he would not be reintubated if he experienced respiratory distress after successful extubation.

Three days later the physicians met with the family, who asked that the physicians allow the patient's death to occur by turning off the respirator "humanely." The doctors agreed to do so by providing the patient with analgesia and sedation to prevent his suffering from air hunger. Three hours after the respirator was turned off the patient died.

Negotiating Autonomy: Who Decides?

Both law and ethics have reiterated the primacy of the competent patient's right to self-determination. In the clinical setting the interaction of the expert physician and the autonomous patient is seen as an ideal model of shared decision-making.[20,21] When a patient lacks capacity for autonomous decision-making, as in Mr. Ortello's case, a surrogate decision maker is designated ([20], p.126-127). Usually the patient's next-of-kin or a close relative is asked to speak for the patient and to reflect the decisions the patient most likely would make. In practice, the surrogate generally acts in consultation with other interested family members and serves as a spokesperson for the family group.

Surrogates are frequently asked to speak for patients in the intensive care unit (ICU) because many of these patients are incapacitated by their illnesses and are unable to share in decisions about their care. However, even in the case of patients who are mentally capacitated, alert, oriented, and able to participate in decision-making, physicians may bypass the patient and discuss treatment options with the family only. In several instances in the ICU it was observed that information about treatment and prognosis was systematically withheld from patients while negotiation and decision-making were undertaken with the family.

Some representative examples of physicians' notes exemplify the importance given to consulting family members in decisions to withdraw technological life supports:

> Lengthy discussion with patient's only son and niece who is a former nurses' aid. Family does not want CPR/cardioversion/defibrillation/dialysis for support in case of cardiopulmonary arrest or worsening liver failure. They are satisfied with current supportive therapy and would also like blood pressure support with medications only as necessary. Orders written as such.

Another example:

> The family has decided to make him DNR and comfort measures only. No lab work. No blood products. No dialysis. No resuscitation. Need to begin withdrawal of dopamine.

Physicians in the ICU are more likely to initiate discussions with family than with the capacitated patient for various reasons. Some physicians believe that a critically ill patient by definition is not aware enough to be consulted about treatment plans and prognosis. Some physicians fear that not discussing the treatment plan with the family will alienate them and perhaps make them more prone to initiate a lawsuit if unexpected complications occur or if the patient dies. Although fears about lawsuits may be unrelated to facts about their actual occurrence, this perceived legal pressure often drives medical decision-making. The saying that "the family remains after the patient dies" expresses the physician's concern to deal with the family instead of the patient directly, not only out of fear of legal repercussions, but also often out of compassion for the distressed family.

Another consideration is that some physicians find it very uncomfortable to confront a patient directly about a poor prognosis or the withdrawal of treatment. Doctors often interpret such discussions as a denial of all hope for survival, which they view as synonymous with failure as a physician and as stripping the patient of hope. A poor prognosis may be disclosed to the patient in steps over time in order to sustain the physician's perception of the patient's need to maintain hope.[22] It has also been suggested that physicians are reluctant to discuss a poor prognosis with a patient because they may believe they have a moral, legal or professional duty to treat any "reversible" medical problem, or because they are reluctant to make decisions based on quality of life considerations.[12]

Although shared decision-making and patient autonomy are said to be important considerations in ethical decision-making, it is often the family's wishes, rather than the patient's, that will be honored. Family members may occasionally disagree among themselves or with a designated surrogate and conflicts may result. But in many cases the family is able to reach an agreement with the physician about the patient's treatment plan. The discussion with family becomes a metaphor for discussion with the patient: The family discussion symbolizes the fulfillment of a moral and legal duty to discuss prognosis and treatment plans directly with the patient. Thus, the negotiation of death is, in most cases, a negotiation between physician and family. The families are presumed to reflect the patient's wishes but in fact may not always do so, as in cases where treatment is continued due to a lack of family consensus about withdrawal, despite the incapacitated patient's previous directives. Or a patient may refuse intubation, but physicians proceed on the basis of "family wishes." In such negotiations for the meaning of the technology and the meaning of the situation, the patient is often the weakest player and the least likely to have his/her meaning prevail.

Negotiating the Meaning of Technologies

The first technology to be bargained over in the negotiation of Mr. Ortello's death was cardiopulmonary resuscitation (CPR). In today's medical climate, CPR is automatically administered for cardiac or respiratory arrest unless a "do-not-resuscitate" (DNR) order has been specified. The physician or family may view CPR as a benefit for the patient, especially in cases where illness is apparently transitory and full recovery is expected. In critical care situations where outcome is uncertain, physicians may be reluctant to consider "do-not-resuscitate" status for a patient because of an association of DNR status with de-escalation of treatment. Although some hospital DNR policies specifically state that a DNR status is compatible with "aggressive" treatment such as chemotherapy or blood transfusions, the initiation of a DNR order often serves as the impetus for discussion of treatment withdrawal in the clinical setting.[3,9] Furthermore, a DNR order may suggest to some physicians and patients the image of "giving up" or abandonment of the patient.

On the other hand, family or physicians may desire a DNR order for a patient. For family, a request for DNR status may mean that their loved one will not be subjected to the pain, violence, and dehumanization that characterize CPR and will be allowed to "die in peace."[18] Physicians who assess a patient's situation as virtually hopeless may view the DNR status as a means of preventing harm to the patient, and may attempt to convince a reluctant patient or family of the benefits of DNR status (a process some resident physicians facetiously refer to as "getting letters"). It is only when the technology holds multiple or conflicting meanings for the physician and family that the situation will be subject to negotiation in order for one meaning to prevail. Davis[23] points out that the physician's control over the meaning of the medical prognosis will affect the patient's or family's interpretation of the patient's situation. The two seemingly paradoxical meanings of DNR, as compatible with aggressive treatment and as a starting point for discussion of further treatment withdrawal provide the physician added control for managing the outcome of the negotiation process.

The family's request for DNR status for Mr. Ortello did not appear problematic, even though the outcome of the patient's treatment at the time of the request was not entirely clear to the physicians. The family did not want to prolong the dying process for their husband and father, so the DNR status appeared reasonable to them. The physicians, who in the beginning maintained some hope for Mr. Ortello's recovery, may have viewed DNR as a concession to the family that would not change any treatment plans -- i.e., they viewed DNR in this instance as compatible with aggressive treatment. Nolan ([24],p.11) notes that because physicians may view the cessation of breathing and heart rate in a concrete way as death, they may feel justified in withholding resuscitation while continuing other therapies. The physician then may believe, says Nolan, that the patient died in spite of everything that was done.

It can also be argued that the DNR status as a concession to the family was unproblematic for the physicians because Mr. Ortello was on a respirator and had an implanted defibrillator. DNR, by definition, is the withholding of CPR, which includes "cardiac, pharmacological, and respiratory intervention."[25] Mr. Ortello was intubated and on a respirator, he was already receiving cardiac medications, and he had an implanted defibrillator. Therefore, he should not have a respiratory arrest because a machine was already breathing for him, and if his heart fibrillated (a cause of many cardiac arrests), his defibrillator would correct the situation. In theory his heart might stop for other reasons, but the medicines he was receiving would make a cardiac arrest less likely.

While the negotiation of the DNR order was unproblematic, the question of initiating the antifungal agent amphotericin B was a source of conflict between family and physicians. In the family's opinion, the risks and discomfort of the treatment for the patient were excessive when compared to the perceived benefits. The physicians viewed Mr. Ortello's infection as potentially reversible and, therefore, felt justified in treating it. The notion of "reversibility" is often invoked by physicians in the ICU setting. During ICU rounds one morning the resident physicians questioned continuing treatment on a patient with multiple organ system failure (a gauge that the patient will most likely die). The response of the staff physician was that "everything here (i.e., the failure of each organ system) is potentially reversible." In another instance, when the senior resident was asked why treatment was continued for a hopelessly ill woman, he replied "her disease has a reversible component." In another clinical setting where decisions regarding the treatment of severely demented patients had to be made, physicians frequently cited potential reversibility of an acute condition as a reason to give full care ([12], p.1982).

The concept of reversibility is related to the physician's belief about the parameters of medical futility as informed by clinical experience and objective medical data. If a condition is deemed reversible, then medical intervention is able to effect change from a pathological state to a normal one. If a condition is deemed irreversible, any medical intervention will be futile -- i.e., unable to return from the pathological state back to the normal one. Reversibility can be seen in reference to the notions of "effect" and "benefit" in futility determinations, as described by Schneiderman *et al.*[26] These authors distinguish between a medical effect, which has a consequence for a limited part of the patient's body, and a benefit, which improves the patient as a whole (p.950). Reversibility, in my interpretation, has at least two usages. The reversibility of a condition is the production of an "effect" under these definitions. A reversible condition is one in which an effect can be produced in a limited part of the body. In their need to treat, many physicians tend to disregard the fact that even if a pathological condition can be reversed, the reversal might not necessarily benefit the patient. A second usage is that "reversibility" is the converse of "futility." The treatment of a reversible condition, in this usage, is standard medical practice.

Although some would argue that parameters of futility can be concretely determined,[26] others acknowledge that multiple meanings inherent in the use of the term prevent a precise determination of futility.[27,28] One common aspect of the concepts of "reversibility" and "futility" is that they can be subjectively interpreted by the physician. As noted previously,[12] some physicians may believe that they have a moral, legal or professional duty to treat any reversible (and, by extrapolation, "non-futile") medical condition. If so, then the physician's subjective interpretation of these terms is crucial to the medical management of the patient. The attribution of either label to a clinical situation provides the criterion and justification that is both medical and moral for continuing or discontinuing aggressive medical treatment. The multivocality of terms such as "futility" and "reversibility" allow fluidity in their application to any particular clinical situation. Again, the physicians' medical expertise enables them to control the meanings of such concepts and provides an advantage in negotiating the definition of the situation.

In Mr. Ortello's case the fungal infection was viewed as a reversible element and treatment with the antifungal medication was justified in the physicians' view. But the patient's illness also manifested other potentially irreversible components: Mr. Ortello's inability to wean from the respirator before the fungal infection began, and the increased number of discharges of the defibrillator, which meant a potentially fatal heart arrhythmia was becoming more frequent. As an isolated entity, the fungal infection might be reversible. In the context of the patient's illness, however, reversing the fungal infection might not change the irreversibility of the other elements. The family's refusal of the antifungal medication, then, prompted further discussions of other means of withdrawing treatment and allowing death to occur. In view of the family's pressing their definition of the situation as hopeless, the physicians also began to accept that definition.

The decision to turn off the defibrillator was an acceptable solution for the family in terms of what they felt the patient wanted and what was most comfortable for the patient. The decision was somewhat more complex for the physicians. It was an acceptable solution for them in that the frequent shocks from the firings of the defibrillator were painful for the patient. Shutting off the device would thus be a comfort measure for him. Turning off the defibrillator also would be an acceptable moral solution for the physicians. The patient would experience fibrillation, and cardiac arrest, which they then would not treat.

In addition, external factors added to the complexity of the situation. The implanted defibrillator was an expensive and somewhat experimental technology. In the view of one physician, Mr. Ortello's prior consent to this treatment should hold and, therefore, he should continue to obtain whatever benefits he might be receiving from the device. In addition, some of the physicians believed that the continuation of this quasi-research was in the interest of society (and the institution, and the individual physician/researcher). The physicians' wish to discontinue the defibrillator for the sake of the patient conflicted with their desire to continue it for the sake of research. The goals of research thus added another dimension to the negotiation of the meaning of the defibrillator and its fate.

In the presence of strong family directives, and an increasing acceptance by the physicians of the dismal prognosis of the patient, the physicians agreed to turn off the defibrillator with the expectation that death would probably occur that same day. When death had not occurred after four days, the physicians may have questioned whether the definition of the situation as hopeless was correct in view of the patient's continued survival. In the medical and moral ambiguity of the situation into which they had been thrust by the patient's survival, and in the face of the family's continued pressing of their definition of the situation as hopeless, the physicians then had to consider how to withdraw treatment further with both medical and moral justification for their actions. An EEG was suggested by one of the residents: if the patient could be declared "brain dead" there would be additional moral justification for stopping the last remaining life-supporting technology, the respirator. The physicians again suggested weaning the patient from the respirator (a process that had been unsuccessful in the past) in order to allow death to occur. If the physicians could get the patient off the respirator for a short time, he would inevitably experience respiratory distress again and they then simply would not reintubate him, a non-action that would lead to his death.

The Locus of Moral Responsibility in Decision-Making

In the negotiation of Mr. Ortello's death, the question emerges as to the locus of moral responsibility for medical decision-making. In each step the family's wishes served to define the situation as one of treatment withdrawal rather than one of continued aggressive treatment. The locus of responsibility for decision-making was shifted to the patient or to the family. When the physicians decided not to treat any future instances of fibrillation and cardiac arrest, and then turned off the patient's defibrillator, they were, in a sense, letting the patient decide his own fate. By attempting to wean Mr. Ortello from the respirator, and then deciding to refrain from reintubating him, they were placing the responsibility for living or dying on the patient.[29] If the physicians had decided to withdraw the respirator without reframing the meaning of their actions as withholding rather than withdrawing treatment, the moral responsibility for allowing death to occur would be theirs.

It is often noted that withdrawing a technology (such as a respirator) that might lead to death is more difficult for physicians than withholding (i.e., not starting) a technology. For example, stopping a respirator for a dying patient who is dependent on this machine to breathe is considered more difficult than not starting this technology when a dying patient comes into the Emergency Room in respiratory distress. Although most ethicists consider the difference between withholding and withdrawing treatment to be morally unimportant, the usual explanation for this difficulty is that withdrawal of treatment is psychologically more difficult than withholding.[20,30,31] I suggest that withdrawing a life-supporting technology is harder for many physicians than withholding it because of the perceived moral responsibility attributed to these actions.

The withdrawal of treatment implies that the physician takes responsibility for allowing death to occur, a meaning that contradicts widely-held beliefs about what a physician is and does, and should do. In withholding treatment the locus of responsibility for the occurrence of death shifts to the patient. It is the patient's physiological state that will determine whether he/she lives or dies. The decision is metaphorically out of the physician's hands. So in Mr. Ortello's case we see the physicians make a difficult decision to withdraw the defibrillator, but at the same time they decide to withhold CPR. On a symbolic level, the patient's physiological state of his heart, not the physician, determines his fate. The physicians try to wean the patient from the respirator, try to enable him to breathe on his own, while deciding they will not reintubate when he inevitably experiences respiratory distress.

Again, (if they had been successful) the patient's physiological status would have determined his fate and the physicians would be morally "off the hook."

A shifting of moral responsibility appears to occur rather frequently in the case of dying patients. (We have already seen it shift to the family.[32]) An expression heard frequently in the ICU exemplifies this displacement of responsibility. When a question of continuing treatment in a potentially futile situation arises, physicians say that "the patient will declare himself." This statement suggests that the patient's physiological signs of an improving or worsening condition will give the physician the moral authority to continue aggressive treatment or to begin its withdrawal. The locus of moral responsibility for decision-making again shifts from the physician to the patient. Moreover, the patient's "declaring" himself as not improving provides the impetus for the physician's redefinition of a reversible condition as an irreversible one, the eventual definition of the situation as "futile" and the moral justification to begin treatment withdrawal.

The difficulty in Mr. Ortello's case was that when the physicians stopped the defibrillator, he did not die, and they failed to wean him from the respirator. They were forced either to accept the responsibility of withdrawing treatment and allowing his death to occur, or to allow him to remain on the respirator indefinitely. The family rejected the latter solution, and the physicians were uncomfortable with both options. The final point for negotiation was the meaning of the respirator: was it a tool for prolonging the patient's life or for prolonging his dying? The meaning of the situation that eventually was accepted by both physicians and family was that Mr. Ortello's situation was hopeless and that continuation of treatment would be futile.

That the family's definition prevailed may have been due to their ability to verbalize assertively their wishes and to ask appropriate questions. A less medically sophisticated family may not have been able to press their desires and the patient might have remained on the respirator until the physicians themselves decided that the pursuit of further medical treatment would be futile. In my interpretation, because the physicians recognized early on that the patient's prognosis was extremely poor, an issue for them in each step of the negotiations was not so much whether treatment was beneficial or futile, but how to allow death to occur without accepting fully the moral responsibility for death that the withdrawal (as opposed to the withholding) of treatment would imply. The negotiations with the family served to share the awesome responsibility of withdrawing treatment and allowing the patient's death to occur. The negotiations also served to reiterate family wishes, thus restraining the felt imperative of the physicians to continue treatment, even in the case of probable futility. Because of the negotiations with the family, the physicians could take comfort in the fact that the moral responsibility for the patient's death was not theirs alone.

Discussion

It has been noted that a decision to withhold CPR is often the stimulus for a re-evaluation of the goals of therapy for a particular patient.[3,8,9,10] The example presented here suggests that treatment limitations after the institution of a DNR order are not necessarily due to a deliberate re-evaluation of treatment goals. Rather, the DNR order is often the starting point of a series of decisions that parallel a "cascade" effect in clinical decision-making. In the cascade effect, one clinical decision inevitably and necessarily leads to a series of other decisions, which in turn leads to others based on the preceding decisions. Those health care professionals caught in the cascade often feel powerless to control it.[33,34] The cascade effect, then, can be interpreted as another means of displacing responsibility from the individual physician to an intangible process. The "system" is to blame, while the individual becomes a tool with little or no control over the system.

In Mr. Ortello's case, each decisional step negotiated between physicians and family "inevitably" led to another decision. The use of the antifungal agent might not have been a question if a DNR order had not been previously negotiated for Mr. Ortello. The forgoing of the use of the antifungal agent then led to the forgoing of the defibrillator and TPN, which eventually led to the withdrawal of the respirator.

In my interpretation, the physicians felt a need to act (i.e., treat) because they were uncomfortable and ambivalent about allowing the "natural" or physiological course of death to proceed. In the physicians' frame of thought the cascade of decisional events should have resulted rather quickly in the patient's death. Instead the process became stalled when the patient survived the withdrawal of the defibrillator, a situation that created the discomfort and ambivalence. If survival of the patient were a possibility, the physicians felt they would have to redefine and renegotiate the meaning of the situation with the family. A medical/moral imperative to restart TPN and to draw blood gases during the weaning process also was felt by the physicians. But these measures would serve to change the meaning of the situation from one of treatment withdrawal to one of continued aggressive therapy. In the perception of the physicians, such actions not only would be a move backwards, but antithetical to what both family and physicians had agreed upon, the patient's cascade toward death. The family's request to withdraw the respirator provided a moral escape route for the physicians: the patient's movement toward death would continue, they would not feel compelled to treat in a situation defined by all as futile, and the moral responsibility for medical failure and death would be shared with the family.

The emphasis placed on patient autonomy and patient rights in the bioethical literature has contributed to an ideology of involving patients and families in clinical decisions that include the forgoing of life-sustaining therapy. As noted previously, decision-making is viewed ideally as shared among physicians, patient and family. For the family (and metaphorically for the patient), the negotiation of death maintains the appearance that the patient's and family's autonomy is being respected, and that they have control over treatment decisions.

The negotiation begins by presenting treatment options, which ostensibly provide the family with choices. But because physicians control medicine and its technology, they also control the choices associated with its use. In the negotiation of the forgoing of life-supporting treatments, physicians offer the patient (or more often, the family) not a real choice, but the illusion of choice.[35] When physicians present families with choices regarding use of life-sustaining technologies, most often they are not offering a choice between death and a restoration to one's previous state of health. The real choice they offer is one between the finality of biological death or the limbo of mechanical prolongation of biological life, between "death now" or "death later."[36] Neither choice is ideal, and a choice is only offered at the point when medical technology is unlikely to fulfill the promise of full restoration to the patient's former state of health.[37]

Offering the illusion of choice empowers the physician both to control in situations of medical uncertainty and to share with the family the moral responsibility for failure in cases of futility. In the face of almost certain failure the negotiated agreement of the family to withdraw treatment provides a sharing of responsibility and an affirmation that the failure is inevitable and acceptable. In ethical decision-making to forgo life-sustaining therapy, then, the question is not medical paternalism versus the patient's right to decide, as it is usually framed in the bioethics literature. Rather, the illusion of choice as offered by the physician begins a negotiation of meanings that allows a sharing of moral responsibility for medical failure and its eventual acceptance by patient, family, and physician alike.

Conclusion

When the use of medical technology, part of the so-called "technological imperative," is considered a moral imperative, then the withdrawal of treatment will become (and has become) a moral question for many physicians. In an era when many individuals are unable to afford basic health care, the use of expensive technology in situations of questionable benefit adds to the moral quandary. As more physicians recognize appropriate situations for the forgoing of life-supporting treatment, the sharing of responsibility for death with the patient (whose physiological state is responsible for his/her death) or with the family (through a negotiation of prognosis and treatment process) may have a positive psychological and emotional effect. Neither the grieving family nor the caring physician has to accept the full moral burden. This sharing of responsibility may be needed especially in today's medical climate where decision-making is no longer a private affair between doctor and patient, but is subject to the scrutiny of strangers.[38]

If the negotiation of death fulfills a need for physicians, family and patient to come to terms with death and the limits of medical technology, then this process supports proposals to include the patient and/or family members in the discussion of futile resuscitation. It has been argued that in cases where CPR would be futile, the initiation of a DNR order need not be discussed with the patient and/or family.[39,40] As demonstrated in this case, a DNR order is usually the first of a "cascade" of decisions to be made in caring for the dying patient. The fact that cardiopulmonary arrest is the last stage in the dying process suggests that the focus on the DNR discussion is misplaced. The entire decisional process of which the negotiation of the DNR order is only a part must be considered or the complexity of the ethical/medical decision-making process remains unexplored.

The negotiation of death also reflects a growing dissatisfaction with the medical control of death. Just as people rallied against medical and technological control of the birthing process in the 1970s through such movements as home birth and midwifery, so too are they becoming more vocal in questioning the medical and technological control of the dying process, as demonstrated by the growth of such organizations as the Society for the Right to Die, Hospice, and the Hemlock Society. The social process of negotiating death is beginning to act as a check on the medical and technological control of the dying process. Eventually it may provide the added effect of leading us to a more realistic appraisal of the limits of medical technology.

Notes

1. Current medical standards exclude direct euthanasia and physician-assisted suicide as options, in spite of recent controversies sparked by the "Debbie" and "Diane" cases, *JAMA* 1988;259(2):272 and *New England Journal of Medicine* 1991;324(10):691-694, respectively), and Dr. Kevorkian's "suicide machine."
2. Delvecchio-Good, *et al.* American Oncology and the Discourse on Hope, *Culture, Medicine and Psychiatry* 1990;14:59-79.
3. Lipton HL. Do-Not-Resuscitate decisions in a community hospital, *JAMA* 1986;256(9):1164-1169. This frequently-quoted statistic is often attributed to the American Hospital Association (AHA) because it appeared in their verbal briefing on the Cruzan case. Lipton's 70% figure is derived from her study of a community hospital, but she notes this incidence figure is similar to that found in studies of some teaching hospitals (p.1168). (I am grateful to the AHA's Resource Center Library for clarifying the source of this information.)
4. Luce JM, Raffin TA. Withholding and withdrawal of life support from critically ill patients, *Chest* 1988;94(3):621-626.
5. Meisel A, *et al.* Hospital guidelines for deciding about life-sustaining treatment: Dealing with health "limbo," *Critical Care Medicine* 1986;14(3):239-246.
6. Ruark JE, Raffin TA, and the Stanford University Medical Center Committee on Ethics. Initiating and withdrawing life support, principles and practice in adult medicine. *New Engl J Med* 1988;318(1):25-30.

7. Wanzer SH, *et al.* The physician's responsibility toward hopelessly ill patients, *New Engl J Med* 1984;310(15):955-959.
8. Smedira NG, *et al.* Withholding and withdrawal of life support from the critically ill, *New Engl J Med* 1990;322(5):309-315.
9. Zimmerman JE. The use and implications of Do-Not-Resuscitate orders in intensive care units, *JAMA* 1986;255(3):351-356.
10. Bedell SE. Do-Not-Resuscitate orders for critically ill patients in the hospital: How are they used and what is their impact? *JAMA* 1986;256(2):233-237.
11. Youngner SJ, *et al.* 'Do Not Resuscitate' orders. Incidence and implications in a medical intensive care unit, *JAMA* 1985;253(1):54-57.
12. Wray N, *et al.* Withholding medical treatment from the severely demented patient. Decisional processes and cost implications, *Arch Intern Med* 1988;148:1980-1984.
13. Beauchamp TL, Childress JF. *Principles of Biomedical Ethics*. New York, NY: Oxford University Press, 1989.
14. Engelhardt HT Jr. *The Foundations of Bioethics*. New York, NY: Oxford University Press, 1986.
15. For examples of the experience-based approach to bioethics see, Zaner RM. *Ethics and the Clinical Encounter.* Englewood Cliffs, NJ: Prentice Hall, 1988; Jonsen AR, Toulmin S. *The Abuse of Casuistry*. Berkeley, CA: University of California Press, 1988; and Reich W, ed. *Experience as a Source of Bioethics*, In progress.
16. Although I examine one case of decision-making in detail, my insights are derived from ten months work in an ethics consultation service and four months of observation during medical rounds in an intensive care unit.
17. Rosen L. The negotiation of reality: Male-female relations in Sefrou, Morocco, In: Beck, L, Keddie, eds. *Women in the Muslim World*. Cambridge, MA: Harvard University Press, 1978.
18. Goodwin JS, Goodwin JM. Second thoughts: CPR, *Journal of Chronic Diseases* 1985;38(8):717-719.
19. Scheff T. Negotiating reality: Notes on power in the assessment of responsibility, *Social Problems* 1968;16:3-17.
20. President's Commission for the Study of Ethical Problems in Medicine and Biomedical and Behavioral Research. *Decisions to Forgo Life-Sustaining Treatment*. Washington, DC: U.S. Government Printing Office, 1983.
21. Katz J. *The Silent World of Doctor and Patient*. New York, NY: The Free Press, 1984.
22. To suffer a prolonged illness or elect to die: A case study. *New York Times* 1984, Dec 16:1, 36.
23. Davis DS. Slim just left town: Decision-making on an intensive care unit, *Connecticut Law Review* 1991;23(2):261-279.
24. Nolan K. In death's shadow: The meanings of withholding resuscitation, *Hastings Center Report* 1987:9-14.
25. Kanoti G, *et al. A Statement of Policy on Do Not Resuscitate*. Cleveland, OH: The Cleveland Clinic Foundation, 1988.
26. Schneiderman LJ, *et al.* Medical futility: Its meaning and ethical implications, *Ann Int Med* 1990;112(12):949-54.
27. Lantos JD, *et al.* The illusion of futility in clinical practice, *Am J Med* 1989;87:81-84.
28. Youngner S. Who defines futility? *JAMA* 1988;260(14):2094-95.
29. Nolan notes a propensity of health care professionals to "blame the victim" in cases of failed resuscitation. See [24], p.11.
30. The Hastings Center. *Guidelines on the Termination of Life-Sustaining Treatment and the Care of the Dying*. Bloomington, IN: Indiana University Press, 1987.
31. Schneiderman L J, Spragg R. Ethical decisions in discontinuing mechanical ventilation, *New Engl J Med* 1988;318(15):984-988.
32. That such a shifting of moral responsibility may be a common occurrence in ICU decision-making is suggested by statements from the documentary "Near Death." This is a film by Frederick Wiseman, aired in January 1990, which portrays actual situations of decision making in an ICU. Nurse: (referring to the impending death of a patient) "I hope this is fast, one way or the other." Doctor: "God decides...these things have a life of their own." The next day a physician reports: "Mr. C. died yesterday. They (the family) felt it was going on too long, so we...turned his FIO2 down to 50% and he flat-lined after that." And in the report given during the same patient's

autopsy: "She (the wife) decided 'no CPR'. Later she made the decision to turn down the FIO2."
33. Mold JW, Stein HF. The cascade effect in the clinical care of patients, *New Engl J Med* 1986;314(8):512-514.
34. Stein HF, Mold JW. Stress, anxiety, and cascades in clinical decision-making, *Stress Med* 1988;4(1):41-48.
35. For an thorough discussion of the illusion of choice in the context of use of the prenatal technology of amniocentesis, see Rothman BK. *The Tentative Pregnancy: Prenatal Diagnosis and the Future of Motherhood*. New York, NY: Penguin Books, 1986.
36. Blackhall LJ. Must we always use CPR? *New Engl J Med* 1987;317(20):1281-1285.
37. This was observed by the author and was also noted by the nurses in the film "Near Death" (see [32]). Quantitative research on the use of DNR orders supports these observations. See, for example, Jonsson PV. The 'Do Not Resuscitate' order: A profile of its changing use, *Arch Intern Med* 1988;148:2373-2375 and [10].
38. Rothman DJ. *Strangers at the Bedside: A History of How Law and Bioethics Transformed Medical Decision Making*. New York, NY: Basic Books Inc., 1991.
39. Murphy DJ. Do-Not-Resuscitate orders: Time for reappraisal in long-term care institutions, *JAMA* 1988;260(14):2098-2101.
40. Hackler JC, Hiller FC. Family consent to orders not to resuscitate: Reconsidering hospital policy, *JAMA* 1990;264(10):1281-1283.

Chapter 63

Care of the Hopelessly Ill -- Proposed Clinical Criteria for Physician-Assisted Suicide

Timothy Quill, Christine Cassel, and Diane E. Meier

One of medicine's most important purposes is to allow hopelessly ill persons to die with as much comfort, control, and dignity as possible. The philosophy and techniques of comfort care provide a humane alternative to more traditional, curative medical approaches in helping patients achieve this end.[1,2,3,4,5,6] Yet there remain instances in which incurably ill patients suffer intolerably before death despite comprehensive efforts to provide comfort. Some of these patients would rather die than continue to live under the conditions imposed by their illness, and a few request assistance from their physicians.

The patients who ask us to face such predicaments do not fall into simple diagnostic categories. Until recently, their problems have been relatively unacknowledged and unexplored by the medical profession, so little is objectively known about the spectrum and prevalence of such requests or about the range of physicians' responses.[7,8,9,10] Yet each request can be compelling. Consider the following patients: a former athlete, weighing 80 pounds (36 kg) after an eight-year struggle with the acquired immunodeficiency syndrome (AIDS), who is losing his sight and his memory and is terrified of AIDS dementia; a mother of seven children, continually exhausted and bed-bound at home with a gaping, foul-smelling, open wound in her abdomen, who can no longer eat and who no longer wants to fight ovarian cancer; a fiercely independent retired factory worker, quadriplegic from amyotrophic lateral sclerosis, who no longer wants to linger in a helpless, dependent state waiting and hoping death; a writer with extensive bone metastases from lung cancer that has not responded to chemotherapy, or radiation, who cannot accept the daily choice he must make between sedation and severe pain; and a physician colleague, dying of respiratory failure from progressive pulmonary fibrosis, who does not want to be maintained on a ventilator but is equally of suffocation. Like the story of "Diane," which has been told in more detail,[11] there are personal stories of courage and grief for each of these patients that force us to take very seriously their requests for a physician's assistance in dying.

Our purpose is to propose clinical criteria that would allow physicians to respond to requests for assisted suicide from their competent, incurably ill patients. We support the legalization of such suicide, but not of active euthanasia. We believe this position permits the best balance between a humane response to the requests of patients like those described above and the need to protect other vulnerable people. We strongly advocate intensive, unrestrained care intended to provide comfort for all incurably ill persons.[1,2,3,4,5,6] When properly applied, such comfort care should result in a tolerable death, with symptoms relatively well controlled for most patients. Physician-assisted suicide should never be

---

Source: Reprinted from *The New England Journal of Medicine*, Vol. 327, pp. 1380-1384, with permission from University Press of America © 1992.

contemplated as a substitute for comprehensive comfort care or for working with patients to resolve the physical, personal, and social challenges posed by the process of dying.[12] Yet it is not idiosyncratic, selfish, or indicative of a psychiatric disorder for people with an incurable illness to want some control over how they die. The idea of a noble, dignified death, with a meaning that is deeply personal and unique, is exalted in great literature, poets; art, and music.[13] When an incurably ill patient asks for help in achieving such a death we believe physicians have an obligation to explore the request fully and under specified circumstances, carefully to consider making an exception to the prohibition against assisting with a suicide.

Physician-Assisted Suicide

For a physician, assisting with suicide entails making a means of suicide (such as a prescription for barbiturates) available to a patient who is otherwise physically capable of suicide and who subsequently acts on his or her own. Physician-assisted suicide is distinguished from voluntary euthanasia, in which the physician not only makes the means available but, at the patient's request, also serves as the actual agent of death. Whereas active euthanasia is illegal throughout the United States, only 36 states have laws explicitly prohibiting assisted suicide.[14,15] In every situation in which a physician has compassionately helped a terminally ill person to commit suicide, criminal charges have been dismissed or a verdict of not guilty has been brought.[14,15] (and Gostin L: personal communication) Although the prospect of a successful prosecution may remote, the risk of an expensive, publicized professional, and legal inquiry would be prohibitive for most physicians and would certainly keep the practice covert among those who participate.

It is not known how widespread physician-assisted suicide currently is in the United States, or how frequently patients' requests are turned down by physicians. Approximately 5,000 deaths per day in the United States are said to be in some way planned or indirectly assisted as probably through the "double effect" of pain-relieving medications that may at the same time hasten death[3,12] or the discontinuation of or failure to start potentially life-prolonging treatments. From 3 to 37 percent of physicians responding to anonymous-surveys reported secretly taking active steps to hasten a patient's death, but these survey data were flawed by low response rate and poor design.[7,8,9,10] Every public-opinion survey taken over the past 40 years has shown support by a majority of Americans for the idea of physician-assisted death for the terminally ill.[16,17,18,19] A referendum with loosely defined safeguards that would have legalized both voluntary euthanasia and assisted suicide was narrowly defeated in Washington State in 1991,[20] and more conservatively drawn initiatives are currently on the ballot in California, before the legislature in New Hampshire, and under consideration in Florida and Oregon.

A Policy Proposal

Although physician assisted suicide and voluntary euthanasia, both involve the active facilitation of a wished-for death, there are several important distinctions between them.[21] In assisted suicide, the final act is solely the patient's, and the risk of subtle coercion from doctors, family members, institutions, or other social forces is greatly reduced.[22] The balance of power between doctor and patient is more nearly equal in physician-assisted suicide than in euthanasia. The physician is counselor and witness and makes the means available, but ultimately the patient must be the one to act or not act. In voluntary euthanasia, the physician provides both the means and carries out the final act, with greatly amplified power over the patient and an increased risk of error, coercion, or abuse.

In view of these distinctions, we conclude that legalization of physician-assisted suicide, but not of voluntary euthanasia, is the policy best able to respond to patients' needs and to protect vulnerable people. From this perspective, physician-assisted suicide forms part of the continuum of options for comfort care, beginning with the forgoing of life-sustaining therapy, including more aggressive symptom-relieving measures, and permitting physician-assisted suicide only if all other alternatives have failed and all criteria have been met. Active voluntary euthanasia is excluded from this continuum because of the risk of abuse it presents. We recognize that this exclusion is made at a cost to competent, incurably ill patients who cannot swallow or move and who therefore cannot be helped to die by assisted suicide. Such persons, who meet agreed-on criteria in other respects, must not be abandoned to their suffering; a combination of decisions to forgo life-sustaining treatments (including food and fluids) with aggressive comfort measures (such as analgesics and sedatives) could be offered, along with a commitment to search for creative alternatives. We acknowledge that this solution is less than ideal, but we also recognize that in the United States access to medical care is currently too inequitable, and many doctor-patient relationships too impersonal, for us to tolerate the risks of permitting active voluntary euthanasia. We must monitor any change in public policy in this domain to evaluate both its benefits and its burdens.

We propose the following clinical guidelines to contribute to serious discussion about physician-assisted suicide. Although we favor a reconsideration of the legal and professional prohibitions in the case of patients who meet carefully defined criteria, we do not wish to promote an easy or impersonal process.[23] If we are to consider allowing incurably ill patients more control over their deaths, it must be as an expression of our compassion and concern about their ultimate fate after all other alternatives have been exhausted. Such patients should not be held hostage to our reluctance or inability to forge policies in this difficult area.

Proposed Clinical Criteria for Physician-Assisted Suicide

Because assisted suicide is extraordinary and irreversible treatment, the patient's primary physician must ensure that the following conditions are clearly satisfied before proceeding. First, the patient must have a condition that is incurable and associated with severe, unrelenting suffering. The patient must understand the condition, the prognosis, and the types of comfort care available as alternatives. Although most patients making this request will be near death, we acknowledge the inexactness of such prognostications[24,25,26] and do not want to exclude arbitrarily persons with incurable, but not imminently terminal, progressive illnesses, such as amyotrophic lateral sclerosis or multiple sclerosis. When there is considerable uncertainty about the patient's medical condition or prognosis, a second opinion or opinions should be sought and the uncertainty clarified as much as possible before a final decision about the patient's request is made.

Second, the physician must ensure that the patient's suffering and the request are not the result of inadequate comfort care. All reasonable comfort-oriented measures must at least have been considered, and preferably have been tried, before the means for a physician-assisted suicide are provided. Physician-assisted suicide must never be used to circumvent the struggle to provide comprehensive care or find acceptable alternatives. The physician's prospective willingness to provide assisted suicide is a legitimate and important subject to discuss if the patient raises the question, since many patients will probably find the possibility of an escape from suffering more important than the reality.

Third, the patient must clearly and repeatedly, of his or her own free will and initiative, request to die rather than continue suffering. The physician should understand thoroughly what continued life means to the patient and why death appears preferable. A physician's too-ready acceptance of a patient's request could be perceived as encouragement to commit suicide, yet it is important not to force the patient to "beg" for assistance. Understanding the patient's desire to die and being certain that the request is serious are critical steps in evaluating the patient's rationality and ensuring that all alternative means of relieving suffering have been adequately explored. Any sign of ambivalence or uncertainty on the part of the patient should abort the process, because a clear, convincing, and continuous desire for an end of suffering through death is a strict requirement to proceed. Requests for assisted suicide made in advance directly or by a health care surrogate should not be honored.

Fourth, the physician must be sure that the patient's judgment is not distorted. The patient must be capable of understanding the decision and its implications. The presence of depression is relevant if it is distorting rational decision-making and is reversible in a way that would substantially alter the situation. Expert psychiatric evaluation should be sought when the primary physician is inexperienced in the diagnosis and treatment of depression, or when there is uncertainty about the rationality of the request or the presence of a reversible mental disorder the treatment of which would substantially change the patient's perception of his or her condition.[27]

Fifth, physician-assisted suicide should be carried out only in the context of a meaningful doctor-patient relationship. Ideally, the physician should have witnessed the patient's previous illness and suffering. There may not always be a preexisting relationship, but the physician must get to know the patient personally in order to understand fully the reasons for the request. The physician must understand why the patient considers death to be the best of a limited number of very unfortunate options, The primary physician must personally confirm that each of the criteria has been met. The patient should have no doubt that the physician is committed to finding alternative solutions if at any moment the patient's mind changes. Rather than create a new subspecialty focused on death,[28] assistance in suicide should be given by the same physician who has been struggling with the patient to provide comfort care, and who will stand by the patient and provide care until the time of death, no matter what path is taken.

No physician should be forced to assist a patient in suicide if it violates the physician's fundamental values, although the patient's personal physician should think seriously before turning down such a request. Should a transfer of care be necessary; the personal physician should help the patient find another, more receptive primary physician.

Sixth, consultation with another experienced physician is required to ensure that the patient's request is voluntary and rational, the diagnosis and prognosis accurate, and the exploration of comfort-oriented alternatives thorough. The consulting physician should review the supporting materials and should interview and examine the patient.

Finally, clear documentation to support each condition is required. A system must be developed for reporting, reviewing, and studying such deaths and clearly distinguishing them from other forms of suicide. The patient, the primary physician, and the consultant must each sign a consent form; a physician-assisted suicide must neither invalidate insurance policies nor lead to an investigation by the medical examiner or an unwanted autopsy. The primary physician, the medical consultant, and the family must be assured that if the conditions agreed on are satisfied in good faith, they will be free from criminal prosecution for having assisted the patient to die.

Informing family members is strongly recommended, but whom to involve and inform should be left to the discretion and control of the patient. Similarly, spiritual counseling should be offered, depending on the patient's background and beliefs. Ideally, close family members should be an integral part of the decision-making process and should understand and support the patient's decision. If there is a major dispute between the family and the patient about how to proceed, it may require the involvement of an ethics committee or even of the courts. It is to be hoped, however, that most of these painful decisions can be worked through directly by the patient, the family, and health care providers. Under no circumstances should the family's wishes and requests override those of a competent patient.

The Method

In physician-assisted suicide, a lethal amount of medication is usually prescribed that the patient then ingests. Since this process has been largely covert and unstudied, little is known about which methods are the most humane and effective. If there is a change in policy, there must be an open sharing of information within the profession, and a careful analysis of effectiveness. The methods selected should be reliable and should not add to the patient's suffering. We must also provide support and careful monitoring for the patients, physicians, and families affected, since the emotional and social effects are largely unknown but are undoubtedly far-reaching.

Assistance with suicide is one of the most profound and meaningful requests a patient can make of a physician. If the patient and the physician agree that there are no acceptable alternatives and that all the required conditions have been met, the lethal medication should ideally be taken in the physician's presence. Unless the patient specifically requests it, he or she should not be left alone at the time of death. In addition to the personal physician, other health care providers and family members should be encouraged to be present, as the patient wishes. It is of the utmost importance not to abandon the patient at this critical moment. The time before a controlled death can provide an opportunity for a rich and meaningful good bye between family members, health care providers, and the patient. For this reason, we must be sure that any policies and laws enacted to allow assisted suicide do not require that the patient be left alone at the moment of death in order for the assisters to be safe from prosecution.

Balancing Risks and Benefits

There is an intensifying debate within and outside the medical profession about the physician's appropriate role in assisting dying.[3,21,29,30,31,32,33,34,35,36,37,38,39,40,41,42] Although most agree that there are exceptional circumstances in which death is preferable to intolerable suffering, the case against both physician-assisted suicide and voluntary euthanasia is based mainly on the implications for public policy and the potential effect on the moral integrity of the medical profession.[35,36,37,38,39,40,41,42] The "slippery slope" argument asserts that permissive policies would inevitably lead to subtle coercion of the powerless to choose death rather than become burdens to society or their families. Access to health care in the United States is extraordinarily variable, often impersonal, and subject to intense pressures for cost containment. It may be dangerous to license physicians to take life in this unstable environment. It is also suggested that comfort care, skillfully applied, could provide a tolerable and dignified death for most persons and that physicians would have less incentive to become more proficient at providing such care if the option or a quick, controlled, death were too readily available. Finally, some believe that physician-assisted death, no matter noble and pure its intentions, would destroy the identity of the medical profession and its central ethos, protecting the sanctity of life. The question, before policy makers, physicians, and voters is whether criteria such as those we have out lined here safeguard patients adequately against these risks.

The risks and burdens of continuing with the current prohibitions have been less clearly articulated in the literature.[21,29,30,31,32,33,34] The most pressing problem is the potential abandonment of competent, incurably ill patients who yearn for death despite comprehensive comfort care. These patients may be disintegrating physically and emotionally, but death is not imminent. They have often fought heroic medical battles only to find themselves in this final condition. Those who have witnessed difficult deaths in hospice programs are not reassured by the glib assertion that we can always make death tolerable, and patients fear that physicians will abandon them if their course becomes difficult or overwhelming in the face of comfort care. In fact, there is no empirical evidence that all physical suffering associated with incurable illness can be effectively relieved. In addition, the most frightening aspect of death for many is not physical pain, but the prospect of losing control and independence and of dying in an undignified, unesthetic, absurd, and existentially unacceptable condition.

Physicians who respond to requests for assisted suicide from such patients do so at substantial professional and legal peril, often acting in secret without the benefit of consultation or support from colleagues. This covert practice discourages open and honest communication among physicians, their colleagues, and their dying patients. Decisions often depend more on the physician's values and willingness to take risks than on the compelling nature of the patient's request. There may be more risk of abuse and idiosyncratic decision-making with such secret practices than with a more open, carefully defined practice. Finally, terminally ill patients who do choose to take their lives often die alone so as not to place their families or care givers in legal jeopardy.[11]

Conclusions

Given current professional and legal prohibitions, physicians find themselves in a difficult position when they receive requests for assisted suicide from suffering patients who have exhausted the usefulness of measures for comfort care. To adhere to the letter of the law, they must turn down their patients' requests even if they find them reasonable and personally acceptable. If they accede to their patients' requests, they must risk violating legal and professional standards, and therefore they act in isolation and in secret collaboration with their patients. We believe that there is more risk for vulnerable patients and for the integrity of the profession in such hidden practices, however well intended, than there would be in a more open process restricted to competent patients who met carefully defined criteria. The medical and legal professions must collaborate if we are to create public policy that fully acknowledges irreversible suffering and offers dying patients a broader range of options to explore with their physicians.

Notes

1. Wanzer Sh, Adelstein SJ, Cranford RE, *et al*. The physician's responsibility toward hopelessly ill patients, *N Engl J. Med* 1984;310:955-9.
2. Wanzer SH, Federman DD, Adelstein SJ, *et al*. The physician's responsibility toward hopelessly ill patients: A socond look, *N Engl J. Med* 1989;320:844-9.
3. Council on Ethical and Judicial Affairs, American Medical Association. Decisions near the end of life, *JAMA* 1992;267:2229-33.
4. Rhymes J. Hospice care in America, *JAMA* 1990;264:369-72.
5. Broadfield L. Evalutaion of palliative care; current status and future directions, *J Palliat Care* 1988;4(3):21-8.
6. Wallston KA, Burger C, Smith RA, *et al*. Comparing the quality of death for hospice and non-hospice cancer patients, *Med Care* 1988;26:177-82.
7. The National Hemlock Society. *1987 Survey of California Physicians Regrading Voluntary Active Euthanasia for the Terminally Ill.* Los Angeles, CA: Hemlock society, 1988.
8. Center of Health Ethics and Policy. *Withholding and Withdrawing Life-sustaining Treatment; A Survey of Opinions and Experienes of Colorado Physicians*. Denver, CO: University of Colorado Graduate School of Public Affairs, 1988.
9. Heilig S. The SFMS euthanasia survey; Results and analyses, *San Francisco Med* 1988:26-6, 34.
10. Overmyer M. National survey; Physicians' views on the right to die, *Physicians Manage* 1991;31(7):40-5.
11. Quill TE. Death and dignity -- A case of individualized decision-making, *N Engl J Med* 1991;324:691-4.
12. Meier DE, Cassel CK. Euthanasia in old age: A case study and ethical analysis, *J Am Geriatr Soc* 1983;31:294-8.

13. Aries P. *The Hour of Our Death*. New York, NY: Vintage Books, 1982.
14. Newman SA. Euthanasia: Orchestrating "the last syllable of ...time," *Univ Pitsb Law Rev* 1991;53:153-91.
15. Glantz LH. Withholding and withdrawing treatment: The role of the criminal law, *Law Med Health Care* 1987/88;15:231-41.
16. Malcolm A. Giving death a hand: rending issue, *New York Times* 1990, Jun 14:A6.
17. Gest T. Changing the rules on dying, *U.S. News & World Report* 1990:22-4.
18. The Hemlock Society. *1990 Roper Poll on Physician Aid-in-Dying, Allowing Nancy Cruzan to Die, and Physicians Obeying the Living Will*. New York, NY: Roper Organization, 1990.
19. Idem. *1991 Roper Poll of the West Coast on Euthanasia*. New York, NY: Roper Organization, 1991.
20. Misbin RI. Physicians' aid in dying, *N Engl J Med* 1991;325:1307-11.
21. Weir Rf. The morality of physician-assisted suicide, *Law Med Health Care* 1992;20:116-26.
22. Glover J. *Causing Death and Saving Lives*. New York, NY: Penguin Books, 1977:182-9.
23. Jecker NS. Giving death a hand; when the dying and the doctor stand in a special relationship, *J Am Geriatr Soc* 1991;39:831-5.
24. Poses RM, Bekes C, Copare FJ, Scott WE. The and to "What are my chances, doctor?" depends on whom is asked: Prognostic disagreement and inaccuracty for critically ill patients, *Crit Care Med* 1989;17:827-33.
25. Charlson ME. Studies of prognosis: Progress and pitfalls, *J Gen Intern Med* 1987;2:359-61.
26. Schonwetter RS, Teasdale TA, Stroey P, Luchi RH. Estimation of survival time in terminal cancer patients: An impedance to hospice admissions? *Hospice J* 1990;6:65-79.
27. Conwell Y, Canine ED. Rational suicide and the right ot die -- reality and myth, *N Engl J Med* 1991;325:1100-3.
28. Benrubi GI. Euthanasia -- the need for procedual safeguards, *N Engl J Med* 1992;326:197-9.
29. Cassel CK, Meier DE. Morals and moralism in the debate over euthanasia and assisted suicide, *N Engl J. Med* 1990;323:750-2.
30. Reichel W, Dyck AJ. Euthanasia: A contemporaty moral quandary, *Lancet* 1989;2:1321-3.
31. Angell M. Euthanasia, *N Engl J Med* 1988;319:1348-50.
32. Rachels J. Active and passive euthanasia, *N Engl J Med* 1975;292:78-80.
33. Lachs J. Humane treatment and the treatment of humans, *N Engl J Med* 1976;294:838-40.
34. van der Maas PJ, van Delden JJM, Pijnenborg L, *et al.* Euthanasia and other medical decisions concerning the end of life, *Lancet* 1991;338:669-74.
35. Singer PA, Siegler M. Euthanasia -- a critique, *N Engl J Med* 1990;322:1881-3.
36. Orentlicher D. Physician participation in assisted suicide, *JAMA* 1989;262:1844-5.
37. Wolf SM. Holding the line on euthanasia, *Hastings Cent Rep* 1989;19(1):Suppl. 13-5.
38. Gaylin W, Kass LR, Pellegrino ED, Siegler M. Doctors must not kill, *JAMA* 1988;259:2139-40.
39. Vaux KL. Debbie's dying: Mercy killing and the good death, *JAMA* 1988;259:2140-1.
40. Gomez CF. *Regulating Death: Euthanasia and the Case of the Netherlands*. New York, NY: Free Press, 1991.
41. Braham D. Euthanasia in Netherlands, *Lancet* 1990;335:591-1.
42. Leenen HJJ. Coma patients in the Netherlands, *BMJ* 1990;300:69.

Chapter 64

The Morality of Physician-Assisted Suicide

Robert F. Weir

In March 1989, 12 physicians published an article on the provision of care to hopelessly ill patients. Unfortunately, many of the substantive points in that article received insufficient attention from readers because the authors' call for appropriate, continually adjusted care for terminally ill patients was overshadowed by a portion of the document in which ten of the authors agreed that "it is not immoral for a physician to assist in the rational suicide of a terminally ill person."[1]

In June 1990, Jack Kevorkian, a retired pathologist in Michigan, gained international media attention by enabling Janet Adkins, a woman in the early stage of Alzheimer's disease, to terminate her life with the help of his "suicide machine."[2] The features of the case were so unusual that physicians, ethicists, and attorneys in health law who were interviewed by journalists were unanimous in judging this particular act of physician-assisted suicide deplorable.[3]

In March 1991, Timothy Quill, an internist in New York, published a detailed account of the suicide of one of his patients identified only as "Diane," a patient with acute myelomonocytic leukemia who requested and received his assistance in killing herself with an overdose of barbiturates.[4] Given the features of this particular case, some of the professionals in medicine, ethics, and law interviewed by the media judged Dr. Quill's action to have been morally acceptable, even if against the law in New York.[5]

The issue of physician-assisted suicide (PAS) is not limited to these well-publicized examples. The American Hospital Association estimates that many of the 6,000 daily deaths in the United States are orchestrated by patients, relatives, and physicians, although how many of these deaths are assisted suicides is unknown.[6] In a 1990 New York Times-CBS poll, taken two weeks after the initial publicity of the Adkins case, 53 percent of the respondents said that physicians should be allowed to assist a severely ill person in terminating his or her own life.[7] Moreover, PAS is beginning to be addressed as a separate ethical issue in the medical literature, without being lumped together with the related but different issue of voluntary euthanasia.[8]

The legal status of PAS is also being tested in an unprecedented manner. The Hemlock Society, having failed three years ago to get "The Humane and Dignified Death Act" on the ballot in California, successfully worked with a coalition called Washington Citizens for Death with Dignity to get Initiative 119 on the ballot in Washington in November 1991. The wording of this initiative, using language that blurs the differences between PAS and voluntary euthanasia, simply asked voters: "Shall adult patients who are in a medically terminal condition be permitted to request and receive from a physician aid-in-dying?"[9]

Source: Reprinted from *Law, Medicine, and Health Care*, Vol. 20:1-2, Spring-Summer 1992, pp. 116-126, with permission from University Publishing Group © 1992.

Given these events, the time has come for a serious discussion of the morality and legality of physician-assisted suicide. I hope to contribute to that discussion by first analyzing the concept of assisted suicide and describing the diversity of possible legal responses to acts of PAS. I will then provide an ethical analysis of PAS by discussing the cases of Janet Adkins and "Diane," sorting out the competing ethical arguments about this issue, and making some recommendations for professional practice and public policy.

The Concept of Assisted Suicide

As is true for all suicides, an assisted suicide involves someone (a person outside a clinical setting, or a patient in a clinical setting) who has suicidal motives, intends to die, does something to cause his or her death, and is noncoerced in deciding to kill himself or herself. However, in contrast to "normal" suicides, an assisted suicide requires aid from a physician, a relative or friend of the person wanting to commit suicide, or some other person who carries out the role of "enabler." The enabler can assist the suicidal person in any number of ways: by supplying information (e.g., from the Hemlock Society) on the most effective ways of committing suicide, purchasing a weapon of self-destruction, providing a lethal dose of pills or poison, giving the suicidal person encouragement to carry out the lethal deed, or helping in the actual act of killing (e.g., by helping the person take the pills, pull the trigger of a gun, close the garage doors, or turn on the gas). Also in contrast to suicide, an act of assisted suicide is an illegal act in many jurisdictions, punishable by fines and/or short-term imprisonment.

Given the surreptitious nature of most physician-assisted suicides, it is reasonable to think that most of these death-enabling acts by physicians are done outside hospitals and nursing homes. However, because cases of PAS can take place inside as well as outside clinical settings, such acts need to be distinguished from: (1) acts of abating life-sustaining treatment; and (2) acts of voluntary euthanasia. The reasons for drawing the distinctions are twofold: to help in accurately describing clinical cases that are conceptually different in important ways, and to provide an explanation for the differing ethical and legal assessment of these three kinds of clinical situations (any of which can, and usually do, result in a patient's death) that is found among physicians, nurses, ethicists, attorneys, legislators, and the rest of our society.

Acts of abating life-sustaining treatment are now a common feature of medical practice, whether the decision to abate treatment involves withholding treatment, decelerating treatment, or withdrawing a modality of treatment (e.g., a ventilator, a feeding tube) that has already been started.[10] From the perspectives of biomedical ethics and the law, a decision by an autonomous patient to abate life-sustaining treatment should be respected and carried out by the patient's physician in virtually all cases. In a similar manner, a reasonable decision by the surrogate of a nonautonomous patient to have life-sustaining treatment stopped should also be respected and carried out by the patient's physician, as long as the decision is based on: (1) the earlier, known preferences of the patient, or (2) a reasonable assessment of the patient's best interests. A physician who abates life-sustaining treatment for either of these reasons, the patient's preferences or the patient's current best interests -- is practicing morally responsible medicine and runs virtually no risk of civil or criminal liability, as demonstrated by a survey of all the relevant case law over the past two decades.[11]

Nevertheless, questions sometimes arise as to whether a patient who refuses life-sustaining treatment is thereby trying to commit suicide, and whether physicians who cooperate with a patient's refusal of life-sustaining treatment could be successfully prosecuted, after the patient's death, for having assisted with the patient's suicide. The answer to both questions is negative, based on existing case law.[12]

Although it is possible that some patients who refuse treatment are suicidal, the judicial cases involving this question have all been decided by the courts in the same way.

Numerous courts, with a unanimous voice, have given two reasons for rejecting claims that patients who refuse life-sustaining treatment are actually engaged in suicide: (1) the patient's intention in refusing treatment, and (2) the "underlying cause" of the patient's death when the patient dies without the treatment. The intention of such patients is not self-destruction, according to the courts, but freedom to control the course of their medical care.[13] In addition, the courts have reasoned that patients who refuse life-sustaining treatment do not thereby cause their deaths, but merely submit to the natural causes that are shutting down one or more critical bodily functions.[14] In the words of the Conroy court:

> Declining life-sustaining medical treatments may not properly be viewed as an attempt to commit suicide. Refusing medical intervention merely allows the disease to take its natural course...In addition, people who refuse life-sustaining medical treatment may not harbor a specific intent to die, rather, they may fervently wish to live, but to do so free of unwanted medical technology, surgery, or drugs, and without protracted suffering...Recognizing the right of a terminally ill person to reject medical treatment respects that person's intent, not to die, but to suspend medical intervention...The difference is between self-infliction or self-destruction and self-determination.[15]

Of course patients are different, and clinical cases almost always differ in important details. Consequently, a physician who cooperates with a patient in abating life-sustaining treatment can be assisting a patient to commit suicide, if the patient is suicidal. However, the clinical cases that have been subjected to judicial analysis in a number of jurisdictions indicate that acts of abating treatment and acts of assisting suicide are usually distinguishable, because of differences in the motivation, intention, and causative role of the person whose life is at stake.

Acts of voluntary euthanasia, when such acts of intentional killing at a patient's request actually occur, are more clearly distinguishable from acts of assisting suicide. The most obvious difference is the difference in final agency. In acts of assisted suicide, the person who does the actual killing is the person who wants to die. In acts of voluntary euthanasia, the person who does the killing is someone (e.g., a physician, a nurse, a relative)/other than the person who wants to die. If a physician is involved, the difference in personal involvement is between providing a suicidal patient with a prescription that would be lethal if taken by the patient in certain amounts, compared with the physician personally administering a lethal injection to the patient at the patient's request.

In addition to this difference, there are other differences that frequently distinguish acts of assisted suicide from acts of voluntary euthanasia. First, a patient who requests to be killed by a physician (or someone else) is usually unable to commit suicide, for either physiological or psychological reasons. The combination of: (1) having decided that death is preferable to the continuation of a personal existence that has become intolerable (e.g., because of intractable pain or extensive paralysis), but (2) being unable to carry out the act of self-destruction means that the patient has to request that someone else do the act of killing if the intended result of death is to occur.

Second, the methods used to do the killing are usually different. The most commonly used method in cases of physician-assisted suicide seems to be sleeping pills, with a physician enabling the suicide to take place by providing the prescription for the drugs and/or discussing the required doses and preferable means of drug administration with the patient. By contrast, virtually any physician who would decide, for reasons of mercy, to kill a patient at the patient's request would choose another method to do it, most commonly an injection of potassium chloride or a bolus of air.

A related difference between acts of assisted suicide and acts of voluntary euthanasia is the certainty of the patient's death as a result of the physician's involvement. A physician who responds to a patient's request for assistance in committing suicide cannot be certain, merely by providing a prescription or discussing dosage, either that the patient will follow through with the attempt at self-destruction or that the attempt at causing his or her death will actually work. By contrast, any physician willing to act on a patient's request to be killed is almost certainly going to have sufficient medical and pharmacological knowledge to ensure that when he or she gives an injection with the intention of killing the patient, the patient's death will be certain and immediate.

A final difference between acts of assisted suicide and acts of voluntary euthanasia, namely the legal liability involved, is also significant. In assisted suicide cases, a physician (or other person) who enables the act of self-killing to be done runs the risk of a relatively mild legal penalty or, in some jurisdictions, no legal penalty at all, a point I will expand on later. By contrast, a physician who kills a patient at the patient's request -- even for reasons of mercy -- runs the risk of being prosecuted for murder or manslaughter.

Assisted suicide, even when the person in the role of "enabler" is a physician, is therefore conceptually different from: (1) treatment abatement, and (2) voluntary euthanasia, although the deaths of patients are the frequent results in each instance. In clinical practice, when the clarity of different concepts can sometimes be blurred, acts of PAS at the very least usually differ from acts of abating life-sustaining treatment, and always differ from acts of voluntary euthanasia. For patients (e.g., some patients with metastatic cancer, or endstage heart or lung or renal disease, or AIDS) who request the assistance of a physician in committing suicide, this difference can be very real: they need more help from the physician than merely abating treatment, but less help than would be required if they were asking the physician to kill them.

The Legal Status of Physician-Assisted Suicide

The cases of Janet Adkins and "Diane," occurring in different states and under very different circumstances, illustrate the legal ambiguity that exists on the issue of assisted suicide. According to early reports of the Adkins case, the specific reason that Jack Kevorkian was willing to use his "suicide machine" in Michigan was his discovery that Michigan was one of the states having no legislative statute that defined assisted suicide as an illegal act.[16] The ensuing controversy about the case in Michigan and elsewhere continued for months, in large part because of the slowness and diversity in response to the case by various legal authorities in the state.

From the outset, attorneys in Michigan acknowledged that the legal status of assisted suicide, whether done by a physician or someone else, was "murky." Not only was there no legislative statute making assisted suicide a crime, there was also no clear case law to provide legal precedent in the state. Two possible precedents, a 1920 Michigan Supreme Court decision and a 1983 Michigan Court of Appeals ruling, were not sufficiently clear to determine the legal consequences that faced Kevorkian.[17]

Nevertheless, some state officials decided that legal steps had to be taken, lest Michigan become a "haven" for persons seeking assistance in killing themselves. The result, acted out over several months, was a series of three events: an unsuccessful attempt to convict Kevorkian of first-degree murder, a successful effort in a civil suit two months later to bar Kevorkian from using his machine again or building another one, and a long-running debate in the Michigan legislature over proposed legislation that would make assisted suicide a crime punishable by a combination of financial penalty and a short prison sentence.[18]

Uncertainty about the legal status of assisted suicide also played a role in the case of "Diane," as indicated by Timothy Quill's published account of the case and the early media reports. Quill's account never specifically states that assisted suicide is illegal in New York, nor does it say that he inquired about the legality of his "'helping Diane to terminate her life. Instead, Quill simply alludes to the legal "boundaries" he was exploring by enabling Diane to kill herself, the possible legal "repercussions" that might occur if a family member had to help her, and his decision not to tell the medical examiner that the cause of the patient's death had been suicide. Quill's final reference to the law is his comment, "I am not sure the law, society, or the medical profession would agree" with the decision to help Diane.[19]

Initial media reports offered differing interpretations of the legal status of assisted suicide in New York. The Rochester (Monroe County) district attorney said, when asked in March about the state statute on assisted suicide, that persons convicted of aiding in a suicide could be sentenced to 1-4 years in prison, but added that he knew of no prosecutions of physicians and had not yet decided whether to submit the case to a grand jury.[20] Three weeks later another report, citing the same district attorney, stated that a person convicted in New York of aiding a successful suicide could be sentenced to as many as 15 years in prison.[21]

The district attorney soon decided not to prosecute Quill, pointing out that, because "Diane" had never been identified, there was no cadaver to be examined medically for evidence of a crime. That decision was rescinded after a journalist discovered Diane's identity and located her dead body in a college anatomy lab.[22] In July, a grand jury in Rochester declined to indict Quill, even though the members of the jury knew that traces of barbiturates had been found in the cadaver.[23] In August, the disciplinary board of the New York State Health Department decided that "no charge of misconduct was warranted" against Quill, noting the longstanding patient-physician relationship in the case and the fact that Quill "himself did not directly participate in any taking of life."[24]

As demonstrated by these cases, the legal status of assisted suicide varies from state to state. In contrast to acts of suicide and attempted suicide, both of which were decriminalized in all the states in the 1970s, acts of assisted suicide remain legally problematic.

Legislative statutes in 26 states make assisted suicide a criminal act, either as: (1) a unique offense governed by a specific statute, or (2) a class (e.g., second degree) of murder or manslaughter.[25] For states having specific statutory prohibitions of assisted suicide, the punishment is usually a fine (in the $1,000-2,000 range) and the possibility of one or more years in prison. In states lacking a specific statute on assisted suicide, anyone assisting in suicide may be legally liable under the state's criminal code for murder or manslaughter or possibly under the common law in the state.

Whether a person, including someone who is a physician, who assists in a suicide will be reported and prosecuted is another question. In particular, the question of prosecution depends on a number of factors related to time, circumstance, and public opinion. It seems reasonable to think, for example, that the publicity and public outcry over the Adkins case made an effort to prosecute Kevorkian unavoidable, even with a weak legal basis for the case.

By contrast, the wide public acceptance of Quill's role in "Diane's" suicide made successful prosecution so unlikely that, even with the legislative statute on assisted suicide, the district attorney initially decided not to file charges. The subsequent decisions by the grand jury and the disciplinary board of the state health department confirmed the political correctness of that initial decision not to prosecute. Nevertheless, a prudent physician in any state should understand that he or she runs some legal risk, however slight, in assisting a patient to commit suicide.

Ethics in the Michigan and New York cases

Even if the criminal law were not a factor in PAS cases, such cases would still be subject to ethical analysis. For that reason, it is important to examine the ethics that seem to have characterized the cases of Janet Adkins and "Diane," at least to the extent we know the facts of the cases as portrayed in published materials. How did the cases differ morally, and what difference do those differences make in an ethical analysis?

In the Adkins case, the first problematic aspect of the case is that Janet Adkins was not a patient of Dr. Kevorkian. She was a 54-year-old woman with a diagnosis of Alzheimer's disease, who lived in Portland and asked her husband to telephone Kevorkian in Detroit after they read about him in a magazine and saw him discuss his "suicide machine" on a television show. The only relationship that existed between them prior to her death was based on two short conversations in Detroit (one at dinner, and one during a 40-minute "consultation") two days before the suicide occurred in the back of Kevorkian's old Volkswagen bus.

Other problematic aspects of the Adkins case involve several steps that Kevorkian failed to take in making an assessment of Adkins' medical condition and providing her with medical advice. Having obtained her medical records from two physicians in Oregon and Washington, he apparently did not consult with any other specialists on Alzheimer's disease, in Detroit or elsewhere, regarding the difficulties of diagnosing this condition, accurately describing the progressive dementia involved, and managing some of the symptoms (e.g., anxiety, depression) that can be treated with medication. He did not, according to media accounts of the videotaped "consultation," make much effort to assess her physical condition or her mental state, and even less effort to ascertain whether she was capable of making a voluntary, informed decision to end her life with his machine. He also did not suggest medical alternatives that she and her husband, who was present at the time, might want to consider. Indeed, his actions did not convey any sense that an act of PAS should be done with great reluctance and as an act of last resort, only when an arduous effort to change the patient's mind has failed.

Finally, given that he was talking with a woman understandably anxious about both the early and longterm disabilities connected with Alzheimer's disease, it is surprising that Dr. Kevorkian did not recommend procedural safeguards to Adkins and her husband before providing her with the means to kill herself with successive intravenous injections of saline, thiopental, and potassium chloride. At the very least, it would have seemed reasonable for him to recommend that she (with her husband, and possibly with her three sons) seek a second medical opinion, psychological counseling, and contact with a local Alzheimer's disease organization or support group before taking the irreversible step that would result in her death.

The case of "Diane" is significantly different, except that both patients committed suicide without their husbands, children, or friends present. "Diane" was a 45-year-old patient of Timothy Quill, and had been his patient for at least 8 years.[26] He knew her medical history, much of her personal history, her husband and college-age son, her virtues and values, her fears and weaknesses, and the importance she placed on avoiding a lingering, suffering death. He knew she had successfully battled against vaginal cancer, alcoholism, and depression, only to develop acute leukemia that, at best, offered her a 25 percent chance of complete remission following chemotherapy and bone marrow transplantation. Quill thought those odds were sufficiently good to recommend treatment; "Diane," after beginning chemotherapy, reached a different conclusion.

As much as anything, "Diane's" case reveals a physician-patient relationship characterized by mutual respect, shared information, numerous conversations, honesty, informed choice, and an emphasis on patient autonomy. Of course the only version we have of the case facts is the version supplied by Dr. Quill. Nevertheless, he clearly indicates that when she refused the chemotherapy, he thought she was making a mistake. Having given her information regarding treatment options and likely outcomes, arranged meetings with two oncologists, and discussed her limited life expectancy in the absence of treatment, he thought she should opt for treatment -- to the point that he did not tell her of the painful deaths of the last four hospital patients with acute leukemia.

When "Diane" refused chemotherapy and subsequently indicated a strong desire to control when and how she died, Dr. Quill took several steps over the course of several months. As a former hospice physician, he helped her understand comfort care and become a hospice patient. He made sure she was not depressed, recommended that she see a psychologist, provided transfusions and antibiotics to her as an outpatient, and encouraged her to say goodbyes to relatives and friends. Fearing that she might botch a suicide attempt and/or involve her family in helping her commit suicide, he told her about suicide information that is available through the Hemlock Society.

When she later asked for barbiturates for sleep, he made sure that she knew the correct amount to use for sleep -- and for suicide. He met with her regularly, and solicited a promise from her to see him one last time before she planned to kill herself. With sadness, he had no doubt that "she knew what she was doing."

What difference do these differences between the two cases make, in terms of the ethics of medical practice? Both physicians say that they understood themselves to be acting outside the realm of currently accepted medical practice, but believed what they were doing was compassionate, beneficent, and necessary. Yet the reported facts of the two cases reveal physicians whose apparent motives, intentions, and actions were drastically different.

Jack Kevorkian seems (according to the reports in the media) to have been insensitive, negligent in several ways, and more interested in publicity than in the person who came for help. Timothy Quill, although acting contrary to conventional medical practice and being liable for criminal prosecution in New York, appears (through his account of the case) to have been genuinely concerned about his patient and her family. Because of that concern, he seems to have given "Diane" reasonable medical options, several informed choices, responsible medical and moral advice, and appropriate palliative care during the terminal phase of her life. In my view, his involvement in enabling her to commit suicide was also morally responsible.

The Case Against Physician-Assisted Suicide

Making a case for an ethical position, especially one that is contrary to traditional moral thinking and current law, requires an analysis of competing arguments and an effort to be as persuasive as possible. I now turn to that dual task by first examining five ethical arguments, some with variant themes, that are sometimes advanced against physician participation in assisted suicide.

(1) *The medical profession is committed to healing*

The most common argument against PAS has two variants, both of which are based on the view that physicians constitute a unique profession that is defined, at least in part, by a traditional group morality stipulating standards of care and of behavior by members of the group. One version of this argument involves a direct appeal to the Hippocratic Oath, dating from the fourth century B.C. In particular, current opponents of PAS appeal to the portion of the Oath that declares: "I will neither give a deadly drug to anybody if asked for it, nor will I make a suggestion to this effect."[27]

The second, more general version of this argument emphasizes the centrality of healing in defining who physicians are and what they do in their professional role.[28] For some persons who advocate this view of medicine, the notion that physicians might, even in rare instances, assist patients to commit suicide is automatically and without exception ruled out of bounds for any member of the medical profession. As stated by David Orentlicher, "Treatment designed to bring on death, by definition, does not heal and is therefore fundamentally inconsistent with the physician's role in the patient-physician relationship."[29]

(2) *Physicians should not cause death*
A related argument asserts that there is no difference between PAS and voluntary euthanasia. Once a physician moves beyond abating life-sustaining treatment, so the argument goes, it does not really matter whether the physician's participation in helping to hasten the patient's death at the patient's request is by prescribing barbiturates or by injecting a lethal agent. Both acts "encourage doctors to use their skills to kill their patients."[30] According to Leon Kass, there is little difference between a physician's role as an accomplice to death or as an agent of death: assisting in a patient's death "is as much in violation of the venerable proscription against euthanasia as were the physician to do it himself."[31]

(3) *Patients should not request physician-assisted suicide*
This argument also has two variants, both of which address the moral responsibility of patients in the relationships they have with physicians. One version, the simpler of the two, states that patients should never ask their physicians to help them commit suicide, given that: (a) many persons regard suicide as an immoral act, and (b) physician participation in enabling that act of self-destruction to occur may constitute criminal action.

The second version of this argument is based on the difference between negative and positive moral rights, as these rights apply to the relationship between a patient and that patient's physician. A decision made by a patient to forgo mechanical ventilation, feeding tubes, or some other life-sustaining treatment involves the negative right (or liberty right) of treatment refusal. A correlate of this negative right is the obligation of the patient's physician not to interfere with or thwart that negative right unless the physician has some overriding obligation of another sort.

By contrast, a request by a patient for a physician's assistance in committing suicide can be interpreted as involving a positive right (or welfare right), or at least a claim to that effect. The difference is important: the patient does not merely request to be left alone by the physician, but tries to impose a moral obligation on the physician to help the patient accomplish the desired end of self-destruction. That claim, whether based on merit or need, is weak, and certainly need not be regarded as imposing an obligation on the physician who receives it.[32]

(4) *Physician-assisted suicide would lead to mistrust and abuses*
This view, a form of the "slippery slope" argument, projects two unfortunate consequences that would follow from the widespread acceptance and/or legalization of PAS. One of these consequences would be damage to the relationship of trust that, one hopes, exists between patients and their physicians. According to David Orentlicher, even a discussion of assisted suicide could damage the patient-physician relationship in two different ways: it could raise questions in the patient's mind about the value the physician attaches to the patient's present life of disability and suffering, and it could raise doubts in the patient's mind about the physician's commitment to provide effective treatment for the patient's current medical conditions. Either way, a physician's willingness even to discuss the possibility of assisted suicide "might seriously undermine" the patient's trust in the physician.[33]

The other consequence, that of abuses by physicians in assisting patients to commit suicide, would be equally serious. As vividly illustrated by the actions of Jack Kevorkian, some physicians would undoubtedly agree to help patients kill themselves without determining whether a given patient is clinically depressed, whether appropriate other medical opinions have been secured, whether the request for help is necessary, whether alternatives to assisted suicide have been explored, or whether relatives and friends who would be psychologically harmed by an unexpected suicide are aware of what may happen. The fact that "Diane's" case was handled in a better manner is of little comfort, according to this argument, since it merely demonstrates that virtually all cases of PAS involve physicians acting alone, with no scrutiny from their peers, the courts, or anybody else.[34]

(5) *Physician-assisted suicide is unnecessary*

Patients turn to their physicians for help in committing suicide for any number of reasons. Chief among these reasons is a desire to avoid the prolonged pain and suffering, both physical and psychological, often involved in the course of a chronic and/or terminal condition. Frequently having witnessed the long, painful deaths of relatives in hospital settings, patients sometimes ask their physicians to help them avoid the same fate. Concerned that physicians will be unable to control the pain or effectively manage the symptoms of their chronic medical conditions, they conclude that suicide, perhaps requiring assistance from a physician or someone else, is their only alternative.

Such reasoning is wrong, according to advocates of hospice programs. In this argument, the availability of hospice care throughout the country precludes the need for patients to seek suicide, thus making the participation of physicians in assisting suicide unnecessary. Some physicians may, out of ignorance regarding effective pain control, "agree with patients that their suffering is intolerable and worthy of assisted suicide when in fact the pain may be easily treatable."[35] A preferable alternative is for physicians to learn how to relieve patients' pain more effectively, manage the symptoms of their conditions more appropriately, and assure them that prolonged suffering need not be the fate that awaits them.[36]

Do these five arguments, taken singly or as a collective argument, make a persuasive case that physicians should never agree to assist their patients in committing suicide? I think not, for the following reasons. Critics of PAS who use the first argument take an undeniably important, defining feature of the medical profession, but emphasize it to the exclusion of other ways of describing who physicians are and what they do professionally. Healing the sick and injured is surely one of the goals of medicine, but not in isolation from other appropriate medical goals. Preventing disease, saving and prolonging lives, relieving pain and suffering, ameliorating disabling conditions, and avoiding undue harm to patients are also important medical goals that represent defining features of medicine as a profession.

Some of these goals of medicine, it is important to note, are appropriate even when patients cannot be healed -- and even when some patients turn to their physicians for help in putting an end to an existence they have come to regard as intolerable. The achievement of these appropriate medical goals is more important than a literal adherence to an ancient oath whose religious and moral framework is of such limited relevance to contemporary medicine that the oath is frequently altered when used in medical school convocations and increasingly replaced entirely by other kinds of oaths, including those written by medical students themselves.

The second argument, the one equating PAS with voluntary euthanasia, is simply misplaced in the debate over PAS. It is true, of course, that euthanasia has for centuries been regarded as contrary to morally responsible medical practice, but the intentional killing of patients is not the ethical issue involved in PAS. Physicians do not cause the deaths of patients in these cases; the patients cause their own deaths, a legal act in all 50 states, subsequent to receiving some type of enabling help from their physicians. Thus critics of PAS who assert that physicians are thereby killing patients are either: (a) mistaken about the differences between assisted suicide and voluntary euthanasia, or (b) intentionally blurring the differences between these two acts to score points with the emotive language of "killing."

The third argument is largely true, in my view, because it appropriately indicates that patients should not make unreasonable demands on physicians. Patients should be hesitant to try to involve their physicians in acts off assisted suicide, just as any of us should refrain from encouraging other persons to participate in actions that may be contrary to their value systems. Equally important, when patients with chronic, progressively deteriorating, or terminal conditions do ask their physicians for help in committing suicide, they should understand that they have no justifiable reason for thinking that their physicians are obligated to render such help. Physician-assisted suicide should be motivated by compassion for a patient, not a misplaced sense of moral obligation.

The last two arguments, the ones stating that PAS is dangerous and unnecessary, are only partially true. Abuses in the name of physician-assisted suicide will undoubtedly take place in the future, as they undoubtedly already do. Whether the abuses will be greater than at present is impossible to say. What is possible to say, however, is that PAS seems to be both necessary and morally justifiable in rare cases and, if handled correctly by morally responsible physicians, need not threaten the foundation of trust that is crucial to patient-physician relationships.

The occasional necessity of PAS is illustrated by the case of "Diane," who requested assistance from Timothy Quill in terminating her life even though she was receiving appropriate medical care as a hospice patient. Unfortunately, even hospice care fails, for some patients, to provide them with sufficient personal control over the terminal phase of their lives. "Diane's" case also suggests that a patient's level of trust in a physician may be increased, not undermined, when a caring physician indicates a reluctant willingness to help the patient bring her or his life to an end.

The Case for Physician-Assisted Suicide

Having provided this critical assessment of arguments against PAS, I will now put forth five arguments that may prove to be persuasive in justifying some cases of physician participation in assisted suicide. Taken together, the arguments claim that PAS is occasionally justifiable as a compassionate way for physicians to respond to current medical reality by alleviating patient suffering, optimizing patient control, and minimizing harm to the patient and other persons important to the patient. Taken individually, the arguments suggest that physicians should, in rare cases, consider assisting their patients to commit suicide, for any of five reasons.

(1) *To respond to current medical reality*

Change is a regular part of medicine, whether the change takes the form of new diagnostic tools, new research discoveries, new victories over old diseases, new diseases, new health problems, new drugs, new life-sustaining technologies, or new concerns over matters pertaining to biomedical ethics, health economics, and health law. Change is surely a factor in the medical problems that patients bring their physicians, with adult patients now presenting more medical problems that are chronic or degenerative in nature than ever before. Added to this factor is another one: patients are living increasingly longer lives, with the combination of chronic medical conditions and extended life expectancy representing the distinct possibility, for some persons, that remaining alive will be regarded as offering nothing other than more disability, more financial and personal hardship, and more suffering.

The good news is that many adults are now capable, with the help of pharmacological and technological advances in medicine, of having long lives with a remarkable health status that would have been unachievable earlier in this century and unimaginable before that. The bad news is that some adults are caught in an existential situation dominated by intractable pain, severe disability, progressive dementia, a deteriorating neurological condition, a terminal condition, or some combination of these that makes life seem not to be worth living. An unknown number of these persons decide that death is a preferable option to the suffering that life holds for them and, for their own personal reasons, ask their physicians to help them end the suffering.

It is this part of medical reality -- the realistic limits of physicians to heal all their patients and effectively relieve suffering -- that represents the ethical core of the debate over PAS. Rather than quoting a passage from the Hippocratic Oath about that physicians cannot do for their patients, contemporary physicians should address medical reality as it currently exists in their patients -- some with terminal conditions, and an increasing number with chronic and degenerative diseases -- and consider again what they might do for that small minority of patients who find their lives to be intolerable and who, perhaps as a last resort, turn to their physicians for help in bringing about death.

(2) *To alleviate patient suffering*

Virtually anyone who is ill suffers from time to time. For some patients, suffering is primarily physical in nature, with the particular forms of suffering including nausea, dyspnea, fever, hunger, thirst, diarrhea, and pain. For other patients, suffering is partially or perhaps primarily psychological in nature, with individuals experiencing anxiety, depression, denial, loneliness, helplessness, anger, and fear. Much of this suffering, whether physiological or psychological in nature, can be effectively managed with empathic support, medications, various other medical and surgical interventions, nursing care, psychological counseling, stress-reduction techniques and rest.

But for Janet Adkins, "Diane," and an unknown number of other patients, the multiple efforts made by themselves, their families and friends, and their physicians to alleviate their suffering ultimately do not work. Janet Adkins, it seems, experienced substantial psychological suffering brought on by thoughts about the losses she had already experienced (she could no longer read literature or play the piano). Additional psychological suffering was undoubtedly created by the anxiety and fear of wondering what her remaining years with Alzheimer's disease would be like for herself and her family.

"Diane" experienced the physical suffering caused by her disease-related bone pain, weakness, infections, fatigue, and fever, but she preferred this suffering to the suffering she would have experienced through hospitalization, chemotherapy, radiation therapy, and bone marrow transplantation. In addition, she seems to have experienced substantial psychological suffering that included anger at an insensitive oncologist, anxiety over losing control of her living and dying, fear about increasing discomfort and dependence, fear about additional pain, and an overwhelming sense of injustice regarding the leukemic condition that struck soon after she had conquered her other health problems.

The ethical challenge that is presented to physicians by such cases is direct and sharp: Should I, having exhausted all other therapeutic possibilities, respond affirmatively to a request for help made by one of my patients? Should I, with the intention of alleviating the life-ruining suffering that my patient is experiencing, be willing to assist the patient in committing suicide? In at least some cases, the appropriate answer is yes.[37]

(3) *To optimize patient control*

The desire to have control over one's living, dying, and death is a factor in assisted suicide cases that matches the desire for suffering to be ended. Janet Adkins was willing to travel from Portland to Seattle for experimental treatment, then to fly (with her husband) to Detroit to make use of the "suicide machine" in order to end her life before it was ravaged further by Alzheimer's disease. Although legitimate questions have been raised about her mental status at the time, there seems to be little doubt that, if she was still autonomous in the days before her death, her choice to kill herself was a choice to control her destiny instead of permitting her disease to control her.

The desire for personal control is even clearer in "Diane's" case. Quill states that "Diane," having overcome her earlier medical problems, "took control of her life" and developed "a strong sense of independence and confidence." When she went against Quill's medical advice and the wishes of her family in refusing chemotherapy, she "articulated very clearly that it was she who would be experiencing all the side effects of treatment." Later, when "Diane" knew she was dying, Quill says that it was "extraordinarily important to "Diane" to maintain control of herself and her own dignity during the time remaining to her.[38] In describing his own participation in the case, Quill states that he felt he was "setting her free to get the most out of the time she had left, and to maintain dignity and control on her own terms until her death."

For physicians in such cases, the option of trying to optimize patient control represents the ultimate challenge of how far one is willing to go to respect the autonomy of patients. If (as seems clear in "Diane's" case, but not Janet Adkins' case) the patient who requests assistance is autonomous, the patient is therefore capable of making an informed, deliberative, and voluntary decision regarding her or his health care. If personal control over one's living and dying is highly valued by the patient, the decisions made about health care will reflect that value. In extreme cases the desire to remain autonomous and in control sometimes includes a request for help from a physician -- a request for help in exercising control over one's final exit.[39]

(4) *To minimize harm to the patient and others*
The ethical principle of non-maleficence has considerable importance in medicine. Throughout the history of medicine, physicians have been expected to avoid intentionally or negligently harming their patients. Given that patients are frequently harmed in a variety of ways in clinical contexts, the ethical requirement placed on physicians is that of trying to ensure that patients are not harmed on balance in the course of efforts to heal them or otherwise promote their welfare.

Traditionally, the ultimate harm to befall a patient has been considered to be death. As a consequence, two longstanding moral rules of medical practice have been derived from this professional aversion to having any intentional (or negligent) role in a patient's death: "do not kill" and "do not assist another person's death."

In the great majority of cases, these moral rules continue to apply. However, patients can be harmed in several significant ways short of death, through the invasion of their important interests, the impairment of their mental or psychological welfare, physical injury, and technological abuse.[40] Moreover, most thoughtful persons have some sort of informal ranking or other cataloging of harmful events that could take place in their lives that would represent, to them, a fate worse than death.

Janet Adkins, "Diane," and unknown other persons have concluded that remaining alive under terrible, worsening circumstances is a fate worse than death. The important question is whether physicians should have any role in facilitating one harmful event (a patient's self-destruction) in order to help the patient avoid other harms (e.g., intractable pain, progressive dementia, loss of personhood, incalculable damage to a family) that the patient regards as worse. In rare cases, the appropriate answer is affirmative, both for the sake of the patient and for persons loved by the patient.

(5) *To act out of compassion*
What counts as a morally responsible motive for physician participation in assisted suicide?

The list of possible motives includes a desire to help the patient, an undervaluing of the quality of the patient's life, a desire to help the family emotionally and financially, a misplaced sense of duty to the patient, a desire for publicity, and so forth.

According to media accounts of the Janet Adkins case, Jack Kevorkian seems to have had several motives, including the desire for publicity and a curious sort of revenge against other persons in the medical profession. By contrast, Timothy Quill seems not to have been motivated by considerations other than the physical and psychological welfare of his patient and her family.

In my view, the only acceptable motive for physicians to have in enabling a patient to commit suicide is that of compassion. In many instances, of course, compassionate physicians decide, for good moral reasons, not to help patients achieve the sort of self-deliverance that they seek. In other, much less frequent instances, compassionate physicians sometimes decide that the plea for help from a patient for whom life has become intolerable is a request that cannot and should not be rejected. Either moral choice, if motivated by compassion, can be correct, depending on the facts of individual cases.

Justifiable Practice and Public Policy

For PAS to be justifiable, several conditions have to be met. First, a morally responsible physician who is asked to assist in a suicide should determine if the patient is suffering from treatable clinical depression and, if so, recommend treatment for that condition. In addition, the physician should try to determine if the patient's pain and other suffering are, in fact, refractory to treatment.

A second condition is for the physician to determine that assisted suicide is a moral last resort, in the sense that there are no effective medical options available that are acceptable to the patient. No medical treatment is available that will reverse or cure the patient's condition, no life-sustaining treatment is being used that could be abated at the patient's request, and no intervention (even hospice care) seems to provide the relief and release the patient desperately seeks.

A third condition consists of several conversations between the physician and the patient, with at least one of the conversations including one or more of the patient's closest relatives and friends. From the physician's perspective, these conversations, whether done within a few days or over several weeks, should have several purposes: to determine that the patient is autonomous and the decision to commit suicide is rational, to recommend a second medical opinion and other appropriate professional help, to make sure that no acceptable alternatives to assisted suicide are available, to determine that the request for assistance is necessary, and to make sure that the patient's close relatives and friends are informed about the prospective suicide. The consent of the patient's family to the contemplated suicide is not required, but they should at least be aware, in general terms, of what may happen so that the psychological harm they experience will be lessened when they find out that the suicide has taken place.

Even when these conditions are met in individual cases, important questions remain as to how PAS cases should be handled in terms of public policy. How should the law respond when a physician or other person helps an individual do something that is legal in every state, when that legal activity is suicide? Should physicians who decide to assist one or more of their patients in committing suicide be criminally liable, either under a specific state statute or a state homicide law? Should assisted suicide, whether done by physicians or other persons, be decriminalized? Should statutes authorizing PAS in certain cases be limited to cases of terminal illness? Should PAS, along with voluntary euthanasia, be legalized as "physician aid-in-dying" under certain conditions?

These questions and many others regarding PAS as a matter of public policy require careful analysis and extensive discussion, much more than can be completed here. However,

I have some tentative recommendations that might contribute to the discussion. A preferable alternative to the current patchwork of state laws on assisted suicide would be for the National Conference of Commissioners on Uniform State Laws (NCCUSL), working with appropriate medical groups, to develop model legislation on PAS that might be adopted throughout the country, so that physicians practicing in any state could have greater certainty regarding the legality (or illegality) of PAS. My hope is that this new legislation will remove PAS from the criminal statutes in all states, so that physicians who decide for reasons of compassion to engage in PAS will no longer have to be secretive and deceptive with their professional colleagues about having done so.

In my view, the legal restrictions on assisted suicide should be lifted only for physicians. Given the ease with which emotionally unstable, demented, and suicidal individuals could be "assisted" in their deaths by numerous other persons with questionable motives, the NCCUSL and/or various state legislatures may decide to maintain the legal liability attached to acts of assisted suicide when performed by persons other than physicians.

Physicians, of course, should not be given a legal blank check. Physicians who receive requests for help in committing suicide with regret and sadness, who give serious consideration to such requests only in carefully limited circumstances, and who meet the conditions for morally responsible PAS should not face legal penalties. By contrast, physicians who are irresponsible in taking requests for PAS, who fail to exercise appropriate care in working with patients seeking PAS, and who are careless in providing patients with the means of self-destruction should face penalties for such negligence, perhaps including losing their licenses to practice medicine.

One final point. The case for PAS has been developed with great reluctance, both because I wish such activity by physicians were unnecessary and because I am uncomfortable advocating an ethical position that departs from much traditional thinking about ethics in medicine. However, I am convinced that PAS is sometimes necessary, that it is an alternative not to be automatically rejected by morally responsible physicians, and that it is, in at least some instances, justifiable as the right and compassionate thing to do.

Notes

1. Wanzer SH, Federman DD, Edelstein SJ, *et al*. The physician's responsibility toward hopelessly ill patients: A second look, *N Engl J Med* 1989;3:844-49
2. Physician aids in suicide. *Chicago Tribune* 1990, Jun 6:Al.
3. As memory and music faded, Oregon woman chose death. *New York Times* 1990, Jun 7:Al.
4. Quill TE. A case of individualized decision-making, *N Engl J Med* 1991;324:691-694.
5. Doctor says he agonized, but gave drug for suicide. *New York Times* 1991, Mar 6:A1
6. Cassel CK, Meier DE. Morals and moralism in the debate over euthanasia and assisted suicide, *N Engl J Med* 1990;323:750-52.
7. Giving death a hand: Rending issue. *New York Times* 1990, Jun 19:A22.
8. Demac AR. Thoughts on physician-assisted suicide, *West J Med* 1988;148:228-30; Orentlicher D. Physician participation in assisted suicide, *JAMA* 1989;262:1844-45; Weir RF. Physicians and assisted suicide, *Iowa Medicine* 1990;80:534; Weir RF. Is assisted suicide justifiable? *Iowa Medicine* 1991;81:27; Weissman DE. Physician assisted suicide, *Bioethics Bulletin* 1991;4:3-4.
9. Gianelli DM. A right to die, *American Medical News* 1991:9.
10. Weir RF. *Abating Treatment with Critically Ill patients*. New York, NY: Oxford University Press, 1989.
11. Weir RF, Gostin L. Decisions to abate life-sustaining treatment for nonautonomous patients, *JAMA* 1990;264:1846-53.
12. Glantz LH. Withholding and withdrawing treatment: The role of the criminal law, *Law, Med & Health Care* 1988;5:231-41.

13. Comissioner of Corrections v. Myers, 399 NE2d 452 (Mass 1979).; Satz v. Perlmutter, 362 So2d 160, 163 (Fla Dist Ct App 1978), Aff'd, 379 So2d 359 (Fla 1980).; Bantling v. Superior Court, 163 CalApp3d 186, 209 CalRptr 220 (1984).; Bouvia v. Superior Court, 179 CalApp3d 1127, 225 CalRptr 297 CalApp2d Dist 1986), Review Denied (Cal June 5, 1986).; In Re Requena, 213 NJ Super 475, 517 A2d 886 (NJ Super Ct Ch Div), Aft'd, 213 NJ Super 443, 517 A2d 869 (Super Ct App Div 1986).; Delio v. Westchester County Medical Center, 129 AD2d 1, 516 NYS2d 677 (App Div 2d Dep't 1987).; In Re Gardner, 534 A2d 947 (Maine 1987).
14. *Ibid.*
15. *In re* Conroy, 98 NJ 321, 486 A2d 1209 (1985).
16. *Chicago Tribune*, *New York Times*, supra notes 2 and 3.
17. Williams M. Ethics, patient's right to die weighed in Kevorkian case, *American Medical News* 1991:18.
18. Michigan judge bars doctor from using suicide machine. *New York Times* 1991, Feb 6:A15; MEA exclusive: Officials knew Kevorkian's plans beforehand, *Med Ethics Advisor* 1991;7:25-27.
19. Quill, supra note 4.
20. *New York Times*, supra note 5.
21. Gianelli DM. NY case reopens debate on doctor-assisted suicide, *American Medical News* 1991:1
22. Doctor who aided patient suicide may be tried. *New York Times* 1991, Jul 22:B12.
23. Jury declines to indict a doctor who said he aided in a suicide. *New York Times* 1991, Jul 27:A1.
24. State won't press case on doctor in suicide. *New York Times* 1991, Jul 17.
25. Smith CK. Assistance in compassionate suicide: Still no legal right, *Hemlock Quarterly* 1990;41:6-7.
26. Quill, supra note 4.
27. *Chicago Tribune*, *JAMA*, supra notes 2 and 8.
28. Gaylin W, Kass LR, Pellegrino ED, Siegler M. Doctors Must Not Kill, *JAMA* 1988;259:2139-40; Kass LR, Neither for love nor money: Why doctors must not kill, *Public Interest* 1989;94:25-46; Brescia FJ. Killing the known dying: Notes of a death watcher, *J Pain Sym Man* 1991;6:337-39.
29. Orentlicher, supra note 8.
30. Rothman DJ. M.D. doesn't mean `more deaths'. *New York Times* 1991, Apr 20:A15.
31. *Chicago Tribune*, supra note 2.
32. Abating Treatment with Critically Ill Patients, supra note to.
33. Orentlicher, supra note 8.
34. *New York Times*, supra note 30.
35. Weissman, supra note 8.
36. Foley KM. The relationship of pain and symptom management to patient requests for physician-assisted suicide, *J Pain Sym Man* 1991;6:289-97.
37. Battin MP. Euthanasia: The way we do it, the way they do it, *J Pain Sym Man* 1991;6:298-305.
38. Institute of Medical Ethics Working Party on the Ethics of Prolonging Life and Assisting Death. Assisted death, *Lancet* 1990;336:610-13; Klagsbrun SC. Physician-assisted suicide: A double dilemma, *J Pain Sym Man* 1991;6:325-28.
39. Quill, supra note 4.
40. Weir, supra note 10.

Chapter 65

The Range of Euthanasia

David C. Thomasma

The idea of euthanasia is very old.[1] It was recommended by Plato, Aristotle, and Luther, among many others.[2] Nonetheless, active euthanasia is legally proscribed and morally suspect in the United States today, as it is in most countries. The only legal ways of ending life at present are abortion, capital punishment, war, and suicide.[3] The morality of these is still open to question.

The situation will no doubt change over the next several years, as increasing discussion of "mercy killing" lays bare some of the major problems facing its opponents.[4] Indeed, in California, where a referendum permitting physicians to employ active euthanasia to relieve patient suffering was being proposed, 23 percent of 600 physicians polled said they helped at least one person die, and 62 percent approved of a physician doing so; 68 percent were in favor of the referendum itself. Half of those polled said they would assist a patient in dying if it were legal and the request were rational.[5]

In the Netherlands, the Hoge Raad (Supreme Court) declared in a case of active euthanasia that a physician may legally commit homicide at the victim's request, given certain stringent conditions, including a medical emergency.[6,7] Nonetheless, physicians rarely encounter rational patients in intractable pain, with supportive families, making clear directives about euthanasia. Instead, they encounter aging patients who are suffering to one degree or another, who have no family, and who are too confused to give directives. For this reason, Dutch physicians are as reluctant as most of their colleagues in other parts of the world to kill patients.[8]

The problems that are currently creating a growing trend toward considering active euthanasia are as follows:

1. Medical technology itself has created a crisis in dying that older generations could not have foreseen. No one seems to have seen the shadow of protracted dying behind all the promises of longevity. A fundamental question that must be answered is, do we not have an obligation to direct this technology to good human ends?[9]

2. If persons suffer more pain and psychological discomfort as a consequence of the success of past medical interventions (for example, controlling infection in burn patients[10]), do we not have a responsibility to address the results of this success?[11]

Source: Reprinted from the *American College of Surgeons Bulletin*, Vol. 73, No. 8, pp. 4-13, with permission from American College of Surgeons.

As Kenneth Vaux observes:

> If biomedical acts of life extension become acts of death prolongation, we may force some patients to outlive their deaths, and we may ultimately repudiate the primary life-saving and merciful ethic itself.[12]

3. If, from time to time, pain control proves fruitless, does not the quality of mercy and compassion compel us to accede to a patient's heartrending request for active euthanasia?[13]

4. Is there any moral difference between omission and commission, if our motive is to help a patient die? Are we not just splitting hairs by arguing that omission permits the "natural course of the disease" to take the patient's life, while commission actively intervenes to kill the patient?[14] Is the distinction between active and passive euthanasia clearly applicable in clinical practice?[15,16]

5. If, as the courts have now consistently affirmed, patients have a constitutional right to determine their own medical care, could the right to privacy and the common law right of self-determination sustain a right to die?[17] Even so, could this right ever require euthanasia from an unwilling physician?

These questions are addressed in the discussion of the range of euthanasia that is currently taking place in the United States.[18]

Definition of Euthanasia

Euthanasia comes from the Greek for "good" or "merciful" death. It is "the art of painlessly putting to death persons suffering from incurable conditions or diseases."[19] Current usage requires the distinction to be made between active and passive euthanasia, although some prefer a distinction between positive and passive euthanasia.[20,21] Active euthanasia is an intentional act that causes death. Passive euthanasia is an intentional act to avoid prolonging the dying process.[22,23,24] Euthanasia itself can be distinguished from murder on the basis of motive. Murder would be killing someone for reasons other than kindness. But the psychology behind both is very complex.

Both active and passive euthanasia aim at the same end, a merciful death. The difference between active and passive forms of euthanasia cannot be sustained on the basis of motive alone. A merciful motive cannot sustain a homicide, for example. Rather, the difference lies in the nature of the act itself. Active euthanasia brings about a kind death through direct intervention. The act performed directly kills the patient. Passive euthanasia, by contrast, is the withholding or withdrawing of life-prolonging and life-sustaining technologies. Death is brought about by the underlying disease or assault on the body. This disease or assault was initially sufficient to kill the patient, but our modern technology and medical skills arrested that process. Withholding or withdrawing such treatment means that the dying process continues unabated.

In any discussion of euthanasia, therefore, death is not considered to be an enemy. Rather it is considered to be a friend for the patient, whose life itself has now become a burden. Thus, the goal of medicine, usually so clearly articulated as the preservation of life, should now be changed.

Medicine should aim at reconstructing life sufficiently to sustain other values. As Engelhardt notes, "One must remember that one prolongs the length of life so that certain values can be realized, not for the mere prolongation itself."[25] These other values include human relationships, working, recreation, study, and contributing to society. When these human values (as defined by the patient) can no longer be sustained because of the physical condition of the patient, then a decision should be made for euthanasia on the basis of the patient's or surrogate's request. One challenge created by the case presented in the article, "It's Over, Debbie," published in the *Journal of the American Medical Association*, is whether the option for euthanasia should be active or passive.[26,27,28,29]

The deepest challenge, however, arises in a clash of values. On one side is the ancient injunction of the Hippocratic ethics that physicians should help the patient, or at least do no harm. In this ethic, a physician may not actively kill patients.[30,31,32,33] On the other side is the growing sense that real harm in the form of terminal suffering does come to patients as a result of the application of current medical and surgical interventions.[34] As a consequence, guidelines for actively terminating the suffering of such patients have been proposed by such groups as the Hemlock Society, following Dutch physician-inaugurated guidelines.[35]

The following discussion uncovers a wider range of options than is usually considered when one encapsulates the choices into the general categories of active and passive euthanasia.

The Range of Euthanasia

Perhaps the most noteworthy feature of modern medical and surgical practice is the clinical blurring of the distinction between active and passive euthanasia. Sometimes physicians and surgeons get involved in what are called "gray areas" that muddy even further the duties and obligations we have toward dying patients. A sketch of some different forms of euthanasia demonstrates this point. This sketch proceeds from clearly active to clearly passive forms of euthanasia:

1. State-sanctioned killing. Some state-sanctioned killing occurs during war, through capital punishment, or when a person resists arrest for a crime such as armed robbery. These forms of taking the lives of others cannot be called euthanasia, since the victims do not request a kind death. Nazi termination of the lives of others for eugenic or economic reasons fall into this category as well.[36] Another form of state-sanctioned killing, however, may possibly be called euthanasia. Such would be the case for individuals like Charles Walker in Illinois who, condemned to death by the courts for murder, request that the sentence be carried out. Walker objected to a stay of execution on April 19, 1988, as the work of "bleeding hearts who should mind their own business."[37] The process of killing such persons in Texas, Illinois, and other states that use death by lethal injection, looks strangely like a form of active euthanasia. Although the American Medical Association (AMA) has strictly ruled out using physicians to push the buttons to inject such patients, doctors are often called upon to determine death in these cases, and thereby assist at a form of active euthanasia. In such cases, the state might be creating "terminal suffering" of persons like Walker by its institution of capital punishment. If he were a free man, would he request this euthanasia?

2. Cryonics. A number of people have become enamored of cryonics. At the Alcor Life Extension Foundation Laboratory in Riverside, CA, an 83-year old woman, Dora Kent, had her head surgically removed from her body and frozen in the hopes that someday she could be brought back to life with a new body. She was apparently still alive when the procedure was started. Her son is a believer in cryonics, and he supervised the removal of his mother's head. The coroner has classified the death a homicide.[38] If active euthanasia is permitted, and a record

were kept that Mrs. Kent consented to this procedure, would this procedure also be permitted?

3. Killing by family members. More and more frequently, one reads about family members who kill their relatives out of love and compassion. On March 8, 1983, Hans Florian shot his wife, who was suffering from Alzheimer's disease. He did so because he was older than she, and he did not want to leave her alone when he died.[39] The Grand Jury refused to indict him. But Roswell Gilbert, who expressed no remorse over killing his wife of 51 years, Emily, is now convicted of murder. He claims he shot her twice in the head because he had to "terminate her suffering."[40] Some observers think that he was convicted precisely because he did not cry about it on the stand. In England, a 38-year-old mother was put on probation for feeding her brain damaged baby Mandrax (a poison) through the baby's feeding tube.[41] Geraldine Sagel tried to kill her retarded dwarf son whom she had cared for in her home for 51 years; her own failing health made her fear that he would be left at the mercy of the world if she died. Nephews who were distraught about the decline of their uncle in a nursing home shot him with a luger. The motive was to provide him with the relief of death. Presumably this motive was based on the previously expressed wishes of the uncle, or upon his presumed wishes.

"In any discussion of euthanasia, death is not considered to be an enemy. Rather it is considered to be a friend for the patient..."

These cases are a form of active euthanasia, but health care professionals are not involved, unless they passively create the conditions that lead to such impulses.

4. Selective abortion. Many people argue that abortion itself is a form of active euthanasia, because it takes innocent human lives -- without the victim's consent. Selective abortion occurs when, through reproductive technology, more fertilized ova begin to gestate in the womb than a couple intended. The additional tragedy of requesting that two out of four fetuses, for example, be aborted so that the others may properly mature, stems from the fact that the couple, until the time of this request, had had fertility difficulties and wanted children desperately. Some physicians have consented to abort such fetuses for the reasons given.[42]

5. Active injection. Active euthanasia by injection is sometimes practiced, but it is legally proscribed in the United States. Euthanasia by injection takes two forms.

In the first instance, the injection is done to "put someone out of his or her misery." But in this form, the injection is administered without the consent of the patient, or with inadequate consent. Thus, a night-shift nurse, Bobbie Sue Dudley Terrell, received a 65-year sentence for killing four elderly patients through injections and strangulation.[43] No one supports this kind of action. If caught, health care professionals who employ this practice are tried for murder.

In the second form, however, the patient has requested death by injection (or other means) so that he or she may be relieved of pain and suffering. If all other means have been exhausted for improving the condition of the patient, and the pain seems tractable, a number of thinkers and physicians have supported active euthanasia based on the patient's own request and a motive of compassion.[44,45] Indeed, some thinkers also support infanticide, or positive killing of persons who are in an irreversibly unconscious state.[46,47,48] Problems regarding informed consent occur in this situation.[49,50,51]

6. Assisted suicide. Sometimes a kind death can be brought about by assisting patients in taking their own lives. This form of euthanasia walks a narrow line between active and passive. It is not, strictly speaking, active euthanasia, since the physician would not directly administer the agent that kills the patient. However, by providing the agent for the patient, the physician clearly is not practicing passive euthanasia either. Thus, a surgeon, having operated on a patient with melanoma and later caring for the patient during the advanced and terminal stages of the disease, may prescribe sufficient pain control medication to kill the patient, and then say, "If things get too bad, take all of this at once." By doing so, the surgeon demonstrates responsibility for reducing the pain and suffering of the patient but leaves the action to the patient. Many people would argue that such an action is comparable to complicity in murder. Others would view this as a good compromise as compared with actively killing the patient.

"Deferring death does not make a life for most people. Persons have a constitutional right to refuse life-sustaining treatment."

7. Court-ordered removal of life-sustaining treatment. Some physicians and hospitals have argued that a court order prohibiting them from providing fundamental "ordinary means," such as nasogastric feeding tubes, gastrostomies, or even IV fluids and nutrition, is tantamount to requiring them to assist at the suicide of patients. Actually, this is a misnomer. Patients who wish to exercise their right of self-determination or privacy, and to decide whether or not to accept medical interventions, are not by that fact committing suicide; nor are their physicians, by helping them carry out their wishes, assisting at their suicides. The reasons are complex. But central to them is the point that the cause of death is the disease the patient suffers, not the act of commission or omission on the part of the patient or physician. Deferring death does not make a life for most people.[52] Persons have a constitutional right to refuse life-sustaining treatment.[53,54]

8. Organ donation. All organ donation is done to benefit others by surrogate decision-makers. Current standards require that the patient, who can no longer participate in this decision, be brain-dead. Nonetheless, American surgeons participated in a case in which the organs of a Canadian-born anencephalic infant were taken to benefit another infant, after which the respirator on which the anencephalic patient was maintained was turned off. This situation constitutes a form of active euthanasia, since an anencephalic is strictly speaking neither brain-dead nor brain-absent. Surgeons in Loma Linda, CA, also attempted to keep three anencephalic infants alive on respirators for the same purpose.[55] It is difficult to draw a conclusion about this category of euthanasia, since anencephalics may not truly be human persons, lacking as they do sufficient physiological brain structure; therefore, taking their lives may not constitute active euthanasia.

What if persons could state in a Living Will that if they ever become permanently comatose or are in a permanent vegetative state, they would want needed organs and tissues (such as eyes and skin, perhaps) taken from them and that they should then be taken off life-support technology? Can persons donate organs even if they are not subsequently brain-dead?[56] It is not possible to do so under current law, but families have begun to request such an action on behalf of loved ones who are in such a state in a clinical setting as a result of an accident or other tragedy.

9. Double-effect euthanasia. Often physicians are faced with undertaking an intervention that has more than one effect. An example would be the administration of increased doses of morphine to control pain with the knowledge that such massive doses will decrease respiration to the extent that the patient will die. There are even subsets of these cases:

    a. The standard example is increasing the IV morphine dosage to control suffering while simultaneously accepting the second dose-dependent effect, which is not a side-effect, of depressing respiration and killing the patient. Many ethicists hold that this action is good and warranted, because one wills only the first effect (pain control) and not the second (the death of the patient. But others wonder why the motive would make any difference if the result is the same. Why would it be wrong if the physician willed both results? Or, as in *JAMA*'s "Debbie" case, where the physician simply willed the second effect (death of the patient) rather than the first (control of pain)?

    b. These questions are brought home when considering a second subset of the double-effect cases, such as a case in which the surgeon who is responsible for the care of a cardiovascular patient who has suffered a massive stroke and is comatose, agrees to the family's request that the respirator be removed from the patient. It is removed, and the physician administers a large dose of morphine shortly thereafter to ensure that the patient does not suffer agonal gasping during his or her dying moments. Perhaps this goal is mixed with compassion for the family as well, since they might suffer from guilt if they witnessed their loved one gasping for breath while dying. Here the motive is to provide a kind death by removing life-sustaining treatment (again at the patient's request through his surrogates), and the cause of death is the underlying disease process. Even though this cause of death is assisted by the morphine or other pain control medication, it seems that the motive was to reduce suffering and not to directly cause death.

    c. How does this case differ from a similar one in which the surgeon, faced with the same conditions, decides to administer the injection before taking the patient off the respirator? This action would be taken to ensure that agonal gasping would be kept to a minimum. There is no doubt, however, that the injection itself would be a primary cause of death. If one objected to this third instance, but not to the second or first, would that not just be a case of "splitting hairs?" What conceivable difference would it make whether the shot was given before or after the patient was removed from the respirator, since the ultimate goal is to help the patient die a comfortable death?

10. Transferring to die. Physicians sometimes transfer patients as a means of providing passive euthanasia. Their motive is that the patient will die during the transfer. Often this occurs by transferring the patient from intensive care to intermediate or ordinary care wings, or by transferring the patient to a less technologically intensive hospital. Actually, this method is one that restricts access to high technology interventions that would only prolong the dying process. Transferring patients to hospices has an explicit goal of passive euthanasia.

"Physicians sometimes transfer patients as a means of providing passive euthanasia. Their motive is that the patient will die during the transfer."

11. Tragic choices. No one holds physicians responsible for the difficult and tragic choices that are involved in some people's diseases. A young patient with severe abdominal pain may be brought to the emergency room. She is operated on for intestinal blockage, but it is found during surgery that her intestines have died as a result of aortic blockage, something rarely seen at her age. The surgeons can remove all of the intestines, put her on hyper-alimentation for a short time, and permit her to speak with her family before her nutritional status is completely compromised and she dies, or they can sew her up, and never permit her to awaken from anesthesia. Both "arms" of the action lead to death. There is nothing that can be done. Which choice leads to the least harm during the dying process?

12. Withholding and withdrawing. While virtually everyone agrees that withholding or withdrawing extraordinary means during the dying process is a form of passive euthanasia that is acceptable, not everyone agrees about what constitutes extraordinary means. The distinction between ordinary and extraordinary has taken on a normative character not originally intended (ordinary = obligatory; extraordinary = optional).

Instead, ethicists and the courts as well have recently stressed the proportion between the intervention and the outcome.[57] The plan should be to reduce burdens and increase benefits. What should be considered extraordinary is anything that adds to the burden of the patient during the dying process. For this reason, "Do-Not-Resuscitate" orders have become common.[58] More common than thought previously, deaths of renal dialysis patients frequently occur because the dialysis was simply stopped.[59] The AMA statement on withdrawing fluids and nutrition also reflects the ethic of not unduly prolonging dying.[60]

13. Social euthanasia. Over 50 million people in the United States cannot gain access to health care because they are uninsured or underinsured. If we continue each day to ignore this problem, are we not just practicing a form of social euthanasia of the passive sort? By restricting access, we are condemning many persons to death who might otherwise benefit from interventions readily available for those who can pay. But this form of passive euthanasia does not count as euthanasia, since it neglects the wishes of patients. As such it comes dangerously close to the eugenics of euthanasia projects of Nazi Germany and Stalin's Russia, in which millions of people were murdered to achieve flimsy social goals.

Death Induction

From the brief descriptions outlined previously, it is clear that there is a broad range of euthanasia practiced in the United States, some forms of which are more acceptable than others. Independent of the many philosophical, theological, social, and political questions is the physician's moral bind: patients often present complications that require compassionate care that borders on killing, yet the physician is committed to preserving the life of the patient. Is there an alternative to active euthanasia?

Inducing death is an alternative to active euthanasia (direct killing) that may be sufficient in all but the most extreme cases in bringing about a good death. Its chief components would be the following:

1. Death should be seen as a kindness for some dying people.

2. Inducing or bringing about death is a virtuous and moral act, especially if it is done in conjunction with the wishes of the patient.

3. Death induction would accept the explicit goal of active euthanasia: A merciful and painless death for the patient, while using passive means to carry out this goal. Among such means would be withholding and withdrawing of technological care at the patient's request, and not instituting antibiotics or fluids and nutrition.

4. Far greater care would be taken than is often the case today to control pain and suffering -- not just physical pain, but also psychological and social suffering. The double-effect would be used to make a commitment to the patient that he or she need not suffer.

5. When and if active euthanasia is permitted by society, the death induction process could be marketed as an alternative that pays attention to fears and concerns of patients who do not wish "to go quickly into that dark night." Evidence exists that very few dying patients want to be dispatched early.[61]

6. Death induction requires a rethinking of the goal of medicine. Medicine's aim in a technological age should be to preserve life as a conditional value -- that is, a good that permits us to pursue higher values, such as love, work, contributions to society, travel, friendship, and the like. When patients themselves, or their surrogates, inform us that their lives no longer have these meanings, it is a cruelty to prolong their lives at all costs while ignoring their statements. The values such patients articulate should be part of the therapeutic plan.

When these values can no longer be achieved, preserving life loses its importance in the therapeutic plan. In the place of preserving life, under these conditions, is the act of bringing about a kind death, death induction.

The increased debate about active euthanasia in our society should be welcomed. It will force the medical profession, ethicists, the legal system, and organized religion to provide better responses to the questions posed at the beginning of this article.

At this time, there is little need for active euthanasia if more attention is paid to controlling pain and suffering, more attention is paid to the patient's value system, much firmer responses are made to patient requests to die, and plans are made with the patient and family about the best way to bring about a kind and merciful death. These are all big "ifs." When I was on a Senior Fulbright Research Fellowship, I surveyed Dutch physicians who independently and unanimously indicated to me the need for far greater attention to the psychological aspects of caring for the dying patient.

Perhaps the greatest argument in favor of active euthanasia is that it is not a form of taking an innocent human life, which is murder, but it is a loving response to an individual's wishes. After all, what possible meaning can a life of suffering and intractable pain have? Especially if that suffering will not go away, but only increase? It is a loving response to our technological patina of care, a patina that brings about increased survival, but sometimes a lower quality of life. Thus, active euthanasia is a way of taking responsibility for our technology, by assuring people who are its subjects that they will not be crucified on a cross of steel operating tables, shunts, and tubes.

The death induction suggestion recognizes this responsibility, but avoids directly killing the patient. This recognition is important, because opponents of active euthanasia, in rejecting the action, appear to be insensitive to patient suffering.

Nonetheless, physicians should not directly take the lives of their patients, although they should help them in the many other ways discussed previously in this article. The reason I object to physicians killing their patients goes beyond professional codes and legal restraints. In all other forms of sanctioned (as opposed to violent and emotional) killing, the person to be killed is made into an enemy or, as in capital punishment, is said to have lost his or her "innocence." Even then, training people like soldiers and executioners to kill takes real work. When soldiers come upon one another as persons rather than as enemies (for example, finding a young "enemy" eating K-rations in a foxhole), they have tremendous difficulty killing each other. Even injecting convicted criminals requires a great deal of impersonality -- one pushes a number of buttons in a box alongside another person, in a room hidden behind the victim. One does not see the convict at all.[62]

A physician who is contemplating active euthanasia is faced with a patient who is not an "enemy" or a "criminal," but a friend who has trusted the physician.

If it is difficult to kill enemies and criminals, how much more difficult is it to kill someone who has trusted in you? There is no social construct available for this action. My own research suggests that physicians who have actively euthanized patients have found it repulsive in just this sense. This opinion was confirmed in an interview with Dr. Borst-Eilers of the Netherlands, who said, "The few doctors I know who have done euthanasia tell me they were miserable for months afterwards. Our doctors are not going to go around killing too easily."[63] Yet, as Weinfeld notes, the meaning of euthanasia is:

> Someone wishing to kill you normally is your enemy; anyone preventing it is your friend. However, there are situations when the opposite is true: he who wishes to kill you is your most precious friend, and anyone preventing it is your worst enemy.[64]

Conclusion

Discussion of active euthanasia should continue. Problems do exist in prolonging suffering.[65,66] These problems must be thoroughly discussed by our professional health care societies and by society at large.[67]

If patients do request active euthanasia, the physician is put on the spot. He or she must make some response to patient needs. The discussion should move beyond proposed guidelines to protect patient wishes, however, to a discussion of professional and social consequences. As Doctors Gaylin, Kass, Pellegrino, and Siegler say, "If physicians become killers or are merely licensed to kill, the profession -- and, therewith, each physician -- will never again be worthy of trust and respect as healer and comforter and protector of life in all its frailty."[68] An additional concern is that in Nazi Germany, physicians began taking lives and were not prosecuted for it.[69] Soon active euthanasia was legalized in medical and nursing facilities.[70] Will the same actions in Dutch and other western societies lead to the same eventuality?[71]

"Patients seem to support active euthanasia by their physicians more than physicians themselves do."

Yet patients seem to support active euthanasia by their physicians more than physicians themselves do, perhaps countervailing the concerns about patients being able to continue trusting physicians.[72,73,74,75] A recent Roper Poll found that 62 percent of Americans support doctors who allow patients to die; the topic of active euthanasia, however, was not addressed as a separate question.[76] There is a real concern, as expressed by Robert Baker, that if physicians do not respond to suffering patients, and instead leave them "howling like dogs," society should not entrust them with the power of mercy killing, because the physicians would have lost all sensitivity to the very meaning of mercy.[77] Offering an alternative like death induction may satisfy physicians and patients alike.

Notes

1. Pounder DJ, Prokopec M, Pretty GL. A probable case of euthanasia amongst prehistoric aborigines at Roonka, South Australia, *Forensic Sci Int* 1983;23:99-108.
2. Weinfeld J. Active voluntary euthanasia -- should it be legalized? *Med Law* 1985;4:101-111.
3. Maguire D. Death: Legal and illegal, *Atlantic Monthly* 1974;233:72-85.
4. Clarke D. Euthanasia and the law, In: Monagle J, Thomasma D, eds. *Medical Ethics: A Guide for Health Professionals*. Rockville, MD: Aspen Publishers, 1988;217-233.
5. Beck J. Californians may be invited to vote on a right to die. *Chicago Trib* 1988, Apr 21; Sec. 1:23.
6. Hoge Raad (Supreme Court), 27 Nov. 1984, Nederlandse Jurisprudentie 1985, No. 106.
7. Scholten HJ. Justification of active euthanasia, *Med Law* 1986;5:169-172.
8. Pence G. Do not go slowly into that dark night: Mercy killing in Holland, *Am J Med* 1988;84:139-141.
9. Van J. `Debbie' case helps euthanasia cause. *Chicago Trib* 1988, Mar 28;Sec. 1:4.
10. Pondelicek I, Koenigova R. The problem of euthanasia and dysthanasia in burns, *Burns Incl Therm Inj* 1983;10:61-63.
11. Kuhse H. The case for active voluntary euthanasia, *Law, Med, Health Care* 1986;14:145-148.
12. Vaux KL. Debbie's dying: Mercy killing and the good death, *JAMA* 1988;259:2140-2141.
13. Clark CB. *Letters, JAMA* 1988;259:2095.
14. Fletcher J. Medical resistance to the right to die, *J Am Geriatr Soc* 1987;35:679-682.
15. Montague P. The mortality of active and passive euthanasia, *Ethics Sci Med* 1978;5:39-45.
16. Rachels J. Active and passive euthanasia, *N Engl J Med* 1975;292:78-80.
17. Wolhandler S. Voluntary active euthanasia for the terrainally ill and the constitutional right to privacy, *Cornell Law Review* 1984;69:363-383.
18. Lundberg G. Editorial: `It's Over, Debbie' and the euthanasia debate, *JAMA* 1988;259:2141-2143.
19. Gillon R. Acts and omissions. Killing and letting die, *Brit Med J* 1986;292:126-127.
20. Gert B, Culver CM. Distinguishing between active and passive euthanasia, *Clin Geriatr Med* 1986;2:29-36.
21. O'Rourke KD. Active and passive euthanasia: The ethical distinctions, *Hosp Prog* (now *Health Progress*) 1976;57:68-73,100.
22. Rachels J. Killing and starving to death, *Philosophy* 1979;54:159-171.
23. Rachels J. Euthanasia, killing and letting die, In: Ladd J, ed. *Ethical Issues Relating to Life and Death*. New York, NY: Oxford University Press, 1979;146-163.
24. Foot P. Euthanasia, *Philosophy and Public Affairs* 1977;6:85-112.
25. Engelhardt HT Jr. The counsels of finitude. Death inside out, *Hastings Cent Rep* 1974;4:119.
26. Anonymous. It's Over, Debbie, *JAMA* 1988;259:272.
27. Krauthammer C. The `death' of 'Debbie'. *Washington Post* 1988, Feb 26.
28. Cohn V. Tales of two dying patients: In one case, the end was painful; in another, drugs eased the way, *Washington Post Health* 1988, Mar 1:15.
29. Bernadin Cardinal J. Action in `Debbie' case was immoral. *Chicago Trib* 1988, Mar 10;Sec. 1:20.
30. Barry R. Killer-doctor. *Chicago Trib* 1988, Feb 14;Sec. C:2.
31. Van J. `It's Over, Debbie' and a doctor takes a life. *Chicago Trib* 1988, Jan 31;Sec. 1:1.
32. Wilkerson I. Essay on mercy killing reflects conflict on ethics for physicians and journalists. *New York Times* 1988, Feb 23;Sec. A:26,1.
33. Siegler M. The AMA euthanasia fiasco. *New York Times* 1988, Feb 26;Sec. A:35,1.
34. Woozley A. Euthanasia and the principle of harm, In: Self DJ, ed. *Philosophy and Public Policy*. Norfolk, VA: Teagle and Little, 1977:93-100.
35. Shaw DC. When patients should be helped to die. *Chicago Trib* 1988, Feb 20;Sec. 1:9.

36. Lifton R. *The Nazi Doctors: Medical Killing and the Psychology of Genocide*. New York, NY: Basic Books, 1986.
37. Judge stays execution of Walker. *Chicago Trib* 1988, Apr 20;Sec. 2:1.
38. Attempt at cryonics is called a homicide. *Chicago Trib* 1988, Feb 25;Sec. 1:4.
39. Will G. When is killing not a crime? *Washington Post* 1983, Apr 14;Sec. A:23.
40. Man convicted of killing wife who begged to die. *New York Times* 1985, May 10;Sec. A:16.
41. Legal Correspondent. Mercy killing and the law, *Brit Med J* 1976;1333-1334.
42. Kolata G. New dilemma: Selective abortion. *Chicago Trib* 1988, Jan 26;Sec. 1:10.
43. Nurse gets 65-year sentence for killing 4 elderly patients. *Chicago Trib* 1988, Feb 25;Sec. I:4.
44. Clark WR. The example of Christ and voluntary active euthanasia, *J Religion Health* 1986;25:264-277.
45. Kuhse H. `Letting die' is not in the patient's best interests: A case for active euthanasia, *Med J Australia* 1985;142:610-613.
46. Rachels J. Active euthanasia with parental consent: Commentary, *Hastings Cent Rep* 1979;9:19-20.
47. Kuhse H. Death by non-feeding: Not in the baby's best interests, *J Med Humanities Bioethics* 1986;7:79-90.
48. Strong C. Positive killing and the irreversibly unconscious patient, *Bioethics Quarterly* 1981;3:190-205.
49. Shepperdson B. Abortion and euthanasia of Down's syndrome children -- the parent's view, *J Med Ethics* 1983;9:152-157.
50. Fletcher J. Abortion, euthanasia, and care of defective newborns, *N Engl J Med* 1975;292:75-78.
51. Lauter H, Meyer JE. Mercy killing without consent. Historical comments on a controversial issue, *Acta Psychiatr Scand* 1982;65:134-141.
52. Quindlen A. Deferring death does not make a life. *Chicago Trib* 1987, Oct 23;Sec. 5:1.
53. Gustaitis R. Right to refuse life-sustaining treatment, *Pediatrics* 1988;81:317-321.
54. Emanuel E. A review of the ethical and legal aspects of terminating medical care, *Am J Med* 1988;84:291-301.
55. Doomed fetus to be organ donor. *Chicago Trib* 1987, Dec 9;Sec. 1:11.
56. Thomasma D. Making treatment decisions for permanently unconscious patients: The ethical perspective, In: Monagle J, Thomasma D, eds. *Medical Ethics: A Guide for Health Professionals*. Rockville, MD: Aspen Publishers, 1988;192-204.
57. Ruark J, Raffin T, and the Stanford University Medical Center Committee on Ethics. Initiating and withdrawing life support, *N Engl J Med* 1988;318:25-30.
58. Zimmerman JE, Knaus WA, Sharpe SM, *et al*. The use and implications of Do-Not-Resuscitate orders in intensive care units, *JAMA* 1986;255:351-360.
59. Neu S, Kjellstrand CM. Stopping long-term dialysis, *N Engl J Med* 1986;314:14-19.
60. O'Rourke K. The AMA statement on tube feeding: An ethical analysis, *America* 1986;321-324.
61. Kotulak R. Study of terminally ill shows most in no hurry. *Chicago Trib* 1986 Feb 9;Sec. 6:5.
62. Gonzales L. The executioners, *Chicago* 1988;37:91-95, 180-185.
63. Otten A. Fateful decision: In the Netherlands, the very ill have option of euthanasia. *Wall Street J* 1987, Aug 21;Sec. 1:1-6.
64. Weinfeld J. Active voluntary euthanasia -- Should it be legalized? *Medicine and Law* 1985;4:101-11.
65. Davis D. Letters, *JAMA* 1988;259:2097.
66. Wilson S. Letters, *JAMA* 1988;259:2097.
67. Thomasma D. Letters, *JAMA* 1988;259:2098.
68. Gaylin W, Kass L, Pellegrino E, Siegler M. Commentaries: Doctors must not kill, *JAMA* 1988;259:2139-2140.
69. Boozer J. Children of Hippocrates: Doctors in Nazi Germany, *Ann Acad Political Social Sci* 1980;450:83-97.
70. Aly G, Roth KH. The legalization of mercy killings in medical and nursing institutions in Nazi Germany from 1938 until 1941: A Commented documentation, *Int J Law Psychiatry* 1984;7:145-163.
71. Barry R. Killer-doctor. *Chicago Trib* 1988, Feb 14;Sec. C:2.
72. Lundberg G. Editorial: `It's Over, Debbie' and the euthanasia debate, *JAMA* 1988;259:2141-2143.

73. Vaux K. If we can bar the door to death, can't we also open it? *Chicago Trib* 1988, Feb 10;Sec. C:23.
74. Shaw D. When patients should be helped to die. *Chicago Trib* 1988, Feb 20;Sec. 1:9.
75. Cantwell R. Dignity in death. Letter. *Chicago Trib* 1988, Apr 21;Sec. 1:22.
76. Euthanasia gains favor. *Chicago Trib* 1986, Jul 17;Sec. 5:2.
77. Baker R. On euthanasia, In: Humbet JM, Almeder RF, eds. *Biomedical Ethics Reviews*. Clifton, NJ: Humana Press, 1983;5-28.

SECTION 9

INSTITUTIONAL ISSUES

Chapter 66

Cases 9.0

Case 9.1: **JOINT VENTURE**

Your hospital is part of a nine-hospital health care system devoted largely to caring for the poor in the inner city. Recently the corporation has been asked to take over another inner city hospital that has been vigorous in providing abortions, sterilizations, and birth-control advice to teenagers, as well as safe-sex advice to the many drug-addicts and homosexuals in the area.

Your corporation is among the 75% of American hospitals that refuse to do abortions, and many of your board members are opposed to the other practices of this inner city hospital. Among them have been rather vicious "throat-cutting" efforts to woo patients away from your more conservatively managed corporate hospitals.

You are aware of current studies that show that not-for-profit hospitals are almost indistinguishable from for-profit because of such joint ventures. A large share of the income from the inner city hospital is in providing the services now in question. If you object to them, what would you do as the chief-of-staff and board member of one of the hospitals in the system?

Case 9.2: **DRUMMING UP ANGIOPLASTIES**

The Chairman of Medicine at a regional medical center in a large midwestern metropolis was recently surprised by a letter he received from a cardiac catherization specialist.

The letter made the following offer:

> As a cardiologist catherization specialist I will offer to train other cardiologists who have not been trained in angioplasty if they will:
>
> 1. Send 75 patients to me.
>
> 2. I will bill them for the procedure.
>
> 3. I will train them on their own patients.
>
> 4. After they do 75 of them, I will give them angioplasty privileges in my practice.

What stunned the Chairman was that this was in effect:

1. A preceptorship based on referral.

2. There was no provision for informed consent for the patients.

3. There was no application/credentialling through a regular department's training program.

4. It seemed like "using" one's patients to gain a skill.

5. The evaluation would be done by a doctor who would be receiving a payment. Lack of objectivity.

Yet, when he thought about it, it seemed that medical education itself involved a lot a experimenting on patients. Patients are not often told that in a medical school, they will be used to train the future physicians. Patients are sometimes billed by the attending when he or she was out of town, and residents performed the procedure.

What should be his response to this letter?

Case 9.3: DOLLARS AND DRUG COMPANIES

In 1987, the American Surgical Association resolved that:

> It is unethical for a surgeon to accept remuneration or material reward for participating in advertising or other product promotional activity of a health care related product with no relationship to professional service rendered by the surgeon. Remuneration or material reward is meant to imply money, gifts, gratuities such as vacation, travel, or other emoluments. Acceptable professional services rendered include legitimate consultations services, legal testimony of qualified specialty consultants, institutionally approved product testing, evaluation, development, experimental and clinical research. Giving papers or lectures at the behest of the health care related industry for the primary purpose of promoting the pharmaceutical or appliance or any other health care supply item is not an acceptable professional service warranting remuneration.

Given the subtleties of defining a relationship between a corporation primarily involved in pharmaceutical manufacture, and a practicing ophthalmologist, what are the ethical issues to be addressed in deciding the following situations that have presented themselves over the last 6 months in the Department of Ophthalmology at the Regional Medical Center? Bear in mind that in 1993, drug corporations spent on average $5,500 per physician in the United States in an effort to influence each physician's clinical decision.

1. A member of the Department is contacted by Firm A to present one evening lecture at a "meeting" organized by the company to foster "good relations" among practitioners in the area. The meeting includes a fly fishing expedition down the beautiful Snake River in Idaho.

2. A member of the Department is contacted by a pharmaceutical industry representative who extends an invitation to attend a four-day conference at the Ritz-Carlton, Laguna Niguel, in order to participate in a "function" and a "seminar" presented by leading authorities in the field. The invitation is also extended to the wife or significant other, and includes an offer to reimburse for all expenses for both parties.

3. Firm B contacts the Department hoping to establish a "special relationship" with the department. The "special relationship" entails the Department's obtaining at minimal cost items of manufacture currently produced and marketed by the company. The

reciprocity of the relationship suggests that the corporation will market their "special" relationship with the Department to enhance their public relations, and add credence to professional acceptance of their manufactured devices.

4. The Department considers organizing and sponsoring a post-graduate course on "recent advances in optic nerve disorders treatments." It is anticipated that the course expenses will exceed the tuition generated. Suggestions are raised by the faculty to contact "related" corporations to "sponsor the program and help offset expected losses."

Used with the permission of B. Katz, M.D.

Case 9.4: LASER SURGERY

The most commonly performed elective surgery in the United States is Gallbladder Surgery. Medical equipment manufacturers have seen the profitability in providing new devices for this, as well as other surgeries.

In the past, removal of the gallbladder was a major operation, necessitating many days hospitalization and home recovery, before returning to work. Some people who had the surgery found that it took them almost 6 months before they really felt "normal" again. With the introduction of laparoscopy, by which surgeons insert a tube into the abdomen and, using television cameras, lights, and cutters through such tubes, root out the offending organ, patients face the possibility of returning home from surgery on the same day, and returning to work much earlier than before. Patients' hospital costs could be dramatically lower than with full-fledged surgery.

No controversy there.

But as patients insisted on laparoscopy, surgeons flocked to learn how to perform this surgery. The problems of the medical-industrial complex, targeted by the editor of *The New England Journal of Medicine* some years ago, began to emerge. By 1994, 80% of all gallbladder surgery will be done using this new procedure. Thus, as the demand for laparoscopy increased, so did the demand for new products.

To delicately remove the gallbladder from the liver, and stop the resultant bleeding, the surgeon can use either an inexpensive electrocauterizer, or an extremely expensive laser. But surgeons who were trained in the new surgery did not know this. Many, taking the courses in laparoscopy, were unaware that these courses were supported by laser companies. In almost all training courses, supported or not by laser companies, the cutting and coagulating was done by lasers. This left the impression that using lasers was the only correct way to perform a laparoscopy.

The problem is that electrocautery equipment costs from $10,000 to $30,000, while laser equipment costs about $200,000 with a $50,000 annual maintenance bill attached. Companies promoting their laser surgery products saw their stock prices soar during the popularity of their products. One company enjoyed a $31.50 stock price until the AMA announced that it saw no advantage in using lasers over the 70-year-old electrocautery process. Then the price dropped to $8.50. The bloom is off the sales of lasers. But while it lasted, the companies were, in the words of Dr. Randolph Seed, "promoting a very expensive device with no patient advantage."[1]

Should patients and/or third party payers pay for the more expensive laser technology when it provides no demonstrated benefit over more traditional cauterizing methods? Should a cost-benefit analysis be applied to all forms of medical technology when other interventions also exist that are equally or nearly equally effective? If health care is to be rationed on the basis of cost, will newer technologies suffer under such an analysis? How can physicians protect themselves and their patients from the sales promotions of new devices? Do not companies have a right to promote their products any way they wish?

Case 9.5: **THE ELDERLY ICU PATIENT**

WP was 103-year-old woman who had been living independently with minimal assistance from her 80-year-old daughter, her closest relative. She enjoyed the company of younger friends who would drop by each day. No home care nursing was needed.

She was admitted with an acute myocardial infarction, and sent to the coronary care unit. Her course was complicated by heart failure and a drop in blood pressure, requiring intubation, ventilator assistance, Foley Catheterization, and multiple intravenous medications. During the course of these complications, the patient became comatose and developed an infective pneumonia requiring antibiotics.

The prognosis is extremely grim, especially for a woman of this advanced age, though she certainly is judged to be a survivor. The conservative estimate of the cost of this patient's care to date has been $184,000. Given the prognosis is it justified to go on? Some questions that bother the staff and the administration of the hospital are:

1. Should the next infection be treated? If not, on what basis would the treatment be withheld? Is this a kind of discrimination against the elderly or the vulnerable?

2. Should this patient should be in intensive care unit, where the rule of the nursing and physician staff is that cardiopulmonary resuscitation will be carried out? The unit will not accept "no code."

3. This patient did not give advance declaration of intent or desire, nor did she assign durable power for health care. Is her 80-year-old daughter empowered to ask the physicians to continue or discontinue therapy?

4. In view of limited health care resources, is this patient's care appropriate? If not, is it ever appropriate to make rationing and allocation decisions at the bedside?

Used with permission of the University of California, Davis Medical Center

---

Case 9.6: **THE TESTS**

A 65-year-old white male presented to the hospital with a 20 pound weight loss over several months, pain in his mid-left abdomen extending to the left flank, a slight fever, and significant weakness. The patient denied any cough or hemoptysis. He denied any change in bowel frequency or caliber or any blood in the stool. He denied any change in urinary habits or any hematuria. He denied any family history of cancer.

Physical examination revealed an emaciated male who appeared somewhat dehydrated and very weak. However, vital signs were within normal limits. Head and neck, heart, and lung exams were normal. The abdominal exam revealed tenderness on palpation of the left abdomen and flank, however, no mass was felt. Muscle strength was markedly diminished. Stool was guaiac negative.

A CT scan of the abdomen was performed which revealed a retroperitoneal mass in the left abdomen, judged to be either renal or adrenal in origin. An ultrasound showed the flank mass to be solid and also demonstrated numerous scattered ectogenic areas distorting the normal liver architecture. These were interpreted as most likely representing tumor metastases. Next, a CT guided biopsy of the left abdominal mass demonstrated poorly differentiated, spindle-shaped cells and also granular cells with large, irregular nuclei, as well as areas of necrosis. Pathology concluded that these indeed represented malignant cells but could not be certain of their histological origin.

The patient's clinical condition continued to worsen. A laparascopic exam of the abdomen was performed which showed the liver surface to contain extensive areas of tumor growth. Upon biopsy of the liver, similar malignant cells were found supporting the likelihood that these were extensive metastases to the liver from the flank mass.

Pathology next proceeded to perform a long battery of expensive immunohistochemical tests on these specimens obtained during the biopsies to determine the exact origin of the malignant neoplasm. Special stains costing about $120 each, according to the pathologist, were performed on the specimens. Some of the stains used in the test battery were kappa and lambda light chains, cytokeratin, vimentin, leucocytic common antigen, CEA, and PSA, etc. This is where the clinical dilemma arises.

Several of the clinicians at a tumor board conference regarding this patient thought that, in view of known facts in the case, since it was already established that this patient had a widely metastatic malignancy and was deteriorating quickly, these expensive immunohistochemical tests were a form of overkill and a waste of money. These clinicians believed that identifying the exact origin of the tumor in this particular case would not benefit the patient or change the treatment plan, which would be mainly palliative regardless of the test results. Others believed that physicians had an obligation to the patient and his family to provide an accurate diagnosis. Still others cited academic reasons for the tests.

The patient's clinical condition deteriorated quickly and he died two weeks later. Which group of physicians were right about the testing? Why?

Submitted by Michael L. Glavin, M.D.

Case 9.7: **HMO'S AND BONE MARROW TRANSPLANTS**

In 1991, Nelene Fox was diagnosed with breast cancer; it had already metastasized to her bone marrow. Mrs. Fox was 38-years-old and the mother of three young daughters. She was covered for medical care under her husband's health insurance policy with Health Net, California's second largest HMO.

Mrs. Fox was determined to be a suitable candidate for a bone marrow transplant, combined with high dose chemotherapy, by her Health Net physician and the Norris Cancer Hospital at the University of South California (a Health Net approved provider).

Although bone marrow transplants are now used routinely in the treatment of some blood related cancers such as leukemia, the procedure has only recently been utilized in treating breast cancer. Clinical trials to examine the efficacy of bone marrow transplant have been implemented by the National Cancer Institute. Nevertheless, some physicians have begun to offer the procedure to patients. Many insurers refuse to cover bone marrow transplantation for breast cancer because they regard it as "experimental" therapy. Some insurers will provide coverage only for patients enrolled in the clinical trials.

Health Net denied coverage for Mrs. Fox, claiming that the procedure was investigational. Mrs. Fox's brother, an attorney, appealed the denial. Health Net agreed to cover the transplant if Mrs. Fox sought a second opinion at the City of Hope Hospital, another Health Net Provider.

Mrs. Fox's family filed suit against Health Net, alleging that Health Net originally approved the procedure, leading them to believe that the procedure would be covered. The suit contended that Health Net knew one of their physicians had already contacted City of Hope Hospital concerning the procedure and that City of Hope had refused to accept her as a patient. Additionally, the suit claimed that the delay caused by having her case reviewed by City of Hope would result in Mrs. Fox's inability to have the procedure done at the Norris Cancer Hospital because of her physical deterioration.

Since they were denied coverage, Mrs. Fox and her family raised $212,000 through public appeals; the drugs required for the bone marrow transplantation were donated. Following the procedure, Mrs. Fox went into remission for a short time, but died in April of 1992, eight months following the procedure.

The suit filed by the Fox family claimed damages for breach of contract, breach of covenant of good faith and fair dealing, intentional infliction of emotional distress and negligent infliction of emotional distress. Additionally, the family claimed financial incentives were created by Health Net for its reviewers in order to encourage them to deny coverage for expensive procedures.

The trial lasted nearly one month. The investigational nature of the bone marrow transplant was not an important issue in the case. The jury found that Health Net had been "reckless" in their denial of coverage and that they had breached the covenant of good faith and fair dealing, causing Mrs. Fox emotional distress. Health Net was ordered to pay $212,000 in medical expenses and the family $12.1 million in compensatory damages and $77 million in punitive damages.

Consider the Following Questions:

1. When a physician works for an HMO, what are his or her obligations to the patients? to the HMO?

2. How do issues related to cost containment and health care rationing affect deliberations concerning medical interventions?

3. Is it right for HMO's to deny coverage for expensive or investigational procedures such as bone marrow transplantation for breast cancer?

4. What kinds of health care reform would you encourage to insure quality care and cost containment? What factors would you consider in your deliberations?

Case 9.8: PRIMARY CARE ENTREPRENEURSHIP

Home health care is the future of modern medicine. As our health care institutions change, they are guided by a complex of values, among them the task of providing cost-conscious but high quality care. Thus, among other values, health care reform demands less expensive, preventive health care. Most medical schools are frantically revising their curricula to reflect an emphasis on primary care. Many regulations, legal rules, and moral arguments are in place regarding secondary and tertiary care issues, but little attention has been paid to moral pitfalls in primary care.

Many private health care providers do not accept Medicare and Medicaid reimbursement, since, on average, such payments fall about 30 to 40 percent short of costs. Caremark International, Inc., unlike such private providers, had a policy of accepting Medicare and Medicaid patients. According to the company, this policy led to an unwelcome three-year investigation by the Justice Department and the Office of the Inspector General of the Department of Health and Human Services. This investigation led to an August, 1994 indictment of Caremark for alleged physician kickbacks. Although the bad publicity about this indictment has hurt sales, the company will take in twice as much money, about 2.8 billion dollars, this year than it did last year.[2]

Caremark makes and distributes home-infusion devices. Transfer of patients from hospitals to their homes with Intravenous therapy is a major cost-saving and patient-oriented technology.

A doctor in Columbus, Ohio was charged with accepting $134,000 in illegal payments for referring Medicaid and Medicare patients to a home-infusion company not officially identified, but informally revealed to be Caremark. According to the government, the "incentives" to the doctor paid by the company were actually a form of kickbacks for referring patients to their home infusion system.

On the negative side, the company is moving toward becoming a comprehensive managed care provider. It already manages three large doctor's groups, a prescription benefit management business, and physical and renal therapy services. There is a lot of opportunity for abuse, since these are $1 billion to $300 million businesses. For example, three middle managers of the company, and the company itself, were indicted in August of 1994 by a federal grand jury on charges of paying kickbacks to induce a doctor to prescribe Genentec Inc.'s synthetic growth hormone Protropin for Medicaid and Medicare patients. Caremark is the main distributor of this product.[3]

In addition to Caremark's reputed transgressions, the rise of "medical fraud" has prompted recent headlines such as "Goodbye Dr. Kildare."[4] A psychiatric hospital chain paid $380 million to federal and state law enforcement agents (in 28 states) to refer arrested individuals to their hospitals, causing millions in unnecessary care. A Georgia doctor referred an old and frail cancer patient across town for radiation therapy to a facility the doctor partially owned, rather than to one two blocks from her house. And Medicaid fraud is rampant.

On the positive side, the company's view is that doctors should be involved in monitoring home infusion services. Were they provided in hospital, they would be far more expensive and doctors would get reimbursed by Medicare and Medicaid. The company feels angry that they accept Medicare and Medicaid patients, like their pioneering efforts to treat AIDS patients at home, and in so doing, they make "substantially less money" than other companies that do not accept such patients. They argue that they are justified in paying physicians to monitor the fluids and/or antibiotic therapies. In its view, "physicians should be compensated for their involvement in overseeing these patients."[5]

Because their image has been tarnished by their association with physicians in this way, the company recently announced that it will be stricter than a new law that went into effect in January, 1994. That law forbids physicians from referring Medicaid and Medicare patients to any company in which the doctor has a financial interest. The law was spearheaded by Fourtney P. Stark (D-Calif.), and was designed to stop the documented expense of physician self-referral. The company will extend the law to referrals of *all* patients, not just those covered by government insurance. Thus, it will discontinue its practice of paying doctors to "quarterback" the care provided by the company to patients at home. Insurance companies and big corporations have already refused to pay doctors for work done in monitoring patients at home.

In analyzing this case, assume one or the other of the following positions:

1. The physician in charge of Caremark's development policies.

2. A home health patient in need of services.

3. A local primary care physician who does not subscribe to Caremark's services or to its policies, and has lost patient care revenue as a result.

Consider, too, the following questions that arise from this case:

1. Should doctors be able to accept money for referrals, especially if this entails saving money from in hospital care?

2. Why physicians cannot be reimbursed for home monitoring of their patients?

3. How can the "unholy alliance" of busines and medicine be more carefully watched?

4. How is professional ethics affected by entrepreneurism in medicine?

5. How does primary care entrepreneurism differ, if at all, from casting about for patients to receive a second or third organ transplant, or soliciting angioplasties for surgical residents, or holding a Christmas or Hannukah party for primary care physicians who refer patients for specialists, or many other referral practices in use today?

6. How is the physician-patient relationship affected by entrepreneurism?

7. What impact do you think present legislation and Caremark's policy might have on the future of what is called the medical-industrial complex?

Notes

1. Morris S. Laser debate cuts into industry sales: Costs weighed of gallbladder removal. *The Chicago Tribune* 1991 Aug 18:Sec.7:3.
2. Morris S. Caremark feels probe effect; growth goes on. *Chicago Tribune* 1994 Sept. 22; Sec 3;1-2.
3. Morris S. Caremark changes its policy on referrals. *Chicago Tribune* 1994 Sep. 26;Sec 3:1.
4. Yates RE, Ryan N. Goodbye Dr. Kildare. *Chicago Tribune* 1994 Oct. 2;Sec 7:1,6.
5. Ibid:2.

Chapter 67

Doctors, Drug Companies, and Gifts

Mary-Margaret Chren, C. Seth Landefeld, and Thomas H. Murray

As usual, many doctors who traveled to the annual American Academy of Dermatology meeting last December enjoyed accommodations, dinners, and entertainment paid for by drug companies. The personal delivery of a $156 check to each senior resident in one training program shortly before the meeting (presumably to cover transportation costs) startled us, however. After the requisite sales pitch for a new anti-acne preparation, we asked the salesman who presented the gift and why his company would give cash to a doctor. The reply was, "Because, doctor, we want you to know that we are thinking of you."

Physicians need to ask, "Are we thinking of our patients?"

Drug companies have made outstanding contributions to modern scientific medicine, such as fostering the development of ß-blockers and other new classes of drugs. Drug companies also provide different sorts of contributions to individual doctors and their organizations, i.e., gifts.

Although this apparently innocuous practice is generally accepted as the norm, we and others[1,2,3,4,5,6,7,8,9] have felt uneasy about its ethical repercussions. Most physicians would agree that direct reimbursement for prescribing a medicine is wrong, as is receiving a free airline ticket for writing a certain number of prescriptions.[1] Are there also ethical repercussions in the less obvious situations that face most of us daily? What about the lunches and dinners hosted by friendly detail people? What about the household objects, tickets to entertainment, even cash that is given "without obligation?" Further, what about the educational endeavors -- the textbooks, journals, research grants, and symposia?

The ethical issues here are complex, and clearly the temptation is to avoid making ethical distinctions because they are hard to make.[2] This article provides a basis for making reasonable ethical judgments about gifts: we describe the phenomenon of gift-giving, consider the ethical implications for physicians, and discuss the need for guidelines for ethical behavior. We propose that the ethical issues may be clarified by recognizing that whenever a physician accepts a gift from a drug company, an implicit relationship is established between the physician and the company or its representative. Inherent in the relationship is an obligation to respond to the gift; this obligation may influence the physician's decisions with regard to patient care or possibly even erode the physician's character.

Contractual and other explicit arrangements between drug companies and doctors raise related but different issues, which we will not address herein. Also, we distinguish the phenomenon of gift-giving from situations that involve more explicit conflicts of interest that arise in the practice of or research in medicine, which have been discussed at length elsewhere.[10,11,12,13]

Source: Reprinted from *The Journal of the American Medical Association*, Vol. 262, No. 24, pp. 3448-3451, with permission from The American Medical Association © Dec. 1989.

The Phenomenon of Gift-Giving

Gift-giving in medicine has moved far beyond the presentation of a notepad or pen embellished by a simple advertisement. Annual specialty society meetings afford ample examples. During the day, long lines form at booths of companies with especially desirable gifts. We counted more than 50 people queued up to receive lip gloss and chic canvas beach bags on "physicians' day" at the Bain de Soleil counter at an American Academy of Dermatology meeting. While more than one person in line confessed to feeling uneasy, the pervasive feeling was that refusing gifts would be stupid, not moral. Indeed, when asked whether they felt there was an ethical conflict in accepting gifts from drug companies, our colleagues all responded, "No, I cannot be bought -- or influenced -- by mere gifts." The sometimes stated corollary was, "If you are concerned that you could be influenced, that's your problem."

The lavish marketing of drugs is not limited to the carnival atmosphere of national meetings, however, and others have lamented what they feel is a ubiquitous attempt to seduce physicians.[1-9] Favors from drug companies -- textbooks, journals, meals, and other gifts that range from travel alarm clocks to travel -- are omnipresent in the daily lives of practicing physicians and residents. Many companies also "give" educational events, often controlling the choice of topic, speaker, and attendance list.[2,14]

Interactions between doctors and representatives from drug companies are inevitable[3,4] and likely to increase because huge profits are at stake. The companies are, of course, motivated by profit, not altruism: "No drug company gives away its shareholders' money in an act of disinterested generosity."[5] Although there are no published studies that document the effect of these drug promotions on prescription-drug sales, the effect of advertising on what physicians prescribe can be independent of scientific drug-performance data.[15] It is reasonable to assume that visits (each of which cost $75 in 1982) (*The Wall Street Journal*, November 8, 1982:1, 25) and gifts from detail persons are used because they improve the bottom line.

Gifts and Their Effects

A physician's acceptance of a gift from a drug company or its representative has at least three major effects independent of any ethical repercussions. First, gifts cost money, and the cost is ultimately passed on to patients without their explicit knowledge. Unlike other forms of marketing, such as advertisements, many gifts are private and are not visible to patients. Second, physicians' acceptance of gifts may contribute to the further erosion of the common perception that the medical profession serves the best interests of patients. This view, and indeed the faith of each patient in his or her doctor, may change if people begin to believe that doctors accept or even solicit gifts from drug companies." Third, and most important to us, is that the acceptance of a gift establishes a relationship between the donor and the recipient, a relationship with vague but real obligations.

The Gift Relationship

The cultural significance of gifts in pre-industrial civilizations has been well documented by anthropologists, especially Mauss,[16] whose book, *The Gift: Forms and Functions of Exchange in Archaic Societies,* is the classic source on the subject. Using the work of other anthropologists, Mauss demonstrated the central importance of gift exchange as a means of initiating and sustaining relationships. In the cultures Mauss described, the relationships were primarily between clans or tribes. Gifts among individuals were of secondary importance, but all gifts were things of social significance.

In contemporary society, we have largely lost sight of the importance of gifts as regulators of human relationships; however, gifts have much greater interpersonal significance than is commonly assumed.[17,18,19] By offering a gift to another, a person is really proffering friendship -- a relationship. For example, in a continuing relationship, gift exchange is used to mark certain events, anniversaries, birthdays, and the like. Failure to give an appropriate gift at one of these expected times is usually taken as a sign that the relationship is not important to the one who did not give. Most of us would agree that declining a gift constitutes a rejection of the relationship.

In addition, accepting a gift is accepting the initiation or reinforcement of a relationship, and it triggers an obligatory response from the recipient that involves a complex web of concerns or sentiments directed toward the giver. By accepting the gift, the recipient generally assumes certain social duties, such as grateful conduct, grateful use, and reciprocation,[19] and responds accordingly. The gift relationship is one of paradox: gifts must be given freely, but they entail an obligation. The giver must not insist on any return, yet a response is required. Gift-giving is an act of generosity; however, it also serves the self-interest of the giver.

Emersons[20] may have captured the negative, potentially manipulative side of gifts most clearly: "It is not the office of a man to accept gifts. How dare you give them? We wish to be self sustained. We do not quite forgive a giver." Not all gifts have this negative side: We distinguish between personal gifts, such as those from drug companies to doctors, and anonymous charitable gifts, such as the donation of blood to the Red Cross. Impersonal gifts, such as anonymous gifts of blood, serve important social values, but they do not establish personal relationships between donor and recipient. In contrast, the receipt of a personal gift does establish such a relationship with its sense of obligation.

How is a physician likely to respond to a drug company or its representative from whom he or she has accepted a gift? While most physicians would consider reciprocation by giving a gift in return unthinkable, we feel obliged to respond in other ways. We might listen to a sales pitch, often in a hurried or social setting not conducive to critical and comparative analyses of drug performance data. We might recognize and favor, however unconsciously, one company's drugs amid a sea of similar products.

Even mundane things (often given to doctors by drug representatives) can have significance when they are gifts[16-19] -- a book is not simply a book if it is used to engender a response. Also, the giving of food plays a central role in many physician-pharmaceutical representative interactions. A special relationship is often formed between people who share food, and a fine -- or at least free -- meal can create an atmosphere of conviviality and agreement.[17]

The value of the gift relationship, with its vague but real obligations, is very clear to companies. Formal contracts between a buyer and seller can be fulfilled or dissolved; the relationship between a giver and receiver endures and is less well defined.[17] Also, the fact that many physicians are not seasoned businesspeople who are aware of subtle, but compelling sales techniques probably contributes to the success of these marketing tactics. Conscientious practitioners, who would shun an explicit commercial relationship with a drug company or its representatives, may be especially vulnerable to the obligation that comes with a gift. The company's ultimate goal in this relationship (because of the responsibilities of corporate management to shareholders) is to increase profits.

Ethical Implications of the Gift Relationship

We have suggested that the use of marketing techniques involving gifts to physicians from drug companies has certain effects: the spending of patients' money without their explicit knowledge or consent, possible alterations in society's perception of the profession, and the establishment of tacit but real obligations on the physician's part that result from the gift relationship with the donor-company (or its representative).

In addition, three sorts of ethical problems arise with respect to gifts from drug companies to doctors. First, some practices may be unjust, because they spend the patient's money for the benefit of the doctor and the drug company, but without the knowledge, consent, or benefit of the patient. Second, obligations that result from gifts may threaten the physician-patient relationship in which the physician's role is that of the patient's agent or trustee whose first consideration is the patient's interests in all clinical decisions, including choice of medications. Last, and most subtle, these gift obligations may affect a physician's character, disturbing the delicate balance that exists in each physician between self-interest and concern for others.[21]

Justice

The first issue is that of distributive justice, which entails the fair allocation of burdens and benefits. We believe it is unjust to have a system in which patients pay for gifts that benefit doctors and drug companies. The burdens (i.e., payment) are the patient's (and perhaps the patient's insurer's), but the benefits (i.e., the beach bag or trip) accrue to the physician, who controls the patient's choice of medication, and to the company, which enjoys the profits. As one of our British colleagues so aptly observed, "... we are being given a meal which many of our patients [who are paying for it in the United States] could not afford but which they would appreciate much more."[7] Furthermore, the injustice to the patient is heightened by the lack of disclosure; most patients probably do not realize that drug companies provide their physicians with valuable gifts.

The Physician-Patient Relationship

Most physicians and accepted professional codes agree that the goal of the physician is to further the patient's welfare.[22] The physician's role is that of a fiduciary who holds the faith, trust, and confidence of the patient and who is empowered to act in the patient's best interests. If gifts from a drug company influence a physician's prescription so that a patient receives a drug that is less optimal or more expensive than an equally safe and effective alternative or a drug when none was needed, then the physician has not acted as the patient's fiduciary, and his actions are ethically questionable. We think gifts sometimes influence physicians' prescriptions; it seems unlikely that drug companies would persist in this expensive practice if it were not profitable. Sound empirical studies of this issue should be conducted.

The Physician's Character: Altruism and Self-Interest

The practice of medicine requires a constant balancing act between altruistic concern for others -- i.e., responding to an emergency call, sacrificing sleep or timetables to serve the patient's needs, and one's innate self-interest and ambition. Jonsen[21] described this tension as "a profound moral paradox" in all physicians; we live with it daily. Our desires to further our careers and to live comfortably are not unethical, and conflicts of interest between altruism and self-concern are inherent in the fee-for-service system of reimbursement, for example, where the patient is fully aware of the arrangement.[10] Our society recognizes that physicians live with this paradox. The fact that physicians have traditionally been entrusted with the regulation of their own practices is an expression of confidence in their ability to maintain an ethical balance.

However, the balance is precarious and "the tension is incessant."[21] Situations that may encourage physicians to satisfy their self-interest without considering their patients' welfare may alter physicians' characters by tipping the balance between self-interest and altruism. Gifts from drug companies feed our human tendencies toward self-interest; they do nothing to foster our concern for our patients. Insofar as such gifts exert a baleful influence on physicians' characters, even subtly, they are ethically suspect.

What About Educational "Gifts?"

The idea of the gift relationship is useful for defining subtle obligations and effects on the physician-patient relationship and/or the physician's character. It is also a useful idea to apply in distinguishing activities of pharmaceutical companies that are laudable from those that are not. The obligations are greatest and most easily maniputable when a relationship is established between two individuals; obligations are minimized when gifts are institutional rather than personal. Therefore, we argue that it is ethically acceptable for drug companies to give money to institutions for educational activities, books, journals, or case records in exchange for only an explicit acknowledgment (for example); this situation poses less of a danger because no personal relationship and no obligation to respond in any way are established between the individual physician and the drug company's representative. Some would argue that the issues of justice and influence by promotion still remain and that institutions also can be corrupted; however, full disclosure, avoidance of extravagance and waste, and the primary goal of improving patient care by physician education make these activities ethically acceptable.

The Need For Guidelines

We have examined gift-giving by drug companies to physicians and have described three ethical implications: injustice in the use of patients' money without their consent or benefit, concrete and symbolic threats to the fiduciary relationship between physician and patient, and alterations in physicians' characters by disrupting the balance between concern for others and self-interest.

Preserving justice, the trusteeship relationship with our patients, and our own altruism are regulative ideals -- that is, standards not always achievable by all of us, but useful templates "against which all efforts can be measured."[23] These standards are especially useful where the potential ethical issues are complex; obviously, gifts vary in value, and the ethical repercussions of using a pocket flashlight are far more subtle (some would argue nonexistent) than those of accepting $156. However, the standards encourage behavior as close to the ideal as possible when the temptation is to avoid making difficult ethical distinctions.[2]

Given the moral complexities and dangers in gift-giving, we feel that professional societies should establish guidelines for physicians' actions in these situations. Written guidelines to address this issue may, in fact, be welcomed by both parties. Many physicians have expressed confusion and discomfort over the present free-for-all,[2,8] and some have suggested that companies may prefer to conduct business with doctors without a currency of gifts and hospitality.[3] Corporations readily recognize the dangers of gifts being used to influence or create obligations in their own employees, and some formally address the issue in codes of business ethics.[24]

Current medical codes of ethics in this country do not specifically mention these subtle issues.[22,25,26] The British have discussed the topic of gifts more widely,[3,5-7,9] and both the Royal College of Physicians and the Association of the British Pharmaceutical Industry have established statements regarding proper conduct. In 1984, the Association of the British Pharmaceutical Industry specifically stated that only "inexpensive gifts" are to be offered to the medical profession[9] and that the hospitality offered by the company should be "...not out of proportion to the occasion [and] not exceed that level which the recipients might normally adopt when paying for themselves."[5] In 1986, the Royal College of Physicians issued a report that attempted to address the acceptance of gratuities and ethical issues that surrounded company sponsorship of continuing medical education. The statement, which was criticized for its vagueness, states categorically that "refreshment" regularly provided by the drug companies at continuing medical education events "degrades" the profession.[9]

In this country, the Accreditation Council for Continuing Medical Education will not accredit programs unless what it stipulates as inappropriate commercial influences are avoided (unpublished data, 1984). The Veterans Administration has issued a detailed document that covers the possible conflicts of interest (or appearance of conflicts of interest) for Veterans Administration employees who interact with pharmaceutical companies (D. Rasinski, MD, JD, written communication, December 1987), and in 1987 the American Surgical Association resolved "that it is unethical for a surgeon to accept...material reward for participating in... product promotional activity...with no relationship to professional service rendered by the surgeon.'"[27]

Although codes such as these may be "castrated by the impossibility of definition,"[5] we feel that properly publicized guidelines can enhance ethical awareness and promote the ideal. These guidelines should provide principles for ethical action, rather than lists of "do's" and "don'ts." We propose that American medical organizations adopt statements about these issues and suggest the inclusion of the following items:

1. The issue: We must acknowledge the ethical dangers inherent in situations in which physicians accept gifts or other favors from drug companies.

2. Minimizing the obligations of gifts: All drug company gifts should be contributions to physicians' education or care of patients and should be made explicitly in ways that avoid the relationship or obligation of the physician to the drug company or its representative. For example, these contributions could be channeled through nonprofit institutions such as professional societies or academic departments. This stipulation applies to both advertising trinkets of minimal value and more expensive items such as books, meals, or cash. To include small personal novelties may seem petty,[27] but, as we have discussed, their value in securing individual relationships may be significant. The key here is not the monetary value of the gift, but whether it is instrumental in fostering a personal relationship. The institution that functions as middleman has ethical responsibilities as well, of course, but the subtle threat to the individual physician's character and duty to his or her patient is minimized by avoiding a personal relationship and its attendant obligation.

3. Continuing medical education: Strict guidelines to ensure the independence of educational events from commercial influences should be followed. Company support for continuing medical education might be in the form of a grant to a society or academic department, which is solely responsible for selection of topics, faculty, and associated social events, perhaps with a simple acknowledgment of the funding source.

4. Disclosure: While potential conflicts of interest are inevitable for the physician, they are more acceptable if the patient is aware of them.[10,13] Similarly, public knowledge of potential conflicts may resolve some ethical dilemmas, or at least guide us in deciding what is "acceptable." The British guidelines cleverly ask the physician, "... would you be willing to have these arrangements generally known?"[9] The public should be made aware of drug company gifts and hospitality to physicians, even if they are funneled through institutions.

5. Responsibilities of teaching programs: Physicians' prescribing patterns should always be guided by available scientific data. Students and physicians in training should be instructed in the ethical dangers inherent in relationships with drug

company representatives, and in the importance of critical consideration of primary data and expert recommendations in the choice of drugs.

Comment

In general, physicians should avoid accepting gifts directly from drug companies: patients' money is spent unfairly; the subtle influence of the gift relationship may alter prescribing practices, thereby threatening the physician's role as patient trustee; and the gift relationship may affect physicians' characters by shifting the balance between self-interest and altruism. We should acknowledge these issues and address them directly.

Notes

1. Graves J. Frequent-flyer programs for drug prescribing, *N Engl J Med* 1987;317:252.
2. Goldfinger SE. A matter of influence, *N Engl J Med* 1987;316:1408-1409.
3. Smith R. Doctors and the drug industry: Too close for comfort, *Br Med J* 1986;293:905-906.
4. Shaughnessy AF. Drug promotion in a family medicine training center, *JAMA* 1988;260:926.
5. Rawlins MD. Doctors and the drug makers, *Lancet* 1984;2:276-278.
6. `Opren scandal.' *Lancet* 1983;1:219-220.
7. Fakes RW. Doctors and the drug industry, *Br Med J* 1986;293:1170-1171.
8. Katz RA. Unhook me, *J Am Acad Dermatol* 1987;17:865-866.
9. The relationship between physicians and the pharmaceutical industry: A report of the Royal College of Physicians, *JR Coll Physicians Lond* 1986;20:235-242.
10. Relman AS. Dealing with conflicts of interest, *N Engl J Med* 1985;313:749-751.
11. Graboys TB. Conflicts of interest in the management of silent ischemia, *JAMA* 1989;261:2016-2017.
12. Healy B, Campeau L, Gray R, *et al*. Conflict of-interest guidelines for a multicenter clinical trial of treatment after coronary-artery bypass-graft surgery, *N Engl J Med* 1989;320:949-951.
13. Relman AS. Economic incentives in clinical investigation, *N Engl J Med* 1989;320:933-934.
14. Chotiner G. Response, *J Am Acad Dermatol* 1987;17:866.
15. Avorn J, Chen M, Hartley R. Scientific versus commercial sources of influence on the prescribing behavior of physicians, *Am J Med* 1982;73:4-8.
16. Mauss M, Cunnison I, trans. *The Gift: Forms and Functions of Exchange in Archaic Societies*. New York, NY: WW Norton & Co Inc, 1967.
17. Murray TH. Gifts of the body and the needs of strangers, *Hastings Cent Rep* 1987;17:30-38.
18. Titmuss RM. *The Gift Relationship*. New York, NY: Pantheon Books Inc, 1971.
19. Camenisch PF. Gift and gratitude in ethics, *J Religious Ethics* 1981;9:1-33.
20. Emerson RW. Gifts, In: *Essays of Ralph Waldo Emerson*. Norwalk, CT: Easton Press, 1979:211-214, Series II.
21. Jonsen AR. Watching the doctor, *N Engl J Med* 1983;308:1531-1535.
22. Ad Hoc Committee on Medical Ethics, American College of Physicians. American College of Physicians ethics manual, part 1: history of medical ethics, the physician and the patient, the physician's relationship to other physicians, the physician and society, *Ann Intern Med* 1984;101:129137.
23. Murray TH. Divided loyalties for physicians: Social context and moral problems, *Soc Sci Med* 1986;23:827-832.
24. Laczniak GR, Murphy PE. *Marketing Ethics: Guidelines for Managers*. Lexington, MA: Lexington Books, 1985.
25. *Drugs and devices: Prescribing. Current Opinions of the Council on Ethical and Judicial Affairs of the American Medical Association-1986*. Chicago, IL: American Medical Association,1986:sect 8.06.
26. American Medical Association House of Delegates. *Substitute Resolution 172-Condemnation of Certain Practices of Pharmaceutical Companies*. Chicago, IL: American Medical Association, 1987.
27. Bricker EM. Industrial marketing and medical ethics, *N Engl J Med* 1989;320:1690-1692.

Chapter 68

The Elderly and High Technology Medicine: A Case for Individualized, Autonomous Allocation

Peter D. Mott

Introduction

Nowhere are the issues about high technology and prolongation of life more fascinating, and more dangerous, than in current debates concerning older persons. Opinions vary from a cost-conscious societal view that would "ration" all expensive, procedurally oriented health care, which would exclude people over age 70 or 80,[1] to the viewpoint that one cannot safely limit any care even if the patient is permanently comatose (among a variety of legal opinions).[2,3,4]

The term "geriatric imperative" applies to these questions, just as it does to the responsibilities of social and educational institutions to provide services and trained professionals to care for more and more older persons. Thus, if mortality rates in the U.S. are now decreasing at 2-1/2% per year, if the well elderly soon will be expected to live normal life spans of 105 to 115 years, and if 25% of our population by the year 2020 will be over age 65, then life and death decisions, and conflicts between the capability of high technology and personal wishes, will be increasingly within the provinces of geriatric medicine. In 1987, we spent $140 billion for the health care of those over 65, with 14% of all Medicare expenditures being spent on the last two months of life. These figures, rapidly increasing each year, have led not only families and physicians but also insurers, both private and public, to involve themselves more and more in the debate. Should such issues be settled in courts, legislatures, or around hospital beds by professionals? Or are they better handled by older persons themselves in private and in advance of mentally incapacitating illness? Should there be general laws or guidelines, such as limitations on the use of high technology by age? Or should each patient's future plan of care be individualized? If so, how should such individualization come about?

Setting costs aside for the moment, and simply putting the question to older persons themselves, their families or surrogates, one is struck by the tremendous variability in the responses. A diversity of responses is also received from ethical, philosophical, and legal experts. The varied responses from older persons is expected, and relates to the well documented heterogeneity of the elderly themselves.[5] Is it reasonable that the master athlete of 85 who has no serious disorders should have the same guidelines for future care as the bedridden, demented, end stage Alzheimer's victim of 70?

Extreme variability also is found in other aspects of the lives of older persons. A group of 75-year-olds may feel entirely differently about whether or not to allow regrafting of their coronary arteries, for example, depending not only upon their varying amounts of disease, but

---

Source: Reprinted from *Theoretical Medicine*, Vol. 11, 1990, pp. 95-102, with permission from Kluwer Academic Publishers © 1990.

also other disorders: e.g., vision, hearing, balance, even the condition of their feet, all of which increasingly affect the quality of life as we age. Their economic well-being may or may not be a factor. More often, the significant factors affecting whether they accept or reject major surgery are their interest in work or play and attachments to family and friends. Apart from their varied interests in items of this life there are, of course, extreme variations in their beliefs -- if any -- about a "next life." How does each person view death? How responsible does each feel for attending to people, pets or affairs that might be left behind? How much do these kinds of concerns influence older people's choices about how aggressive and high tech should be their future care?

Because of the almost limitless variability in these components of decision-making, it appears to be irrational and arbitrary for courts to decide or legislatures to determine rules governing our distribution of expensive, life-extending technologies. Moreover, the idea that an outside individual such as a physician, should take it upon him or herself to make such a determination also would appear to be arbitrary and irrational.

Ethicists refer to the individualized approach as preference utilization: i.e., that one way to allocate resources, in order to get the greatest possible good (or the least possible harm) to the greatest number of people, is by eliciting individual preferences. Advocates believe that this is preferable to a traditional utilitarian view that such resources should be distributed more uniformly, based on agent-neutral values. In this paper the argument will be that individual preference should be the basis for allocations of health services, not an arbitrary distribution based on such a criterion as age (e.g., that no high tech services would go to those over age 70 in order to increase the benefit to all those under 70).

How, then, would older persons decide such issues? Would the resultant pattern of distribution of services be as varied as one might expect? Would the results be affordable to society? At this point both studies of populations and individual case studies become important.

Studies of Patient Preference

Despite a vast literature about ethical decision-making in regard to high technology, prolongation of life, resuscitation, etc., there is comparatively little information about how people themselves choose among alternatives. Danis *et al.*[6] interviewed 193 patients over age 55 admitted to an intensive care unit during a one year period. Obviously a select group, favoring those who agreed to be admitted to an intensive care unit, they found that 70% were willing to repeat the experience, even if only to achieve one month of survival. This result was not significantly affected by such factors as age, functional status, severity of illness, or perceived quality of life.

Finucane *et al.*[7] interviewed 34 patients, finding varying responses to the presentation of different scenarios. Thus, in the event of Alzheimer's disease severe enough to preclude self-feeding, 25 were against resuscitation (CPR) if their hearts were to stop. Seven favored CPR and two didn't know. Twenty-one (62%) would refuse a feeding stomach tube, eight would favor it and five didn't know. Moreover, if their hearts were to stop right then, during the interview, all but six would want CPR.

In another study, Bedell and Delbanco[8] interviewed 24 competent patients who survived CPR, another very select population. Of the 24, 15, if they had been asked, would have favored CPR, eight would not, and one was ambivalent. Of those who would have refused CPR, all stated six months after successful CPR that they still would not want it repeated.

Pearlman and Uhlmann[9] found that patients' perceptions of their quality of life differed significantly from physicians' impressions. The patients' feelings were related to health, social, and economic factors. The physicians underestimated their patients' own views of their quality of life.

Thus, while not enough is yet known about how the elderly make such decisions, it is clear that they can decide when offered the chance, and that responses vary greatly among individuals. These findings support the proposition that many older persons, but not all, would limit their use of high tech procedures, and that informed individual preference could provide a rational basis for allocating resources. What we don't know are: (a) how best to inform and allow patient choice, (b) the numbers of people likely to choose each path, and (c) whether services (and costs) for society would increase or decrease over the currently varied, usually unorganized ways of dealing with or -- more often ignoring these concerns.

Case Studies

The stories of three differing people are presented. Each demonstrates in its own, individualized way how the elderly can and do make rational health care decisions.

Case 1

Mrs. A.U., 67-years-old, with severe chronic lung disease, short of breath for 11 years, requiring cortisone for eight years, receiving continuous oxygen for three, and nursing home care for two years. In her final two years of life she was bed -- and chair -- bound for one month out of three by an acute respiratory infection. However, between those episodes, she was able to propel herself around the building in an electric wheelchair and to visit relatives' homes supported by her portable oxygen unit.

Two years before her death and upon entering the nursing home, Mrs. A.U. stated that she wanted fully aggressive medical care, including intensive care unit (ICU), but she did not want cardio-pulmonary resuscitation (CPR) in the event of a cardiac arrest. Nor did she want to be intubated, even if a breathing tube placed in her throat was felt to be necessary to save her life.

She survived the first year of acute flare-ups without hospitalization. Nine months before death, however, she had a severe pneumonia and became progressively more hypoxic, cyanotic, exhausted, and delirious. As her arterial blood gases showed steadily worsening oxygen and carbon dioxide levels, her physician and nearest relative agreed that her decision against resuscitation would be observed. But they were not certain that she had fully understood the pros and cons of temporary intubation. The patient was by then unable to make any rational decision. The nearest relative and the physician agreed to override Mrs. A.U.'s previously expressed wish not to be intubated. A tube was placed in her larynx and she was transferred to a hospital ICU where she made a rapid recovery. The tube was gradually removed over a one week period, and she returned to the nursing home.

On return she was able to resume her activities, but she made her wishes clear -- at a time when she was not depressed -- that intubation was never to be repeated. Thus, nine months later and with recurrent pneumonia, she was hospitalized but not intubated. She gradually weakened, was kept comfortable, visited with family and friends, discussed with all her desire to die, and then expired.

Case 2

Mr. P.V. is an 88-year-old man living in an intermediate care facility (ICF) who has had repeated episodes of a life-threatening cardiac arrhythmia. He had a history of hypertension with two myocardial infarctions, a ventricular aneurysm, congestive heart failure and chest pains and, after admission, two small strokes. He remained mentally clear, able to walk, and to take care of himself.

Three months after admission he collapsed, remained conscious, and was found to be in ventricular tachycardia. He received one electric shock by the cardiac defibrillator, which returned his heart to normal rhythm. Hospitalized for one week, on return he stated that he not only didn't want to be resuscitated in the event of another cardiac arrest but also he did not want to "go through that [defibrillation] again." After psychiatric consultation, he was treated with a tricyclic antidepressant which improved his mood. He decided he would like any treatment short of resuscitation for a cardio-pulmonary arrest. The same arrhythmia recurred one year later, despite anti-arrhythmic therapy. After a second defibrillation, hospitalization, and recovery he repeated the same wish to have similarly aggressive therapy if it happened again. On several occasions, however, when more depressed, he has stated that he wanted to die, only to change his mind when he returned to his usual state of mind. Currently he is independent in his daily functions, walking, mentally alert, mildly depressed, but deriving some definite pleasure from activities around him.

Case 3

Mr. O.H. is a 79-year-old man who has lived in an intermediate care facility (ICF) for nine months. He is alert except for chronic mild confusion and disorientation. He walks and cares for himself and enjoys visits. With a background of hypertension, diabetes, and two strokes he developed abdominal pain and blood was found in his bowel movements. After he consented to a full gastrointestinal work-up, a biopsy via gastroscopy proved the presence of stomach cancer. A computerized tomographic (CT) scan showed only the local mass with no visible spread of the cancer outside the stomach wall.

In discussing medical options with Mr. O.H., he was told that he had a cancer. He was informed that pain and bleeding were controlled only temporarily, and that without surgery, he would die. He was further told that surgery is the only type of treatment for his type of cancer, that there is a 25% chance of cure. The patient thinks he would like to undergo surgery, although he does not want to be resuscitated if he has a cardio-pulmonary arrest. It is unclear whether he understands the surgical odds. His family feels he is too confused to understand his medical choice fully. They are adamantly opposed to surgery, "He has suffered enough."

Discussion

The case presentations reveal both similarities and differences among the three. In all three cases the patients chose not to be resuscitated if heart and lung functions were to cease (i.e., to be "Do-Not-Resuscitate" or "DNR"). In each case, however, the patient chose to have a certain amount of high technology. Mrs. A.U. wanted every chance to survive short of laryngeal intubation. Mr. P.V. wanted electro-cardioversion and hospitalization for any cardiac arrhythmia that was not immediately fatal. Mr. O.H. appears to want extensive surgery for his cancer, even with poor odds, because he has no chance to live without it. If it is decided, with planned psychiatric consultation and mental testing, that he is not competent to decide this for himself, then his family would refuse the surgery. The question of resuscitation at the time of death appears to be either easier to understand or simpler to decide than the issues of how aggressive care ought to be before death. For one thing, many feel -- despite the facts -- that a cardiopulmonary arrest is a natural death rather than an event reversible by resuscitation. For another, these three patients were made aware of the poor record of CPR attempts in older persons.[10]

All three patients, when counseled about options, designed future plans for themselves which allowed certain amounts of aggressiveness of care. None wanted unlimited, aggressive, high tech care. All had set some limits on its use.

Not only were the responses varied, but both of the first two patients' wishes changed over time. Thus, Mrs. A.U. became more adamant, or more convincing, in refusing a second intubation after receiving the first. Mr. P.V.'s opinions varied with the amount of his depression. In the case of Mr. O.H. another variable may be the amount of guilt the family may feel about not caring for him at home. It is possible they are exaggerating the amount of confusion they think he has and the amount of suffering they think he has experienced.

It appears from these experiences and the literature that, if older persons themselves decide how aggressive and high tech their future medical care will be, a kind of individualized and autonomous allocation will result. In many cases (perhaps a majority, but the quantity is unknown), this type of rationing would result in a reduction in current rates of hospitalization,[11] surgery and cardio-pulmonary resuscitation. Such individualized, autonomous rationing could limit aggressive and high tech care in a myriad of cases which are often felt to be excessive, unnecessary, even inhumane. On the other hand, if informed patient preference becomes the criterion, there would also be many who would not want to be excluded or "rationed" from aggressive medical care simply on the basis of age.

Conclusion

In the U.S. most older persons do not yet have the chance to participate in decisions about how aggressive and high tech should be their future medical care. Health planners are increasingly interested in containing the rapidly increasing costs of care but are also concerned with the lack of services (e.g., long-term care) for many elderly people. At the same time, debates are heating up about potential conflicts between growth in the use of high tech procedures and both the quality-of-life and dignity-of-death of older persons. Proposals to deal with these issues vary from increasing services to all by a re-direction of funds from other sectors (e.g., the defense budget) to proposals by others that expensive, especially high tech services, should be allocated by age alone (e.g., no one over age 70 would receive intensive care).

An alternative approach, which appears to be objective and rational, is for all persons above age 70, for example, or earlier if they have serious chronic diseases, to be fully and sensitively counseled and given the chance to determine for themselves just how much high technology they want used in their future medical care. The large majority of older persons have the mental capacity to make such decisions. Most of those without such capacity have relatives or surrogates who could decide.

What percentages of the population would choose which approaches to future care? Can society afford to let individual-preference determine the future distribution of expensive services? This needs further study including more information on how people are best counseled, what procedures lead to the most consistent patient choices, far more data than is now available about the actual choices elderly people would make and, finally, the implications for society in regard to needed services and costs. At this time we do not have enough information to answer the crucial question: i.e., if everyone made informed choices, and health care professionals carried out individual care plans based on those choices, would services (and costs) for the elderly increase or decrease? Proponents of the alternative method of allocation of resources based on age also lack such data.

If the course of patient preference is to be followed, then the role of health professionals will be to provide the facts, to counsel, to be sure their patients or their surrogates understand fully and have the chance to change their minds over time. It is unclear whether the physician should be neutral and non-directive in such decision-making. The role of the clergy in such cases includes helping the decision-maker -- the patient -- set the boundaries around the decision; for example, how current quality-of-life is judged in relation to one's past and one's view of the future, including both life, death, and whatever may come after death.

An individualized, autonomous, flexible approach to such difficult decisions would protect all of us from two other factors. One is our current ignorance about such basic items as how healthy the elderly will be in later life as life span extends to over 100 years. This is not yet known. Therefore, we ought not to jump to the false conclusion that being older automatically means requiting more high tech, aggressive care. Secondly, this approach would allow the individual to protect him or herself against the growing influence of high technology itself over our health professions, our budgets and ourselves.

Notes

1. Callahan D. *Setting Limits: Medical Goals in an Aging Society*. New York, NY: Simon and Schuster, 1987.
2. Emanuel EJ. A review of the ethical and legal aspects of terminating medical care, *Am J Med* 1988;84:291-301.
3. Barondess JA, Kalb P, Weil WB, Cassel C, Ginsberg E. Clinical decision-making in catastrophic situations: the relevance of age, *J Am Geriatr Soc* 1988;36:919-37.
4. Ruark JE, Raffin TA. Initiating and withdrawing life support. Principles and practice in adult medicine, *N Engl J Med* 1988;318:25-30.
5. Rowe JW. Health care of the elderly, *N Engl J Med* 1985;312:827-35.
6. Danis M, Patrick DL, Southerland LI, Green ML. Patients' and families' preferences for medical intensive care, *JAMA* 1988;260:797-802.
7. Finucane TE, Shumway JM, Powers RL, *et al*. Planning with elderly outpatients for contingencies of severe illness, *J Gen Intern Med* 1988;3:322-5.
8. Bedell SE, Delbanco TL. Choices about cardiopulmonary resuscitation in the hospital, *N Engl J Med* 1984;310:1089-93.
9. Pearlman RA, Uhlmann RF. Quality-of-life in chronic diseases: Perceptions of elderly patients, *J Gerontol* 1988;43:25-30.
10. Murphy DJ. Do-not-resuscitate orders: Time for reappraisal in long-term care institutions, *JAMA* 1988;260:2098-101.
11. Mott PD, Barker WH. Hospital and medical care use by nursing home patients: the effect of patient care plans, *J Am Geriatr Soc* 1988;36:47-53.

Chapter 69

The Doctor as Double Agent

Marcia Angell

In eariler times -- that is, before 1980 -- it was generally agreed that the doctor's sole obligation was to take care of each patient. The doctor was the patient's fiduciary or agent, and the doctor was to act only in the patient's interest. Now all that has changed. Many of us -- economists, governmental officials, corporate executives, even ethicists, and yes, even many doctors themselves -- now believe that doctors have other obligations that compete with their obligation to the patient. In particular, they believe that doctors have acquired an obligation to save resources for society. Doing so requires doctors to practice with one eye on costs, which may mean sometimes denying beneficial care that they would surely have provided in earlier times.

According to the new view, doctors are no longer simply agents for their patients. They are now agents for society's needs as well. They are, in short, double agents, expected to decide whether the benefits of treatment to their patients are worth the costs to society. Many distinguished ethicists have enthusiastically embraced this new ethic (Callahan 1990; Morreim 1991). To them, keeping an eye on the price tag means saving scarce resources for other, more important uses.

How did this extraordinary shift in our view of doctors' obligations come about? Is it just coincidence that it began with our first realization -- roughly in the mid-1970s -- that our seemingly endless resources were in fact, finite? And is it just coincidence that it accorded with the wishes of the third-party payers -- who discovered during the 1980s that they had severe and growing budgetary problems? In short, can it be that the ethical underpinnings of the practice of medicine have been scrapped in a single decade for financial reasons? Is economics driving ethics?

I'll begin with my conclusions. I believe that doctors are now asked to be double agents and that their dual obligation is a recent construct, which arose out of the economic difficulties of the large third-party payers. I will argue that we embrace this new ethic at our peril. Even if we as a society decide that health care should take a smaller piece of the national economic pie, there are ways to do this that do not entail rebuilding -- and perhaps destroying -- almost overnight, the ethical underpinnings of the profession.

Historical Reivew

First, a quick review of how we got here. This requires an economic analysis, since my thesis is that economics is now driving ethics. The economic history of health care in the United States can be divided into three phases. First, there was the phase of the true market, lasting until roughly World War II. Patients paid doctors out-of-pocket for their medical care. If the

---

Source: Reprinted from *Kennedy Institute of Ethics Journal*, Vol. 3, No. 3, pp. 279-286, with permission from Kennedy Institute of Ethics © 1994.

price was too high, the doctor was confronted with an unhappy patient. Even after private insurance companies began to flourish in the 1930s, the premiums were still paid out-of-pocket and so patients continued to feel the costs, although the pain was blunted. Fortunately, medical care was fairly inexpensive. Unfortunately, it was also relatively ineffective, compared with the power of modern medicine.

The second phase was marked by the entry of big business into the health care picture. Big business began to offer health insurance as a fringe benefit in order to evade the wage and price controls in effect during World War II. Offering health insurance was tantamount to increasing wages, and furthermore, it was not taxed. The connection between employment and health insurance was thus an historical accident that haunts us still. But the important effect of this connection for the discussion here is that it insulates patients from the costs of medical care. Neither doctors nor patients had to worry any longer about the costs of medical care. With the enactment of Medicare and Medicaid in 1966, this insulation from costs spread to the poor and, most importantly, to the elderly -- a politically powerful group. By the end of the 1960s, anything resembling a true market in health care had vanished. Nearly everyone was covered by third-party payers -- government, business, and private insurance companies. And medical care was becoming both more expensive and more effective. Despite the increasing costs, the third parties happily paid the charges, with few questions asked.

The third phase began with the realization that health care costs were consistently rising far more rapidly than the GNP. Now that patients and doctors and hospitals were insulated from accountability, there were no limits on the expansion of the health care industry in this country. It was open-ended and nearly risk-free, absorbing an ever greater share of our domestic spending. While national expenditures for other social goods, such as education, stagnated or declined, expenditures for health care rose rapidly -- from roughly 6 percent of the GNP in 1965 to nearly 10 percent in 1980 to 13 percent in 1991 (Stoline and Weiner 1993).

Not only was there nothing to stop the inflation, but there were features that virtually guaranteed it. These included the piecework, fee-for-service reimbursement system that is greatly skewed toward high-technology procedures and specialists. Doctors, of course, act as both providers and purchasing agents, so these highly paid specialists could easily generate their own business. For example, the cardiologist who recommends coronary angiography to a patient also bills for it.

Cost Containment

In the 1970s, the Arab oil embargo made Americans realize that our resources were finite. Health care costs began to occupy the attention of some experts and policy-makers. By the 1980s, it became clear to nearly everyone that we could not indefinitely sustain rising health care costs, and for the first time, efforts were made to control them. "Cost containment" crept into the lexicon, and by the end of the 1980s the *New England Journal of Medicine* probably received more manuscripts about cost containment than about cancer. The efforts to control costs were spearheaded by the major third parties -- government and big business. They were responding essentially to budgetary problems, not to moral problems. They went about cost containment in a number of ad hoc, uncoordinated ways, as briefly mentioned below. None of them was notably successful. In fact health care costs rose even faster -- I believe, because of cost containment efforts, not despite them.

Regulation by third parties, including managed care, simply led to the growth of an expensive and intrusive new bureaucracy. Efforts to foster competition led to increased marketing, not to lower prices. And attempts to limit demand through higher deductibles and co-payments simply shifted costs and limited care, primarily to the most vulnerable. Efforts by insurers to avoid risks also shifted costs. In general, savings to one part of the system were costs to another. In fact, the dominant characteristic of the American health care system is that there is no system. There is just a hodgepodge of arrangements, existing independently, often working at cross purposes, and generating enormous administrative costs. Indeed, administrative costs -- billing, marketing, underwriting, claims processing, utilization review -- now consume more than 20 cents of the health care dollar (Woolhandler and Himmelstein 1991).

Why do I recapitulate this sorry history of the economics of the American health care system? I do so because it is important to understand the context in which doctors are being invited to act as double agents. They are invited to do so in an open-ended, inherently inflationary system (or, rather, nonsystem) that spends roughly 40 percent more per citizen on health care than the next most expensive health care system in the world and at least twice as much on administrative costs. Further, this system is embedded in a society that routinely spends billions and billions on such goods as tobacco, television ads, and cosmetics. Clearly, we as a society are not facing scarcity; instead we are facing the inefficient and frivolous use of vast resources.

Saving For Third Parties

What precisely is the doctor supposed to do as double agent? In a nutshell, doctors are supposed to tailor their care of patients to save money for third parties. For example, under the DRG system of hospital reimbursement for Medicare patients, doctors are supposed to be agents for the hospital, discharging patients as rapidly as possible and keeping services to a minimum so that the hospital can game the system. In many HMOs doctors are expected to keep costs as low as possible, and some HMOs even directly reward doctors with bonuses when the HMO comes out ahead. They may also withhold a portion of doctors' salaries if they refer patients to specialists too often or use too many tests and procedures. Thus, doctors are agents for the HMO and have a direct incentive to undertreat their patients, just as in the fee-for-service system they have an incentive to overtreat them. Other forms of managed care also deter doctors from delivering care. Those that require utilization review often make it so complicated and difficult to get approval for hospitalization or procedures that the doctor is reluctant even to try. And it should be noted that nearly all medical care these days is managed in one way or another, by which I mean it is subject to efforts of insurers to limit care.

In essence, then, doctors are increasingly being asked, in one way or another, to save money for a third party -- and sometimes for themselves -- by scrimping on the medical care they deliver. But the pressure is seldom described in these terms. Instead, it is described as practicing "cost-effective" medicine. "Cost-effective" is the new watchword. It used to be a technical term that referred to the least expensive of two equally effective alternatives, or to the most effective of two equally costly ones. Now it is simply a shorthand for any attempt to save money. The word sounds fine, and who can object to it?

Jusitification For Double Agents

But how can we justify asking doctors to deprive their patients of care, including clearly beneficial care that in other circumstances they would not hesitate to provide? Just as the problem is new, so are the ethical justifications.

First, it is claimed that limiting care is what society wishes, and that the medical profession has an obligation not only to accept the will of society but to further it. Doctors are simply anticipating and delivering what is expected of them by the body politic, despite the fact that individual patients may want something else when they are sick.

Second, it is argued that because third parties now pay for nearly all medical care, they have gained a legitimate voice -- indeed, the overriding voice -- in how much medical care patients should receive. I find this a peculiarly American argument. Essentially the message is that whoever pays the piper calls the tune. The purest example of this view is the Oregon plan for rationing the care received by Medicaid patients. This is often described as a decision to allocate scarce resources rationally and justly, but it is, of course, nothing of the sort. It is instead a matter of taxpayers deciding to limit the care received by the poor, on the grounds that the taxpayers are funding it. Those who drew up the priority list of medical services are not those to whom it would apply. Even if we were to accept the idea that paying for medical care confers the right to limit it, we should remember that most patients do in fact still pay for their medical care, just as they always did. They simply pay in advance and indirectly, through their work or their taxes. The third parties are not using their own money.

The third justification for doctors to be double agents is the most compelling. It appeals to the doctor as good citizen or, more dramatically, to the doctor as occupant of a metaphorical lifeboat with limited supplies. According to this view, resources saved in denying patients expensive medical care could be used to provide less expensive care to a larger number of patients. Or it could be used for even more important public purposes, such as education. This line of argument has been put forward most persuasively by Dan Callahan (1990) who contends that Americans have overvalued individual health care compared with other social goods.

Arguments Against Double Agents

Despite these justifications, I see five serious problems with the view that doctors should act to contain costs, patient by patient. First and most simply, this view of the role of doctors is based on the premise that resources in our health care system are in fact scarce. But, of course, they aren't. The mere fact that we spend so much more on health care than all other advanced nations is proof that our health care resources are plentiful. Given that in 1990 we spent about $2,566 on every man, woman, and child in the United States, and Canada spent only $1,770, we can hardly claim inadequate resources (Schieber, Poullier, and Greenwald 1992). And since Americans and Canadians are subject to the same ailments and have roughly the same outcomes, we must assume that our system is grossly inefficient. Clearly, the answer to an inefficient system is not to stint on care, but rather to restructure the system to make it more efficient.

Second, enlisting doctors as ad hoc rationers presumes that resources saved by denying health care would be put to better use. But in our system there is absolutely no reason to think that it would. As Norman Daniels (1986) has pointed out, in the United Kingdom or Canada, resources saved by denying care would be used for presumably more valuable health care, but that is not the case here. In the U.S., we do not have a closed system in which funds taken from one form of health care are diverted to another that is deemed to be more important. Instead, funds not used for health care may find their way into any sector of the larger economy, to be used for anything -- e.g., defense, education, farm subsidies, or personal savings. Furthermore, even funds that remain within the health care system might not be used for more effective care; instead, money saved on, say, heart transplantation may very well find its way to a hospital's public relations office or to higher salaries for administrators. Under these circumstances, it is very difficult to sustain an ethical argument for doctors acting as double agents. The only principled way to ration health care is to close the system and establish limits that apply to everyone -- not just to the poor.

Third, asking doctors to be double agents overlooks an important symbolic function of health care. Our society was founded on the principle that individuals enjoy a set of basic rights that cannot be denied them. As medicine has become increasingly effective in preserving life, medical care has come to be counted among these rights. Thus, doctors are seen to preserve a basic human right, namely life, just as criminal lawyers are seen to preserve liberty by defending their clients. Lawyers do not decide part way through a trial to call it quits because it's just too expensive to go on with it. In both situations, there has been a consensus that the single-minded focus on the patient or the client serves the broader interests of society. This argument is particularly compelling in a society as unequal as ours. People will tolerate the vast inequities in income and privilege in this country only if they feel assured that their irreducible set of rights is truly protected. It has been suggested that high technology medicine may serve precisely such a reassuring function in our society. And public opinion polls tend to support this view (Blendon 1991). The public, in contrast to the third-party payers, does not feel that we are spending too much on health care, only that we are not getting our money's worth.

Fourth, when doctors act as double agents, they are merely acting on their own particular prejudices. They are deciding that this or that medical service costs too much. This is not a medical judgment, but a political or philosophical one. Another doctor (or a plumber or electrician) might make quite a different judgment. This is no way to allocate health care.

And fifth and perhaps most important, the doctor as double agent is not honest. Sick people need and expect their doctors' single purpose to be to heal them. The doctor-patient relationship would not survive a candid statement by the doctor that only care that seems to the doctor to be worth the money will be provided. Anything short of full efforts to heal the individual patient, then, must involve a hidden agenda-man ethically indefensible position.

Conclusion

In sum, we should be loath to abandon or modify the patient-centered ethic, and we should be wary of ethical justifications for doing so. Unfortunately, history shows us that ethics in practice are often highly malleable, justifying political decisions rather than informing them. Necessity is the mother of invention, in ethics as well as in other aspects of life. For example, in 1912, when the AMA thought salaried practice was a threat to the autonomy of the profession, its Code of Ethics pronounced it unethical for physicians to join group practices. Now, some 80 years later, we are again hearing that it is a matter of ethics for the medical profession to carry out what is essentially a political agenda. But ethics should be a little more stable than that. Ethics should be based on fundamental moral principles governing our behavior and obligations toward one another. If a doctor is ethically committed to care for the individual patient, that commitment should not be abridged lightly. And it should not be nullified by a budgetary crunch. Doctors should continue to care for each patient unstintingly, even while they join with other citizens to devise a more efficient and just health care system. To control costs effectively will in my view require a coherent national health care system, with a global cap and a single payer (Angell 1993). Only in this way can we have an affordable health care system that does not require doctors to be double agents.

Notes

1. Angell M. How much will health care reform cost? *New England Journal of Medicine* 1993;328:1778-79.
2. Blendon RJ. The public view of medicine, *Clinical Neurosurgery* 1991;37:2563-65.
3. Callahan D. *What Kind of Life? The Limits of Medical Progress*. New York, NY: Simon & Schuster, 1990.
4. Daniels N. Why saying no to patients in the United States is so hard: cost containment, justice, and provider autonomy, *New England Journal of Medicine* 1986;314:1380-83.
5. Morreim EH. *Balancing Act: The New Medical Ethics of Medicine's Economics*. Boston, MA: Kluwer Academic Publishers, 1991.
6. Schieber GJ, Poullier JP, Greenwald LM. U.S. health expenditure performance: An international comparison and data update, *Health Care Financing Review* 1992;13(4):1-15.

7. Stoline AM, Weiner JP. *The New Medical Marketplace: A Physician's Guide to the Health Care System in the 1990s*. Baltimore, MD: Johns Hopkins University Press, 1993.
8. Woolhandler S, Himmelstein D. The deteriorating administrative efficiency of the U.S. health care system, *New England Journal of Medicine* 1991;324:1253-58.

CONTRIBUTORS

Gene G. Abel, M.D.
Chapter 24
Professor of Psychiatry
Emory University School of Medicine
Behavioral Medicine Institute of Atlanta
Atlanta, Georgia

S. James Adelstein, M. D.
Chapter 35

Steven R. Alexander, M.D.
Chapter 43

Marcia Angell
Chapter 69
Executive Editor
New England Journal of Medicine
Boston, Massachusetts

George J. Annas, J.D., MPH
Chapter 12
Edward Utley Professor of Health Law
Boston University School of Medicine and Public Health
Boston, Massachusetts

Drue H. Barrett, Ph.D.
Chapter 24
Behavioral Medicine Institute of Atlanta
Atlanta, Georgia

William G. Bartholome, M.D., MTS
Chapter 13
Associate Professor of Pediatrics and Clinical Ethicist
Department of History and Philosophy of Medicine
The University of Kansas Medical Center
Kansas City, Kansas

William E. Benitz
Chapter 16
Pediatric Division of Neonatology
Stanford University Medical School
Palo Alto, California

Jeffrey Blustein
Chapter 22
Bioethicist
Weiler Division of Montefiore Medical Center
New York, New York
Associate Professor of Philosophy
Mercy College
Dobbs Ferry, New York

E. Ann Braun, MSc, M.D.
Chapter 46
see Molloy

Philip W. Brickner, M.D.
Chapter 45
Department of Community Medicine
St. Vincent's Hospital and Medical Center
New York, New York

Dan W. Brock, Ph.D.
Chapter 30
Professor of Philosophy and Biomedical Ethics
Department of Philosophy
Brown University
Providence, Rhode Island

Laurel A. Burton, Th.D., F.C.O.C.
Chapter 18
Bishop Anderson Professor of Religion and Medicine
DE of Psychology & Social Sciences
Rush-Presbyterian St. Luke's MC
Chicago, Illinois

Daniel Callahan, Ph.D.
Chapter 53
President
The Hastings Center
Briarcliff Manor, New York

Christine K. Cassel, M.D.
Chapters 35, 63
Chief, Section of Internal Medicine
Department of Medicine
The University of Chicago
Chicago, Illinois

Eric J. Cassell, M.D.
Chapters 33, 58
Professor of Public Health
Cornell University Medical Center
New York, New York

Edwin Cassem, M.D.
Chapter 35

Mary-Margaret Chren, M.D.
Chapter 67
Department of Dermatology
University Hospitals of Cleveland
Cleveland, Ohio

Roger M. Clarnette, MB, BS, FRACP
Chapter 46
see Molloy

James C. Corby, M.D.
Chapter 27

June Corwin, Ph.D.
Chapter 45
Department of Psychiatry
New York University School of Medicine
New York, New York

Madeleine Crain
Chapter 45
Department of Psychology
New York University
New York, New York

Ronald Cranford, M.D.
Chapter 35

Gabriel M. Danovitch, M.D.
Chapter 43

Laurie Dornbrand, M.D.
Chapter 55

James F. Drane, Ph.D.
Chapter 28
Department of Philosophy
Edinboro University of Pennsylvania
Edinboro, Pennsylvania

Martin R. Eisemann, Ph.D.
Chapter 46
see Molloy

Ellen Elpern
Chapter 18
see Yellen

Daniel D. Federman, M.D.
Chapter 35

Peter S. Gardos, M.A.
Chapter 24
Behavioral Medicine Institute of Atlanta
Atlanta, Georgia

Thomas G. Gutheil, M.D.
Chapter 25
Massachussetts Mental Health Center
Bolston, Massachusetts

J. Chris Hackler, Ph.D.
Chapter 54
Div Director for Medical Humanities
University of Arkansas
College of Medicine
Little Rock, Arkansas

Dallas M. High, Ph.D.
Chapter 47
Prof Sanders Brown Center on Aging
Department of Philosophy
University of Kentucky
Lexington, Kentucky

F. Charles Hiller, M.D.
Chapter 54
U. of Arkansas for Medical Sciences
Little Rock, Arkansas

Edward W. Hook, M.D.
Chapter 35

Nancy S. Jecker, Ph.D.
Chapter 61
Associate Professor
Dept of Medical History and Ethics
U of Washington School of Medicine
Seattle, Washington

David H. Johnson, J.D.
Chapter 56
University of New Mexico Law School
Albuquerque, New Mexico

Rodney Johnson, J.D.
Chapter 27

Albert R. Jonsen, Ph.D.
Chapter 48, 57
Prof of Ethics and Medicine
Chairman: Dept History, and Ethics
University of Washington
Seattle, WA

Lawrence Kahana, M.D.
Chapter 43

Joseph Kambe, M.D.
Chapter 31

Bertram L. Kasiske, M.D.
Chapter 43

F. Russell Kellogg, M.D.
Chapter 45
Dept of Community Medicine
St. Vincent's Hospital & Med Center
New York, New York

Seth Landefeld, M.D.
Chapter 67
Department of Medicine
University Hospitals of Cleveland
Cleveland, Ohio

Lawrence R. LaPalio, M.D.
Chapter 50
Dept of Geriatrics
LaGrange Memorial Hospital
LaGrange, Illinois

Bernard Lo, M.D.
Chapters 35. 55
Assistant Professor
Division of General Internal Medicine
U of California Medical Center
San Francisco, California

Erich H. Loewy, M.D.
Chapters 19, 32
Professor of Medicine
Director, Clinical Ethics
Department of Medicine
U of Illinois School of Medicine
Peoria, Illinois

Michael J. McNamee, M.D.
Chapter 31

Marianne Culkin Mann, M.D.
Chapter 31

Susan S. Mattingly, Ph.D.
Chapter 7
Associate Professor of Philosophy
Lincoln University
Jefferson City, Missouri

Diane E. Meier, M.D.
Chapter 63
Associate Professor of Geriatrics and Internal Medicine
Mount Sinai School of Medicine
New York, New York

Charles Miller, M.D.
Chapter 39
see Rhodes

Charles G. Moertel, M.D.
Chapter 35

David W. Molloy, MB, BCh, MRCPI, FRCP(C)
Chapter 46
Hamilton Civic Hospitals
Henderson General Division
Hamilton, Ontario, Canada

Peter D. Mott, M.D.
Chapter 68
Geriatric Medicine Unit
Monroe Community Hospital
Rochester, New York

Thomas H. Murray, Ph.D.
Chapter 67
Dir. of Center for Biomedical Ethics
Case Western Reserve University
School of Medicine
Cleveland, Ohio

John F. Neylan, III, M.D.
Chapter 43

Christine Overall, Ph.D.
Chapter 8
Associate Professor
Queen's University
Kingston, Ontario, Canada

John J. Paris, S.J.. J.D.
Chapter 60
Department of Theology
Boston College
Chestnut Hill, Massachusetts

Robert A. Pearlman, M.D., MPH
Chapter 48
Assistant Professor of Medicine
Geriatric Reserach Education and Clinical Center
VA Medical Center
Seattle, Washington
University of Washington

Edmund D. Pellegrino, M.D.
Chapters 14, 20
John Carroll Professor of Medicine and Medical Ethics
Director: Center for Clinical Ethics
Georgetown University
Washington, D.C.

Henry S. Perkins, M.D.
Chapter 41

Ruth B. Purtilo, Ph.D.
Chapter 40
Professor of Clinical Ethics
Center for Health Policy and Ethics
Creighton University
Omaha, Nebraska

Timothy Quill, M.D.
Chapter 63
Department of Medicine
Genesee Hospital
Rochester, New York

Thomas A. Raffin, M.D.
Chapter 36
Associate Professor
Division of Respiratory Medicine
Department of Medicine
Stanford University Medical Center
Stanford, California

Frank E. Reardon
Chapter 60

Warren Thomas Reich, S.T.D.
Chapter 11
Professor of Bioethics
Center for Clinical Ethics
Georgetown U School of Medicine
Washington, D.C.

Rosamund Rhodes, Ph.D.
Chapter 39
Director, Bioethics Education
Medical Education
Mt. Sinai School of Medicine
New York, New York

Robert R. Riggio, M.D.
Chapter 43

John A. Robertson, J.D.
Chapter 6
School of Law
University of Texas
Austin, Texas

Peter Safar, M.D.
Chapter 35

Lee M. Sanders
Chapter 36

Steven Schenker, M.D.
Chapter 41
Department of Medicine
Division of Gastroenterology
U of Texas Health Science Center
San Antonio, Texas

Lawrence J. Schneiderman, M.D.
Chapter 61
Professor
University of California
San Diego, California

Myron Schwartz, M.D.
Chapter 39
See Rhodes

Edwin Shneidman, Ph.D.
Chapter 26
Neuropsychiatric Institute
U.C.L.A.
Los Angeles, California

Evelyne Shuster, Ph.D.
Chapter 37
VA Medical Center, ACC
Philadelphia, Pennsylvania

Richard Singelenberg
Chapter 34
Department of Cultural Anthropology
University of Utrecht
Utrecht, The Netherlands

Jacquelyn Slomka, Ph.D.
Chapter 62
Department of Bioethics P-31
The Cleveland Clinic Foundation
Cleveland, Ohio

B. Sneiderman, BA, LLB, LLM
Chapter 46
see Molloy

Michael F. Sorrell, M.D.
Chapter 41

Alan Stone, M.D.
Chapter 35

Robert J. Sullivan, Jr., M.D., MPH
Chapter 51
Department of Medicine
Duke University Medical Center
Durham, North Carolina

Owen S. Surman, M.D.
Chapter 40
Behavior Therapy and
Psychopharmacology
Want Ambulatory Care Center
Boston, Massachusetts

Martha Swartz, J.D.
Chapter 9
University Counsel
Thomas Jefferson University
Philadelphia, Pennsylvania

David C. Thomasma, Ph.D.
Chapters 42, 49, 59, 65
The Fr. Michael I. English, S.J.,
Professor of Medical Ethics
Dir, Medical Humanities Program
Loyola U Stritch School of Medicine
Maywood, Illinois

Jan van Eys, M.D.
Chapter 35

Robert M. Veatch, Ph.D.
Chapter 21
Director: The Joseph & Rose Kennedy
Institue of Ethics
Georgetown University
Washington, D.C.

John Votto, D.O.
Chapter 31
Pulmonary Disease
New Britain Memorial Hospital
New Britain, Connecticut

Sidney H. Wanzer, M.D.
Chapter 35
Harvard School of Health Sciences
Cambridge, Massachusetts

Robert F. Weir, Ph.D.
Chapters 15, 64
Dir of Program in Biomedical Ethics
Professor of Pediatrics and
Religious Studies
University of Iowa
College of Medicine
Iowa City, Iowa

Martin G. White, M.D.
Chapter 43
Dallas Nephrology Associates
Dallas, Texas

Suzanne B. Yellen, Ph.D.
Chapter 18
Clinical Director
Division of Psychosocial Oncology
Rush Cancer Center
Rush-Presbyterian-St. Luke's
Medical Center
1725 West Harrison, Suite 820
Chicago, Illinois 60612

Ernlé W. D. Young, Ph.D.
Chapter 27
Stanford University
Center for Biomedical Ethics
Palo Alto, California